BLOOD COMPATIBLE MATERIALS and DEVICES

HOW TO ORDER THIS BOOK

BY PHONE: 800-233-9936 or 717-291-5609, 8AM–5PM Eastern Time

BY FAX: 717-295-4538

BY MAIL: Order Department
Technomic Publishing Company, Inc.
851 New Holland Avenue, Box 3535
Lancaster, PA 17604, U.S.A.

BY CREDIT CARD: American Express, VISA, MasterCard

BLOOD COMPATIBLE MATERIALS and DEVICES

Perspectives Towards the 21st Century

Edited by

CHANDRA P. SHARMA, Ph.D.
MICHAEL SZYCHER, Ph.D.

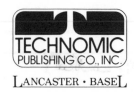

TECHNOMIC
PUBLISHING CO., INC.
LANCASTER · BASEL

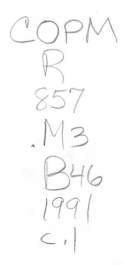
Blood Compatible Materials and Devices
a **TECHNOMIC**®publication

Published in the Western Hemisphere by
Technomic Publishing Company, Inc.
851 New Holland Avenue
Box 3535
Lancaster, Pennsylvania 17604 U.S.A.

Distributed in the Rest of the World by
Technomic Publishing AG

Printed in the United States of America
10 9 8 7 6 5 4 3 2 1

Main entry under title:
   Blood Compatible Materials and Devices: Perspectives Towards the 21st Century

A Technomic Publishing Company book
Bibliography: p.

Library of Congress Card No. 90-71281
ISBN No. 87762-733-9

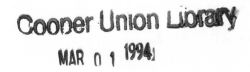

Contents

Preface

The purpose of this volume is to review the present status of biomaterials and devices and to project the possible pattern of research extending to the beginning of the next century. We hope to stimulate the fundamental thought process among graduate students and to challenge professionals in the health care industry to utilize this information for the introduction of improved medical devices. Such a difficult blend has been missing in available texts; this blend has been a major objective of the present volume. The task has been difficult, but I believe we have been moderately successful.

I acknowledge the contribution of Prof. M. S. Valiathan and the help of Mr. A. V. Ramani in providing me with the required facilities for this project. I also wish to thank the many reputed visitors to our Institute who inspired me to start this book, namely Prof. D. F. Williams, Liverpool; Dr. D. Annis, Liverpool; Prof. A. W. Neumann, Toronto; Dr. J. W. Boretos, NIH, U.S.A.; Dr. V. L. Gott, Johns Hopkins, U.S.A.; Dr. R. E. Baier, HIDI, U.S.A.; and Prof. P. K. Bajpai, U. Dayton, U.S.A.

Lastly, I am also thankful for the encouraging correspondence I frequently had with Prof. W. J. Kolff, Utah, U.S.A.; Dr. L. Vroman, N.Y., U.S.A.; as well as the many colleagues involved in the completion of this project—directly or indirectly.

Chandra P. Sharma, D.Sc.
Trivandrum, India

The field of biomaterials, encompassing the traditional sciences (chemistry and physics), as well as the more modern engineering sciences (chemical, mechanical and biomedical), is the gentlest and most humanitarian of all disciplines.

As the most humanitarian discipline, one would expect that Biomaterials Science would transcend national barriers, being truly international in scope, with contributions from all parts of the globe. This book is a striking example of international cooperation in the field of biomaterials and its applied art: medical devices. The book was co-edited in India and the U.S. and contributions originated in Canada, India, Italy, UK, France, Ireland, as well as the U.S.

We can only hope that this book will contribute towards the worldwide dissemination of knowledge and encourage the development of improved medical devices for the benefit of mankind.

Michael Szycher, Ph.D.
Burlington, MA, USA

CHAPTER 1

An Overview of Biomaterials

R. E. BAIER, Ph.D.

Many factors are important for the blood compatibility and proper healing of tissue around implanted prosthetic devices.

Of major importance are the nature, degree of attachment and surface properties of the first deposited biomacromolecules at both the blood-implant and implant-tissue interfaces. The surface qualities of the original implant material are especially critical in determining the adsorbed configuration of these earliest biofilms. The biofilm qualities, in turn, determine whether contacted living cells remain rounded, unaffected and poorly adhesive or whether they passively spread— maximizing their surface areas and attaching tenaciously. Cell spreading and adhesive processes transduce metabolic signals across cell membranes to cytoplasmic and, perhaps, nuclear levels to stimulate mitogenesis and subsequent cell proliferation. DEPOSITION AND ORGANIZATION OF THE FIRST PRIMARY FILMS AND ADJACENT CELL LAYERS DETERMINE WHETHER THE IMPLANT WILL BE CLOSED BY THROMBOSIS, "WALLED OFF," OR TISSUE-INTEGRATED.

Proper attention to implant surface preparation presents excellent possibilities to influence the adhesion, aggregation and differentiation of blood and tissue cells. Such decisions require, first, understanding, prediction, and control of the surface energy, surface charge, and surface texture of the implants *as they enter the host anatomies*. CONTROL OF THESE PROPERTIES AT MANUFACTURING STAGES ONLY IS NOT ADEQUATE, SINCE HANDLING, PACKAGING, STERILIZATION, AND STORAGE OFTEN SIGNIFICANTLY MODIFY THE SURFACE QUALITIES. Experimental and clinical data suggest that modulation of the surface energy state of implants shows the greatest promise for selecting, in advance, the desired degree of adhesion, activation and differentiation of the contacted blood or tissue elements.

Although surface texture, surface charge, and surface chemistry (energy) are all important, surface chemistry— as it relates to the state of cleanliness of the implant and to its potential for strong adhesion—is the most important property to control. With such control, one can achieve passive thromboresistance, early patency, external tissue acceptance and eventually immobilization in the surrounding tissue bed. Later events are more influenced by other factors such as compliance and fluid impedance, therefore significant knowledge of the biomechanical properties of implant materials in the host environment is also required.

Many specific physical and chemical characterization techniques are helpful in this context.

Nondestructive determination of the operational surface energy state of all of the boundaries of the implants is particularly relevant. This determination can be done by direct measurement of contact angles of pure, diagnostic test fluids on the surfaces of interest. Often, nonreactive fluids can be applied, even to the devices about to be emplaced, with no compromise of the clinical result. Inspection of the surface textures of test units, at the scanning electron microscopic level (together with energy-dispersive x-ray analysis for elemental determinations), is also recommended. Final biomechanical testing of prepared devices over long periods (one week) in aqueous electrolyte solutions is a useful means to detect likely *in vivo* degradation problems that are, otherwise, not revealed when implants are tested by only short-term (minutes to hours) static methods.

As the knowledge base increases, it will be useful to determine such additional surface features as presence of specific molecular groupings or radicals that can participate in strong biomaterial interactions to either the benefit or detriment of the host acceptance.

Both implant structural design and implant site preparation also influence the initial compatibility, long-term stability, and stress-transfer relations between implant and tissue.

Implant site preparation is of extreme importance. Meticulous technique is required to minimize damage to sensitive proteins and cells of the host anatomy. Implant design should minimize cul-de-sacs where inadequate flow or difficult penetration of host tissue will allow the sequestering of aggregates or retention of necrotic or infective agents.

With adequate attention to surface cleanliness, surface energy, and gross contouring of the devices—sufficient short-term and long-term blood compatibility and tissue stability can be achieved with "smooth" implants. Surface augmentation (e.g., providing deliberate pores, or roughening) may be unnecessary and possibly even detrimental.

Complete knowledge and control of the state of surface receptivity to host bio-macromolecules and cells should make it clear that it is more of a disadvantage than a benefit to create highly irregular textures for blood contact surfaces. Once such knowledge and control are obtained, one can proceed more confidently to the enhancement of surface areas—if that is required for cell anchorage, load-bearing, or stress-transfer applications.

Additional attention can then also be given to placing stress relief layers of elastomeric materials between solid cardiovascular implants and the delicate tissues with which they mate.

An important task in all implant evaluation trials is selection of appropriate preparation methods that will not compromise the surface qualities of otherwise carefully controlled test materials. The suitability of different base materials, or of the same materials displaying different surface chemical, energetic, or textural states for particular applications in biomedical devices, must be judged in tests where the final sterilization event does not change the test surface from its design condition. The different surface properties selected for screening usually prevent any single sterilization protocol from being suitable for all test specimens, even if their bulk properties are identical. This problem remains to be addressed by the biomaterials community.

CHAPTER 2

Role of Plasma Protein Adsorption in the Response of Blood to Foreign Surfaces

J. L. BRASH, Ph.D.[1]

INTRODUCTION

The adsorption of plasma proteins plays a key role in the interactions of blood with foreign surfaces, and knowledge of these phenomena can be expected to lead to improvements in blood-compatible materials. It is generally believed that plasma protein adsorption is the first event to occur following blood–surface contact and that subsequent phenomena are to a large extent determined by interactions of the blood with the adsorbed protein layer. The major normal "end point" of blood–foreign surface contact consists of coagulation, thrombus formation, and embolization. These are potentially catastrophic events and may well be the kind of events responsible for the occurrence of strokes in recent artificial heart recipients. Other blood–surface effects have also been noted. For example, it is now known that cellulosic hemodialysis membranes activate complement which leads to transient white cell depletion [1]. Thrombocytopenia with extra-corporeal circulation has been noted in either hemodialysis or heart lung bypass [2,3]. Calcification has also been observed in recent years as a relatively late complication of implanted materials, particularly those of biological origin such as porcine bioprosthetic heart valves [4]. However, the principal limiting blood–material interactions are those involved in thrombotic complications. Such complications are responsible for most of the failures in vascular grafts, external AV shunts for blood access in hemodialysis, prosthetic heart valves, heart assist devices, and artificial hearts.

An outline of the mechanisms of thrombogenesis at foreign surfaces is shown in Figure 1. Various "pathways" are distinguished, mainly as a pedagogic convenience, since, as shown, there are many interactions among them. Most of the effects, although not considered in detail here, will be discussed in later sections of this chapter. The initiation and central role of protein adsorption is emphasized in this figure. It is assumed that the adsorption of proteins, which is commonly observed to occur in a few seconds [5,6], is responsible for the initiation and propagation of the plasma coagulation system. In addition, the platelets and other cells arriving later at the surface must interact with the protein layer and not with the material itself. Thus, since it is well established that different protein layers show varying adhesivity toward platelets [7,8,9], the characteristics of protein adsorption on a material determine its platelet reactivity.

The objective of this chapter is to review current knowledge of protein–solid surface interactions, as embodied in Figure 1, and then to suggest how such knowledge may be useful in pointing the way to surfaces of improved blood compatibility. Background material is first provided on fundamental physicochemical aspects of these interactions through a phenomenological description of protein adsorption to solids as derived from studies of single proteins. Adsorption from protein mixtures, plasma and blood is then reviewed. This discussion covers the major plasma proteins, the contact phase of coagulation, complement activation, fibrinolytic involvement, and knowledge of the development and evolution of the protein layers on different surfaces. Finally, in the spirit of "perspectives toward the twenty-first century," and of exploiting knowledge of protein adsorption to bring about improvements, adsorption "control" is discussed. The central thesis of this chapter is that protein adsorption is the initial and "fate determining" event in blood material interactions and that to control these interactions we must be able to control adsorption. Examples of such control are selective adsorption of a particular protein from a

[1]Departments of Chemical Engineering and Pathology, McMaster University, Hamilton, Ontario, Canada

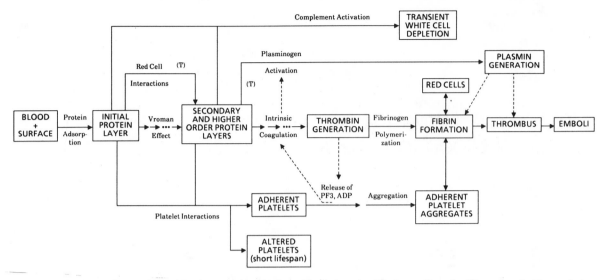

Figure 1. Sequence of events during blood–material interactions. The designation T indicates "tentative." Reproduced with permission from Annals of New York Academy of Sciences, 516:206 (1987).

mixture, minimization of adsorption, and specific spatial orientation of adsorbed proteins. Control of adsorption may be envisaged at the level of surface properties or at the level of "process variables" such as temperature, flow, and the like. The latter are not to any great extent the choice of the designer of blood contact devices, so that the burden of adsorption control falls on control of surface properties.

FUNDAMENTALS OF PROTEIN ADSORPTION: SINGLE PROTEINS

In view of the context of this article, the discussion will be limited to the solid–solution interface although the reader should be aware of the considerable literature which exists on protein behaviour at the air–solution interface [10]. A vast literature also exists on the phenomenology of adsorption of gases and other relatively simple molecules. The adsorption of proteins differs from these other species mainly in that proteins are large and chemically heterogeneous: they contain hydrophobic regions, electrically charged regions (both negative and positive), and polar regions. These domains exist in the surface as well as the interior of the protein [11]. Generally speaking, the surfaces of solids are also heterogeneous and contain a similar variety of surface chemical domains so that a number of different protein–surface binding mechanisms are possible.

The relatively large size of proteins means that adsorption of a single molecule may involve several types of binding sites. Also, since native proteins have well-defined, but not generally symmetric shapes or conformations, they can exist in the adsorbed state in a number of distinct orientations with respect to the solid surface; in

particular, for proteins that have a rod-like conformation, "end-on" and "side-on" orientations may be distinguished. With these general points in mind, we now discuss various aspects of the phenomenology of protein adsorption.

Kinetics

As in all interfacial phenomena, an important question in any protein adsorption system is whether the rate is reaction-controlled or transport-controlled. For this discussion, it is assumed that the surface is "macroscopic" and relatively smooth and that no phenomena such as pore diffusion intervene. There is general agreement that protein adsorption is rapid and that in the initial stages of the process, when fractional surface coverage is low (less than perhaps 10%), the rate is transport-controlled. In this context, distinction must be made between static and flow systems. For static systems, transport to the surface is by diffusion alone and the rate of adsorption equals the flux to the surface, given by:

$$\frac{d\Gamma}{dt} = C_o \left(\frac{D}{\pi t} \right)^{1/2} \tag{1}$$

so that

$$\Gamma = 2C_o \left(\frac{Dt}{\pi} \right)^{1/2} \tag{2}$$

where Γ = surface concentration; C_o = solution concentration; D = diffusivity; and t = time. Equation [2] predicts the often-observed $t^{1/2}$ dependence of adsorption.

Under flow conditions, convective as well as diffusive mass transport occurs. In this case, the correct form of the convective–diffusion equation must be formulated and solved. The form of the equation depends on geometry and flow regime; an example of a protein adsorption system involving laminar flow through a rectangular slit has been given by Lok et al. [12]. In general, for transport control the adsorption rate is dependent on flow parameters such as surface shear rate. For example, if the steady-state concentration and velocity profiles are established, the solution of the convection diffusion equation (Levesque solution) predicts that adsorption rate should vary as shear rate to the one-third power. Lok et al. [12] have found this to be true for the initial rate of adsorption of albumin and fibrinogen to silicone rubber at shear rates up to 400 s⁻¹ at a concentration of 1 mg/ml.

In the later stages of adsorption, when surface coverage exceeds about 10%, it has generally been observed that adsorption is reaction-controlled; the rate law is then of the mass action type:

$$\frac{d\Gamma}{dt} = f(C_o, T) \qquad (3)$$

where T = temperature. Under these conditions, the rate is independent of flow conditions. Data obtained in the present author's laboratory illustrate this point with respect to the glass–fibrinogen system [13]. Adsorption was studied in glass tubes under laminar flow conditions. It was found that the amount of fibrinogen adsorbed at a given time from 5 to 300 minutes was independent of surface shear rate from 0 to 2100 s⁻¹. Surface coverage, even after 5 minutes, was of the order of 75%, indicating an intrinsically rapid adsorption at the concentration studied (1 mg/ml or 3 μM).

Equilibria and Isotherms

The use of the term "equilibria" in connection with protein adsorption is somewhat questionable, since it is frequently found that the adsorption is irreversible with respect to dilution on a realistic time scale [14–16]. It seems likely that this apparent irreversibility has kinetic origins due to the multi-site attachment of adsorbed proteins and consequently slow desorption rates. Based on observations of adsorption hysteresis, Jennissen has proposed the existence of a series of metastable states arising from conformational changes to explain apparent irreversibility [17].

Despite the pedagogic difficulty with the terms "isotherm" and "equilibria", it has been found nevertheless that plots of adsorbed amount versus bulk solution concentration are well-defined and show plateaux or quasi-plateaux similar to small molecule adsorptions [18–20]. Most adsorption data agree reasonably well with the Langmuir or Freundlich equations. Furthermore, adsorbed amounts at saturation are generally in the range corresponding to

monolayers. For example, fibrinogen (MW = 340,000) may be modeled as a rod with dimensions of 450 Å long and 60 Å diameter, and close packed monolayers should range from 0.2 μg/cm² (side-on orientation) to 1.8 μg/cm² (end-on). We have found plateau values of adsorption from 0.02 to about 1.2 μg/cm² for various (mostly polymeric) materials [21]. In a few studies, surface concentrations beyond the monolayer range have been found. A notable example is the recent work of Williams on the adsorption of albumin and fibrinogen to metal surfaces [22]. In these studies several metals adsorbed very large amounts of both proteins; particularly high surface concentrations were seen on silver, gold and copper. The authors noted that these metals are all Group IB elements and suggested that chemical binding between metal and protein might be involved.

The "isotherm" for adsorption of fibrinogen to glass as determined in the present author's laboratory [13,23], shown in Figures 2 and 3, exhibits the shape of a high-affinity Langmuir isotherm with a well-defined plateau at about 0.7 μg/cm². The low concentration region nonetheless shows a "measured" increase suggesting equilibrium properties for the phenomena involved. On the assumption of true equilibrium, it may be deduced from Figure 3 that the free energy of adsorption is about 7 kcal/mole [24]. This is a relatively low value, particularly if it is considered that multi-site binding is involved, and suggests that initially adsorbed molecules are bound via hydrophobic or other weak interactions.

Desorption and Exchange

As already noted, the vast majority of protein adsorption studies have concluded that adsorption is irreversible to dilution, but that adsorbed protein may be desorbed by various eluents. Again, using the glass–fibrinogen system as an example, Figure 4 shows that over a five hour period

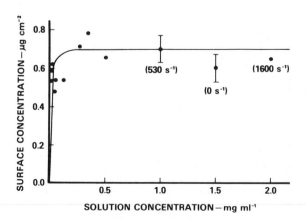

Figure 2. *Adsorption isotherm of fibrinogen on glass in high concentration regime. When not specified, data were obtained at 1060 sec⁻¹. Reproduced with permission from Ref. 13.*

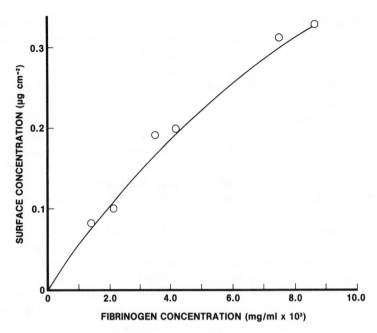

Figure 3. *Adsorption isotherm of fibrinogen on glass in low concentration regime. Reproduced with permission from Ref. 23.*

no fibrinogen is desorbed from a monolayer in contact with the original buffer. However, when the buffer molarity is increased from 0.05 to 1.0 M, rapid desorption of 80% of the layer takes place, suggesting a strong role for electrostatic interactions. The remaining 20% may be eluted by sodium dodecylsulfate, a surfactant which is in general an excellent protein eluent.

Another phenomenon relevant to reversibility is exchange between adsorbed and dissolved protein without change in surface concentration. Such an effect has been found in a number of studies [12,13,25–27]. Figure 5 shows exchange data for fibrinogen on glass obtained using radiolabelled protein. Initial adsorption was done with ^{125}I-labelled protein. After attainment of steady state, [131]I-

labelled protein at the same concentration was introduced and an exchange of isotopes occurred. The rate and extent of exchange are generally found to vary with bulk concentration, but the extent is usually less than 100%.

It may be considered paradoxical that desorption does not occur, while exchange, which must involve a desorption step, does. A definitive explanation for this apparent anomaly is still lacking, but it may be that a concerted process involving interaction of bulk and surface protein is involved. Such a process has been described by Andrade

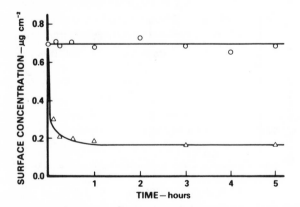

Figure 4. *Desorption of fibrinogen from glass at pH 7.35 and 1060 sec⁻¹; (○) 0.05M Tris; (△) 1.0M Tris, pH 7.35. Reproduced with permission from Ref. 13.*

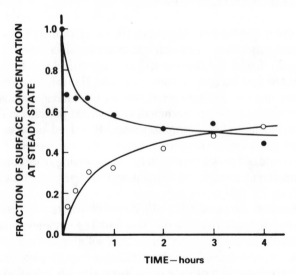

Figure 5. *Exchange between dissolved and adsorbed fibrinogen on glass. Fibrinogen concentration 2.0 mg ml⁻¹, 0.05M Tris, pH 7.35, 1060 sec⁻¹. ¹²⁵I-labeled fibrinogen (●); ¹³¹I-labeled fibrinogen (○). Reproduced with permission from Ref. 13.*

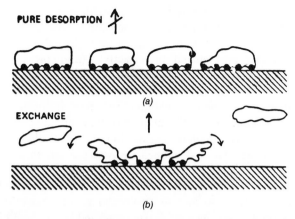

Figure 6. Cartoon showing: *(a) low probability of desorption for a protein adsorbed via several binding sites; (b) concerted cooperative mechanism of exchange between bulk and adsorbed protein. Reproduced with permission from Ref. 28.*

[28] and is schematized in Figure 6. Alternatively, a simple thermodynamic argument based on a high surface–protein affinity, which necessitates that the surface remain covered, may suffice.

Effect of Surface Type

In the broader context of this chapter, it is of surpassing interest to know how surface properties affect protein adsorption from blood. Unfortunately, the present state of knowledge does not permit a definitive treatment of this topic, and it can be dealt with only piecemeal, as opposed to systematically (see the sections on adsorption from plasma and blood). Since information on single protein systems is more extensive, it seems appropriate to attempt a more systematic treatment of surface dependence here.

One convenient classification of surfaces is in terms of hydrophobic and hydrophilic, i.e., surfaces on which water respectively does not and does exhibit a zero contact angle. Protein adsorption is generally considered to be greater and to involve stronger binding on hydrophobic than on hydrophilic surfaces. For example, Chuang et al. [29] reported that plasma proteins have greater affinity for polyvinylchloride (hydrophobic) than for cuprophan dialysis membrane (hydrophilic), and Waugh et al. [30,31] have shown that thrombin binds more strongly to polymethylmethacrylate than to glass. Data from the present author's research also support this point of view [21]. An important caveat must be mentioned in connection with this generalization: namely, that adsorption is more readily and rapidly reversible on hydrophilic than on hydrophobic surfaces [14,15,21]. Therefore, if measurement of adsorption involves rinsing the surface before determining the quantity of bound protein, it is likely that for hydrophilic surfaces protein will be lost, and artificially low values will be obtained. Only "in situ" techniques

(i.e., techniques not requiring surface–solution separation to measure adsorption) are not subject to this problem. Using solution depletion as an in situ method, MacRitchie [15] has shown that the energy associated with adsorption of albumin is greater for hydrophobic than for hydrophilic silica. More recently, Elwing et al. [32] have studied protein adsorption to surfaces having a hydrophobicity gradient. Using ellipsometry, an in situ method, they observed that fibrinogen adsorbed significantly more at the high hydrophobicity end of the gradient.

Hydrogels are a special class of hydrophilic materials which absorb large amounts of water into their structures. Such materials generally show minimal protein interaction. This property is exploited in the use of polyacrylamide gels as protein electrophoresis media, and of Sepharose gels for size exclusion chromatography of proteins where absence of interactions is a "sine qua non." Horbett and Hoffman [33] showed that fibrinogen adsorption was less on Silastic grafted with polyhydroxyethyl methacrylate (HEMA) than on Silastic itself. Gregonis et al. [34] found that IgG and serum protein adsorption to quartz is greatly reduced by surface attachment of polyethylene oxide. Similarly, Golander et al. [35] found minimal albumin adsorption onto polymer surfaces grafted with polyethylene oxide. A number of studies of adsorption to soft contact lens materials (e.g., HEMA) have been reported [36–38]. Such studies are motivated by the hypothesis that development of lens opacity over time is related to protein adsorption from tear fluids [39], implying that although protein adsorption may be reduced on these materials relative to hydrophobic surfaces, it still occurs to a significant extent. Indeed, there are some reports of multilayer quantities of protein being adsorbed on HEMA-based hydrogels. For example, Castillo et al. [36] have found albumin surface concentrations of 2.0 $\mu g/cm^2$, equivalent to about 10 layers, on HEMA contact lenses. Horbett and Hoffman [33] have pointed out that high adsorption to such gels may be associated with methacrylic acid residues which may cause electrostatic repulsion. Horbett has recently reviewed adsorption of proteins to hydrogels [40], and a perusal of this review suggests that generalizations claiming that adsorption is always low on hydrogels should be viewed with caution.

Another useful basis for surface classification is electrical charge. The earlier literature on blood–material compatibility was replete with suggestions that since the vast majority of blood components, including proteins, have a net negative charge at blood pH, then they should be repelled from negatively charged surfaces. This point of view, of course, ignores the fact that secondary minima (attractive interactions) can exist in the interaction potential energy curves due to local heterogeneities in both surface and protein. Weiss [41] has expressed this point of view particularly well in relation to cell–surface interactions where microheterogeneities of surface charge are even more pronounced than in proteins. Attractive interactions between surfaces and proteins of the same charge sign can also be explained by ion bridging between the surface and the protein. In this connection Norde and Lyklema [42] have shown that extensive charge redistribution may occur upon adsorption, involving incorporation of small ions into the adsorbed layer. The conclusion is that negative–negative or positive–positive interactions are possible. There have not been many systematic studies on the effect of charge on protein adsorption, but the conclusions from such studies as exist [20,24,43,44] suggest that surface charge is relatively unimportant as a determinant of whether, and to what extent, adsorption will occur. As an example, we have recently shown that similar amounts of fibrinogen are adsorbed on a series of polyelectrolyte complexes of varying charge (ion exchange capacity from $+1.21$ to -1.33 meq/g) [24].

A frequent observation in studies of single protein adsorption is that the adsorbed amount is a maximum at the protein's isoelectric point (IEP). It is tempting to assume that this effect is related to electrical charge. If so, this effect may well be more a manifestation of protein–protein than protein–surface interactions. Norde [45] has ascribed the IEP maximum to structural changes in the protein as a function of pH.

Compared to polymers, there has been less work on adsorption to other types of solids such as metals and ceramics. Of course, such materials, since they are mechanically less suitable for vascular implants, are of lesser interest than polymers in the blood compatibility area. A number of studies in the older literature have been reviewed by the present author [46]. This older work suggested that protein monolayers generally formed on metals [47]. However, a recent study by Williams et al. [22] has shown that very thick layers of albumin and fibrinogen were adsorbed to Group IB metals such as silver, copper and gold. There is a possibility that chemical bond formation is involved in these interactions. Protein adsorption to metals is of greater interest for surface fouling in food processing [48]. An interesting, recently recognized phenomenon, is the acceleration of metal corrosion by protein adsorption [49]. Adsorption of proteins to metal and metal oxide surfaces has recently been discussed by Ivarsson et al. [50].

ADSORPTION FROM MIXTURES, PLASMA AND BLOOD

As already indicated, proteins are universally surface active; however, there are differences in surface activity from one protein to another. This is reflected in the tendency of a given protein to adsorb preferentially in the presence of other proteins. These tendencies are important in determining the composition of protein layers adsorbed from complex fluids such as blood. Also important are protein–protein interactions and the relative concentrations of proteins in the fluid, and it is the balance between concentration and surface activity (more precisely, free energy of adsorption) which determines the equilibrium composition of the adsorbed layer. Kinetic factors will also intervene at conditions away from equilibrium.

To be able to predict layer compositions, the free energies of adsorption on the surface in question would need to be known. These quantities are available only through experiment, and even qualitative estimates of relative affinity are difficult, since proteins are so complex and their structures so diverse. Molecular weight should be important, however, and this is supported by the data of Zsom [51], who has found that albumin dimers and higher oligomers adsorb preferentially to monomeric albumin.

The discussion in this section, then, is based on the notion of adsorption competition resulting in a characteristic protein composition at the surface. The organization is based on the adsorption environment, beginning with simple plasma simulants and progressing to whole blood.

Mixtures of Plasma Proteins

Because of the complex nature and relative difficulty in handling plasma and blood, a number of studies have been conducted using simple compositional models of plasma. These models have generally consisted of the three abundant proteins, albumin, IgG and fibrinogen, in varying proportions. Data generated in the present author's laboratory [18,21] for mixtures of albumin and fibrinogen showed, using a variety of surfaces, that fibrinogen is preferentially adsorbed, and that the degree of fibrinogen preference correlates with platelet reactivity [21]. Subsequently, using albumin, IgG and fibrinogen in the same proportions as are found in plasma, we showed that the relative abundance of the proteins adsorbed on the surface is reversed compared to the solution [23]. Fibrinogen was dominant, IgG was present in small amounts ($\sim 5\%$ of total) and albumin was undetectable. Other work supports the conclusion that fibrinogen is more surface active than albumin and IgG. For example, Lee, Adamson and Kim [52] showed that fibrinogen was preferred over albumin and γ-globulin on teflon, silicone rubber and a segmented polyether–urethane–urea. Horbett and Hoffman [33] studied competitive adsorption between albumin–fibrinogen and γ-globulin–fibrinogen on Silastic and on Silastic grafted with HEMA and N-vinylpyrrolidone (NVP) hydrogels. Again, it was found in all cases that fibrinogen was strongly preferred. From these studies it is tempting to infer that in blood, fibrinogen would be a major component of the adsorbed protein layer, but as is discussed below, such extrapolations from simple media to blood cannot be made.

There is also evidence from simple competitive adsorption experiments that in addition to fibrinogen, hemoglobin has strong surface affinity [53], and it was estimated that relative protein affinities for polyethylene are in the order: hemoglobin $\gg$ fibrinogen $>$ albumin $\cong$ γ-globulin. Chen et al. [54] have shown differences in the adsorption of oxy- and deoxy-hemoglobin and have formulated a "hemoglobin hypothesis" to explain the difference between venous and arterial behavior of implants. Work in the present author's laboratory suggested strong differences in surface activity between oxyhemoglobin and methemoglobin [55]. While free hemoglobin is not a major component of normal plasma (concentration $\sim$ 0.003 mg/ml), its concentration will undoubtedly increase in implant situations due to device-stimulated hemolysis. Thus, it seems likely that it may be of some importance as an adsorbed component in blood–material contact situations. In this regard, it has been noted by Coleman et al. [56] that the pumping chambers of the Jarvik 7 heart retrieved from Barney Clark were discolored, and it was speculated that this may have been hemoglobin-related.

Plasma

The use of plasma represents an intermediate step between single proteins and simple mixtures on the one hand and whole blood on the other. Plasma may be stored frozen for relatively long periods without serious deterioration and is therefore more convenient to work with than whole blood. While a considerable number of studies of adsorption from plasma have been reported, their content and focus have varied widely. For example, some studies have been concerned with elucidation of the plasma coagulation mechanism, others have been motivated by the need to separate and isolate plasma proteins by chromatographic means, and others again have been aimed directly at the protein adsorption phase of blood–material interactions. Such a diverse body of data is difficult to organize for the purpose of drawing conclusions about the protein layer composition on different surfaces. Organization based on protein type has been chosen for this presentation.

Fibrinogen, Albumin and IgG

In the blood–material interactions field there has been a tendency to assume that the "big three" proteins of plasma, namely albumin, IgG and fibrinogen, with plasma concentrations of 500 to 800 μM, 50 to 120 μM and about 9 μM, respectively, must be important components of adsorbed layers. Surprisingly, other proteins that are at least as abundant as fibrinogen, and in some cases more abundant, have been neglected. Among these are lipoproteins,

transferrin (about 40 μM), α_1-antitrypsin (about 50 μM), haptoglobin (about 20 μM) and complement C3 (about 6 μM). One may speculate that neglect of these components, which should have about the same probability as fibrinogen of being adsorbed from plasma, is due to experimental difficulties and to their relative unavailability in pure form.

In any event, it now seems clear that abundance or relative concentration in plasma has very little to do with adsorption tendency. For example, work in the present author's laboratory has shown that albumin, although present on most surfaces exposed to human plasma, is not a major adsorbed component [57]. On hydrophobic surfaces such as polyethylene and silicone, surface concentrations of about 0.1 μg cm^{-2}, i.e., partial "monolayers", were found, while on hydrophilic surfaces such as glass, essentially no albumin was found. Horbett et al. [58], working with bovine plasma, found similar "equilibrium" concentrations of albumin on various polymers both hydrophobic, e.g., polyethylene and polyethylmethacrylate (EMA), and hydrophilic, e.g., polyhydroxyethyl methacrylate (HEMA). Later work in the same laboratory [59] led to the conclusion that albumin is not a major constituent of the protein layer deposited on a series of copolymers of EMA and HEMA and indeed is considerably depleted in the surface relative to the bulk phase [60]. Surface concentrations, while varying with hydrophilicity, were again of the order of 0.1 μg cm^{-2}. In recent studies by Sevastianov et al. [61,62], very high albumin adsorption levels from plasma were reported. These levels correspond to multilayers of very large proportions.

IgG also appears to be present on all surfaces exposed to plasma [57,59,60], but again it cannot be considered as a major constituent of the layer. For example, we have found surface concentrations of the order of 0.1 μg cm^{-2} or less, representing relatively small fractions (10 to 30%) of the total capacity of the surfaces for IgG [57]. Horbett [60] reported similar values of surface concentration for the HEMA/EMA copolymer series and also observed that relative abundance in the adsorbed layer versus the bulk showed either slight enrichment or slight depletion, depending on the particular surface examined.

Fibrinogen adsorption from plasma to a wide variety of surfaces has been observed by a number of investigators [57–60,63,64] and is without doubt a highly significant event in blood–material interactions. Aside from its potential involvement in clotting, adsorbed fibrinogen has also been shown to be highly reactive to platelets [7–9,65]. It has been found [64,66–68] that fibrinogen adsorption from plasma is transient and that initially adsorbed fibrinogen is replaced by other proteins, notably high molecular weight kininogen (HMWK), within a few minutes of contact (see below for a more detailed discussion). Therefore, it is essential to specify contact time when discussing fibrinogen adsorption. (This is probably true for all protein adsorption from plasma.) We have found [57,66] that absolute values of surface concentration on glass and polyethylene after exposures of 30 minutes are, respectively, about 0.01 and 0.04 μg cm^{-2}. At the adsorption maximum (occurring at a contact time of less than 1 minute) the values are about 0.1 μg cm^{-2}. Horbett has found similar surface concentrations on a HEMA/EMA copolymer series after two hours of contact with bovine plasma. These values compare to surface capacities obtained from single protein experiments of the order of 1.0 μg cm^{-2} [18]. On the question of amounts of fibrinogen in the layer relative to other proteins, recent work in our laboratory [69] has shown that on glass even at long times, fibrinogen is present and appears to be a significant layer constituent. Horbett's data [60] suggest that fibrinogen relative to albumin, IgG and hemoglobin is enriched in the surface compared to the plasma phase by factors of 2 to 3 depending on the surface.

There are a number of other reports describing adsorption of these proteins from blood or plasma [63,68,70–74]. These reports are either qualitative in nature or, if quantitative, give adsorbed amounts not as absolute values, but in terms of some uncalibrated measure related to the protein detection method. Examples of the latter are absorbance of infrared bands [71,72] or color formed by a chromogenic substrate of an enzyme-conjugated antibody [68]. Such results are difficult to relate to data from other techniques (e.g., to the absolute surface concentrations discussed above), but sometimes allow conclusions regarding relative abundance. For example, Breemhaar et al. [68] concluded that "only small adsorption of the major blood proteins occurs from plasma."

Other Abundant Plasma Proteins

It seems likely from the known capacities of surfaces for proteins and the relatively small adsorption of the "big three" proteins that other proteins are present in the layer. Evidence is beginning to accumulate to support this point of view. For example, we have been studying the adsorbed layer qualitatively with the objective simply of identifying these other proteins [69]. This work involves the use of packed columns with the surface of interest in the form of small particles to provide a relatively large surface-to-volume ratio. After appropriate contact with plasma the adsorbed proteins are eluted and separated by polyacrylamide gel electrophoresis. Identifications of eluates are based on estimates of molecular weights from the gels and on immunochemical evidence.

On glass in addition to some albumin, IgG and fibrinogen we have shown there are many other proteins. Constituents so far identified are plasminogen, transferrin, and considerable plasmin-induced fibrinogen degradation products (FDP). We hypothesize that FDP are produced via adsorption of plasminogen followed by its activation to plasmin (see Figure 1). This activation appears to be related to the contact phase of the blood coagulation system since FDP are reduced when factor XII-deficient plasma is used. These findings call attention to the role of surface in fibrinolysis, an aspect of blood–material interactions that has been largely ignored.

We have also carried out preliminary studies of the "heparin like" materials of Jozefowicz et al. using this column elution technique [75]. These are crosslinked polystyrenes that have been modified by sulfonation and attachment of amino acids via sulfonamide bonds [76]. They have been shown to possess anticoagulant properties and might thus be expected to behave differently from glass, a highly procoagulant surface. Again, a multiplicity of proteins are eluted and many remain to be identified. There are some similarities to glass: for example, FDP and plasminogen are present. However, considerably more intact fibrinogen appears to be adsorbed compared to glass, suggesting that initially adsorbed fibrinogen is less readily displaced on such materials. In the sense that fibrinogen may be replaced by contact phase clotting factors and since these materials do have anticoagulant properties, it may be that retention of initially adsorbed fibrinogen is desirable. This interpretation is discussed further below.

Elution-type studies have been done in other laboratories and have revealed the presence of other proteins in adsorbed layers. Horbett et al. [59,77] have used in situ radiolabelling followed by elution to show that hemoglobin, probably prothrombin and a number of unidentified components are adsorbed to various HEMA/EMA copolymers. Also, Limber et al. [73,74] found that a number of proteins could be eluted from cuprophane hemodialysis membrane after contact with plasma. In addition to albumin and IgG, they tentatively identified α_1-lipoprotein, β-lipoprotein, haptoglobin, IgA, IgM and IgD.

Other proteins have been proposed as likely candidates for adsorption because of their potential to act as "adhesives" for cells. Grinnell [78] has reported on the adsorption of fibronectin from plasma to both wettable and nonwettable surfaces. The von Willebrand/factor VIII protein complex has been shown to increase platelet adhesion when pre-adsorbed to solid surfaces [79], and Horbett and Counts [80] have found that, despite its low plasma concentration (about 10 μg ml^{-1}) this protein is nonetheless adsorbed to a number of surfaces. Although the absolute levels are low (e.g., 0.001 μg cm^{-2} on polyethylene), there is considerable enrichment in the surface relative to the plasma. Similarly, we have recently shown that plasminogen (plasma concentration 0.20 mg/ml) is adsorbed from plasma to all surfaces so far studied [81]. Again, the surface concentrations are in the low range from 0.0002 to 0.04 μg/cm^2. However, if adsorbed plasminogen is activated to plasmin, these small amounts may become significant as agents of surface-associated fibrinolytic activity.

Such activation is suggested by the finding that fibrinogen adsorbed from plasma undergoes degradation to FDP [69].

Proteins of The Contact Phase of Blood Coagulation

The literature of blood coagulation contains many references to the role of "negatively charged surface" in triggering the early or "contact" phase of this process (see reference [82] for a review). Clearly, such effects are germane to a discussion of plasma protein layer composition since adsorption of some of the contact phase proteins is implied, and since surface induced coagulation is perhaps the most critical problem in blood–material interactions.

The activation of the contact system is a complex process involving an interplay among factors XII and XI, prekallikrein, HMWK and the surface. At the present time this process is only partially understood. Factor XII activation is generally considered as the first step in the intrinsic coagulation pathway and much attention has been focussed on this protein. There is little doubt that factor XII is adsorbed from plasma to glass and other clot-promoting surfaces, as has been demonstrated by Revak et al. [83]. Several authors have proposed an "autoactivation" mechanism for activation of factor XII [84,85], as well as a mechanism involving activation by kallikrein. Autoactivation involves a reaction between inactive factor XII and activated factor XII (XII_a) to form two molecules of XII_a. However, as recently emphasized by Colman "The origin of the trace XII_a remains controversial" [86]. Griffin has shown [87] that binding of factor XII to kaolin surface "greatly enhances its susceptibility to cleavage" by kallikrein, plasmin and factor XI_a. He attributes the effect of the surface to a conformational change in adsorbed factor XII. However, it could also be that the surface merely concentrates factor XII, thereby producing a much more rapid rate of cleavage than in the bulk plasma phase.

HMWK is also surface active and its role in contact activation appears to be to transport prekallikrein and factor XI (with both of which it exists as equimolar complexes in plasma [90,91]) to the surface and facilitate their adsorption [90]. In support of this hypothesis, it has been shown [91] that factor XI is adsorbed from normal plasma to kaolin but not from HMWK-deficient plasma. Similar effects have also been reported for a glass surface by Margalit and Schiffman [92]. As will be discussed in more detail below, HMWK (or HMWK complexes with prekallikrein and factor XI) also has the effect of removing initially adsorbed fibrinogen from surfaces exposed to plasma.

No specific surface-related role in contact activation has yet been assigned to prekallikrein. As already stated, this molecule is transported by HMWK to the surface where it exerts a reciprocal proteolytic activation effect on factor XII.

Most of the work described so far on contact factor adsorption has been carried out by hematologists and biochemists more from the point of view of the blood than of the surface. Recent work by Matsuda et al. [93] has generated data on the degree of contact activation induced by various surfaces. The technique used measures (a) contact activation by determining kallikrein generation using a fluorogenic substrate, and (b) contact factor adsorption by an immunoassay method. It was found that glass is a more potent activator than silicone polymers and that negative charges increase, while positive charges decrease activation. Activation was found to correlate with the amounts of factor XII and HMWK adsorbed on the various surfaces.

As already noted it is conventional in the blood coagulation literature to imply that negative charge is required for a surface to have contact activation activity. However, it is clear that all surfaces, with perhaps the exception of normal vascular endothelium, have the ability to initiate coagulation. A more accurate statement may be that negatively charged surfaces have greater activity than either neutral or positive surfaces. It is interesting to note that a number of surfaces which appear to have some degree of blood compatibility are also negatively charged [76,94, 95], implying that even if the contact phase is strongly activated, the later phases of coagulation can be inhibited to give an overall anticoagulant effect.

Time Variation in Adsorbed Layer Composition: The Vroman Effect

Numerous references to the irreversibility of protein adsorption can be found in the literature dealing with single protein adsorption [14,15,20], although this is probably more a question of slow reversibility than thermodynamic limitation. Irreversibility would imply that once formed, the layer would remain fixed in composition. However, it has been shown repeatedly that surface–solution exchange occurs and in a complex fluid such as plasma or blood, initially adsorbed proteins can later be exchanged with others due to differences in concentration and in the kinetic and thermodynamic parameters for adsorption of the various components. For example, an abundant, rapidly adsorbing protein having low surface affinity might be exchanged with a low concentration, slowly adsorbing protein having high affinity. Such exchange would lead to changes in layer composition with time. From this point of view, ultimate equilibrium might be attained only slowly over hours or even days, rather than minutes. This idea is incorporated in Figure 1 through the concepts of primary, secondary and higher order protein layers.

Perhaps the most extensive observations of time dependence of adsorption from plasma come from the work of Vroman et al. They have reported observations of transient fibrinogen adsorption dating from 1969 [6]. Initially, they showed that on several surfaces, both wettable and

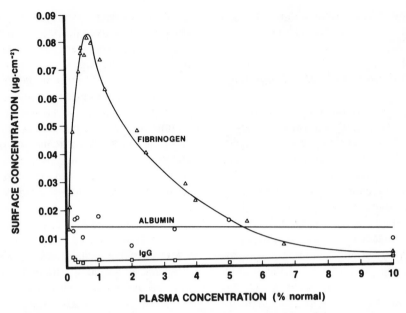

Figure 7. Adsorption of proteins to glass from plasma as a function of plasma concentration. Plasma was diluted with isotonic Tris, pH 7.35 and adsorptions were for 5 minutes. Reproduced with permission from Ref. 66.

nonwettable, fibrinogen could be immunochemically identified up to several minutes after plasma contact, but not at longer times. Subsequently, they showed that initially adsorbed fibrinogen is replaced by HMWK [64]. This conclusion is supported by experiments showing that in circumstances where insufficient HMWK is available, e.g., in "narrow spaces" [96] or in highly diluted plasma

[66,97], initially adsorbed fibrinogen remains on the surface. A reasonable alternative explanation, that adsorbed fibrinogen is enzymatically digested by plasmin (perhaps formed via activation of factor XII), has been ruled out on the basis that fibrinogen displacement still occurs in plasminogen-free plasma [98].

The transient nature of fibrinogen adsorption has been

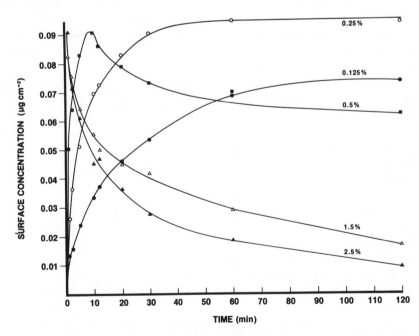

Figure 8. Kinetics of adsorption of fibrinogen to glass from plasma at varying plasma dilutions. Plasma concentrations are indicated on curves. Reproduced with permission from Ref. 66.

observed in other laboratories on an extensive range of surfaces [57,66–68] and appears to be a general phenomenon which has been designated the "Vroman Effect" [66,67]. We have shown, for example, on glass, siliconized glass and polyethylene, that although relatively small amounts of fibrinogen are adsorbed from normal plasma, adsorption increases considerably when the plasma is diluted and reaches a maximum at a dilution of about 100:1 (1% normal). This effect is shown in Figure 7.

These data can be explained by postulating, in agreement with Vroman, that low concentration components of plasma are in competition with fibrinogen for adsorption sites. As the plasma is diluted, the concentration of competitor becomes insufficient to replace fibrinogen. Kinetics data at high dilution support this interpretation in that they do not show maxima (Figure 8). The plasma concentration at maximum adsorption is surface dependent and generally increases with surface hydrophobicity [66,67, 97], suggesting that the binding strength of fibrinogen increases with hydrophobicity. We have now shown, in agreement with Vroman et al., that the main competitive species is HMWK since if plasma deficient in HMWK is used, the concentration-dependent maximum is greatly attenuated [99]. It appears also from our work [99], that factor XII is involved, although perhaps in an indirect fashion, i.e., by activating kallikrein which in turn converts HMWK from a procofactor to an active cofactor form. Experiments related to plasminogen–plasmin involvement were inconclusive. Breemhaar et al. [68] have also observed maximum fibrinogen adsorption as a function of plasma concentration and have suggested that high density lipoprotein is the competitive species.

The significance of the Vroman Effect in relation to surface thrombogenesis is not entirely clear, but as already discussed it is known that HMWK is a cofactor in the contact phase of blood coagulation and is required for the full expression of factor XII procoagulant activity [86]. The characteristics of the Vroman Effect, e.g., fibrinogen displacement rate and extent, vary considerably from surface to surface [66,67,97]. Whether these variations are significant in relation to the thrombogenic potential of the surfaces remains to be ascertained. If the key surface property is inertness toward activation of coagulation, and if displacement of fibrinogen leads to adsorption and activation of coagulation factors, then fibrinogen retention, i.e., minimal Vroman effect, may be desirable. If, on the other hand, inertness to platelets is the most important property for non-thrombogenicity, then since adsorbed fibrinogen is generally believed to be platelet-reactive, fibrinogen displacement and a vigorous Vroman effect should be desirable.

Indications that transiency of adsorption may not be unique to fibrinogen are given by recent observations of Vroman et al. [100] that there is a tendency in general for more abundant plasma proteins to be adsorbed initially and to be replaced later by less abundant proteins. Clearly, relative surface affinities, as well as concentrations of the proteins must play a role. Such "sequential" effects may reflect a change from kinetic to thermodynamic control at longer times.

Grinnell and Phan [78] have recently reported a "dilution" effect in the adsorption of fibronectin from plasma to polystyrene. This result is probably also due to competitive adsorption, although the competing species are not identified.

Whole Blood

Ex Vivo and Clinical Studies

Knowledge of protein adsorption from whole blood has come mostly from so-called ex vivo experiments in which a device is connected directly to an animal or patient but is not implanted. Based on such experiments, Baier and Dutton [5] and Brash and Lyman [14] were among the first to suggest that protein adsorption is the initial event during whole blood contact. These experiments were crude in the sense that no details about the types of protein adsorbed were obtained.

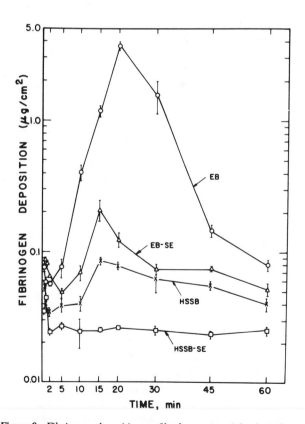

Figure 9. Fibrinogen deposition profiles for commercial polyurethanes with and without solvent extraction. Note the peaks at about 1 min (Vroman Effect?) and 20 min (embolization). Reproduced with permission from Ref. 102.

In recent years, the most extensive data on adsorption from whole blood ex vivo have been obtained by Cooper et al. using an AV shunt experiment in dogs [9,63,79] or subhuman primates [101]. Labelled proteins and labelled platelets are given to the animal, and accumulations of these components on the material of the shunt are measured with time. A common observation from these studies is that fibrinogen adsorption passes through an early maximum at less than one minute and then through a second peak at about 10–20 minutes [102]. Figure 9 shows typical data. The first peak may relate to the Vroman Effect, already discussed in relation to plasma interactions. The second fibrinogen peak coincides with a peak in platelet deposition. The platelet and fibrinogen peaks are undoubtedly interrelated, although it is difficult to determine whether the platelets or the fibrinogen constitute the primary agonist. It may be that the second fibrinogen peak really represents fibrin strands which enmesh the platelets and are secondary to platelet activation since the animals are not always heparinized. The second fibrinogen peak is believed to be caused by initial thrombus build-up followed by embolization. Indeed, there are sometimes third and fourth peaks [101,103] indicating a cycle of build-up and embolization events. This experiment has been performed using a variety of materials and wide variation in blood response has been found. It is rare that the initial peak of fibrinogen adsorption exceeds 0.1 μg/cm^2, a value similar to that found for plasma in vitro [66,67,97]. The second peak is higher, ranging up to 10 μg/cm^2 on oxidized polyethylene and, as mentioned, may be due to fibrin formation secondary to platelet deposition. On a series of polyurethanes including Biomer®, the material used in the Jarvik 7 artificial heart [56], fibrinogen deposition varied with the polymer structures (soft segment, hard segment type and content, whether solvent extracted) but was generally in the low range of values. The deposition of both platelets and fibrinogen on Biomer decreased markedly after solvent extraction.

Adsorption kinetics of other proteins has also been investigated in this experiment [79]. For this purpose, the dogs were heparinized and adsorption of albumin, γ-globulin, fibrinogen and fibronectin was measured over a 2-hour period on Silastic and PVC. In all cases, adsorption kinetics showed early maxima which were particularly marked for fibrinogen and fibronectin. However, in contrast to the in vitro plasma experiments discussed above [66,67,97] these data showed that substantial amounts of fibrinogen (and other proteins) remained adsorbed at long times. Surface concentrations ranged between 0.1 and 1.0 μg/cm^2. Albumin adsorption was higher on Silastic than on PVC and it was suggested this might account for the more benign blood response of the former.

Another group of investigators have studied protein adsorption ex vivo using FTIR spectroscopy. With this method it is difficult to distinguish one protein from another, but total protein deposition can be monitored. In one study [72] it was found that, independent of the surface, total protein adsorption followed similar kinetics. A substantial fraction of the adsorption was completed in 30 to 90 secs. Slower increases then followed, and a plateau was reached after about 30 minutes (Figure 10). From analysis of the spectra there was evidence of early albumin adsorption, subsequent exchange of one protein for another, and later deposition of cell-derived glycoproteins.

Horbett [104] has studied the ex vivo adsorption of fibrinogen in a baboon AV shunt model using radiolabelled fibrinogen. On some surfaces adsorption was in two phases: an early phase (up to 10 mins) where adsorption was low (~0.02 μg/cm^2) and a later phase where adsorption was much higher (~1 μg/cm^2). The second phase was inhibited by heparin and was attributed to fibrin formation. As in the studies of Cooper et al., there was evidence of the embolization of the second phase (fibrin) deposit and a correspondence of this phase with platelet response (in this work measured as steady-state platelet consumption with the shunt in place [105]). On other materials there was a relatively constant low level of fibrinogen deposition with no second phase. Surfaces such as polyethylene, which give a strong Vroman Effect with plasma in vitro [67], did not exhibit second phase (thrombotic) deposition of fibrin, whereas materials such as polyurethanes and EMA/HEMA copolymers, which showed low fibrinogen adsorption in vitro and only a mild Vroman effect, had strong second phase fibrin deposition.

Seifert and Greer [106] and Matsuda et al. [107] have also reported ex vivo animal studies of blood–material interactions. In the work of Seifert and Greer a series of HEMA or PVP-grafted Silastic materials of varying hydrophilicity were examined as AV shunts in dogs. Protein deposition was examined by FTIR but only a single (15 minute) ex situ measurement was made in contrast to the real-time continuous measurements of Gendreau et al. [72]. It was found that less protein was deposited on the more hydrophilic materials. Only an indication of total protein was obtained and no attempt was made to identify individual proteins. Since thrombus was consistently generated, the protein deposits undoubtedly consisted mainly of fibrin and cellular protein. Insight into initial or intermediate protein events are thus not readily available from this work.

The recent work of Matsuda et al. [107] was based on implantation of diaphragm-type LVAD's in non-anticoagulated goats. After two-month implantations with no thrombotic complications, the polyurethane pump surfaces were found to be coated with a uniform protein layer of thickness about 1 μm, suggesting multimolecular layers. Again, no information on the protein composition of the layer was obtained. It was hypothesized that this layer acted as a passive surface and inhibited any subsequent thrombotic events.

In addition to the animal studies described above, a few

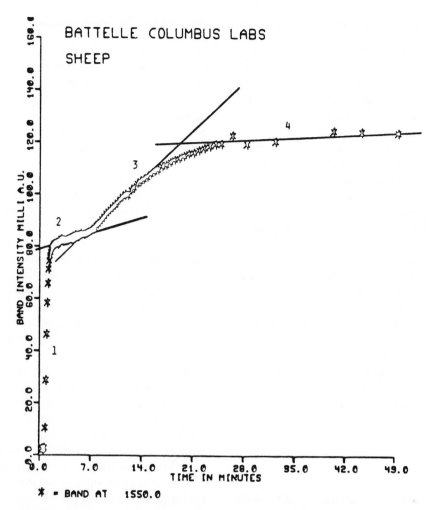

Figure 10. *Plot of amide II (1550 cm⁻¹) band intensity vs time of blood flow showing total amount of protein adsorbed in the time period indicated. Spectra collected every 5s for initial period (49 min). Reproduced with permission from Ref. 72.*

investigations have been conducted based on data from human subjects. These clinical data were obtained through the use of extracorporeal blood circulation procedures such as hemodialysis and heart-lung bypass. Chuang [108] has measured quantities of fibrinogen adsorbed to cuprophan membranes following a 6-hour dialysis procedure. Quantities of the order of 0.2 μg/cm² were found. Only a tenth of this amount was observed on in vitro exposure to heparinized plasma after 30 minutes (Vroman Effect) and about one fifth using a triple mixture of albumin, fibrinogen and IgG at the same concentrations as in plasma. The area distribution of protein deposition on the clinical membranes was non-uniform, and it was speculated that the relatively high surface concentrations may have been due to fibrin thrombi.

A recent study by Owen et al. [109] identified albumin and hemoglobin as the major proteins adsorbed to the surfaces of blood oxygenators during short-term heart-lung bypass. In addition to these two proteins, IgG was found in abundance on oxygenator surfaces during long-term extracorporeal membrane oxygenation (ECMO).

A relatively recent phenomenon that has been identified in blood material interactions is the activation of the complement system. This phenomenon was first reported in connection with extracorporeal circulations and has been studied mainly in the context of hemodialysis [1] and cardiopulmonary bypass [110]. It is probably not directly involved in thrombogenesis, but in extracorporeal circulation leads to clinical manifestations such as transient neutropenia and pulmonary dysfunction. Different materials activate complement to different degrees; for example, cellulose membranes are potent activators while polyacrylonitrile-based membranes cause virtually no complement activation [111]. It seems likely that complement activation begins with complement adsorption, suggesting that certain components of the complement system are selectively adsorbed to cellulose. Interestingly, it has also been found [111] that reused cuprophane (cellulose) dialyzers have greatly reduced complement activation capacities. This observation suggests that the original complement binding sites on the membrane are irreversibly saturated during the initial blood exposure and are not available for activation during subsequent dialysis. Chenoweth suggested [111] that C3b is the irreversibly adsorbed complement component. Thus, complement activation provides another example of selective protein adsorption. Subsequent to these discoveries based on in vivo studies, a number of investigations of complement activation in vitro using plasma have been reported [61,62,112, 113]. Ward et al. [112] have shown that air microbubbles trapped in the surface roughness of materials are partly responsible for complement activation, suggesting that air–interface adsorption may be involved. Sevastianov et al. [61] demonstrated an inverse relationship between complement activation and albumin adsorption for a series of commercial polymers including polyurethanes, silicones and polyethylene. These data lead to the interesting hypothesis that complement activation depends on the composition of the protein layer adsorbed from blood to the material (see Figure 1). This is analogous to the widely held belief that thrombogenesis is also controlled by the adsorbed protein layer. Horbett and Payne [113] showed that complement activation may be directly related to surface hydroxyl content so that cellulose and hydroxylethylmethacrylate copolymers are potent complement activators. Elwing et al. [114] have shown that C3 is adsorbed from human serum onto both hydrophilic and hydrophobic silica.

Red Cell Effect

An obvious difference between blood and plasma is the respective presence and absence of cells. Work in our laboratory has attempted to determine the role of red cells in protein adsorption. We have consistently found that with solutions of single proteins, addition of red cells inhibits adsorption [55,115], and we have attributed this "red cell effect" to the fact that red cell–surface contact results in deposition of membrane components [55], producing a new surface that is relatively nonadsorptive. We have recently shown that red cells deposit integral membrane proteins on contacting surfaces without being lysed [116], implying a type of nonhemolytic partial membrane extrusion onto the surface. If important in vivo, this effect will contribute to the protein layer composition (see Figure 1). There is little doubt that in a flowing whole blood situation involving a foreign surface, some hemolysis will occur [117], thereby increasing the local concentration of free hemoglobin in the plasma. Since hemoglobin is known to possess high surface activity [53,55] it seems likely that hemoglobin will be adsorbed. Hemoglobin has, in fact, been found on the membranes of clinically used blood oxygenators [109] and on surfaces of an explanted Jarvik 7 artificial heart [56], as discussed above. Whether the particular "red cell effect" found in our laboratory is important in whole blood contact situations has not been determined. In agreement with the red cell effect, Horbett has found reduced fibrinogen adsorption levels in ex vivo studies using baboons [104], whereas Chuang [108] has found higher levels of fibrinogen after clinical use of cuprophan dialysis membranes compared to in vitro plasma exposure. Fibrinogen may not be the best choice of protein in this connection since, as well as being adsorbed, it may be deposited in the form of fibrin secondary to platelet activation.

TOWARDS THE FUTURE: CONTROL OF ADSORPTION

Many investigators, including the present author, have argued that blood-compatible materials will only be realized when sufficient understanding of surface associated thrombogenesis, including protein adsorption effects, is achieved. Although our present understanding certainly falls short of being sufficient in this sense, it may be useful to try to identify preliminary "signposts" towards thromboresistance of surfaces.

What seems to emerge from current knowledge (see Figure 1) is that protein adsorption controls thrombogenesis. It therefore seems clear that to control thrombogenesis we must control protein adsorption. This strategy has already been used either explicitly or implicitly in a number of approaches to blood compatibility [34,118,119, 120]. In a broad sense, control of protein adsorption has a number of aspects such as: selective adsorption of a particular protein, minimization or prevention of adsorption, and control of the surface orientation of adsorbed proteins. All of these aspects have some relevance to blood–material compatibility, but it is perhaps the first two that have attracted the most attention. These are now discussed in turn.

Selective Adsorption

Protein chromatography provides some of the best examples of selective protein adsorption. There are several types of protein chromatography currently in general use, but the most spectacular selectivities are obtained with affinity chromatography, based on specific chemical or biochemical interaction between the protein and the chromatographic surface. The latter generally consists of agarose particles to which are bound "ligands" having specific high affinity for the protein to be "captured." Some examples of ligands and captured proteins are shown in Table 1.

Many affinity matrices have only partial, as opposed to absolute, specificity and will merely enrich a particular protein, not "select" it. A good example is the ligand Cibacron-Blue F3GA, a complex aromatic blue dye. This

TABLE 1. Examples of Ligands and Corresponding Proteins in Affinity Chromatography[121-124]

Ligand	Protein Selectively Bound
Protein A	Immunoglobulins
Lysine	Plasminogen
Heparin	Antithrombin III
Gelatin	Fibronectin
Octyl	Caseins, Lactalbumin

ligand was at one time believed to selectively remove albumin from blood plasma [125]. More recently [126], it has been shown that, depending somewhat on conditions, as many as 27 proteins are adsorbed out of plasma by this material.

The ligand protein A has recently become the basis of the new biomedical technology known as immuno adsorption. This technology involves the selective removal from a patient's blood of antibodies or immune complexes which accumulate in certain disease states. Protein A is a material present in the cell walls of certain bacteria and has been found to bind specifically to the Fc portion of immunoglobulin G [121]. An example of the application of this material in clinical medicine is the selective removal of "blocking factor" from the blood of patients with certain types of cancer. Blocking factor is an unidentified agent (probably an immune complex) which prevents the natural cytotoxic immune response of the host to the cancer; its removal by immuno adsorption on protein A immobilized to silica led to regression of tumors in a significant number of patients suffering from breast and pancreatic cancer [127].

The example of surface-bound heparin as an affinity matrix for antithrombin III (AT III) is particularly relevant to blood compatibility. Many attempts have been made to prepare heparinized surfaces [128–132] for thromboresistance and indeed some short-term success has been achieved. The effectiveness of heparinized surfaces has been attributed to a number of mechanisms as discussed elsewhere [132]. This is still an area of debate, and mechanisms include anticoagulation of blood locally near the surface and catalysis of the thrombin–AT III reaction at the surface with the formation of thrombin–AT III complexes which are released from the surface leaving it available for further thrombin neutralization [130]. The use of heparin as an affinity ligand for AT III suggests that heparinized surfaces can be looked on simply as materials which preferentially adsorb AT III.

A number of modifications of the heparinized surface approach have also been developed in recent years. Among these are the heparin-like surfaces of Jozefowicz et al. [76,94] and the albumin–heparin conjugates proposed by Kim and Feijen [119]. The materials of Jozefowicz et al. do not contain heparin itself, but incorporate structural features, e.g., sulfonate, and amino sulfamide

linkages which attempt to mimic the active sites of heparin. Some of these materials are heparin-like in the sense that they catalyze the thrombin–AT III reaction. They may well act by selective, though not necessarily exclusive, adsorption of AT III [133]. In Kim and Feijen's approach, covalent complexes of albumin–heparin are synthesized and pre-adsorbed (presumably via the albumin component) onto hydrophobic materials [119]. The rationale for this approach is to use the albumin as a long "spacer arm" for heparin so that it becomes "more available for complex formation with AT III" [134], a tacit acknowledgement of the AT III adsorption mechanism of heparinized surfaces.

The principle of selective, controlled adsorption is perhaps best exemplified by the work of Eberhart et al. [118]. This work is based on the hypothesis that adsorbed albumin provides passivation of blood contacting surfaces since albumin layers interact minimally with platelets [7,8]. Therefore, attempts have been made to develop surfaces that selectively bind albumin from blood. The approach of Eberhart et al. is based on the natural affinity of albumin for lipid-like materials such as long chain fatty acids [135]. Thus, for example, they have "grafted" long chain alkyl groups of chain length 8 to 30 carbon atoms, to the surface of polyurethanes. These "derivatized" materials have been found to increase the retention of albumin in contact with plasma compared to underivatized controls [118]. A number of in vitro and in vitro studies by Eberhart et al. support the hypothesis that these materials selectively adsorb albumin and show a degree of thromboresistance [136].

The example of Sepharose–lysine as an affinity matrix for plasminogen focuses attention on another approach to blood compatibility, namely the promotion of fibrinolysis at the surface. It could be argued that this approach also depends on control of protein adsorption, in this case the fibrinolytic proteins plasminogen and plasmin. Kusserow et al. [137] were the first to suggest that surface thromboresistance might be imparted by the ability to promote fibrinolysis. Their approach was to immobilize the enzyme urokinase, a potent activator of the plasminogen–plasmin conversion. The enzyme would be available at the surface for activation of plasminogen, a natural consituent of any small clots that might be formed. The plasmin formed would then lyse the incipient clots. This approach has recently been revived by Senatore et al. [138,139]. They have attempted to develop a small diameter vascular graft with fibrinolytic properties by immobilizing urokinase in dacron-reinforced collagen. Compared to controls lacking urokinase these grafts showed a higher degree of patency and increased fibrinolytic activity.

It has long been known to coagulation specialists that surfaces are associated with fibrinolytic activity, although it is not clear whether this is a direct effect or if it occurs via the surface-induced formation of factor XIIa, which is a known plasminogen activator. Recent work in our labo-

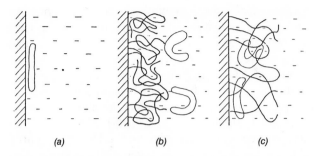

Figure 11. *Schematic models of different surfaces interacting with protein in aqueous solution: (a) rigid surface with denatured protein; (b) diffuse surface with intact protein; (c) diffuse surface intermixed with protein. Reproduced with permission from Ref. 120.*

ratory has shown that when surfaces are incubated with either solutions of "pure" fibrinogen containing a trace of plasminogen or plasma, considerable plasmin-induced degradation of adsorbed fibrinogen occurs [69,75,140]. We believe this indicates that surfaces may have the ability to facilitate the plasminogen–plasmin conversion and that the approach of maximizing fibrinolysis should be further investigated. Clearly, for this to succeed surfaces must be found that will selectively adsorb plasminogen.

Minimization of Adsorption

In principle, protein adsorption should not occur if the interfacial free energy of the solid–solution interface is identical to that of the adsorbed protein–solution interface. This idea is implicit in the usual approaches to minimization involving what may be called minimally interacting hydrogels, i.e., materials which imbibe large quantities of water, usually swelling in the process, and which have generally low interfacial tensions with aqueous media.

Ikada et al. [120] have investigated polyethylene–acrylamide grafted surfaces in which the original rigid hydrophobic polyethylene is converted to a "diffuse" hydrophilic polyacrylamide surface. In addition, polyacrylamide is chemically unreactive to proteins, a fact which is taken advantage of in its use as a medium for electrophoresis of proteins. The rationale is schematized in Figure 11. The polyethylene rigid surface is seen as denaturing the adsorbed protein. The grafted surfaces prevent access of the protein to the rigid substrate, and in the aqueous milieu of the grafted region adsorption is minimal. The graft density must be optimized to achieve the desired result: if too high, the graft itself becomes adsorbent, if too low, the protein is able to penetrate to the rigid substrate.

A second example of hydrogel use to minimize adsorption is provided by the work of Gregonis et al. [34], in which polyoxyethylene, the hydrophilic polymer, is "coated" on the rigid substrate, in this case glass. This approach is based on the observation that there can be a sig-

nificant decrease in concentration of enzyme solutions (generally of low initial concentration) because of adsorption to the walls of containers. Furthermore, it has been reported [141] that such "losses" can be prevented by addition of polyethylene oxide (PEO) to the solutions. The mechanism by which PEO achieves this effect is still in dispute, and recently [142], it has been suggested that it is merely the rate of adsorption which is diminished. Based on the idea that a PEO "surface" itself should be minimally adsorbent, Gregonis et al. have developed methods to chemically bind PEO to glass using the binding agent aminopropylsilane, and have shown, using total internal reflection fluorescence (TIRF), that adsorption of several proteins is drastically reduced. It was also found that protein adsorption decreased with increasing MW of the PEO. This may indicate a steric repulsion mechanism similar to that described for stabilization of colloids by adsorbed polymers [143]. Golander et al. [35] have also reported a strong reduction of adsorption on surfaces to which PEO has been grafted.

CONCLUSION

Knowledge of protein adsorption in relation to blood compatibility, as summarized in this chapter, has developed impressively over the past decade. During this period, studies of single proteins and simple mixtures have been supplemented by investigations using plasma and blood. Both areas must continue if adequate understanding and information are to be obtained.

The thesis is advanced in this chapter that control of protein adsorption may be the key to blood compatibility. This notion may seem trite since it ultimately means that surface properties must be controlled—so what else is new? However it seems to the present author that such an idea sharpens and focuses our thinking. Certainly most investigators have already accepted that we must control surface properties, but we now know a bit more about how and in what sense they should be controlled. This knowledge will expand further as we learn more in the coming years about protein adsorption kinetics and protein layer compositions adsorbed from blood as a function of surface properties.

ACKNOWLEDGEMENTS

The author wishes to thank the Medical Research Council of Canada, the Heart and Stroke Foundation of Ontario, and the Natural Sciences and Engineering Research Council of Canada for financial support of his research in the area of this article.

NOTE ADDED IN PROOF

The writing of this article was completed in 1986. Since that time publication of data on protein adsorption has continued at a brisk pace, and a number of new methods of studying adsorption have been developed. Advances in understanding have also been made though probably not in proportion to the expansion of the data base. It is perhaps appropriate to mention some of this more recent work but it must be emphasized that no more than a selection of what the present author considers to be the highlights will be indicated. The reader is also referred to two recent publications containing considerable information on protein adsorption [144,145].

Observations of the Vroman effect have continued to be made [146–151]. Most surfaces appear to undergo this effect and it is now established that it occurs in whole blood as well as in plasma [150]. The broader view of the Vroman effect as a general phenomenon whereby low concentration, high surface affinity proteins displace low affinity, high concentration proteins is becoming generally accepted. In support of this view, Horbett et al. have shown that proteins in binary mixtures can be adsorbed and then displaced [149,151], and work in the author's laboratory has shown that IgG as well as fibrinogen undergoes the Vroman effect [152]. IgG is adsorbed and displaced more rapidly than fibrinogen, suggesting that fibrinogen may displace IgG. This observation supports the earlier conclusions of Vroman and Adams referred to above (Reference [100], main text). Modeling of the Vroman effect has been attempted by Cuypers et al. [146] and by Slack and Horbett [153]. The former authors used a modified Langmuir model and formulated adsorption rate constants which include terms for interaction with other proteins already adsorbed. This model predicts sequential adsorption in binary protein systems. Slack and Horbett also used a modified Langmuir model in which the plasma was approximated to a binary protein system with fibrinogen as one protein and all the others combined as a second. This second "protein" is assumed to be able to displace adsorbed fibrinogen. The experimentally observed adsorption behavior was predicted qualitatively but not quantitatively by the model.

Recent work by Horbett et al. has focused on transitions in adsorbed proteins, particularly fibrinogen, as a function of time [154]. Adsorbed fibrinogen was found to become less elutable, less reactive to platelets, and less able to recognize anti-fibrinogen antibody, with increasing residence time on a polyurethane surface. This work suggests that protein layers are continuously evolving in biological and physical properties as well as in composition.

Among the methods recently developed to study protein adsorption, one should mention various immunochemical techniques. Cooper et al. [155] have reported on methods of mapping adsorbed proteins using gold-antibody markers which can be visualized in the electron microscope. Anderson et al. [156] have developed a double antibody method using a radiolabeled second antibody to quantify proteins adsorbed from blood. We have used immunoblotting methods qualitatively to identify proteins adsorbed from plasma or blood to surfaces [157].

A new method reported by Andrade et al. [158] is also worthy of note with respect to blood–surface interactions. These authors are using 2-dimensional electrophoresis of plasma before and after surface contact to determine quantitatively the adsorption of various proteins. This is essentially a depletion technique.

Considerable interest has also been generated recently by the possibility of using scanning–tunneling microscopy and atomic force microscopy to image individual adsorbed protein molecules in situ [159,160]. These techniques appear to hold considerable promise although for the moment it seems likely that they will be applicable to single proteins rather than plasma and blood.

REFERENCES

1 CRADDOCK, P. R., J. Fehr, A. P. Dalmasso, K. L. Brigham and H. S. Jacob. "Hemodialysis Leukopenia: Pulmonary Vascular Leukostasis Resulting From Complement Activation by Dialyzer Cellophane Membranes," *J. Clin. Invest*, 59:879–888 (1977).

2 LYNCH, R. E., R. M. Bosl, A. J. Streifel, J. P. Ebben, S. M. Ellers and C. M. Kjellstrand. "Dialysis Thrombocytopenia: Parallel Plate Versus Hollow Fiber Dialyzers," *Trans. Am. Soc. Artif. Int. Organs*, 24:704–707 (1978).

3 LAVAL DE, M., J. D. Hill, H. Mielke, M. L. Bramson, C. Smith and F. Gerbode. "Platelet Kinetics During Extracorporeal Circulation," *Trans. Am. Soc. Artif. Int. Organs*, 18:355–357 (1972).

4 FISHBEIN, M. C., R. J. Levy, V. J. Ferrans, L. C. Dearden, A. Nashef, A. P. Goodman and A. Carpentier. "Calcification of Cardiac Valve Prostheses," *J. Thorac. Cardiovasc. Surg.*, 83:602–609 (1982).

5 BAIER, R. E. and R. C. Dutton. "Initial Events in Interactions of Blood With a Foreign Surface," *J. Biomed. Mater. Res.*, 3:191–206 (1969).

6 VROMAN, L. and A. L. Adams. "Identification of Rapid Changes at Plasma-Solid Interfaces," *J. Biomed. Mater. Res.*, 3:43–67 (1969).

7 PACKHAM, M. A., G. Evans, M. F. Glynn and J. F. Mustard. "The Effect of Plasma Proteins on the Interaction of Platelets With Glass Surfaces," *J. Lab. Clin. Med.*, 73:686–697 (1969).

8 WHICHER, S. J. and J. L. Brash. "Platelet-Foreign Surface Interactions: Release of Granule Constituents From Adherent Platelets," *J. Biomed. Mater. Res.*, 12:181–201 (1978).

9 YOUNG, B. R., L. K. Lambrecht, R. M. Albrecht, D. F. Mosher and S. L. Cooper. "Platelet-Protein Interactions at Blood-Polymer Interfaces in the Canine Test Model," *Trans. Am. Soc. Artif. Int. Organs*, 29:442–446 (1983).

10 MACRITCHIE, F. "Proteins at Interfaces," *Adv. Protein Chem.*, 32:283–326 (1978).

11 KLOTZ, I. M. "Comparison of Molecular Structure of Proteins:

Helix Content, Distribution of Apolar Residues," *Arch. Biochem. Biophys.*, 138:704–706 (1970).

12 LOK, B. K., Y. -L. Cheng and C. R. Robertson. "Protein Adsorption on Crosslinked Polydimethyl Siloxane Using Total Internal Reflection Fluorescence," *J. Colloid Interface Sci.*, 91:104–116 (1983).

13 CHAN, B. M. C. and J. L. Brash. "Adsorption of Fibrinogen on Glass: Reversibility Aspects," *J. Colloid Interface Sci.*, 82:217–225 (1981).

14 BRASH, J. L. and D. J. Lyman. "Adsorption of Plasma Proteins in Solution to Uncharged Hydrophobic Polymer Surfaces," *J. Biomed. Mater. Res.*, 3:175–189 (1969).

15 MACRITCHIE, F. "The Adsorption of Proteins at the Solid-Liquid Interface," *J. Colloid Interface Sci.*, 38:484–488 (1972).

16 BRYNDA, E., M. Houska, Z. Pokorna, N. A. Cepalova, Y. V. Moiseev and J. Kalal. "Irreversible Adsorption of Human Serum Albumin Onto Polyethylene Film," *J. Bioeng.*, 2:411–418 (1978).

17 JENNISSEN, H. P. and G. Botzet. "Protein Binding to Two-Dimensional Hydrophobic Binding-Site Lattices: Adsorption Hysteresis on Immobilized Butyl Residues," *Int. J. Biolog. Macromolecules*, 1:171–179 (1979).

18 BRASH, J. L. and V. J. Davidson. "Adsorption on Glass and Polyethylene From Solutions of Fibrinogen and Albumin," *Thromb. Res.*, 9:249–259 (1976).

19 WEATHERSBY, P. K., T. A. Horbett and A. S. Hoffman. "Adsorption of Fibrinogen to Surfaces of Varying Hydrophilicity," *J. Bioeng.*, 1:395–409 (1977).

20 NORDE, W. and J. Lyklema. "The Adsorption of Human Plasma Albumin and Bovine Pancreas Ribonuclease at Negatively Charged Polystyrene Surfaces. I. Adsorption Isotherms. Effect of Charge, Ionic Strength and Temperature," *J. Colloid Interface Sci.*, 66:257–265 (1978).

21 BRASH, J. L. and S. Uniyal. "Dependence of Albumin-Fibrinogen Simple and Competitive Adsorption on Surface Properties of Biomaterials," *J. Polym. Sci.*, C66:377–389 (1979).

22 WILLIAMS, D. F., I. N. Askill and R. Smith. "Protein Adsorption and Desorption Phenomena on Clean Metal Surfaces," *J. Biomed. Mater. Res.*, 19:313–320 (1985).

23 BRASH, J. L., S. Uniyal, B. M. C. Chan and A. Yu. "Fibrinogen-Glass Interactions: A Synopsis of Recent Research," *Amer. Chem. Soc. Symp. Ser.*, 256:45–61 (1984).

24 SCHMITT, A., R. Varoqui, S. Uniyal, J. L. Brash and C. Pusineri. "Interactions of Fibrinogen With Surfaces of Varying Charge and Hydrophobic-Hydrophilic Balance. I. Adsorption Isotherms," *J. Colloid Interface Sci.*, 92:25–34 (1983).

25 CHENG, Y. L., S. A. Darst and C. R. Robertson. "Bovine Serum Albumin Adsorption and Desorption Rates on Solid Surfaces With Varying Surface Properties," *J. Colloid Interface Sci.* 118:212–223 (1987).

26 BRASH, J. L., S. Uniyal, C. Pusineri and A. Schmitt. "Interactions of Fibrinogen with Solid Surfaces of Varying Charge and Hydrophobic–Hydrophilic Balance. II. Dynamic Exchange Between Surface and Solution Molecules," *J. Colloid Interface Sci.*, 95:28–37 (1983).

27 JENNISSEN, H. P. "The Binding and Regulation of Biologically Active Proteins on Cellular Interfaces: Model Studies of Enzyme Adsorption on Hydrophobic Binding Site Lattices and Biomembranes," *Adv. Enzyme Regul.*, 19:377–406 (1981).

28 ANDRADE, J. D. "Surface and Interfacial Aspects of Biomedical Polymers," *Protein Adsorption, Vol. 2*, New York:Plenum Press (1985).

29 CHUANG, H. Y. K., W. F. King and R. G. Mason. "Interaction of

Plasma Proteins With Artificial Surfaces: Protein Adsorption Isotherms," *J. Lab. Clin. Med.*, 92:483–496 (1978).

30 WAUGH, D. F., L. J. Anthony and H. Ng. "The Interactions of Thrombin With Borosilicate Glass Surfaces," *J. Biomed. Mater. Res.*, 9:511–536 (1975).

31 WAUGH, D. F., J. A. Lippe and Y. R. Freund. "Interactions of Bovine Thrombin and Plasma Albumin With Low Energy Surfaces," *J. Biomed. Mater. Res.*, 12:599–625 (1978).

32 ELWING, H., S. Welin, A. Askendal, U. Nilsson and I. Lundstrom. "A Wettability Gradient Method for Studies of Macromolecular Interactions at the Liquid/Solid Interface," *J. Colloid Interface Sci.*, 119:203–210 (1987).

33 HORBETT, T. A. and A. S. Hoffman. "Bovine Plasma Protein Adsorption Onto Radiation Grafted Hydrogels Based on Hydroxyethyl Methacrylate and N-Vinyl Pyrrolidone," *Amer. Chem. Soc. Adv. Chem.*, 145:230–254 (1975).

34 GREGONIS, D. E., D. E. Buerger, R. A. Van Wagenen, S. K. Hunter and J. D. Andrade. "Poly(ethylene glycol) Surfaces to Minimize Protein Adsorption," *Trans. Soc. Biomaterials*, 7:266 (1984).

35 GOLANDER, C. -G., S. Johnsson, T. Vladkowa, P. Stenius and J. C. Eriksson. "Preparation and Protein Adsorption Properties of Photopolymerized Hydrophilic Films Containing N-Vinylpyrrolidone, Acrylic Acid or Ethylene Oxide Units," *Colloids and Surfaces* (to be published).

36 CASTILLO, E. J., J. L. Koenig and J. M. Anderson. "Characterization of Protein Adsorption on Soft Contact Lenses. I. Conformational Changes of Adsorbed Human Serum Albumin," *Biomaterials*, 5:319–325 (1984).

37 RATNER, B. D. and T. A. Horbett. "Protein Adsorption to Contact Lens Material," *Trans. Soc. Biomaterials*, 7:76 (1984).

38 BASZKIN, A., J. E. Proust and M. M. Boissonnade. "Adsorption of Bovine Submaxillary Mucin on Silicone Contact Lenses Grafted With Poly(vinyl pyrrolidone)," *Biomaterials*, 5:175–179 (1984).

39 TRIPATHI, R. C., B. T. Tripathi and R. Montague. "The Pathology of Soft Contact Lens Spoilage," *Am. Acad. Opthalmol.*, 87:365 (1980).

40 HORBETT, T. A. "Protein Adsorption to Hydrogels," in *Hydrogels in Medicine and Pharmacy*. N. A. Peppas, ed. Boca Raton:CRC Press Inc., pp. 127–171 (1986).

41 WEISS, L. "Studies on Cellular Adhesion in Tissue Culture. X. An Experimental and Theoretical Approach to Interaction Forces Between Cells and Glass," *Exp. Cell. Res.*, 53:603–614 (1968).

42 NORDE, W. and J. Lyklema. "Adsorption of Human Plasma Albumin and Bovine Pancreas Ribonuclease at Negatively Charged Polystyrene Surfaces. III. Electrophoresis," *J. Colloid Interface Sci.*, 66:277–284 (1978).

43 ORESKES, I. and J. M. Singer. "The Mechanism of Particulate Carrier Reactions. I. Adsorption of Human γ-globulin to Polystyrene Latex Particles," *J. Immunol.*, 86:338–344 (1961).

44 NORDE, W. and J. Lyklema. "Adsorption of Proteins From Aqueous Solution on Negatively Charged Polystyrene Surfaces," in *Ions in Macromolecular and Biological Systems*. D. H. Everett and B. Vincent, eds. Bristol:Colston Research Society, pp. 11–40 (1978).

45 NORDE, W. "Adsorption of Proteins at Solid Surfaces," in *Adhesion and Adsorption of Polymers, Part B*. L. H. Lee, ed., New York:Plenum Publishing Corp., pp. 801–825 (1980).

46 BRASH, J. L. and D. J. Lyman. "Adsorption of Proteins and Lipids to Nonbiological Surfaces," in *The Chemistry of Biosurfaces, Vol. 1*. M. L. Hair, ed. New York:Marcel Dekker, pp. 177–232 (1971).

47 MATHOT, C. and A. Rothen. "Adsorption of Purified Serum Pro-

teins on Metalized Glass Slides and Their Significance for the Immunoelectroadsorption Method," *J. Colloid Interface Sci.*, 31: 51–60 (1969).

48 ARNEBRANT, T. and T. Nylander, "Sequential and Competitive Adsorption of β-lactoglobulin and χ-Casein on Metal Surfaces," *J. Colloid Interface Sci.*, 111:529–533 (1986).

49 CLARK, G. C. F. and D. F. Williams. "The Effects of Proteins on Metallic Corrosion," *J. Biomed. Mater. Res.*, 16:125–134 (1982).

50 IVARSSON, B., P. -O. Hegg, I. Lundstrom and U. Jonsson. "Adsorption of Proteins on Metal Surfaces Studied by Ellipsometric and Capacitance Measurements," *Colloids and Surfaces*, 13:169–192 (1985).

51 ZSOM, R. L. J. "Dependence of Preferential Bovine Serum Albumin Oligomer Adsorption on the Surface Properties of Monodiperse Polystyrene Latices," *J. Colloid Interface Sci.*, 111:434–445 (1986).

52 LEE, R. G., C. Adamson and S. W. Kim. "Competitive Adsorption of Plasma Proteins Onto Polymer Surfaces," *Thromb. Res.*, 4:485–490 (1974).

53 HORBETT, T. A., P. K. Weathersby and A. S. Hoffman. "The Preferential Adsorption of Hemoglobin to Polyethylene," *J. Bioeng.*, 1:61–77 (1977).

54 CHEN, J., J. D. Andrade and R. Van Wagenen. "Oxy- and Deoxy-haemoglobin Adsorption Onto Glass and Polymer Surfaces," *Biomaterials*, 6:231–236 (1985).

55 UNIYAL, S., J. L. Brash and I. A. Degterev. "Influence of Red Blood Cells and Their Components on Protein Adsorption," *Amer. Chem. Soc. Adv. Chem.*, 199:277–292 (1982).

56 COLEMAN, D. L., H. L. C. Meuzelaar, T. R. Kessler, W. M. McLennen, J. M. Richards and D. E. Gregonis. "Retrieval and Analysis of a Clinical Total Artificial Heart," *J. Biomed. Mater. Res.*, 20:417–431 (1986).

57 UNIYAL, S. and J. L. Brash. "Patterns of Adsorption of Proteins From Human Plasma onto Foreign Surfaces," *Thromb. Haemostas*, 47:285–290 (1982).

58 HORBETT, T. A., P. K. Weathersby and A. S. Hoffman. "Hemoglobin Adsorption to Three Polymer Surfaces," *Thromb. Res.*, 12:319–329 (1978).

59 HORBETT, T. A. and P. K. Weathersby. "Adsorption of Proteins from Plasma to a Series of Hydrophilic-Hydrophobic Copolymers. I. Analysis With the In Situ Radio Iodination Technique," *J. Biomed. Mater. Res.*, 15:403–423 (1981).

60 HORBETT, T. A. "Adsorption of Proteins from Plasma to a Series of Hydrophilic-Hydrophobic Copolymers. II. Compositional Analysis with the Prelabeled Protein Technique," *J. Biomed. Mater. Res.*, 15:673–695 (1981).

61 SEVASTIANOV, V. I. and E. A. Tseytlina. "The Activation of the Complement System by Polymer Materials and Their Blood Compatibility," *J. Biomed. Mater. Res.*, 18:969–978 (1984).

62 SEVASTIANOV, V. I. and O. V. Laksina. "Adsorption-Desorption Processes of Proteins at Solid-Blood Interfaces," *J. Colloid Interface Sci.*, 112:279–289 (1986).

63 IHLENFELD, J. V. and S. L. Cooper. "Transient In Vivo Protein Adsorption onto Polymeric Biomaterials," *J. Biomed. Mater. Res.*, 13:577–591 (1979).

64 VROMAN, L., A. L. Adams, G. C. Fischer and P. C. Munoz. "Interaction of High Molecular Weight Kininogen, Factor XII, and Fibrinogen in Plasma at Interfaces," *Blood*, 55:156–159 (1980).

65 MASON, R. G., M. S. Read and K. M. Brinkhous. "Effect of Fibrinogen Concentration on Platelet Adhesion to Glass," *Proc. Soc. Exp. Biol. Med.*, 137:680–682 (1971).

66 BRASH, J. L. and P. ten Hove. "Effect of Plasma Dilution on Adsorption of Fibrinogen to Solid Surfaces," *Thrombos. Haemostas*, 51:326–330 (1984).

67 HORBETT, T. A. "Mass Action Effects on the Adsorption of Fibrinogen from Hemoglobin Solutions and from Plasma," *Thrombos. Haemostas*, 51:174–181 (1984).

68 BREEMHAAR, W., E. Brinkman, D. J. Ellens, T. Beugeling and A. Bantjes. "Preferential Adsorption of High Density Lipoprotein from Blood Plasma onto Biomaterial Surfaces," *Biomaterials*, 5:269–274 (1984).

69 BRASH, J. L. and J. A. Thibodeau. "Identification of Proteins Adsorbed from Human Plasma to Glass Bead Columns: Plasmin-Induced Degradation of Adsorbed Fibrinogen," *J. Biomed. Mater. Res.*, 20:1263–1275 (1986).

70 LYMAN, D. J., L. C. Metcalf, D. Albo, K. F. Richards and J. Lamb. "The Effect of Chemical Structure and Surface Properties of Synthetic Polymers on the Coagulation of Blood. III. In Vivo Adsorption of Proteins on Polymer Surfaces," *Trans. Amer. Soc. Artif. Int. Organs*, 20:474–478 (1974).

71 GENDREAU, R. M. and R. J. Jakobsen. "Blood-Surface Interactions: Fourier Transform Infrared Studies of Protein Surface Adsorption from Flowing Blood Plasma and Serum," *J. Biomed. Mater. Res.*, 13:893–906 (1979).

72 WINTERS, S., R. M. Gendreau, R. I. Leininger and R. J. Jakobsen. "Fourier Transform Infrared Spectroscopy of Protein Adsorption from Whole Blood: II. Ex Vivo Sheep Studies," *Applied Spectroscopy*, 36:404–409 (1982).

73 LIMBER, G. K. and R. G. Mason. "Studies of Proteins Elutable from Cuprophane Exposed to Human Plasma," *Thromb. Res.*, 6:421–430 (1975).

74 LIMBER, G. K., C. H. Glenn and R. G. Mason. "Studies of Proteins Elutable from Certain Artificial Surfaces Exposed to Human Plasma," *Thromb. Res.*, 5:735–746 (1974).

75 BOISSON-VIDAL, C., J. Jozefonvicz and J. L. Brash. "Interactions of Proteins in Plasma with Modified Polystyrene Resins," *J. Biomed. Mater. Res.* (submitted).

76 FOUGNOT, C., J. Jozefonvicz, M. Samama and L. Bara. "New Heparin-Like Insoluble Materials: Part I," *Ann. Biomed. Eng.*, 7:429–439 (1979).

77 WEATHERSBY, P. K., T. A. Horbett and A. S. Hoffman. "A New Method for Analysis of the Adsorbed Plasma Protein Layer on Biomaterial Surfaces," *Trans. Amer. Soc. Artif. Int. Organs*, 22:242–251 (1976).

78 GRINNELL, F. and V. Phan. "Deposition of Fibronectin on Material Surfaces Exposed to Plasma," *J. Cell Physiol.*, 116:289–296 (1983).

79 YOUNG, B. R., L. K. Lambrecht, S. L. Cooper and D. F. Mosher. "Plasma Proteins: Their Role in Initiating Platelet and Fibrin Deposition on Biomaterials," *Amer. Chem. Soc. Adv. Chem.*, 199:317–350 (1982).

80 HORBETT, T. A. and R. B. Counts. "von Willebrand Factor/Factor III Adsorption to Surfaces from Human Plasma," *Thromb. Res.*, 36:599–608 (1984).

81 WOODHOUSE, K. A. and J. L. Brash. "Adsorption of Plasminogen from Plasma to Solid Surfaces" (manuscript in preparation).

82 GRIFFIN, J. H. "Surface Dependent Activation of Blood Coagulation," in *Interaction of the Blood with Natural and Artificial Surfaces*. E. W. Salzman, ed. New York:Marcel Dekker, pp. 139–170 (1981).

83 REVAK, S. D., C. G. Cochrane and J. H. Griffin. "The Binding and Cleavage Characteristics of Human Hageman Factor During Contact Activation. A Comparison of Normal Plasma with

Plasmas Deficient in Factor XI, Prekallikrein, or High Molecular Weight Kininogen," *J. Clin. Invest.*, 59:1167–1175 (1977).

84 WIGGINS, R. C. and C. G. Cochrane. "The Autoactivation of Rabbit Hageman Factor," *J. Exp. Med.*, 150:1122–1133 (1979).

85 SILVERBERG, M., J. T. Dunn, L. Garen and A. P. Kaplan. "Autoactivation of Human Hageman Factor. Demonstration Using A Synthetic Substrate," *J. Biol. Chem.*, 255:7281–7286 (1980).

86 COLMAN, R. W. "Surface-Mediated Defense Reactions. The Plasma Contact Activation System," *J. Clin. Invest.*, 73:1249–1253 (1984).

87 GRIFFIN, J. H. "The Role of Surface-Dependent Activation of Hageman Factor (Factor XII)," *Proc. Natl. Acad. Sci. USA*, 75:1998–2002 (1978).

88 MANDLE, R., R. W. Colman and A. P. Kaplan. "Identification of Prekallikrein and High Molecular Weight Kininogen as a Complex in Human Plasma," *Proc. Natl. Acad. Sci. USA*, 73:4179–4183 (1976).

89 THOMPSON, R. E., R. Mandle and A. P. Kaplan. "Studies of the Binding of Prekallikrein and Factor XI to High Molecular Weight Kininogen and Its Light Chain," *Proc. Natl. Acad. Sci. USA*, 76:4862–4866 (1979).

90 GRIFFIN, J. H. and C. G. Cochrane. "Mechanisms for the Involvement of High Molecular Weight Kininogen in Surface-Dependent Reactions of Hageman Factor (Coagulation Factor XII)," *Proc. Natl. Acad. Sci. USA*, 73:2554–2558 (1976).

91 WIGGINS, R. C., B. N. Bouma, C. G. Cochrane and J. H. Griffin. "Role of High Molecular Weight Kininogen in Surface Binding and Activation of Coagulation Factor XI and Prekallikrein," *Proc. Natl. Acad. Sci. USA*, 74:4636–4640 (1977).

92 MARGALIT, R. and S. Schiffman. "Factor XI Adsorption to Surface: Interaction of High Molecular Weight Kininogen (HMWK) and a Plasma Adsorption Inhibitor," *Blood*, 56:168–172 (1980).

93 MATSUDA, T., T. Toyosaki and H. Iwata. "Adsorption and Activation Processes of Contact Phase of Intrinsic Coagulation on Polymer Surfaces," *Trans. Soc. Biomat.*, 7:8 (1984).

94 FOUGNOT, C., J. Jozefonvicz, M. Samama and L. Bara. "New Heparin-Like Insoluble Materials: Part II," *Ann. Biomed. Eng.*, 7:441–450 (1979).

95 BOFFA, M. C., B. Dreyer and C. Pusineri. "Plasma Contact Activation and Decrease of Factor V Activity on Negatively Charged Polyelectrolytes," *Thromb. Haemostas*, 51:61–64 (1984).

96 ADAMS, A. L., G. C. Fischer, P. C. Munoz and L. Vroman. "Convex-Lens-on-Slide: A Simple System for the Study of Human Plasma and Blood in Narrow Spaces," *J. Biomed. Mater. Res.*, 18:643–654 (1984).

97 WOJCIECHOWSKI, P., P. ten Hove and J. L. Brash. "Phenomenology and Mechanism of the Transient Adsorption of Fibrinogen from Plasma (Vroman Effect)," *J. Colloid Interface Sci.*, 111:455–465 (1986).

98 SCOTT, C. F., L. D. Silver, M. Schapira and R. W. Colman. "Cleavage of Human High Molecular Weight Kininogen Markedly Enhances Its Coagulant Activity. Evidence That This Molecule Exists as a Procofactor," *J. Clin. Invest.*, 73:954–962 (1984).

99 BRASH, J. L., C. F. Scott, P. ten Hove, P. Wojciechowski and R. W. Colman. "Mechanism of Transient Adsorption of Fibrinogen from Plasma to Solid Surfaces: Role of the Contact and Fibrinolytic Systems," *Blood*, 71:932–939 (1988).

100 VROMAN, L. and A. L. Adams. "Adsorption of Proteins Out of Plasma and Solutions in Narrow Spaces," *J. Colloid Interface Sci.*, 111:391–402 (1986).

101 LAMBRECHT, L. K., M. D. Lelah, C. A. Jordan, M. E. Pariso, R. M. Albrecht and S. L. Cooper. "Evaluation of Thrombus De-

position onto Polymeric Biomaterials in a New Subhuman Primate Ex Vivo Series Shunt Model," *Trans. Am. Soc. Artif. Int. Organs*, 29:194–199 (1983).

102 LELAH, M. D., T. G. Grasel, J. A. Pierce and S. L. Cooper. "Ex Vivo Interactions and Surface Property Relations of Polyether Urethanes," *J. Biomed. Mater. Res.*, 20:433–468 (1986).

103 LELAH, M. D., T. G. Grasel, J. A. Pierce, L. K. Lambrecht and S. L. Cooper. "Effect of Silastic Tubing Wall Thickness on Ex Vivo Thrombus Formation in a Series Shunt," *Trans. Am. Soc. Artif. Int. Organs*, 30:411–416 (1984).

104 HORBETT, T. A. "The kinetics of Baboon Fibrinogen Adsorption to Polymers: In Vitro and In Vivo Studies," *J. Biomed. Mater. Res.*, 20:739–772 (1986).

105 HANSON, S. R., L. A. Harker, B. D. Ratner and A. S. Hoffman. "In Vivo Evaluation of Artificial Surfaces With a Nonhuman Primate Model of Arterial Thrombosis," *J. Lab. Clin. Med.*, 95:289–304 (1980).

106 SEIFERT, L. M. and R. T. Greer. "Evaluation of In Vivo Adsorption of Blood Elements onto Hydrogel-Coated Silicone Rubber by Scanning Electron Microscopy and Fourier Transform Infrared Spectroscopy," *J. Biomed. Mater. Res.*, 19:1043–1071 (1985).

107 MATSUDA, T., H. Takano, K. Hayashi, Y. Jaenaka, S. Takaichi, M. Umezu, T. Nakamura, H. Iwata, T. Nakatini, T. Tanaka, S. Takatani and T. Akutsu. "The Blood Interface with Segmented Polyurethanes: Multilayered Protein Passivation Mechanism," *Trans. Amer. Soc. Artif. Int. Organs*, 30:353–357 (1984).

108 CHUANG, H. Y. K. "In Situ Immunoradiometric Assay of Fibrinogen Adsorbed to Artificial Surfaces," *J. Biomed. Mater. Res.*, 18:547–559 (1984).

109 OWEN, D. R., C. M. Chen, J. A. Oschner and R. M. Zone, "Interactions of Plasma Proteins with Selective Artificial Surfaces," *Trans. Am. Soc. Artif. Int. Organs*, 31:240–243 (1985).

110 CHENOWETH, D. E., S. W. Cooper, T. E. Hugli, R. W. Stewart, W. H. Blackstone and T. W. Kirklin. "Complement Activation During Cardiopulmonary Bypass: Evidence for Generation of C3a and C5a Anaphylatoxins," *New Eng. J. Med.*, 304:497–503 (1981).

111 CHENOWETH, D. E. "Biocompatibility of Hemodialysis Membranes. Evaluation with C3a Anaphylatoxin Radioimmunoassays," *Asaio J.*, 7:44–49 (1984).

112 WARD, C. A., A. Koheil, W. R. Johnson and P. N. Madras. "Reduction in Complement Activation from Biomaterials by Removal of Air Nuclei from the Surface Roughness," *J. Biomed. Mater. Res.*, 18:255–269 (1984).

113 PAYNE, M. S. and T. T. Horbett. "Complement Activation by Hydroxyethylmethacrylate-Ethylmethacrylate Copolymers," *J. Biomed. Mater. Res.*, 21:843–859 (1987).

114 ELWING, H., B. Ivarsson and I. Lundstrom. "Complement Deposition from Human Sera on Silicon Surfaces Studied In Situ by Ellipsometry. The Influence of Surface Wettability," *Eur. J. Biochem.*, 156:359–365 (1986).

115 BRASH, J. L. and S. Uniyal. "Adsorption of Albumin and Fibrinogen to Polyethylene in Presence of Red Cells," *Trans. Am. Soc. Artif. Int. Organs*, 22:253–256 (1976).

116 BORENSTEIN, N. and J. L. Brash. "Red Blood Cells Deposit Membrane Components on Contacting Surfaces," *J. Biomed. Mater. Res.*, 20:723–730 (1986).

117 BLACKSHEAR, P. L. in *The Chemistry of Biosurfaces, Vol. 2*, M. L. Hair, ed., New York:Marcel Dekker, pp. 523–562 (1972).

118 MUNRO, M. S., R. C. Eberhart, N. J. Maki, B. E. Brink and W. J. Fry. "Thrombo Resistant Alkyl Derivatized Polyurethanes," *Asaio J.*, 6:65–75 (1983).

119 HENNINK, W. E., S. W. Kim and J. Feijen. "Inhibition of Surface-Induced Coagulation by Pre-adsorption of Albumin-Heparin Conjugates," *J. Biomed. Mater. Res.*, 18:911–926 (1984).

120 SUZUKI, M., Y. Tamada, H. Iwata and Y. Ikada. "Polymer Surface Modification to Attain Blood Compatibility of Hydrophobic Polymer," in *Physiochemical Aspects of Polymer Surfaces*, K. L. Mittal, ed. New York:Plenum, pp. 923–942 (1983).

121 GOUDSWARD, J., J. A. van der Donk and A. Noordzij. "Protein A Reactivity of Various Mammalian Immunoglobulins," *Scand. J. Immunol.*, 8:21–28 (1978).

122 DEUTSCH, D. G. and E. T. Mertz. "Plasminogen: Purification from Human Plasma by Affinity Chromatography," *Science*, 170:1095–1096 (1977).

123 ENGVALL, E. and E. Rhuoslahti. "Binding of Soluble Form of Fibroblast Surface Protein, Fibronectin, to Collagen," *Int. J. Cancer*, 20:1–5 (1977).

124 FAROOQUI, A. A. "Purification of Enzymes by Heparin-Sepharose Affinity Chromatography," *J. Chromatog.*, 184:335–345 (1980).

125 TRAVIS, J. and R. Powell. "Selective Removal of Albumin from Plasma by Affinity Chromatography," *Clin. Chim. Acta*, 49:49–52 (1973).

126 GIANAZZA, E. and P. Arnaud. "A General Method for Fractionation of Plasma Proteins. Dye-Ligand Chromatography on Immobilized Cibacron Blue F3-GA," *Biochem. J.*, 201:129–136 (1982).

127 KINET, J. -P., W. I. Bensinger, F. Frankenne, G. Hennen, J. Foidart and P. Mahieu. "Immunoadsorption with Staphylococcal Protein A in Human Neoplasms." in *Selective Plasma Component Removal*. A. A. Pineda, ed. Mount Kisco, N.Y.:Futura, pp. 105–137 (1984).

128 LEININGER, R. I. "Polymers as Surgical Implants," *Crit. Rev., Bioengineering*, 1:333–381 (1972).

129 KIM, S. W., C. D. Ebert, J. Y. Lin and J. C. McRea. "Nonthrombogenic Polymers. Pharmaceutical Approaches," *Asaio J.*, 6:76–87 (1983).

130 HATTON, M. W. C., G. Rollason and M. V. Sefton. "Fate of Thrombin and Thrombin-Antithrombin III Complex Adsorbed to a Heparinized Biomaterial: Analysis of the Enzyme-Inhibitor Complexes Displaced by Plasma," *Thromb. Haemostas*, 50:873–877 (1984).

131 ARNANDER, C., M. Dryjski, R. Larson, P. Olsson and J. Swendenborg. "Thrombin Uptake and Inhibition on Endothelium and Surfaces with a Stable Heparin Coating: A Comparative In Vitro Study," *J. Biomed. Mater. Res.*, 20:235–246 (1986).

132 PLATÉ, N. "On the Mechanism of Enhanced Thrombo Resistance of Polymeric Materials in Presence of Heparin," *Biomaterials*, 4:14–20 (1983).

133 FOUGNOT, C., M. Jozefowicz and R. D. Rosenberg. "Affinity of Purified Thrombin or Antithrombin III for Two Insoluble Anticoagulant Polystyrene Deriatives: I. In Vitro Adsorption Studies," *Biomaterials*, 4:294–298 (1983).

134 HENNINK, W. E., L. Dost, J. Feijen and S. W. Kim. "Interaction of Albumin-Heparin Conjugate Pre-absorbed Surfaces with Blood," *Trans. Am. Soc. Artif. Int. Organs*, 29:200–205 (1983).

135 PERTER, T., Jr., H. Taniuchi and C. B. Anfinsen, Jr. "Affinity Chromatography of Serum Albumin with Fatty Acids Immobilized on Agarose," *J. Biol. Chem.*, 248:2447–2451 (1973).

136 RICCITELLI, S. D., R. G. Schlattarer, J. A. Hendrix, G. B. Williams and R. C. Eberhart. "Albumin Coatings Resistant to Shear-Induced Desorption," *Trans. Am. Soc. Artif. Int. Organs*, 31:250–256 (1985).

137 KUSSEROW, B. K., R. Larrow and J. Nichols. "The Urokinase-Heparin Bonded Synthetic Surface. An Approach to the Creation of a Prosthetic Surface Possessing Composite Antithrombogenic and Thrombolytic Properties," *Trans. Am. Soc. Artif. Int. Organs*, 17:1–5 (1971).

138 SENATORE, F., F. Bernath and K. Meisner. "Clinical Study of Urokinase-Bound Fibrocollagenous Tubes," *J. Biomed. Mater. Res.*, 20:177–188 (1986).

139 SENATORE, F. and F. Bernath. "Lysis Time and FDP Immunoprecipitation by Soluble and Immobilized Urokinase," *J. Biomed. Mater. Res.*, 20:189–203 (1986).

140 BRASH, J. L., B. M. C. Chan, P. Szota and J. A. Thibodeau. "Degradation of Adsorbed Fibrinogen by Surface-Generated Plasmin," *J. Biomed. Mater. Res.*, 19:1017–1029 (1985).

141 WASIEWSKI, W., M. J. Rasco, B. M. Martin, J. C. Detwiler and J. W. Fenton. "Thrombin Adsorption to Surfaces and Prevention with Polyethylene Glycol 6000," *Thromb. Res.*, 8:881–886 (1976).

142 HORNE, McD. K. "The Adsorption of Thrombin to Polypropylene Tubes: The Effect of Polyethylene Glycol and Bovine Serum Albumin," *Thromb. Res.*, 37:201–212 (1985).

143 NAPPER, D. H. *Polymeric Stabilization of Colloidal Dispersions*, London:Academic Press (1983).

144 "Proteins at Interfaces," Brash, J. L. and T. A. Horbett, eds., *Amer. Chem. Soc. Symp. Ser., Vol. 343, ACS Books, Washington, D.C.* (1987).

145 "Blood in Contact with Natural and Artificial Surfaces," Ann. N.Y. Acad. Sci., Vol. 516 (1987)

146 CUYPERS, P. A., G. M. Willems, H. C. Hemker and W. T. Hermens. "Adsorption K. Kinetics of Protein Mixtures: A Tentative Explanation of the Vroman Effect," Ann. N.Y. Acad. Sci., 516:244–252 (1987).

147 ELWING, H., K. Askendal and I. Lundstrom. "Competition between Adsorbed Fibrinogen and High Molecular Weight Kininogen on Solid Surfaces Incubated in Human Plasma (the Vroman Effect): Influence of Solid Surface Wettability," *J. Biomed. Mater. Res.*, 21:1023–1028 (1987).

148 LINDON, J. N., G. McManama, L. Kushner, E. W. Merrill and E. W. Salzman. "Does the Conformation of Adsorbed Fibrinogen Dictate Platelet Interactions with Artificial Surfaces," *Blood*, 68:355–362 (1986).

149 SLACK, S. M., J. L. Bohnert and T. A. Horbett. 1987. "Effects of Surface Chemistry and Coagulation Factors on Fibrinogen Adsorption from Plasma," Ann. N.Y. Acad. Sci., 516:223–243 (1987).

150 BRASH, J. L. and P. ten Hove. "Transient Adsorption of Fibrinogen on Foreign Surfaces: Similar Behavior in Plasma and Whole Blood," *J. Biomed. Mater. Res.*, 23:157–169 (1989).

151 SLACK, S. M. and T. A. Horbett. "Physicochemical and Biochemical Aspects of Fibrinogen Adsorption from Plasma and Binary Protein Solutions onto Polyethylene and Glass," *J. Colloid Interface Sci.*, 124:535–551 (1988).

152 CORNELIUS, R. M. and J. L. Brash. "Real Time Analysis of Protein Adsorption," *Colloid and Surface Science Symposium, Seattle, Washington, 1989*, abstr. #134.

153 SLACK, S. M. and T. A. Horbett. "Changes in the Strength of Fibrinogen Attachment to Solid Surfaces: An Explanation of the Influence of Surface Chemistry on the Vroman Effect," *J. Colloid Interface Sci.*, 133:148–165 (1989).

154 CHINN, J. A., S. E. Posso, T. A. Horbett and B. D. Ratner. "Residence Time Effects on Surface Bound Fibrinogen as Indicated by Changes in SDS Elutability, Antibody Binding, and Platelet Adhesion," *Trans. Soc. Biomat.*, 13:242 (1990).

155 PITT, W. G., K. Park and S. L. Cooper. "Sequential Protein Ad-

sorption and Thrombus Deposition on Polymeric Biomaterials," *J. Colloid Interface Sci.*, 111:343–362 (1986).

156 ZIATS, N. P., B. P. Tierney, N. Topham, O. D. Ratnoff and J. M. Anderson. "Protein Adsorption on Biomedical Polymers from Whole Human Blood," *Trans. Soc. Biomat.*, 13:268 (1990).

157 MULZER, S. R. and J. L. Brash. "Identification of Proteins Adsorbed to Hemodialyzers during Clinical Use," *J. Biomed. Mater. Res.*, 23:1483–1504 (1989).

158 HO, C. H., V. Hlady, J. D. Andrade and K. D. Caldwell. "Solution Depletion and Two Dimensional Gel Electrophesis—A Method for the Study of the Competitive Adsorption of Plasma Proteins," *Trans. Soc. Biomat.*, 13:137 (1990).

159 LEWIS, K. B. and B. D. Ratner. "Scanning Tunneling Microscopic Study of Fibrinogen Adsorption on Gold Surfaces," *Trans. Soc. Biomat.*, 13:94 (1990).

160 LIN, J. N., B. Drake, A. S. Lea, P. K. Hansma and J. D. Andrade. "Real Time Imaging of Immunological Adsorption on Mica Using the Atomic Force Microscope," *Trans. Soc. Biomat.*, 13:135 (1990).

CHAPTER 3

Surface Modification:
Blood Compatibility of Small Diameter Vascular Graft

CHANDRA P. SHARMA, Ph.D.[1]

ABSTRACT: An attempt is made to explain the blood. material interactions on the basis of surface energy parameters. The changes at the interface caused by various drugs and antiplatelet agents are also discussed. The relevance of such concepts in the development of small diameter vascular graft is stressed.

INTRODUCTION

For biomedical applications, particularly small diameter vascular graft (<4mm inner diameter), it is imperative that a material is nontoxic, sterilizable, noninflammatory, mechanically stable with matching compliances, nondegradable, noncarcinogenic, and fabricable [1]. These properties, however, do not guarantee the prolonged life of the material inside the body, nor do they ensure hemostasis in the cardiovascular environment [2].

Since prosthetic–blood interaction is dependent on the nature of the surface (e.g., surface charge [3–5], surface free energy [2,5], chemical group distribution, heterogenicity, surface texture, porosity [7–8], smoothness, and flow conditions [9]), various surfaces may behave differently. Some surfaces, for example, may adsorb certain proteins much more than others under the same physiological conditions. It is possible to take advantage of this phenomenon and prepare and modify the surfaces in such a way that they adsorb a desired protein, e.g., albumin, much more than others, because it has been suggested that platelets adhere where they find adsorbed fibrinogen [10,11].

Albumin is chosen because it discourages platelet adhesion, which is one way of encouraging antithrombogenicity [12,13]. We must mention here that thrombosis is a very complex process, and our efforts are limited to a few parameters only. These efforts are, in fact, part of an endeavour to understand the physicochemical nature of thrombosis.

BACKGROUND AND CURRENT STATUS

Significant efforts have been made for developing the vascular graft, and various solutions have emerged since 1942. These solutions include the homograft [14,15], autogenous saphenous vein [16], autogenous arteries [17], endarterectomy [18,19], dacron (polyester) prostheses [20,21] PTFE grafts [22], autogenous endothelial coated grafts [23,24], polyurethane grafts (electrostatically spun) [25,26], and grafts from biological origins [27,28] (e.g., umbilical cord graft, glutaraldehyde starch tanned umbilical vein [29] surrounded with a dacron net (Dardick graft), Johnson bovine biograft [30] and glutaraldehyde tanned negatively–charged graft developed by Sawyer and associates). However, it seems none of the solutions is final with regard to the nonthrombogenicity of the grafts.

The prediction that surface properties are related to blood compatibility has been made from very early times [1,2]. Andrade [31] postulated that material surfaces which tend to have an interfacial energy of zero will be highly thromboresistant. The fact that materials with a minimal interfacial energy, like hydrogels, do possess a low thrombus adherence enhances the validity of this theory. Similarly, the surface free energies of many polymers have been calculated by contact angle measurements [32–34]. It was also observed that a polymer having

[1]Division of Biosurface Technology, Biomedical Technology Wing, Sree Chitra Tirunal Institute for Medical Sciences and Technology, Poojapura, Trivandrum–695012, India

a critical surface tension of around 20–30 dynes/cm is highly blood–compatible [35], but exceptions have been reported—as in the case of LTI carbons ($\gamma c = 50$ dynes/cm).

Further surface characterization has been done by Kaelble and Moacanin [36]. They have indicated that dispersion $\alpha_s = \sqrt{\gamma_s^d}$ and polar $\beta_s = \sqrt{\gamma_s^p}$ components of polymer surfaces play an important role in interfacial interactions. They reached this conclusion on the basis of their surface energy analysis of 190 biological and implant surfaces (more than about twenty different types). It was found that low dispersion–high polar surfaces, typified by surface–treated Stellite 21 with $\alpha_s = 5.0$ (dynes/cm)$^{1/2}$ and $\beta_s \geq 5.0$ (dynes/cm)$^{1/2}$, provide surface energies that appear to favor weak adsorption and retention of plasma protein, i.e., a poor surface from the compatibility point of view. Again, high dispersion–low polar surface energy for the implant, e.g., low temperature isotopic (LTI) carbon with $\alpha_s \geq 6.0$ (dynes/cm)$^{1/2}$ and $\beta_s \leq 2.0$ (dynes/cm)$^{1/2}$, provide surface energetics favoring stable plasma protein film retention. They indicated this case as an excellent surface for blood compatibility. Recent experimental observations and theoretical calculations have also suggested an optimum α_s of 4.7 (dynes/cm)$^{1/2}$ and β_s of 3.0 (dynes/cm)$^{1/2}$ for a possible blood–compatible surface [6]. This conclusion is based on observations on Biomer, PU-1025, and avcothanes.

It is also noted that such surfaces may adsorb albumin preferentially, on the basis of the dispersion and polar components of the protein interacting with the surface. With this logic, not only can we explain why LTI carbons are blood–compatible [37] (due to increased adsorption of albumin), but we can also explain the cell adhesion onto nonbiological substrates [38], although this is only one parameter and our explanation is certainly not complete. The surface energy of platelets, γ_{PV}, has been evaluated [39] to be 69.7 ergs/cm². We can express γ_{PV} as follows:

$$\gamma_{PV} = \gamma_{PV}^d + \gamma_{PV}^p = \alpha_P^2 + \beta_P^2 = 69.7 \text{ ergs/cm}^2 \quad (1)$$

where

$$\alpha_P = \sqrt{\gamma_{PV}^d} \text{ and } \beta_P = \sqrt{\gamma_{PV}^p}$$

Note that γ_{PV}^d and γ_{PV}^p are dispersion and polar components, respectively, of γ_{PV}.

The work of adhesion, W_{PL}, can be written as

$$W_{PL} = \gamma_{LV} (1 + \cos \theta_L)$$

The contact angle, θ_L, of saline water on platelets is determined to be 16.3° and the surface tension of water, γ_{LV}, is 72.5 ergs/cm². These values yield

$$W_{PL} = 72.5 (1 + \cos 16.3°) = 142 \text{ ergs/cm}^2 \quad (2)$$

Work of adhesion can also be expressed as:

$$W_{PL} = 2 (\alpha_P \alpha_L + \beta_P \beta_L) \leq 2 \gamma_{LV} \quad (3)$$

For water we know [6] $\alpha_L \cong 4.67$ (dynes/cm)$^{1/2}$ and $\beta_L \cong 7.14$ (dynes/cm)$^{1/2}$. We then use Equations (1), (2) and (3) to evaluate α_p and β_p as 4.4 (dynes/cm)$^{1/2}$ and 7.1 (dynes/cm)$^{1/2}$, respectively. Now by using these dispersion and polar components of platelets, their interaction at the interface with any artificial surface can be understood as has been described for LTI carbons earlier in the case of proteins [37]. In case of blood contact with LTI carbons, adhesion of cells is minimized by albumin adsorption on the surface by similar considerations [37].

Since platelets, cells, and proteins tend to have net negative charges, as does the blood vessel wall (which has a negative zeta potential of -8 to -13 mV [5,40]), surface charge is also thought to be important in thrombosis. Therefore, the repulsion between the blood constituents and the blood vessel wall may be the factor that prevents coagulation. Electrets with a negative surface charge have been found to show better blood compatibility than a nonpolarized polymer surface. Recent observations have predicted that a very high negative charge (-40 to -120 mV, zeta potential) on the surface may prove beneficial for developing a nonthrombogenic surface [40]. However, the view that a highly charged surface will not adsorb protein and, therefore, will remain nonthrombogenic is dubious because such surfaces that never form passivating layers will always remain active. In such cases, even if protein adsorption is not taking place, blood components may still be suffering damage. This damage may cause the implant to be unsuccessful in the long term.

On the other hand, if the surface is not very highly charged, certain proteins may be adsorbed and form a passivating layer, which may ultimately make the material less adverse toward blood components and hence relatively more blood–compatible. Therefore, surfaces should be modified in such a way that they adsorb certain proteins, such as albumin, preferentially and form a good, blood–compatible passivating layer.

Further conformational changes in protein structure during interaction with an implanted surface [41,42] may be due to local variations in dispersion and polar components of surface energy and these changes may encourage other interactions with blood components. Fibrinogen has platelet–adhering sites [43] that may have different surface–energy parameters than the rest of the segment. These sites may be suitable for encouraging preferential platelet adherence.

However, when fibrinogen is adsorbed on polyacrylonitrile, no increased adhesion of platelets is observed [44]. That is, either all active sites participate in interaction with the surface, or the protein has become inactive after adsorption due to conformational variations.

The initial phase of clotting has been well studied and reported by various groups and laboratories led by Ratnoff [45], Cochrane [46], Kaplan [47], Davies [48] and Colman [49]. Surface contact under physiological conditions induces activation of Factor XII. According to Ratnoff [45], acceleration of the interaction of Factors IX and VIII and of Factors X and V by altered platelets also reflects a surface–mediated effect of platelet phospholipids (platelet Factor III). These aspects constitute the intrinsic coagulation system for which surface effects are significant. It has been indicated [50,51] that the inhibition of blood coagulation on a negatively charged graphite surface could be enhanced by adsorption of a cationic detergent followed by ionic bonding of heparin. Similar aspects have been reviewed earlier [52,53]. In fact, when heparin is dissolved in blood, it does not block the activation of Factor XII, and unless it is present in very high concentrations, it does not inhibit the adhesion or aggregation of platelets, except that induced by thrombin [50]. However, further evidence suggests that dissolved heparin may activate Factor XII, but the adsorption of plasma proteins to surface-bound heparin apparently occurs without activation of coagulation. Clotting tests employing Factor–XII-deficient plasma and assessment of plasma esterase activity indicate that heparinized surfaces fail to activate Factor XII—a feature very important in their compatibility with blood. Platelets have been found not to adhere to heparinized surfaces [50]. Fibrinogen adsorption is highly retarded, but the stability of the ionically bound heparin, using TDMAC (tridodecyl methyl ammonium chloride) or benzalkonium chloride, is still a matter of controversy. Covalent coupling has resulted in the denaturation of heparin, resulting in limited antithrombogenic character. It is also believed that leaching of heparin from the surface may be the reason for the resultant anticoagulant action [50]. However, it seems that blood compatibility can be further enhanced if a slow release of antithrombogenic agents from polymer surfaces is effected. Heparin–type structures possessing sulfamate and carboxylate groups have also been synthesized [54,55]. For example, polyelectrolytes synthesized from natural rubber have shown good blood compatibility properties when fixed on polyetherurethane surfaces [56].

Structural regularity also seems to play an important role in the protein adsorption process of synthetic polymers [57]. Various proteins and polymers exhibit electrical conduction and semiconduction properties that may be affected by structural regularity. Furthermore, to provide a blood–compatible surface under physiological flow conditions, the polymer surface should generate a water structure similar to that in the adjacent layers of the endothelial surface. This is true especially in the case of hydrogels where the water content (nearly 17%) has been found to produce the least thrombus in the case of a HEMA–EMA graft [58]. A hydrogel-like combination of polycations and polyanions has also been proved to have good antithrombogenicity [59].

In our laboratory we have attempted to graft hydroxyethyl methacrylate (HEMA) on polyetherurethanes to adjust the dispersion and polar components for encouraging preferential adsorption of albumin [60–62]. It seems that about fifteen minutes' exposure in N_2 atmosphere of HEMA to our grafts (fabricated by precipitation on glass rods), with about two–and–one–half hours' exposure of Co^{60} source (total dosage 0.275 Mrad) brings the surface close to optimization, i.e., encouraging albumin adsorption (as evaluated by I^{125}-labelled albumin and fibrinogen adsorption–desorption kinetics) from a mixture of proteins [62] containing 25 mg% albumin, 15 mg% γ-globulin and 7.5 mg% fibrinogen.

Similar work in progress elsewhere [63] relates to the monomer (e.g., tetrafluoroethylene) grafting on the polymer substrate (e.g., dacron). Actually, the monomer gas is introduced into a vacuum system containing the substrate material and is subjected to an electric discharge to generate the active species that covalently bond to the substrate's surface. In the ex vivo femoral shunt baboon model, improved patency has been observed for the above small diameter vascular grafts. However, it seems we still are not close enough to have a satisfactory small diameter vascular graft.

Another approach is to develop a biological substrate on the polymer surface using albumin. Polyetherurethane urea (PEUU), synthesized in our laboratory, and biomer (Ethicon) were used for modification studies [64–66]. Albumin was adsorbed on the PEUU grafts and was permanently fixed by γ-irradiation. Since the first layer of protein may be denatured by the irradiation, a second layer of albumin was adsorbed that was crosslinked with glutaraldehyde. The unlinked aldehyde groups were utilized to immobilize a third layer of albumin with minimal conformational change. The stability of the albumin layers was studied using I^{125}-labelled protein [67].

In the natural vessel, prostacyclin released from the intima prevents the thrombus formation [68]. Because prostaglandins such as PGI_2, PGE_1 and PGD_2 are potent inhibitors of platelet adhesion and aggregation [68,69], we immobilized PGE_1 on albuminated polyurethane substrate via glutaraldehyde coupling [65]. The platelet adhesion was discouraged on these surfaces. The albumin to fibrinogen mole ratio for adsorption was found to be high, favoring antithrombogenicity [67]. Immobilized urokinase on albuminated polyurethane or collagenated polyurethane also demonstrated good results towards nonthrombogenicity [70].

Since γ-irradiation may affect the bulk properties of the polymer, we have attempted to crosslink albumin by glow–discharge treatment with nitrogen plasma [71]. The exposure time was standardized ($\sim$ 15 minutes) on the basis of contact angle measurements. Glow discharge treatment was also employed to couple polyelectrolytes (synthesized from natural rubber, Hevea Brasiliensis "para rubber"), which possess proven anticoagulant and antiplatelet properties. Natural prostaglandins like PGI$_2$ and PGE$_1$ have a very short half life; hence, an attempt was made to immobilize a synthetic analog of PGI$_2$ in combination with polyelectrolyte on albuminated PEUU employing the glow discharge technique [72]. The results were very encouraging. The surfaces thus modified showed negligible platelet adherance, and the fibrinogen to albumin mole ratio was low compared to the unmodified surface. These results prompted us to select a combination of PGI$_2$ analog and heparin for immobilization on albuminated PEUU [73]. Here the fibrinogen adsorption was relatively high compared to the bare surface, while the platelet adherance remained low. These observations suggest that when interpreting the fibrinogen–platelet interrelationship towards thrombogenicity, the antiplatelet activity of the immobilized molecules should also be given consideration.

Some surfaces exhibit increased adsorption of albumin simultaneously with antiplatelet activity. Typical examples are PGE, immobilized surfaces [67], c-AMP adsorbed surfaces [74], and some drug adsorbed surfaces, particularly Sembrina [75] (Methyl Dopa). We think that there may be a general pattern of biological interactions as antiplatelet biomolecules either encourage albumin adsorption onto artificial surfaces or indirectly mediate the fibrinogen molecules away from platelet receptor sites by preferentially promoting albumin at the interface. This possibility needs to be explored further.

These studies provide some insight into the development of nonthrombogenic polymer surfaces. Some in vivo tests on albuminated PEUU grafts (inner diameter ~ 5 mm) as a replacement for iliac arteries in mongrel dogs showed short–term (~ 18 days) encouraging results. However, it seems that initiation of thrombus function is usually at the junction. Preliminary efforts to develop a new fabrication procedure to avoid this problem are underway.

The polymer (polyetherurethane urea) is dissolved in dimethylformamide. Several glass rods of proper diameter (say 4 mm) are washed with chromic acid cleaning mixture, then rinsed with copious amounts of distilled water. The clean glass rods are then rotated vertically with appropriate speed in the polymer solution and then in distilled water. These glass rods are then dried in a hot air oven at 60°C for ~ 30 min. The procedure is repeated only once more to keep this layer thin (~ 0.1 mm). About 1 cm from each end, several layers of aluminum foil (approximately equal to the wall thickness of natural artery) are wrapped, and the above procedure is repeated again (usually three times) to get the appropriate thickness of ~ 0.3 mm. The rods are left overnight in distilled water, and the next day the graft is removed easily. The

aluminum foil is also removed. The double layer at the ends can be used for adjusting the natural artery ends. The artery is sutured in between these two layers. This procedure can help inhibit the platelets from contacting the freshly cut artery, i.e., collagen, and also facilitate the blood flow rather smoothly. To produce a kink–resistant graft, reinforcement with a coil of any thin (~ 0.2 mm diameter) soft wire [76] that is noncorrosive and nonmagnetic can be accomplished during the procedure. The preferred wire is either titanium or a chromium–cobalt–molybdenum alloy such as MP-35 N (Wayne Metals, Inc., Indiana).

We have also observed that Vitamin C discourages platelet adhesion [77] and encourages albumin adsorption [78]. An attempt is being made to develop a suitable combination which can help improve the long-term blood compatibility of implants without causing many side effects. From in vitro observation it seems that 0.5 mg% aspirin + 1.5 mg% Vitamin C + 0.15 mM Vitamin B$_6$ + 2 mg% Vitamin E, significantly decreases platelet adhesion and enhances albumin adsorption [79]. Blood compatibility was also observed to improve if the implant stored in glutaraldehyde was rinsed with Vitamin B$_6$ solution. The effect of antibiotics (namely neomycin, gentamycin, penicillin–G, streptomycin and ampicillin) on polymer fibrinogen binding was also studied using I^{125}–labelled protein [80]. It was observed that antibiotics inhibit fibrinogen–surface binding in variable degrees, whereas lymphocyte infusion extends the surface–fibrinogen bonding beyond two hours of incubation. Antibiotics may bind to the fibrinogen molecule and prevent its surface from binding, but they may modulate the lymphocyte membrane and extend their absorption to polymer substrates. The above observations may have clinical implications. Since complementary proteins are important from the allergic and immune response point of view [81], we have also attempted to understand the interaction of these proteins (e.g., C$_1$, C$_{1q}$, C$_2$, C$_3$ and C$_4$) with artificial surfaces like polycarbonate, teflon and cellophane [82,83]. We have observed that C$_1$ and C$_{1q}$ discourage platelet adhesion much more than C$_2$, C$_3$ and C$_4$. Lipid and enzyme interactions are also important and should be considered before the final choice is made [84].

Currently, in addition to having a pharmaceutical modification of blood by vitamins and drugs, and surface modification of the graft, a release of c-AMP is also maintained [85]. Such a release of c-AMP onto PGE$_1$ immobilized, albuminated surfaces will further enhance the albumin adsorption from the blood with minimal adherence of platelets. Since albumin encourages the cell growth, this will create a suitable condition for the growth of intima within the physiological environment.

Attempts are also being made to induce normal endothelial cells to grow to confluence [86] over the surface, utilizing human vascular endothelial cells. Some success has been achieved, although Saphenous vein still seems to be the standard choice.

FUTURE OUTLOOK

Since the success of a small diameter vascular graft is dependent upon its interaction with various blood components, the material used should be able to initiate preferential interaction to create biological manifestations in favor of antithrombogenicity, e.g., quickly evolving the conditions for the formation of neointima. In the last decade, although much knowledge has been accumulated, and it seems as if we are fairly close to the solution, true success is still elusive due to our present limitations in relation to the complex nature of the problem. Obviously, a great deal of fundamental and applied research is still required in order to obtain a surface closer in character to the natural surface of an artery. The most promising possibilities are the development of new materials and new physicochemical and biological techniques for surface modification.

REFERENCES

1 LYMAN, D. J. "Polymers in Medicine and Surgery," in *Polymer Science and Technology, Vol. 8*, R. L. Kronenthal, ed. New York: Plenum (1975).

2 SHARMA, C. P. "Surface Interface Changes of Polymers and Biocompatibility," *J. Sci. Ind. Res.*, 39:453 (1980).

3 SAWYER, P. N., B. Stanczewski and F. D. Mistry. "Current Appraisal of Negatively Charged Glutaraldehyde–Tanned Grafts," in *Biologic and Synthetic Vascular Prostheses*, J. C. Stanley et al., eds. New York:Grune & Stratton (1982).

4 SAWYER, P. N. "Electrode–Biologic Tissue Interactions at Interfaces—A Review," *Biomat. Med. Dev. Art. Org.*, 12:161–196 (1984–85).

5 SAWYER, P. N. and J. W. Pate. "Bioelectric Phenomena as an Etiologic Factor in Intravascular Thrombosis," *Surg.*, 34:491–500 (1953).

6 SHARMA, C. P. "Surface Energy and Interfacial Parameters of Synthetic Polymers to Blood Compatibility," *Biomaterials*, 2:57–59 (1981).

7 BORETOS, J. W. "Cellular Polymers for Medical Use. The Vital Role of Porosity and Permeability," *Cellular Polymers*, 3:345–358 (1984).

8 WESOLOWSKI, S. A., C. C. Fries, K. E. Karlson, J. DeBakey and P. N. Sawyer. "Porosity: Primary Determinant of Ultimate Fate of Synthetic Vascular Grafts," *Surgery*, 50:91 (1961).

9 VROMAN, L. "Problems in the Development of Materials That are Compatible with Blood," *Biomat. Med. Dev. Art. Org.*, 12:307–323 (1984–85).

10 VROMAN, L., A. L. Adams and M. Klings. "Interactions Among Human Blood Proteins at Interfaces," *Fed. Proc.*, 30:1494–1501 (1971).

11 VROMAN, L., A. L. Adams, G. C. Fischer, P. C. Munoz and M. Stanford. "Proteins, Plasma and Blood in Narrow Spaces of Clot–Promoting Surfaces," *Adv. in Chemistry Series*, 199:266–276 (1982).

12 LYMAN, D. J., K. G. Klein, J. L. Brash, B. K. Fritzinger, J. D. Andrade and F. Bonomo. "Platelet Interaction with Protein Coated Surfaces: An Approach to Thrombo–Resistant Surfaces," *Thromb. Diath. Haemorr (Supp)*, 42:109–114 (1971).

13 PACKHAM, M. A., G. Evans, M. F. Glynn and J. F. Mustard. "The Effect of Plasma Proteins on the Interactions of Platelets with Glass Surfaces," *J. Lab. Clin. Med.*, 73:686–697 (1969).

14 PATE, J. W., P. N. Sawyer, R. A. Deterling, W. Blunt and M. S. Parshley. "Early Results in the Experimental Use of Freeze–Dried Arterial Grafts," *Surg. Forum Am. Col. Surg.*, 3:147 (1952).

15 HUFNAGEL, C. A., P. J. Rabil and L. Reed. "A Method for the Preservation of Arterial Homo– and Heterografts," *Surg. Forum*, 4:162 (1953).

16 SZILAGYI, D. E. et al. "Autogenous Vein Grafting in Femoro-popliteal Atherosclerosis: The Limits of Its Effectiveness," *Surgery*, 86:836 (1979).

17 URSCHEL, H. C. et al. "Aorta to Coronary Artery Vein Bypass Graft for Occlusive Disease," *Ann. Thorac. Surg.*, 8:114 (1969).

18 SAWYER, P. N. and M. J. Kaplitt. "Gas Endarterectomy: Clinical Applications in Cardiovascular Therapy," A. N. Breast, ed. Philadelphia:F. A. Davis (1969).

19 SOBEL, S., M. J. Kaplitt, M. Reingold and P. N. Sawyer. "Gas Endarterectomy," *Surgery*, 59:517 (1966).

20 DEBAKEY, M. E. et al. "Clinical Application of a New Flexible Knitted Dacron Arterial Substitute," *Arch. Surg.*, 77:713 (1958).

21 WESOLOWSKI, S. A. "Evaluation of Tissue and Prosthetic Vascular Grafts," Springfield, Ill.:Charles C. Thomas (1962).

22 FLORIAN, A., L. H. Cohn, G. J. Dammin and J. J. Collins. "Small Vessel Replacement with Gore-Tex (Expanded Polytetra Fluoroethylene)," *Arch. Surg.*, 3:267 (1976).

23 HERRING, M. B., R. Dilley, R. A. Jersild, Jr., L. Boxer, A. Gardner and J. Glover, "Seeding Arterial Protheses with Vascular Endothelium. The Nature of the Lining," *Ann. Surg.*, 190:84 (1979).

24 SALZMAN, E. W. and E. W. Merril. "Interaction of Blood with Artificial Surfaces," in *Hemostasis and Thrombosis—Basic Principles and Clinical Practice*. R. W. Colman, J. Hirsk, V. J. Marker and E. W. Salzman, eds. Philadelphia:J. B. Lippincott, p. 931 (1982).

25 ANNIS, D., A. Bornat, R. O. Edwards, A. Higham, B. Loveday and J. Wilson. "An Elastomeric Vascular Prothesis," *Trans. Amer. Soc. Artif. Inter. Org.*, 24:209 (1978).

26 LYMAN, D. J., F. J. Fazzio, W. Voornees, G. Robinson and D. Albo. "Compliance as a Factor Effecting the Patency of a Copolyurethane Vascular Graft," *J. Biomed. Mater. Res.*, 12:337 (1978).

27 DARDIK, H. and I. Dardik. "Successful Arterial Substitution with Modified Human Umbilical Vein," *Ann. Surg.*, 183:252 (1976).

28 ROSENBERG, N. et al. "The Use of Arterial Implants Prepared by Enzymatic Modification of Arterial Heterografts. II. The Physical Properties of the Elastica and Collagen Components of the Arterial Wall," *AMA Arch. Surg.*, 74:89 (1957).

29 BAIER, R. E. "Physical Chemistry of Blood–Surface Interface," in *Biologic & Synthetic Vascular Prostheses*. J. C. Stanley, W. E. Burkel, S. M. Lindenauer, R. H. Bartlett and J. G. Turcotte, eds. New York:Grune & Stratton, p. 83 (1982).

30 ROSENBERG, N. "The Modified Bovine Arterial Graft," *Arch. Surg.*, 3:272 (1976).

31 ANDRADE, J. D., H. B. Lee, M. S. John, S. W. Kim and J. B. Hibbs, Jr. "Water as a Biomaterial," *Trans. Amer. Soc. Artif. Int. Org.*, 19:1 (1973).

32 HOLLY, F. J. and M. F. Refojo. "Wettability of Hydrogels. 1. Poly(2-hydroxyethyl methacrylate)," *J. Biomed. Mater. Res.*, 9:315–326 (1975).

33 ANDRADE, J. D., R. N. King, D. E. Gregonis and D. J. Coleman. "Surface Characterization of Poly(hydroxyethyl methacrylate) and Related Polymers. I. Contact Angle Methods in Water," *J. Polym. Sci. Polym. Symp.*, 66:313 (1979).

34 HOLLY, F. J. and M. F. Refojo. "Hydrogels for Medical and Related Applications," *Amer. Chem. Soc. Symp. Series.* J. D. Andrade, ed. 31:252 (1976).

35 BAIER, R. E., V. L. Gott and A. Furuse. "Surface Chemical Evaluation of Thromboresistant Materials Before and After Venous Implantation," *Trans. Amer. Soc. Artif. Int. Org.*, 16:50–57 (1970).

36 KAELBLE, D. M. and J. Moacanin. *Proceedings of the 1st Cleveland Symposium on Macromolecules: Structure and Properties of Biopolymers, October 1976, Polymer*, 18:475 (1977).

37 SHARMA, C. P. "LTI Carbons: Blood Compatibility," *J. of Colloid. Inter. Sci.*, 97:585–586 (1984).

38 SHARMA, C. P. "Protein and Platelet Interaction with Polymer Surfaces—A Comment," *Biomat. Med. Dev. Art. Org.*, 12:267–271 (1984–85).

39 NEUMANN, A. W., O. S. Hum, D. W. Francis, W. Zingg and C. J. Van Oss. "Kinetic and Thermodynamic Aspects of Platelet Adhesion from Suspension to Various Substrates," *J. Biomed. Mat. Res.*, 14:499 (1980).

40 THUBRIKAR, M., T. Reich and I. Cadoff. "Study of Charge of the Intima and Artificial Materials," *J. Biomechanics*, 13:663 (1980).

41 MORRISSEY, B. W. "The Adsorption and Conformation of Plasma Proteins: A Physical Approach," *Ann. N.Y. Acad. Sci.* Leo Vroman and E. F. Leonard, eds. 283:50–64 (1977).

42 MORRISSEY, B. W., L. E. Smith, R. R. Stromberg and C. A. Fenstermaker. "Ellipsometric Investigation of the Effect of Potential on Blood Protein Conformation and Adsorbance," *J. Colloid Inter. Sci.*, 56:557–563 (1976).

43 MARGUERIE, G. A., E. F. Plow and T. S. Edgington. "Human Platelets Possess an Inducible and Saturable Receptors Specific for Fibrinogen," *J. Biol. Chem.*, 254:5357–5363 (1979).

44 CHUANG, H. Y. K., T. R. Sharpton, S. F. Mohammad, N. C. Sharma and R. G. Mason. "Reactivity of Human Fibrinogen Adsorbed on Two Different Types of Hemodialysis Membranes," (Abstract), *VIIth International Congress on Thrombosis and Haemostasis*, 46:304 (1981).

45 RATNOFF, O. D. "Surface–Mediated Reactions of Blood Clotting and Related Phenomena," *Nouv. Rev. Hematol.*, 21:75–79 (1979).

46 WIGGINS, R. C. and C. C. Cochrane. "The Autoactivation of Rabbit Hageman Factor," *J. Exp. Med.*, 150:1122–1133 (1979).

47 SILVERBERG, M., J. T. Dunn, L. Garen and A. P. Kaplan. "Autoactivation of Human Hageman Factor," *J. Biol. Chem.*, 255:7281–7286 (1980).

48 HEIMARK, R. L., K. Kurachi, K. Fujikawa and E. W. Davie. "Surface Activation of Blood Coagulation, Fibrinolysis and Kinin Formation," *Nature*, 286:456–460 (1980).

49 SCOTT, C. F., E. P. Kirby, P. K. Schick and R. W. Colman. "Effects of Surfaces on Fluid–Phase Prekallikrein Activation," *Blood*, 57:553–560 (1981).

50 ROSENBERG, R. D. and L. H. Lam. "Heparinized Surfaces—A Comment," *Annals New York Acad. Sci.*, 283:404–418 (1977).

51 GOTT, V. L. "The Second Decade of Biomaterials Development and Evaluation: A Time To Apply the Scientific Method," *Bull. N.Y. Acad. Med.*, 48:216–224 (1972).

52 SHARMA, C. P. and T. Chandy. "Surface Modification of Polymers, Blood Compatibility of L-Ascorbic Acid: Understanding and Challenges," *Polym. Plast. Tech. Eng.*, 23:119–131 (1984).

53 SHARMA, C. P., V. K. Krishnan and M. S. Valiathan. "Perspectives and Problems of Blood Compatible Polymers," *Polym. Plast. Tech. Eng.*, 18:233 (1982).

54 VANDER DOES, L., T. Beugeling, P. E. Froehling and A. Bantjes. "Synthetic Polymers with Anticoagulant Activity," *J. of Polym. Sci. Polym. Symp.*, 66:337–348 (1979).

55 SHARMA, C. P., T. Chandy and P. V. Ashalatha. "Surface Modification of Polycarbonate with Synthetic Polyelectrolyte—Anticoagulant Activity," *Biomat. Med. Dev. Art. Organs*, 12:215–233 (1984–85).

56 SHARMA, C. P. and P. V. Ashalatha. "Surface Modification—Blood Compatibility," *Cellular Polymers*, 3:325–343 (1984).

57 SHARMA, C. P. "Proteinated Surfaces at Solid–Water–Octane Interface," *Polym. Journal*, 14:1007 (1982).

58 RATNER, B. D., A. S. Hoffmann, S. R. Hanson, L. A. Harker and J. D. Whiffen. "Blood Compatibility—Water Content Relationships for Radiation–Grafted Hydrogels," *J. Polym. Sci. Polym. Symp.*, 66:363–375 (1979).

59 VOGEL, M. K., R. A. Cross, H. J. Bixler and R. J. Guzman. "Medical Use for Polyelectrolyte Complexes," in *Biomedical Polymers*, A. Rembaum and M. Shen, eds. pp. 181–197 (1971).

60 SHARMA, C. P. "Radiation–Induced Modification of Polyurethane with Hydroxyethyl Methacrylate," *Bull. Mat. Sci.*, 7:71 (1985).

61 SHARMA, C. P. and A. K. Nair. "Radiation Induced HEMA Grafted Polyurethane Surfaces: Platelet Adhesion," *J. Colloid. Inter. Sci.*, 104:277 (1985).

62 NAIR, A. K. and C. P. Sharma. "Interaction of Proteins and Platelets with HEMA Grafted Polyurethane Surfaces," *Current Science*, 4:185 (1985).

63 GARFINKLE, A. M., A. S. Hoffman, B. D. Ratner, L. O. Rynolds and S. R. Hanson. "Effect of a Tetrafluoroethylene Glow Discharge on Patency of Small Diameter Dacron Vascular Grafts," Presented at the annual meeting of the Am. Soc. for Artificial Internal Organs, Washington, D.C. (May 1984), Transactions of the ASAIO, 30 (1984).

64 SHARMA, C. P. and G. Kurian. "Radiation Induced Albuminated Surfaces—Their Modifications Towards Blood Compatibility," *J. Colloid. Int. Sci.*, 97:38 (1984).

65 SHARMA, C. P. and G. Joseph. "Surface Immobilized PGE₁ and Albumin Towards Blood Compatibility: Platelet Adhesion Changes Due to Aspirin—Vitamin C," *Polym. Plast. Tech. Eng.*, 24:297–307 (1985).

66 SHARMA, C. P. and N. V. Nirmala. "Protein–Polyelectrolyte–PGE₁–Modified Biomer—Platelet Adhesion," *J. Colloid Inter. Sci.*, 101:591 (1984).

67 SHARMA, C. P. and G. Joseph. "Proteins Adsorption on PGE₁ Immobilized Albuminated Biomer," *J. Colloid Inter. Sci.*, 3(2):534 (1986).

68 MONCADA, S. and J. R. Vane. "The Role of Prostacyclin in Vascular Tissue," *Fed. Proc.*, 38:66–71 (1979).

69 BONNE, C., B. Martin, M. Watada and F. Regnault. "The Antagonism of Prostaglandins I₂, E, and D₂ by Prostaglandin E₂ in Human Platelets," *Thromb. Res.*, 21:13–22 (1981).

70 SHARMA, C. P. and M. C. Sunny. "Changes in Protein Adsorption/Desorption on Albuminated Surfaces due to c-AMP Release," *Poly. Plastics Tech. & Eng.*, 26(2):83–93 (1987)

71 JOSEPH, G. and C. P. Sharma. "Platelet Adhesion to Surfaces

Treated with Glow Discharge and Albumin," *J. Biomed. Mat. Res.*, 20:677 (1986).

72 JOSEPH, G. and C. P. Sharma. "Prostacyclin Immobilized Albuminated Surfaces," *J. Biomed. Mat. Res.*, 21:937 (1987).

73 SHARMA, C. P. and G. Joseph. "Fibrinogen/Platelet Interaction with PGI₂ Analog—Heparin Immobilized Albuminated Polyurethane," *ACS Proceedings on Polymeric Materials Sc. & Engg., Fall Meeting, Chicago, Illinois*, p. 423 (1985).

74 CHANDY, T. and C. P. Sharma. "Protein–Polymer Interaction — Changes with Plasma Components, Vitamins and Antiplatelet Drugs at the Interface," *Polymer Plast. Tech. Eng.*, 26:143–227 (1987).

75 SHARMA, C. P. and T. Chandy. "Changes in Albumin/Platelet Interaction with an Artificial Surface," *Artificial Organs*, 12:143–151 (1988).

76 SHARMA, C. P. and M. C. Sunny. "Fabrication Techniques for Thin–Walled, Kink–Resistant Tubular Structures for Use in Medical Devices—A Simplified Method," *Current Science*, 55(17):846 (1986).

77 CHANDY, T. and C. P. Sharma. "Platelet Adhesion on Polycarbonate Changes Due to L-ascorbic Acid," *J. Colloid. Int. Sci.*, 92:102–104 (1983).

78 CHANDY, T. and C. P. Sharma. "Changes in Protein Adsorption on Polycarbonate Due to L-ascorbic Acid," *Biomaterials*, 6:416–420 (1985).

79 CHANDY, T. and C. P. Sharma. "Protein/Platelet Interaction with an Artificial Surface: Effect of Vitamins and Platelet Inhibitors," *Thromb. Research*, 41:9–22 (1986).

80 CHANDY, T. and C. P. Sharma. "Antibiotics Reversal of Surface–Fibrinogen Interaction: Changes with Lymphocytes," *Artificial Organs*, 205:969–976 (1986).

81 PORTER, R. R. and K. B. M. Reid. "The Biochemistry of Complement," *Nature*, 275:699–704 (1978).

82 SHARMA, C. P. and T. Chandy. "Artificial Surface—Complement Proteins—L-ascorbic Acid: Platelet Interaction at the Interface—An Understanding," *Current Science*, 54:615–618 (1985).

83 CHANDY, T. and C. P. Sharma. "Platelet Adhesion to an Artificial Surface: Interactions by C₁ᵩ, C₄ Complement Proteins and Vitamin C," *Thromb. Research*, 32:245–251 (1983).

84 CHANDY, T. and C. P. Sharma. "Lipid–Protein Interaction at the Blood–Polymer Interface—Changes Due to L-ascorbic Acid," *J. of Colloid. Int. Sci.*, 108:104 (1985).

85 SHARMA, C. P. and M. C. Sunny. "Albuminated Surfaces with Cyclic-AMP Release: Blood Compatibility," *Second National Symposium on Surfactants: Emulsions and Biocolloids*, IIT Delhi, pp. 22–24 (December 1985), *Polymer Plast. Tech. Engg.*, 26:83–93 (1987).

86 CALLOW, A. D. "New Thoughts on Arterial Substitutes: The Biologic Period IInd World Congress on Biomaterials," Washington, D.C., *Transactions*, 7:292 (1984).

CHAPTER 4

Biostability of Polyurethane Elastomers: A Critical Review

MICHAEL SZYCHER, Ph.D.[1]

HISTORICAL

Nineteen eighty-seven marked the 50th anniversary of the introduction of polyurethanes. Professor Otto Bayer was synthesizing polymer fibers to compete with nylon when he developed the first fiber-forming polyurethane in 1937.

His invention ranks among the major breakthroughs in polymer chemistry, but the polymer was dismissed as impractical by his superiors at I.G. Farberindustrie. For more than 20 years Germany had been at the forefront of synthetic fibers technology, beginning with the introduction of polyvinyl-chloride fibers in 1913.

Germany remained pre-eminent in this field until 1935 when Carothers discovered the nylons; E. I. du Pont in America introduced and began marketing nylon fibers, protected by a barrage of patents which proved impossible to overcome. Nothing as versatile and practical as the polyamides was available, prompting Bayer to investigate similar polymers, not covered by the impenetrable DuPont patents.

At the end of January, 1938, Rinke and collaborators were successful in reacting an aliphatic 1,8 octane diisocyanate with 1,4 butanediol to form a low-viscosity melt from which they were able to draw fibers. These early efforts resulted in what are now known as polyurethanes: the esters of carbamic acid. These polyurethanes could be spun from the melt; yarns and monofilaments that could be made from their new polymer were of high quality. Rinke and associates were awarded the first U.S. patent on polyurethanes in 1938 [1].

Like many developments, polymer chemistry, which began as a small specialized branch of organic chemistry,

began to grow rapidly and adopted a new nomenclature, much as biochemistry had done before. Table 1 presents the recognized names of two important linkages found in polymers, comparing classical organic chemistry nomenclature to that used in polymer chemistry and biochemistry.

The first I.G. Farberindustrie polyurethane had a melting point of 185°C, and became available under the trade names Igamid U for synthetic fabrics, and Perlon U for producing artificial silk or bristles. A softer version was also available under the trade name Igamid UL. Foams were also produced by adding water to isocyanates in the presence of hydroxyl-terminated polyesters, to form carbonamides and release carbon dioxide as the blowing agent. These foams, named Troporit M were used to produce aircraft propeller blades, and rigid, foam-filled landing flaps and skis.

Not to be outdone, DuPont was also at the forefront of polyurethane technology in the U.S., receiving patents in 1942 covering the reactions of diisocyanates with glycols, diamines, polyesters and certain other active hydrogen-containing chemicals. From these humble beginnings emerged the polyurethanes, the most versatile polymers in the biomaterials armamentarium.

Table 2 summarizes some of the most important events in the historical development of the polyurethanes, with emphasis on biomedical applications.

POLYURETHANE ELASTOMERS

The dictionary defines "elastomer" as a "material which at room temperature can be stretched repeatedly, and upon immediate release will return to its approximate original length." Since natural rubber was the original elastomer, in polymeric nomenclature, synthetic materials that approximate or exceed cured natural rubber in

[1]Chairman, Chief Technical Officer, PolyMedica Industries, Inc. Burlington, Massachusetts 01803, U.S.A.

TABLE 1. Recognized Nomenclature of Some Important Polymers

Linkage	Organic Chemistry	Polymer Chemistry	Biochemistry
H O | || −N−C−	Amide	Nylon	Peptide
H O | || −N−C−O− |	Carbamate	Urethane	Not applicable

physical properties are called "elastomeric." Because natural rubber exhibits such an excellent combination of physical properties (i.e, tensile strength: 4000 psi, 400 to 600 percent ultimate elongation), the term "elastomeric grade" is frequently used to characterize and describe those synthetic materials with the highest physical performance.

Among the highest performing biomedical-grade elastomers are the polyurethanes. Polyurethanes are block copolymers containing blocks of low molecular weight polyesters or polyethers linked together by a urethane group:

$$\left(\!\!\begin{array}{ccc} N & - & C & - & O \\ | & & \|\| \\ H & & O \end{array}\!\!\right)$$

These have the versatility of being either rigid, semi-rigid, or flexible. They have also demonstrated excellent blood compatibility [9], outstanding hydrolytic stability [10,11,12], superior abrasion resistance, excellent physical strength and high flexure endurance. No wonder the polyurethanes enjoy such great popularity among producers of medical prostheses.

However, the use of the generic term "polyurethane" is deceiving in that all useful polyurethane polymers contain a minority of urethane functional groups. Thus, polyurethane is a term of convenience rather than accuracy, since these polymers are not derived by polymerizing a monomeric "urethane" reactant, nor are they polymers containing primarily urethane linkages. In fact, other groups such as ethers, amides, biurets, and allophanates are the majority linkages in the molecular chain. Although urethane linkages represent the minority of functional

TABLE 2. Historical Development of Polyurethane Elastomers

Year	Event	Reference
1937	I.G. Farbenindustrie applies for first polyurethane patent	
1938	First U.S. Patent awarded to Rinke, et al.	1
1942	Introduction of Igamid U, Perlon U and Igamid UL in Germany	
1943	Linear polyesters introduced to polyurethane reaction, leading to production of Vulcollan elastomers	
1954	Patent on Lycra® awarded to Langerak	2
1955	Patent on Estane awarded to C. Schollenberger (B.F. Goodrich)	3
1960	Patent on Lycra awarded to Steuber (DuPont) U.S. Patent No. 2,929,804	
1971	Patent on Avcothane awarded to E. Nyilas (Avco)	4
1972	Lycra T-126, subsequently renamed Biomer, researched by J.W. Boretos	5
1977	Family of thermoplastic elastomers introduced under the trade name Pellethane (Upjohn)	6
1979	Second generation aliphatic polyurethanes disclosed by Szycher, et al.	7
1984	Patent on thermoplastic elastomers awarded to M. Szycher	8

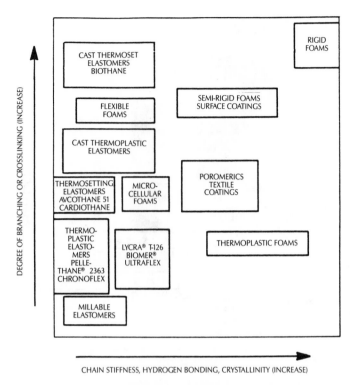

Figure 1. *Structure–property relationships in polyurethanes.*

groups, as long as the polymers contain a significant number of urethane linkages, the name polyurethane is correctly ascribed to these polymers.

The polyurethanes are a heterogeneous family of polymers, unlike PVC, polyethylene, and polystyrene. The polyurethanes comprise an array of different products, ranging from rigid foams to soft, millable grains.

Figure 1 presents a summary of structure–property relationship for polyurethanes; branching/cross-linking is plotted on the ordinate, and intermolecular forces on the abscissa. Under these conditions, we can encompass all the commercially available polyurethanes, and define which elastomeric products are of the greatest importance in biomedical applications. At the right corner, representing extreme branching and chain stiffness, are the rigid urethane foams. Therefore, at this extreme, the thermoset rigid foams occupy the highest rank of cross-linking and chain stiffness.

None of the polyurethanes listed at either extreme of Figure 1 have attained any sort of clinical significance. The same can be said for the flexible foams, semi-rigid foams, and microcellular foams. Thin thermoplastic polyurethane films are widely used in semi-occlusive wound dressings, and a cast thermoset elastomer, trade-named Biothane has been used for many years with success. However, none of these polymers are implantable grade; they are used only paracorporeally.

Thermoplastic polyurethane elastomers are by far the most important *implantable-grade* polyurethanes used in

medical applications. Another polyurethane elastomer, Biomer, is listed next to the thermoplastic elastomer. However, because of the presence of substituted urea linkages in the molecular backbone and the concomitant high degree of interchain hydrogen bonding, Biomer is a virtual thermoset. Biomer has been the most extensively tested implantable polyurethane; it is widely considered the yardstick by which all other polyurethanes are measured.

By the time that Biomer was being investigated as a possible new biomaterial, another polymer had been widely used and accepted by the biomaterials community: the silicones. The silicones had shown exceptional biostability, remarkable blood compatibility and good flexure endurance. However, the silicones could only be produced in the low-durometer hardness range, whereas many prosthetic applications required polymers with higher hardness. The polyurethanes could be produced in hardnesses ranging from a low of Shore 75A, to a high of Shore 75D, as shown in Figure 2.

In addition, the tensile strength of the polyurethanes was nearly six times greater than that of the silicones, permitting the manufacture of thinner catheters, which became a necessity when dual pacemaker leads were introduced. Finally, the polyurethanes displayed unprecedented flexure endurance, opening the way for the fabrication of artificial heart diaphragms which could reliably flex 500 million times or more [13].

Focusing our attention specifically on the polyurethane

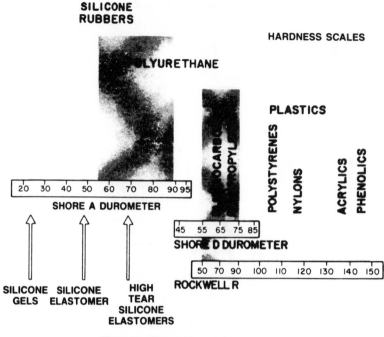

DUROMETER CONVERSIONS

A	B	C	D	O	OO
100	89	77	58		
95	81	70	46		
90	76	59	39		
85	71	52	33		
80	66	47	29	84	98
75	62	42	25	79	97
70	56	37	22	75	95
65	51	32	19	72	94
60	47	28	16	68	93
55	42	24	14	65	91
50	37	20	12	61	90
45	32	17	10	57	88
40	27	14	8	53	86
35	22	12	7	48	83
30	17	9	6	42	80
25	12			35	76
20	6			28	70
15				21	62
10				14	53
5				8	45

Figure 2. Polyurethanes—the bridge between silicon rubbers and plastics.

elastomers, these polymers are based on three monomers: (1) an isocyanate source, (2) a macroglycol, and (3) a chain extender, or curative. As shown in Table 3, the isocyanates can be either aromatic or aliphatic and, as subsequent data will show, there is a profound difference between polymers made from either of these materials.

The macroglycols represent perhaps the single most important choice in the synthesis of medical-grade polyurethanes. The final physical and biological properties we associate with the polyurethanes depend for the

most part on what type of macroglycol is used in the synthesis of medical-grade elastomers. We will critically discuss these crucial monomers in greater detail in subsequent sections.

Among chain extenders, there are two choices: either difunctional or multifunctional monomers. For the production of linear elastomers, only difunctional chain extenders are used; of these, diols and diamines are by far the most important.

We will now discuss the three monomers that comprise

TABLE 3. Urethane Elastomers

Technology Based on Three Monomers

- Isocyanate Source $\left[\begin{array}{l} \text{Aromatic} \\ \text{Aliphatic} \end{array}\right.$

- Macroglycol
  - Polyester
  - Polyether
  - Polycaprolactone
  - Poly Butadiene
  - Castor Oil

- Chain Extender $\left[\begin{array}{l} \text{Diols} \\ \text{Diamines} \end{array}\right.$

the polyurethane elastomers, starting with the isocyanate sources. Figure 3 presents the chemical structure of the prototype aromatic isocyanate example, methylene diphenyl diisocyanate, better known in the industry as MDI. MDI is a very quick reacting isocyanate; in fact, it is so reactive that in many cases, a catalyst is not required for synthesis if a diamine chain extender is used. On a practical basis, commercially available aromatic polyurethanes reacted with diols contain small amounts of a catalyst.

One disadvantage of the aromatic polyurethanes is that polymers based on aromatic isocyanates will yellow upon exposure to ultraviolet radiation. The chemical equation that shows the basic fundamental principle of how these materials yellow is shown at the bottom of Figure 3. As shown, MDI has been reacted with a hydroxyl group. We have an NH−CO−O group, so there is a urethane linkage on either side of the aromatic group.

Under the influence of UV and oxygen, there is a molecular rearrangement where the methylene group that is between the two benzene groups loses its hydrogen. The nitrogen also loses its hydrogen, forming water, and a diquinone imide structure is formed. This di-quinone imide structure is a chromophoric group, a group that absorbs all colors except yellow. Therefore, as an aromatic polyurethane, when it is exposed to UV radiation (say from fluorescent light), it tends to get more yellow with the passage of time. No true physical properties are reduced as a result of the formation of di-quinone imide structures, but yellowing does take place and that may, in fact, be objectionable under certain circumstances. Fortunately, the biocompatibility of the aromatic polyurethanes has never been shown to be compromised as the result of the formation of these chromophoric groups.

Perhaps the greatest single disadvantage of the aromatic polyurethanes resides in the possibility of formation of highly toxic aromatic anilines during improper thermal processing or excessive steam sterilization. In 1978, Darby et al. [14], reported that Pellethane 2363-80A, an aromatic-based polyurethane elastomer, contained an aromatic amine analog of MDI, namely 4,4′ diamino diphenylmethane, better known by the trivial name of methylene dianiline (MDA). This landmark study identified MDA as aqueous extracts of Pellethane, while also alerting the biomedical community of the mutagenic potential of MDA. MDA is a known carcinogen [15,16], mutagen [17], teratogen [18] and displays immediate cell toxicity [19].

MDA can be formed by two independent mechanisms. Szycher and coworkers [20] proposed a thermal degradation mechanism which produces small amounts of MDA, and a second, two-step thermohydrolytic degradation which results in substantial amounts of MDA. Figure 4 represents the thermal degradation, and Figure 5 is the postulated thermohydrolytic degradation sequence.

Thermohydrolytic degradation leading to trace amounts of MDA can be generated when aromatic polyurethanes are subjected to a single steam sterilization cycle at 120°C [21]; MDA can be generated in the 3–5 ppb range under prolonged steam autoclaving [22]. Szycher et al., were able to consistently detect MDA in Biomer following processing and excessive steam sterilization at levels of 10 to 25 μm MDA per gram of polymer. MDA was extracted with methylene chloride, since this amine is sparsely soluble in water.

The important message regarding the aromatic polyurethanes boils down to this simple admonition: to prevent formation of MDA, aromatic polyurethane pellets should

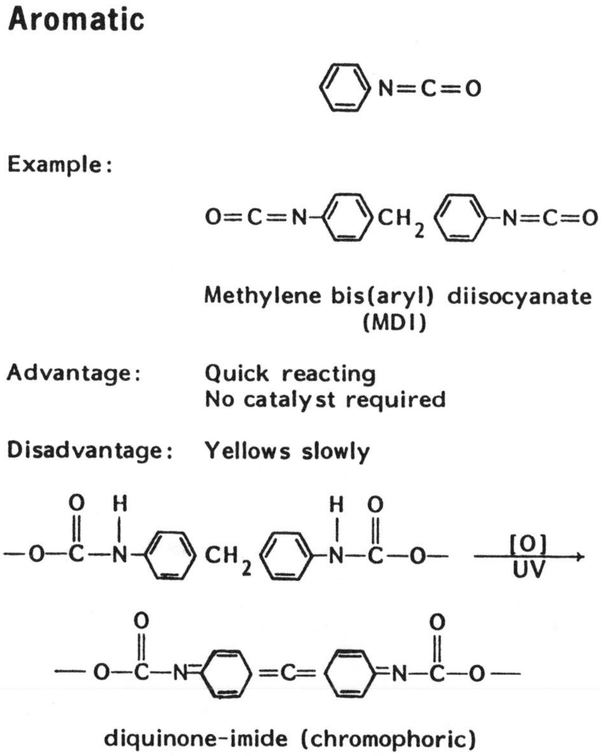

Aromatic

Example:

Methylene bis(aryl) diisocyanate (MDI)

Advantage: Quick reacting
No catalyst required

Disadvantage: Yellows slowly

diquinone-imide (chromophoric)

Figure 3. Isocyanate sources.

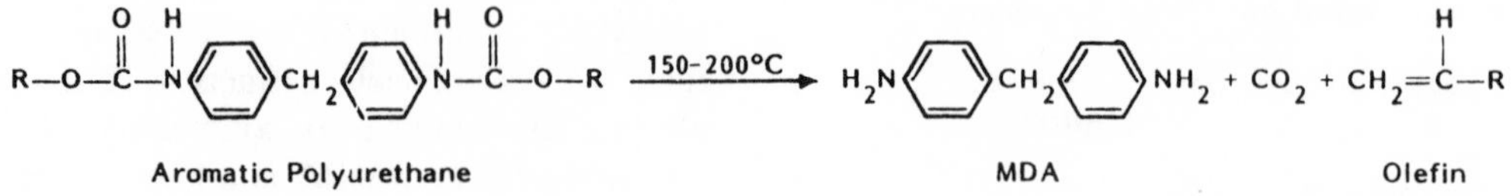

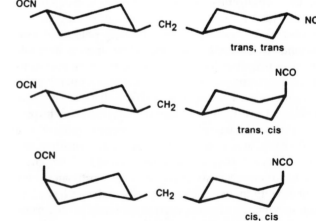

Figure 4. *Thermal degradation of aromatic-based polyurethanes, leading to formation of methylene dianiline (MDA).*

STEP 1

Aromatic Polyurethane → 150–200°C → Free Aromatic Diisocyanate + Precursor Alcohol

STEP 2

Aromatic Diisocyanate + H_2O → 150–200°C → MDA + CO_2

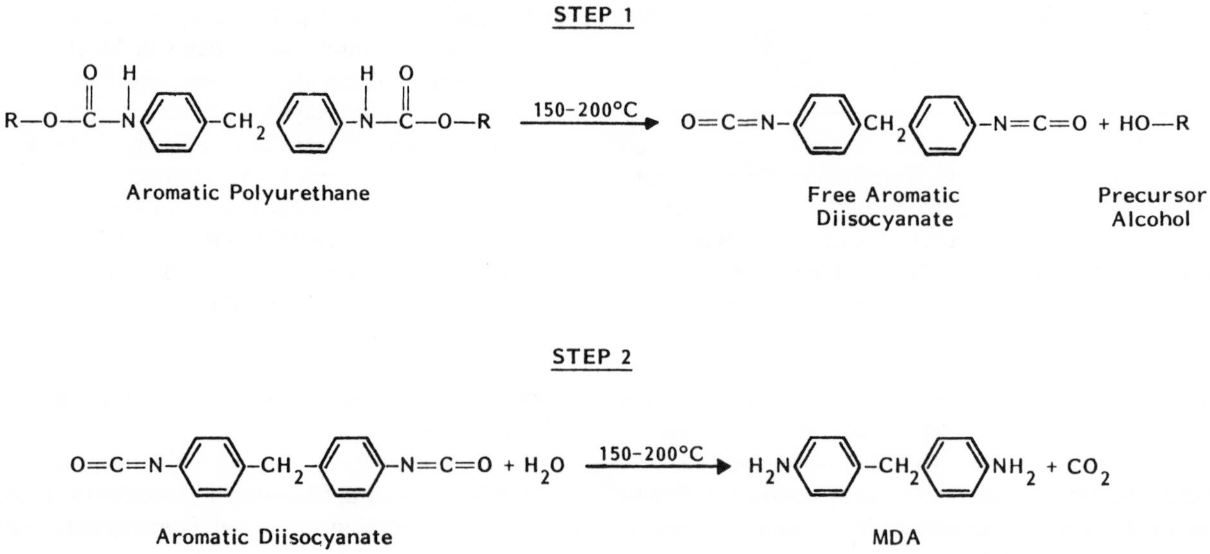

Figure 5. *Postulated thermohydrolytic degradation of aromatic-based polyurethanes, leading to accelerated formation of methylene dianiline (MDA).*

Aliphatic

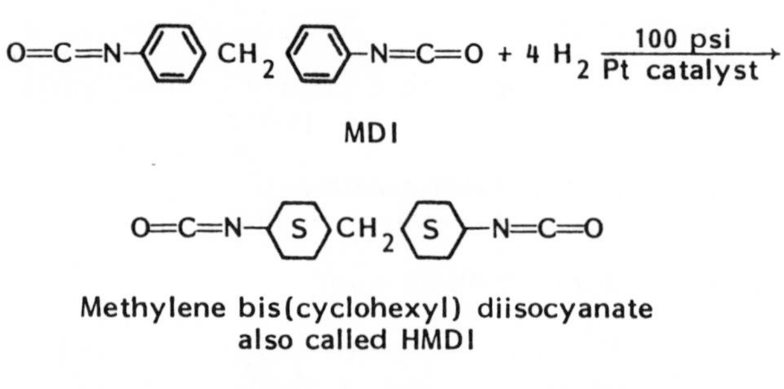

MDI + 4 H_2 →(100 psi / Pt catalyst)→

Methylene bis(cyclohexyl) diisocyanate
also called HMDI

Advantage: Non-yellowing

Disadvantage: Low cure rate: 100°C, 3 hrs

Figure 6. *Isocyanate sources.*

trans, trans

trans, cis

cis, cis

Figure 7. *Isomers of 1,1'-methylenebis (4-isocyanatocyclohexane) (Desmodur W = 30% trans-trans; 65% trans-cis and 5% cis-cis isomer mixture).*

TABLE 4. Diisocyanate Monomers Capable of Yielding Color-Stable Polyurethanes

Acronym	Chemical Name	Chemical Structure	Trade Name and Supplier
HDI	1,6 Hexamethylene Diisocyanate	CH_2—CH_2—CH_2—N=C=O CH_2—CH_2—CH_2—N=C=O	Desmodur H Bayer Chemie
HMDI	4,4' Methylene bis Cyclohexyl Diisocyanate	O=C=N⟨ ⟩—CH_2—⟨ ⟩—N=C=O	Desmodur W Mobay Chemical
TMDI	Trimethyl-Hexamethylene Diisocyanate	O=C=N—CH_2—C(CH_3)(CH_3)—CH_2—CH(CH_3)—CH_2—CH_2—N=C=O 2,2,4 O=C=N—CH_2—CH(CH_3)—CH_2—C(CH_3)(CH_3)—CH_2—CH_2—N=C=O	TMDI (Isomeric mixture) Veba Chemie
IPDI	Isophorone Diisocyanate	H_3C, H_3C ⟨ ⟩—N=C=O H_3C CH_2—N=C=O	IPDI Veba Chemie
XDI	Xylene Diisocyanate	CH_2NCO ... CH_2NCO (m-) CH_2NCO ... CH_2NCO (p-) (70%) m— (30%) p—	Takenate 500 (70/30 mixture of meta and para) Takeda Chemical

be well dried prior to thermal processing, and the finished product should not be subjected to prolonged steam sterilization cycles.

Aliphatic urethanes, on the other hand, do not show the embrittlement, weakening and progressive darkening of the aromatic-based urethanes. This led to the search for nonyellowing isocyanate sources. In the mid-1960s, research at Allied Chemical Corp. resulted in the solution to the degradation/yellowing problem of the aromatic polyurethanes. At that time Allied introduced a cycloaliphatic diisocyanate H_{12}MDI, which produced color-stable polyurethanes, designated as Nacconate H-12. DuPont also supplied H_{12}MDI, trade named Hylene W, but stopped production in 1980. At present, Mobay Chemical Corp. is the sole supplier of H_{12}MDI, trade named Desmodur W. Other diisocyanates capable of yielding color-stable polyurethanes are presented in Table 4.

We decided to concentrate on the synthesis of medical-grade polyurethanes based on H_{12}MDI. This cycloaliphatic isocyanate is derived from an aromatic precursor which is fully hydrogenated to form the cyclohexyl aliphatic final product composed of a mixture of isomers, as shown in Figures 6 and 7. The aliphatic isocyanates produce elastomers that are somewhat inferior in physical properties to the aromatic equivalents, and are significantly more expensive. The higher cost of the aliphatic-based polyurethanes can be traced to higher raw materials cost, and a long cure time, 100°C for a minimum of 3 hours.

Although the isocyanate monomer plays an important role, many of the properties associated with the polyurethanes are derived from the macroglycol portion of the chain and, depending on the choice of macroglycol, the polyurethanes have been found to perform differently in varying clinical applications [23]:

- The polyester-based polyurethanes undergo rapid hydrolysis when implanted in the human body, and thus should not be used in medical applications.
- The polyether-based polyurethanes are the polymers of choice in medical applications, since they are virtually insensitive to hydrolysis, and are thus very stable in the physiological environment.
- The polycaprolactone-based polyurethanes, due to their quick crystallization, can be used advantageously as medical, solvent-activated, pressure-sensitive adhesives.
- The polybutadiene-based polyurethanes have been evaluated, but no medical application has been found to date.
- The castor oil-based polyurethanes can be used as potting and encapsulating compounds, but due to their poor tear resistance, find limited use in medical applications.

Ninety percent of all polyurethane elastomers used commercially are polyester-based products. The reason that polyester-based polyurethane elastomers are used is

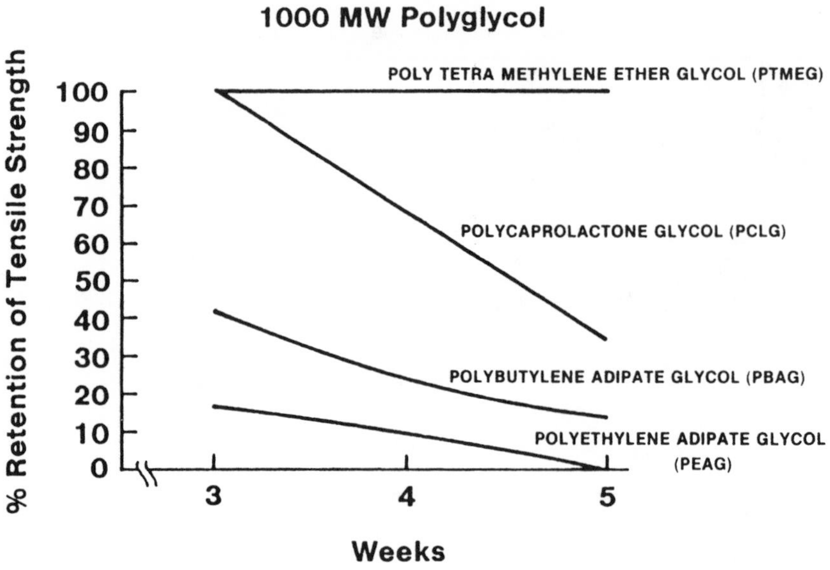

1000 MW Polyglycol

Figure 8. *Polyurethane performance (MDI/BDO) humidity aging at 80°C/95% RH (tested 1 week after removal).*

that they have very high tensile strength, very high tear strength, and are easy to fabricate. They have excellent abrasion resistance and are relatively low in cost. However, they should not be used for medical applications because they undergo hydrolytic degradation when implanted in the body. They can only be used in applications where a prosthesis is implanted for very short periods of time (one to three hours). For applications where implantation of a week or longer is likely to be required, the polyester-based polyurethane should not be used because they will depolymerize, and a variety of physiological implications will result from that degradation, as shown in Figure 8.

As Figure 8 shows, two polyester-based polyurethanes, polybutylene adipate glycol and polyethylene adipate glycol, have retained only 40 and 18 percent of their respective initial strength when aged at high temperature and humidity for 3 weeks. A polycaprolactone-based elastomer loses 50 percent of initial tensile strength after 4.5 weeks. By contrast, the polyether-based polyurethane remains unchanged for the duration of the study.

Therefore, we conclude that, for medical applications, the polyether-based polyurethanes, particularly those based on polytetramethylene ether glycol (PTMEG) seemed the best choice. And, indeed, all commercially available medical-grade polyurethanes—Avcothane, Biomer, Pellethane and Tecoflex—are PTMEG-based. However, for chronic implantation, the PTMEG-based polyurethanes are known to microcrack, especially when subjected to stress. The polybutadiene macroglycols are used primarily as encapsulants for electronic applications. However, they are practically never used in the medical field because the polybutadienes still contain double bonds on the butadiene chain, and these double

bonds are very susceptible to oxidation. When implanted in the body these materials tend to oxidize very quickly; as a result, practically no one uses polybutadienes for implantable medical prostheses.

The castor-oil-based polyurethanes have very good hydrolytic stability and very good oxidation stability. However, they are only used as encapsulants (such as in hemodialysis machines). As encapsulants they perform a very good function because they have very good compression set and are very balancing materials. However, they are precluded for use in those applications where tear strength and tear propagation are important because they have very poor tear resistance.

Regarding chain extenders, urethane elastomers can be synthesized from either diamines or diols. If diamines are used, the high hydrogen bonding attraction between substituted urea linkages render these materials as thermosets; Biomer which is chain extended with diamines can only be obtained from solvent solutions. Any attempt to extrude Biomer will result in thermal degradation.

To synthesize thermoplastic polyurethanes, the chain extenders must be linear diols. If a branched diol, such as ethylene-oxide-capped trimethylol propane is used, crosslinking occurs, and the polymer is no longer capable of being processed by thermal methods. The chemical structure of these chain extenders is shown in Figure 9.

Of the available chain extenders, 1,4 butane diol is the universal choice for medical applications. This chain extender produces thermoplastic polyurethanes with high physical properties, excellent processing conditions and clear polymers. Butane-diol-extended polymethanes display the best combination of physical properties, as presented in Figure 10.

One reason for the excellent physical properties dis-

- ## Linear Diol

$$HO—CH_2CH_2CH_2CH_2—OH$$

1,4 Butane Diol

- ## Branched Diol

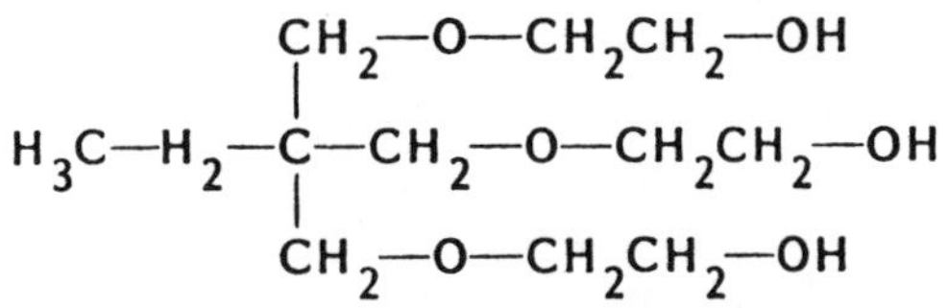

$$
\begin{aligned}
&\quad\quad\quad CH_2—O—CH_2CH_2—OH\\
&\quad\quad\quad\ |\\
H_3&C—H_2—C—CH_2—O—CH_2CH_2—OH\\
&\quad\quad\quad\ |\\
&\quad\quad\quad CH_2—O—CH_2CH_2—OH
\end{aligned}
$$

Ethylene-Oxide Capped
Trimethylol Propane

- ## Amines

$$H_2N—CH_2—CH_2—NH_2$$

Ethylene Diamine

Figure 9. Chain extenders.

GLYCOL	TENSILE (PSI)	ELONGATION (%)	MODULUS (PSI)	TEAR (LB/IN.)	HARDNESS SHORE B
ETHYLENE	6500	500	2000	230	61
1,3 PROPANEDIOL	6600	600	950	270	61
1,4 BUTANEDIOL	7900	600	1000	270	61
1,6 HEXANEDIOL	7400	500	850	170	60
1,5 PENTANEDIOL	7100	600	900	280	62

Figure 10. Physical properties of polyurethane elastomers as influenced by glycols.

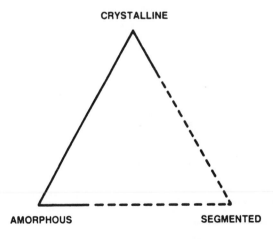

Figure 11. States of intermolecular order.

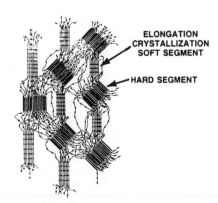

Figure 12. Strain-induced elongation crystallization of polyether soft segments in a segmented polyurethane elastomer by elongating it to 200% extension. [From Bonart, R. J. Macromol. Sci. Phys., *32:115* (1968).]

played by butane-diol-extended polymer is their tendency to pack themselves into tight, stereoregular molecular chains, a phenomenon referred to as crystallinity. A crystalline polymer is usually the opposite of an amorphous polymer; however, it is now known that polyurethane elastomers consist of a mixture of crystalline and amorphous domains, a state described as segmentation.

Polymer Science characterizes intermolecular order as the geometrical relationship between adjacent polymer molecules and their arrangement in the total mass of polymeric material. At present we recognize three distinctly different states of intermolecular order as shown in Figure 11.

When polymer molecules are arranged in completely random, intertwined coils, the unordered structure is known as the amorphous state. When polymer molecules are so neatly arranged that each atom falls into precise position in a tightly packed repeating regular structure, this highly oriented structure is described as the crystalline state. Polyurethane elastomers are a two-phase structure, where the hard segments separate to form discrete domains in a matrix of soft segments. This arrangement is termed segmented.

Polyurethane elastomers are segmented polymers. The rigid segments act as bridges, and as filler particles, reinforcing the soft segment matrix.

An example of this type of structure is in the segmented polyurethane elastomers obtained from polyether [poly-(oxytetramethylene)] and polyester (a copolyester) based elastomers incorporating MDI and extended with ethylene diamine. In the relaxed state, spatially separated hard and soft segments can be shown (by x-ray diffraction) to exist in the material. The hard segments are considered held together in discrete domains through the action of Van der Waal's forces and hydrogen bonding interactions. This concept is demonstrated in Figure 12, where the crystallization of soft segments is accomplished by elongating the polymer by 200 percent. Even greater crystallization is observed at 500 percent elongation as shown in Figure 13.

Once crystallinity has been achieved, an additional phenomenon occurs within the polyurethane chains — hydrogen bonding. Polyurethanes contain basic electronegative ions with semiavailable unshared pairs of valence electrons, such as nitrogen and oxygen ions. Nitrogen and oxygen donate these valence electrons to the hydrogen atoms of adjacent molecules to produce hydrogen bonding between the two molecules. Hydrogen bonding between adjacent polymer chains significantly increases the physical properties of polyurethane elastomers. This gives rise to a three-dimensional, "virtually cross-linked" molecular domain structure.

Interchain attractive forces between rigid segments are far greater than those present in the soft segments, due to the high concentration of polar groups and the possibility of extensive hydrogen bonding. Hard segments significantly affect mechanical properties, particularly modulus, hardness and tear strength. The performance of elastomers at elevated temperatures is very dependent on the structure of the rigid segments and their ability to remain associated at these temperatures. Rigid segments are considered to result from contributions of the diisocyanate and chain extender components.

The lateral effect of all the foregoing states, and forces, particularly crystallinity and hydrogen bonding, is to tie together or "virtually cross-link" the linear primary polyurethane chains. That is, the primary polyurethane chains are cross-linked in effect, but not in fact. Concurrently, of course, the virtual linkages also lengthen the primary polyurethane chains. The overall consequence is a labile infinite network of polymer chains that displays the superficial properties of a strong rubbery vulcanizate over a practical range of use temperatures.

Virtual cross-linking is a phenomenon that is reversible with heat and, depending upon polymer composition, with solvation, offers many attractive processing alternatives for thermoplastic polyurethanes. Thermal energy great enough to (reversibly) break virtual cross-links, but too low to appreciably disrupt the stronger covalent chemical bonds that link the atoms in the primary polymer chains, can be used to extrude or mold the polymers, and a solvent that solvates the polymer chains, reversibly insulating the virtual cross-links, carries the primary polymer chains into solution separate and intact for such application as coatings or adhesives.

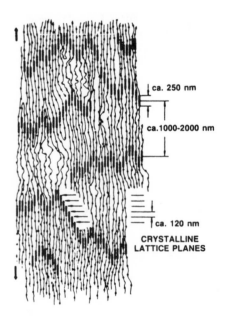

Figure 13. Segmented polyurethane elastomer at 500% extension and placed in warm water at 80°C. [From Bonart, R. J. Macromol. Sci. Phys., 32:115 (1968).]

TABLE 5. Common Polymers Classified as Either Crystalline or Amorphous*

Crystalline	Amorphous
Polyacetal	ABS
Polyamide	Polyamide
Polybutylene terephthalate	Polyacrylate
Polyethylene terephthalate	Polycarbonate
Polyetherether ketone	Polyetherimide
Polyphenylene sulfide	Polyphenylene oxide
Polyethylene	Polysulfone
Polybutylene terephthalate	
Polypropylene	
Nylon 6/6	

*Note: Polyurethane elastomers are a mixture of crystalline and amorphous regions. Therefore, they are classified as segmented polymers.

Present views on the morphology and structure of segmented polyurethane polymers are as follows:

- Because the hard and soft blocks are partly incompatible with each other, the elastomers show a two phase morphology, although there is a significant level of mixing of the hard and soft blocks.
- The soft segments containing the macroglycol form an amorphous matrix in which the hard segments are dispersed.
- The hard domains containing the chain extender act as multi-functional cross-link sites or "virtual cross-links," resulting in elastomeric behavior.

- Hydrogen bonding can occur between hard and soft blocks although the extent to which this is responsible for physical properties is not certain.
- Hydrogen bonding occurs between individual hard blocks giving rise to a three-dimensional molecular domain structure.
- These domains may themselves be in a larger, ordered arrangement including both soft and hard blocks, the hard blocks being built up in a transverse orientation to their molecular axis leading, in cases, to the appearance of spherulites in the polymer.
- The morphology is unstable with respect to temperature and is dependent on both the chemical constitution and thermal history of the polymer.

In summary, crystallinity refers to any highly ordered arrangement of atoms. Polymers can be visualized as long meandering chains of atoms that occasionally find themselves in patterns of highly oriented, close proximity.

These small regions of high order are referred to as spherulites or crystallites. Regions containing randomly oriented and widely spaced chains are described as being amorphous. The degree of crystallinity is a measure of the frequency of these highly ordered crystallites. It is important to emphasize that no polymer is totally crystalline and that an amorphous material can exhibit crystalline characteristics. In practice, polymers are classified as being amorphous, segmented, or crystalline according to their various degrees of crystallinity and their tendencies to form crystallites as shown in Tables 5 and 6.

The probability that a given polymer will exhibit crystalline structure is determined primarily by the chemical nature of the polymer chains. Polymer chains of low molecular weight, or that possess high flexibility, favor

TABLE 6. Selected Characteristics of Crystalline and Amorphous Polymers

Crystalline	Amorphous
High strength	More pronounced glass-transition temperature
Increased stiffness	
Increased density	Transparency
Resistance to organic solvents	Reduced mold shrinkage (0.8 ± 0.4 vs. 2.0 ± 1.0)
Opacity	More uniform mold shrinkage
Resistance to dynamic fatigue	Decreased dimensional response to temperature gradients
Increased temperature range with reinforcement	Low density
Pronounced melting point	Good impact strength
Low viscosity melt	Melting range
Chemical resistance	

TABLE 7. Commercially Available Biomedical-Grade Polyurethane Elastomers

Name	Supplier	Description	Structure	Advantage	Disadvantage
ANGIOFLEX	Abiomed Danvers, MA	Silicone-urethane CoPolymer	MDI-PTMEG BD-Sil	Good blood compatibility	Difficult to fabricate
BIOMER	Ethicon Somerville, NJ	Aromatic Co(polyether-urea)	MDI-PTMEG EDA	Outstanding flex endurance	Research use only
CARDIOTHANE	Kontron, Inc. Everett, MA	Silicone-urethane CoPolymer	MDI-PTMEG BD-Sil	Good blood compatibility	Difficult to fabricate
CHRONOFLEX	PolyMedica Burlington, MA	Aliphatic Non-ether	HMDI-???-BD	Biostable	Needs to be qualified
HEMOTHANE	Sarns, Div 3M Ann Arbor, MI	Similar to Biomer	Similar to Biomer	Similar to Biomer	Internal use only
MITRATHANE	PolyMedica Burlington, MA	Similar to Biomer	Similar to Biomer	Similar to Biomer	Commercially available
PELLETHANE	Dow Chemical La Porte, TX	Aromatic ether-based	MDI-PTMEG BD	Thermoplastic elastomer	Microcracks
SURETHANE	Cardiac Control Palm Coast, FL	Purified Lycra	MDI-PTMEG EDA	Similar to Biomer	Commercially available
TECOFLEX	Thermedics Inc. Woburn, MA	Aliphatic ether-based	HMDI-PTMEG BD	Thermoplastic elastomer	Microcracks

MDI—Methylene-bis-phenyl diisocyanate (aromatic).
PTMEG—PolyTetraMethylene Ether Glycol.
HMDI—Hydrogenated MDI (aliphatic).
BD—1,4-Butane Diol.
EDA—Ethylene DiAmine.
???—unpublished structure.
Sil—silicone.

crystallinity. For example, polyphenylene sulfide is composed of many flexible sulfide linkages adding to its tendency toward crystallinity. Other flexible units include ether and ester linkages. Polyurethane elastomers are mixtures of crystalline and amorphous regions.

If the polymer is capable of forming intermolecular bonds and if these bonds are advantageously distributed along the polymer chain, crystallinity is more likely. These forces include hydrogen bonding, as in polyurethane. Homopolymers present more ideal conditions for crystalline structure than random copolymers, whose chemistry will result in an uneven distribution of intramolecular forces.

Because crystallites consist of closely packed chains, it is correct to assume that polymer chains containing bulky side groups (as in polystyrene), or branching (as in low-density polyethylene), would inhibit close packing and interfere with the formation of crystallites. This is also known as hindrance.

Crystallinity is an important parameter in polyurethane biostability. In general, as the elastomer becomes more crystalline the biostability becomes greater under any given set of circumstances.

At present, only five biomedical-grade segmented polyurethanes are used in the manufacture of medical devices: Angioflex, Biomer, Cardiothane, Pellethane and Tecoflex, as shown in Table 7.

POLYURETHANE TECHNOLOGY

Current activities of materials suppliers, designers, manufacturers, and physicians clearly indicate that devices manufactured from synthetic polymers have become an integral part of health-care technology. Initially focused on life-threatening situations, their clinical uses now include permanent implantation (e.g., artificial hearts, hip prostheses, intraocular lenses), intermediate applications (e.g., contact lenses, removable dental prostheses, renal dialyzers), and transient applications (e.g., cardiopulmonary bypass, over-the-needle catheters, diagnostic and therapeutic catheters) [24]. The polymers used most often in these applications are the silicone elastomers, the acrylics, polyvinyl chloride, fluorinated ethylene propylene, and the polycarbonates.

In the past ten years, research work on the artificial heart has stimulated interest in this new family of polymers, the segmented polyurethane elastomers. Originally developed for commercial applications, these polymers exhibit high flexure endurance, high strength, and inherent nonthrombogenic characteristics, and are expected to have a positive effect on future medical applications. While the polyurethanes can be predicted to have maximum impact in medical prostheses, the most immediate and promising applications appear to be in the cardiovascular area, where chronic, nonthrombogenic in-

TABLE 8. Current Biomedical Applications of Polyurethanes

Blood bags, closures, fittings

Blood oxygenation tubing

Breast prostheses

Cardiac assist pump bladders, tubing, housing, coatings

Catheters

Dental cavity liners

Endotracheal tubes

Heart pacemaker connectors, coatings, lead insulators, fixation devices

Hemodialysis tubing, membranes, connectors

Leaflet heart valves

Mechanical heart valve coatings

Orthopedic splints, bone adhesives

Percutaneous shunts

Reconstructive surgery materials

Skin dressing and tapes

Surgical drapes

Suture material

Synthetic bile ducts

Vascular grafts and patches

terfacing with circulating blood is of paramount importance, as shown in Table 8. The purpose of this section is to report on some of the physicochemical properties displayed by these new polymers, and to examine their performance characteristics when used in the manufacture of chronically implantable medical devices.

Polymer Configuration

As we have seen, the generic term polyurethane is very deceiving in that useful compositions rarely contain a majority of urethane functional groups. In fact, ether, ester, urea and other groups generally outnumber urethane linkages on the molecular chains of "polyurethane" elastomers.

While an infinite number of polyurethane structures are theoretically possible, two medical-grade thermoplastic polyurethane elastomers have attained commercial importance: the thermoplastic urethanes (TPU). A nonthermoplastic polyurethane elastomer, Biomer, has been extensively investigated; however, since Biomer is not commercially available, several companies have developed equivalent versions for captive use. Surethane (Cardiac Control Systems), Mitrathane (PolyMedica) and Hemathane (Sarns, 3M) are believed to be similar in chemical composition to Biomer.

Perhaps the best known, and certainly the most tested, of all the polyurethane elastomers has been Biomer. Biomer can be fully described as a linear, segmented, aromatic, polyether-based polyurethane that is ethylenediamine chain extended. In terms of fabrication, Biomer-based devices can only be made by solution casting methods. The presence of diurea linkages in the molecular backbone results in very high degrees of hydrogen bonding, thus turning the polymer into a nonthermoplastic. Thus, Biomer is only available as a 30-percent

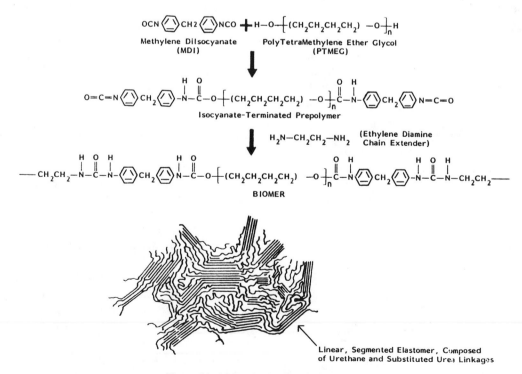

Figure 14. Molecular architecture of Biomer.

TABLE 9. Stiffness vs. Hardness

Hardness - Resistance to Penetration

Stiffness - Resistance to Bending Under Stress
            Within the Elastic Limit = Modulus of Elasticity = $\frac{\sigma}{\epsilon}$

solids solution in dimethyl acetamide. The molecular structure and synthesis route is shown in Figure 14.

The molecular architecture of the Pellethane Series 2363, shown in Figure 15, is a family of materials ranging from a Shore-A Hardness of 80, to a Shore-D hardness of 75. These are linear, segmented, aromatic polyether-based polyurethanes, chain extended with butane diol, and are thus thermoplastics.

The molecular architecture of a typical aliphatic ether-based TPU is shown in Figure 16.

Although the durometer hardness of aromatic Pellethane 2363-80A and aliphatic 80A are identical, there are substantial differences in stiffness, processing conditions and solvent resistance. These differences will be discussed in detail in subsequent sections.

Hardness Versus Stiffness

What is the difference between hard and stiff? In mechanical terms, hardness refers to resistance to penetration, and stiffness refers to resistance to bending. As illustrated in Figure 17, material "A" is said to be harder than material "B" since a stylus penetrates deeper into "B," under an equal local of one pound.

As presented in Table 9, stiffness is measured indirectly by the term modulus of elasticity, as defined by Hooke's Law. The modulus of elasticity is most easily calculated from a typical stress-strain diagram, shown in Figure 18. In this figure, material "A" is said to be stiffer than material "B," since the ratio of stress (σ) to strain (ϵ) is greater in "A" than "B."

Hardness and stiffness are important parameters in medical catheters. Figure 19 graphically illustrates that 70 Shore A C-Flex (a butadiene-styrene copolymer by Concept Inc.) is similar to aliphatic 80A, whereas Pellethane 80A is much stiffer. By comparison, the stiffness of a very soft 45 Shore A silicone rubber is also shown on the graph.

A catheter made of MDX 4-4514 would require thick walls to allow for penetration into the body because it lacks the necessary stiffness. On the other hand, for the same stiffness, catheters made of Pellethane could have significantly thinner walls (i.e., smaller outer diameter), and thus could be more easily inserted by the physician.

Ideally, a catheter should be initially stiff to allow for easy insertion and permit torque transmission, but after insertion should lose stiffness to prevent mechanical trauma to delicate body tissues. The segmented polyurethanes display such ideal characteristics, as illustrated in Figure 20, where aliphatic TPU's can be seen losing more than half their original stiffness as the polymer reaches body temperature and attains equilibrium in the aqueous environment.

The degree of softening, expressed as a percentage decrease of the modulus is significant, reversible and dependent on the ratio of hard-to-soft segment and the extent of microphase separation [25].

In a myriad of special performance advantages of the TPU (thermoplastic urethane) based biomaterials, the ability to soften without degradation when exposed to the body environment is held very dearly. This controllable softening can be used to adjust, for example, the compliance of an artificial vascular graft to that of the vessel to be repaired. The importance of such adjustment for the patency of small-diameter vascular grafts is well established [26,27]. In the area of vascular catheterization, the ability of TPUs to soften in the vessel upon insertion reduces the potential of vessel wall irritation and consequent thrombus formation and phlebitis [28]. Furthermore, the ability to control softening by the selection of reactive precursors [29] opens the door for even more exciting applications.

The polyurethanes owe their special performance characteristics to their multiphase nature. It is now accepted that the TPUs are $(AB)_n$ block copolymers. The hard segments are composed of relatively immobile regions containing short polyurethane sequences. These regions are connected by polyether or polyester soft segments which provide the flexible character to the polymer. By selection of various hard and soft segment intermediates the TPUs can be formulated to have a broad range of physical/mechanical properties. A pre-selected composition leads to a particular morphology dominated by its two-phase nature. The degree of separation between the soft and hard segments, the nature and shape of hard and soft segment domains, the domain purity and the nature of continuous and dispersed phases will impart unique characteristics to the polymer and will affect its response to the biological environment.

In a landmark study, Zdrahala [30] concluded that softening is dependent on polymer morphology; i.e., since the soft segment is already in its rubbery state, the softening must be due to plasticization of the interface layer connecting the hard and soft domains. This layer, composed of a blend of the soft and hard segments can be plasticized by both water and heat. The added water molecules occupy the available hydrogen bonding sites while the heat increases the kinetic energy which in turn increases chain mobility. Both of these factors weaken the interconnecting forces between and among the respective domains which softens the material.

By definition, the hard segment weight percentage is

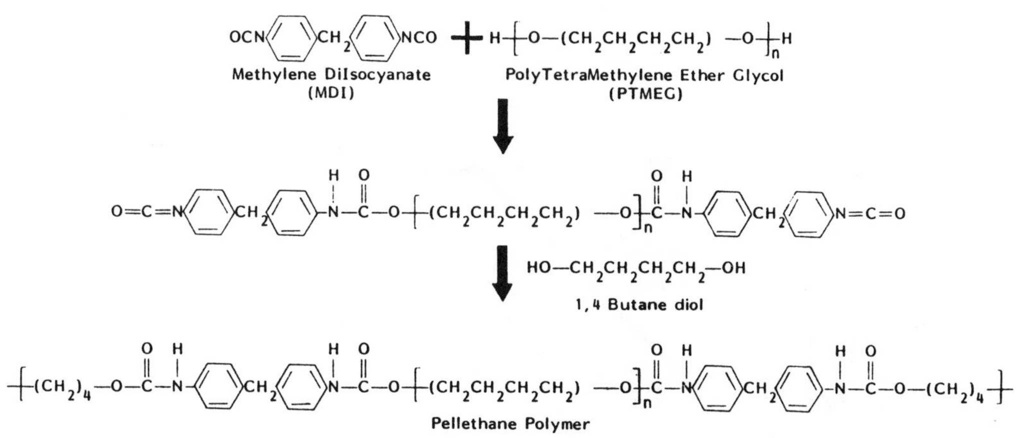

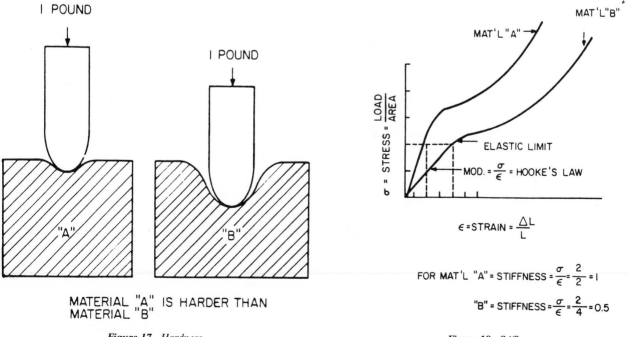

Figure 15. *Molecular architecture of Pellethane.*

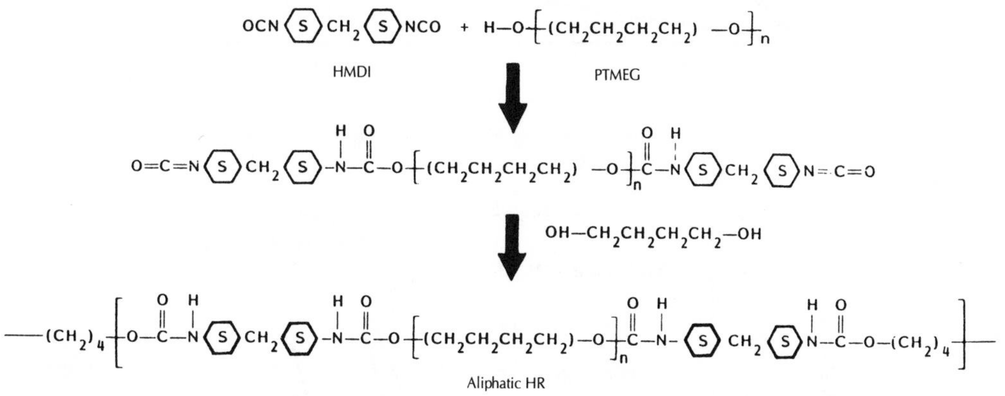

Figure 16. *Molecular architecture of aliphatic elastomer.*

I POUND

I POUND

"A"

"B"

MATERIAL "A" IS HARDER THAN
MATERIAL "B"

Figure 17. *Hardness.*

$\sigma = STRESS = \dfrac{LOAD}{AREA}$

MAT'L "A"

MAT'L "B"

ELASTIC LIMIT

MOD. $= \dfrac{\sigma}{\epsilon} =$ HOOKE'S LAW

$\epsilon = STRAIN = \dfrac{\triangle L}{L}$

FOR MAT'L "A" = STIFFNESS $= \dfrac{\sigma}{\epsilon} = \dfrac{2}{2} = 1$

"B" = STIFFNESS $= \dfrac{\sigma}{\epsilon} = \dfrac{2}{4} = 0.5$

Figure 18. *Stiffness.*

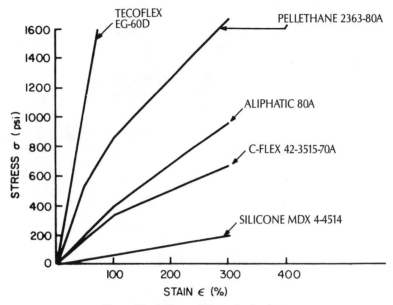

Figure 19. *Stiffness of biomedical polymers.*

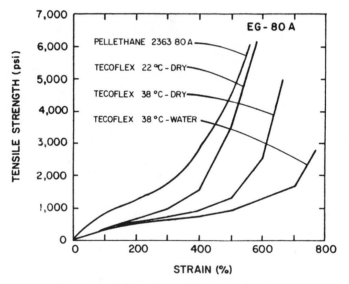

Figure 20. *Stiffness change following implantation.*

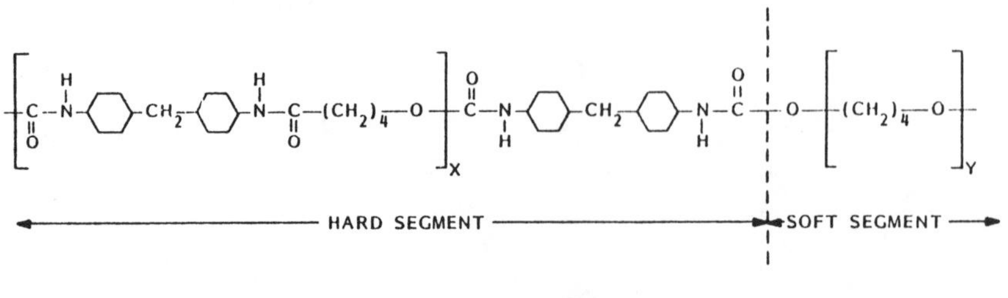

Figure 21. *Schematic diagram of an aliphatic, PTMEG, BD polyurethane elastomer.*

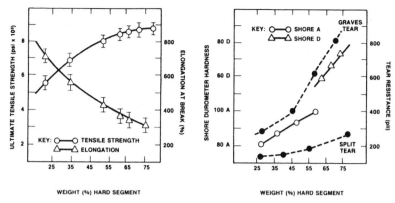

Figure 22. *Relationship between weight percent hard segment and some physico chemical characteristics of aliphatic PU elastomers.*

calculated as the weight of isocyanate plus chain extender; by extrapolation, the weight percentage of the soft segment is simply the weight of macroglycol in the formulation. Thus, segmented polyurethane compositions can be expressed as weight percentage of hard segment, schematically shown in Figure 21.

Many observed physicochemical characteristics of segmented polyurethanes can be explained by expressing the polymer composition in terms of weight percentage of hard segment. This concept is illustrated in Figure 22.

The softening of both hardness and stiffness of polyurethane elastomers in the biological environment is likewise a linear relationship to weight percentage of hard segment, as presented in Figure 23. However, it must be emphasized that PTMEG molecular weight is a major determinant in this behavior, where softening is a linear function of hard segment if the molecular weight of the PTMEG is 1000 or 2000 Dalton units for aliphatic PU; the softening bears a complex relationship to hard segment content when the PTMEG molecular weight is 2000 Dalton units or above.

Processing Conditions

Processing conditions can have a significant impact on the eventual biostability of polyurethane-based prostheses. Residual stresses on polyurethane tubing accelerates *in vivo* surface microfissuring, and residual stresses can be induced in tubing by inappropriate stretching during extrusion (we recommend a draw-down ratio of 1.5:1.0 or lower). Residual stresses can also be induced in the tubing if the temperature in the water bath is too cold (we recommend a water bath temperature between 70 and 80°F throughout the year).

The equipment recommended for extruding medical-grade Pellethane 2363 resins includes a single-stage nonvented, 24/1 L/D extruder with a heavy duty, dc variable speed, high torque drive. For example, a 2-1/2-inch extruder should have a 40 to 50 hp drive. Screw design is the metering type (typically: 6 flights feed-9 flights transition-9 flights metering) with a 2.6–3.1 compression ratio. Mixing and barrier screws can be used for maximizing melting with low energy input and high uniform

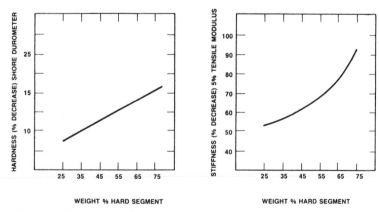

Figure 23. *Influence of 37°C saline on hardness/stiffness of aliphatic 1000 MW PTMEG polyurethane elastomers.*

TABLE 10. General Processing Conditions, and Physical Properties of Pellethane 2363 Series TPU Elastomers

Grade	2363-80AE	2363-80A	2363-90A	2363-55D	2363-65D	2363-75D
Barrel: Rear, °F	350	370	380	390	400	390
Middle, °F	360	380	390	400	410	400
Front, °F	370	390	400	410	420	410
Adapter, °F	390	390	400	410	425	420
Die, °F	380	390	400	410	425	425
Melt, °F	380-400	400-420	410-430	415-435	420-435	420-435

Grade	80AE	80A	90A	55D	65D	75D**
Hardness, Shore	83A	83A	93A	55D	62D	75D
Specific Gravity, g/cc	112	113	114	115	117	121
Tensile Modulus, psi at:						
50% elongation	530	550	1100	1800	2500	----
100% elongation	850	850	1530	2500	3000	4650
300% elongation	1450	1650	4100	4500	5000	6570
Tensile Strength, psi	4120	6000	6750	6500	6520	7240
Elongation at Break, %	600	550	500	430	420	340
Tear Strength, Die C, pli	450	475	575	650	1100	1470
Clash Berg Modulus, T_F, °C	-58	-58	-46	-21	-22	-9
Taber Abrasion H-22 Wheel mg loss	<0.03	<0.02	<0.01	<0.01	<0.10	<0.06

throughput. The employment of breaker plates and screen packs is standard operating procedure with polyurethane resins. The use of screens up to 325 mesh is common with these materials. Barrel temperatures are generally cooler at the rear depending on the extrusion product (film, sheet, or profile) and hotter at the die end to ensure good mixing and positive metering in the barrel. Extrusion dies are like those used for flexible PVC and are streamlined with land lengths 10 to 15 times the die opening.

The takeup equipment is usually longer than that used for PVC with the profile passing through a warm bath (70 to 90°F) to eliminate residual surface tack and blocking on windup. Vacuum sizers and internally cooled mandrels are not recommended because of the soft, tacky nature of the thermoplastic polyurethane materials, especially those less than 55 Shore D hardness. Sheet extrusion is best carried out with a coathanger manifold die with stock temperatures running higher than for shape extrusion. A standard three-roll stack with roll temperatures decreasing progressively from 120°F to 80°F is used for takeup. The 2363-80A and 80AE resins are the only grades that are suitable for cast- or blown-film extrusion. All others are suitable for profile work only. General processing conditions for the extrusion of Pellethane resins, and their physical properties are presented in Table 10.

Aliphatic polyurethanes, should be processed at significantly lower temperatures than corresponding aromatic polyurethanes, as shown in Table 11. Since aliphatic TPU's grades are hygroscopic (they attract and hold chemisorbed water) the pellets must be dried before extrusion using a desiccant-type hopper drier for a minimum of four hours at 150°F and a dew point of -40°C.

For single-stage screw applications, a 24:1 L/D extruder is recommended, with a 12-6-6 screw for softer grades, and a 6-9-9 screw for the harder grades. Since urethanes are heat sensitive compounds, caution is ad-

vised during startup or shutdown when the compound may be heated for long periods of time. Extruders should be purged with low-density polyethylene (such as USI Brand type NA 301) to clean any heat decomposed material from the screw flights and ancillary dies.

In general, melt temperatures (measured at the breaker plate or at the tip of the metering section) may be increased when large throughputs and short dwell times are used; conversely, temperatures should be decreased when small products or oversized machines are used. Typical extruder screw conditions are shown in Figures 24 and 25, and physical test data in Tables 12 and 13.

As we have already mentioned, aliphatic polyurethanes are extruded at significantly lower temperatures than aromatic polyurethanes as shown in Figure 26. Other thermoplastic resins are included in the figure for comparison. For biomedical applications, in general, the lower the thermoforming temperatures the lower the thermodegradation of polymers, since degradation follows Arrhenius' law; i.e., the rate of degradation doubles for each increment of 10°C. It follows that lower extrusion temperatures are advantageous in minimizing potential surface degradation which may be detrimental in the biological environment.

Another important consideration in the production of precision medical tubing is the extruder diameter. As the diameter increases the output increases, with a substantial reduction in cost; however, as the output increases, tolerances and surface finish are compromised. The relationship between output and extruder diameter is a parabolic function, as shown in Figure 27. Commonly the larger-diameter extruders are used for the production of larger tubing (Table 14). Manufacturers typically utilize 1-inch diameter, 24:1 L/D extruders for the production of precision, small-bore medical tubing, utilizing 500-mesh screen packs for maximum filtering of the melt.

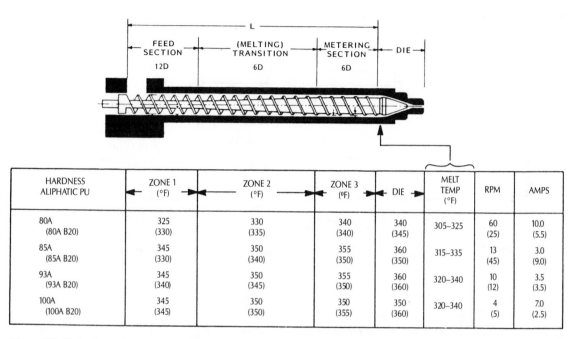

HARDNESS ALIPHATIC PU	ZONE 1 (°F)	ZONE 2 (°F)	ZONE 3 (°F)	DIE	MELT TEMP (°F)	RPM	AMPS
80A (80A B20)	325 (330)	330 (335)	340 (340)	340 (345)	305–325	60 (25)	10.0 (5.5)
85A (85A B20)	345 (330)	350 (340)	355 (350)	360 (350)	315–335	13 (45)	3.0 (9.0)
93A (93A B20)	345 (340)	350 (345)	355 (350)	360 (360)	320–340	10 (12)	3.5 (3.5)
100A (100A B20)	345 (345)	350 (350)	350 (355)	350 (360)	320–340	4 (5)	7.0 (2.5)

Figure 24. *Typical extruder screw conditions (conditions will vary with tubing size). B20 = 20% barium sulfate by weight.*

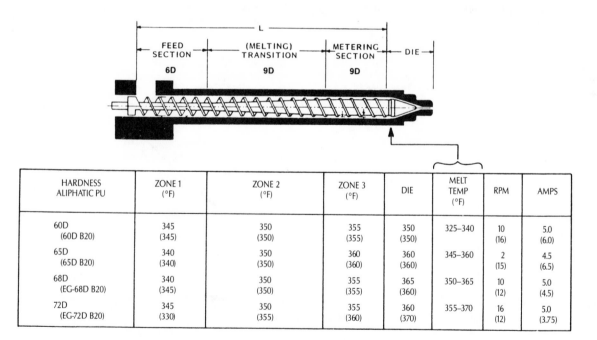

HARDNESS ALIPHATIC PU	ZONE 1 (°F)	ZONE 2 (°F)	ZONE 3 (°F)	DIE	MELT TEMP (°F)	RPM	AMPS
60D (60D B20)	345 (345)	350 (350)	355 (355)	350 (350)	325–340	10 (16)	5.0 (6.0)
65D (65D B20)	340 (340)	350 (350)	360 (360)	360 (360)	345–360	2 (15)	4.5 (6.5)
68D (EG-68D B20)	340 (345)	350 (350)	355 (355)	365 (360)	350–365	10 (12)	5.0 (4.5)
72D (EG-72D B20)	345 (330)	350 (355)	355 (360)	360 (370)	355–370	16 (12)	5.0 (3.75)

Figure 25. *Typical extruder screw conditions (conditions will vary with tubing size). B20 = 20% barium sulfate by weight.*

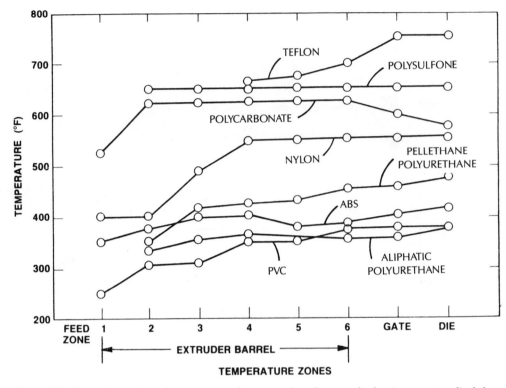

Figure 26. Comparison of extruder temperature between polyurethanes and other important medical thermoplastics.

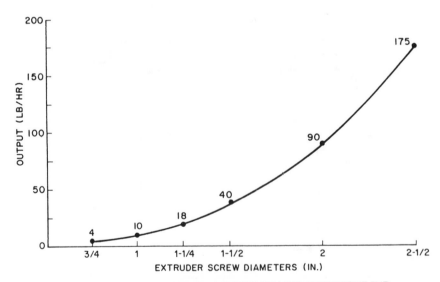

NOTE: OUTPUTS ARE BASED ON ALIPHATIC-80A WITH OPEN FRONT END,
RUNNING AT FULL SCREW SPEED.

Figure 27. Relationship between output and extruder diameter.

TABLE 11. Recommended Melt Temperature Ranges for Extrusion of Aliphatic TPU Elastomers

Material Shore A,D	Melt-Temperature
-80A	305-325°F
-85A	315-335°F
-93A	320-340°F
-100A	320-340°F
-60D	325-340°F
-65D	345-360°F
-68D	350-365°F
-72D	355-370°F

Finally, we recommend the use of 4140 tool steel for the screws, and either 303 or 304 stainless-steel for dies used in the extrusion of aliphatic TPU's. These materials represent a good compromise between cost and purity of the tubing. Several other possible materials of construction are shown in Table 15 with appropriate comments regarding their possible use when extruding Tecoflex resins.

Solvent Resistance

The use of the "wrong" solvent could materially affect the surface characteristics of polyurethanes. Some solvents are innocuous, while others produce surface fissuring, crazing and tack. Obviously, the biostability of these polymers can be severely compromised by the use of inappropriate solvents during prostheses manufacture and/or assembly.

Which solvent is best for any given polymer? This question has puzzled technologists for decades; the property of solubility (or insolubility) is fundamental in the selection of adhesives, coatings, swelling agents and surface cleaners. Thus, a basic discussion of the concepts of solubility parameters and their application to the production of urethane-based prostheses is essential.

As an approximation, the old expression that "like dissolves like" provides a good insight. Polystyrene is soluble in benzene and uncured rubber is soluble in aliphatic solvents; yet, there is no way that polymer solubilities can be predicted with assurance except for laborious trial and error.

The unreliability of "like dissolves like" and another rule of thumb "polarity" is demonstrated in Tables 16 and 17. Obviously, a scientific way to predict solubility would be invaluable to prostheses manufacturers. Ideally, this system might involve simple numerical constants, fundamental in nature, like density, molecular weight or boiling point. By comparing such constants for solvents and polymers we could determine whether a given solvent would dissolve a polymer, swell the polymer, or have absolutely no effect.

This section discusses the development of the solubility parameter concept by Hildebrand [31]. The theoretical background and derivation of the constants are described to better illustrate the practical applications to polymer solubility and swelling.

The polymer dissolution process may be pictured as occurring when a thermal movement of a segment of the

TABLE 12. Aliphatic Polyether-Based Polyurethane—Clear Grades Physical Test Data

Test Material Shore A,D	Vicat Softening Point D1525	Flexural Modulus D790 psi MPa	Specific Gravity D792	Ultimate Tensile D412 psi	Ultimate % Elongation D412	Hardness (Durometer) After Injection Molding
1. EG 80A	53.5°C	1040 7.3	1.04	5640	709	72A
2. EG 85A	60.0°C	2300 15.9	1.05	6935	565	77A
3. EG 93A	57.0°C	3210 22.1	1.08	7127	423	87A
4. EG 100A	48.0°C	10,400 71.3	1.09	8282	370	94A
5. EG 60D	45.0°C	13,200 90.8	1.09	7829	363	51D
6. EG 65D	45.5°C	37,000 255.0	1.10	8074	335	60D
7. EG 68D	57.4°C	45,900 316.4	1.10	8686	332	63D
8. EG 72D	49.0°C	92,400 636.9	1.11	7739	307	67D

These testing results are based on small samples of TECOFLEX polyurethane and do not necessarily represent average results from larger testing samples.

This information should NOT be used for establishing engineering specifications or manufacturing guidelines.

TABLE 13. Aliphatic Polyether-Based Polyurethane—Radiopaque Grades Physical Test Data

Test Material Shore A,D	Vicat Softening Point D1525	Flexural Modulus D790 psi MPa	Specific Gravity D792	Ultimate Tensile D412 psi	Ultimate % Elongation D412	Hardness (Durometer) After Injection Molding
9. EG 80A B 20	53.0°C	1240 8.6	1.24	5571	715	73A
10. EG 85A B 20	58.0°C	2700 15.6	1.25	5282	632	83A
11. EG 85A B 40	50.5°C	3650 25.2	1.51	5093	559	84A
12. EG 100A B 20	48.0°C	17,200 118.8	1.29	7104	369	93A
13. EG 100A B 40	57.0°C	21,700 149.7	1.54	5607	360	96A
14. EG 60D B 20	48.0°C	27,400 188.5	1.32	7484	370	55D
15. EG 65D B 20	53.5°C	81,900 564.5	1.32	6986	321	63D

These testing results are based on small samples of TECOFLEX polyurethane and do not necessarily represent average results from larger testing samples.

This information should NOT be used for establishing engineering specifications or manufacturing guidelines.

TABLE 14. Larger Diameter Extruders Are Commonly Utilized to Produce Bigger Tubing Profiles

Extruder Screw Size (inches)	Range of Tubing O.D. (inches)	Range of Line Speed (ft/min)
3/4	0.010 to 0.090	30 to 300
1	0.040 to 0.125	20 to 200
1-1/4	0.090 to 0.250	50 to 500
1-1/2	0.125 to 0.400	75 to 300
2	0.200 to 1.000	75 to 200
2-1/2	0.375 to 2.000	75 to 200

TABLE 15. Recommended Materials of Construction for the Extrusion of Aliphatic Tubing

Material	Strength	Corrosion Resistance	Cost
4140 Tool Steel	Excellent	Poor	Low (Recommended for Tecoflex)
17-4PH Stainless Steel	Good	Fair	Low
Hastalloy C-276	Poor	Excellent	High
4140 Chrome Plated	Excellent	Fair to Good	Low
4140 Electroless Nickel Plated	Good	Good	Low
4140 With Hard Facing (Stellite #6) (Colmonoy 56)	Excellent	Fair to Good	Intermediate
Recommended Construction Material for Dies			
303/304 Stainless Steel	Fair	Excellent	Low

TABLE 16. Like Dissolves Like (?)

Polymer	Is Soluble In	But Insoluble In
Cellulose	70% H_2SO_4	Water
Polystyrene	Butyl acetate	Methylcyclohexane
Ester gum	Mineral spirits	Glycerol
"Epon" Epoxy	Butyl acetate	Ether
Phenolic (BR17620)	Cellosolve acetate	Xylol
Polyvinyl acetate	Bromonaphthalene	Ethanol

polymer molecule makes a "hole" in space which instantly becomes occupied by a more mobile solvent molecule. This process continues until the entire polymer molecules become separated and "solution" is effected. If the molecules are cross-linked, the movement of the segments is limited. A lightly crosslinked polymer will swell or "dissolve solvent" until the osmotic or diffusional forces are balanced by the elastic contractile forces of the stretched molecules, but it will not dissolve to form a mobile solution. As such it might be said to exhibit partial miscibility or partial solubility. A highly cross-linked polymer cannot permit much segmental motion and, therefore, will not absorb much liquid; it will not swell or dissolve. Crystalline forces existing between molecules may be strong enough and abundant enough to prevent solution by acting as a type of secondary valence crosslink. We may, therefore, postulate that a solvent must exist for every noncrystalline, non-cross-linked polymer.

If we apply the familiar free energy equation in its simplest form to the process of mixing or dissolving a solvent and polymer we may write:

$$\Delta F = \Delta H - T\Delta S$$

This equation says that the change in free energy on mixing is equal to the heat of mixing minus the product of temperature and entropy change. The value of the free energy equation is to predict whether a given process will go. If the free energy has a negative value, the process will proceed. Therefore, it is apparent that whether or not a polymer will dissolve (or more correctly), whether the solvent and polymer will be miscible) depends on a balance of the heat factor, the entropy change and the temperature. It is well recognized that increasing the temperature favors solution. This is predicted by the free energy equation since increasing T tends to make ΔF more negative. However, for the purposes of our discussion we will assume the temperature remains constant.

The Entropy Factor

In considering the entropy factor, it is well to have a clear conception of the meaning of the term. Entropy is a measure of disorder or randomness or it may be considered as freedom of motion. If a molecule is so restricted that it can move in only a limited way, it will have a limited entropy as, for example, a molecule occupying a site within a crystal. On the other hand, a gas molecule, being free to move about would have high entropy. Likewise molecular processes tend to proceed toward conditions in which the molecules may possess greater entropy. This too is predicted by the free energy equation, since a large value of ΔS would make ΔF more negative.

TABLE 17. Solubility Compared with Polarity

Solvent	Dipole Moment	Dielectric Const.	Nitrocellulose	Polyvinyl Acetate	Polystyrene	Butylated Urea Resin
Butane	0	1.8	Insoluble	Insoluble	Insoluble	Insoluble
Hexane	0	1.87	Insoluble	Insoluble	Insoluble	Insoluble
Benzene	0	2.29	Insoluble	Soluble	Soluble	Insoluble
Carbon tetrachloride	0	2.24	Insoluble	Soluble	Soluble	Insoluble
Chloroform	1.1	5.0	Insoluble	Soluble	Soluble	Insoluble
Diethyl ether	1.1	4.3	Insoluble	Insoluble	Insoluble	Insoluble
Methanol	1.7	34	Soluble	Soluble	Insoluble	Insoluble
Ethanol	1.7	26	Insoluble	Insoluble	Insoluble	Insoluble
Butanol	1.7	18	Insoluble	Insoluble	Insoluble	Soluble
Methyl acetate	1.7	7.3	Soluble	Soluble	Soluble	Soluble
Water	1.8	80	Insoluble	Insoluble	Insoluble	Insoluble
Butyl chloride	2.0	9.6	Soluble	Insoluble	Soluble	Insoluble
Ethylene glycol	2.3	41	Insoluble	Insoluble	Insoluble	Insoluble
Diethyl ketone	2.7	17	Soluble	Soluble	Soluble	Insoluble
Acetone	2.8	21	Soluble	Soluble	Insoluble	Insoluble
Nitromethane	3.0	39	Soluble	Soluble	Insoluble	Insoluble
Acetonitrile	3.2	39	Soluble	Soluble	Insoluble	Insoluble

Let us consider what this means in the process of solution of a polymer. In a solid particle of amorphous polymer the molecules are so long and intertwined that the probability of an entire molecule moving past its neighbors is very low (otherwise the substance would be a liquid). Molecular motion is, therefore, limited to segmental Brownian movement. Although the entire molecule cannot move as a whole, groups of atoms along a chain may exhibit thermal or kinetic energy by moving away from the molecular axis temporarily. Such segmental motion would be much more free to take place and a whole new degree of freedom of motion would develop if the polymer molecules could be untangled from their neighbors. The new freedom of motion would include not only translatory movement of the molecule as a whole, but also the possibility of a large, linear, flexible molecule assuming innumerable "contortions." In this respect, polymer molecules are susceptible to much greater entropy increase than are low-molecular-weight molecules. In fact, the increase in configurational entropy would start as soon as the molecular separation started and would not be dependent on complete molecular separation. Consequently, the total entropy will be increased by any process tending to separate the polymer molecules from one another.

The solution process may be considered as occurring somewhat as follows: When the solid polymer particle is immersed in a solvent, the segmental motion of the molecules permits mobile solvent molecules to diffuse into the particle by vacating successive sites for the progressive movement of the solvent molecules. Thus, the concept of solvent dissolving into the polymer is not wholly fictional. Of course, as solvent molecules penetrate, the particle swells.

The Heat Factor

Since the entropy change is invariably large, the magnitude of the heat term ΔH is the deciding factor in determining the sign of the free energy change. It is the study of the heat term which gives us the clue to solubility. Many theoretical treatments of this factor have been made, but that proposed by Hildebrand is most useful for our purpose. Hildebrand stated:

$$\frac{\Delta H_M}{V_M \phi_1 \phi_2} = \left[\left(\frac{\Delta E_1}{V_1} \right)^{1/2} - \left(\frac{\Delta E_2}{V_2} \right)^{1/2} \right]^2$$

where

ΔH_M = overall heat of mixing, calories
V_M = total volume of the mixture, cc
ΔE = energy of vaporization of component 1 or 2, calories
V = molar volume of component 1 or 2, cc

ϕ = volume fraction of component 1 or 2 in the mixture, dimensionless

The expression $(\Delta E/V)$ is the energy of vaporization per cc. Thus it can variously be described as the "internal pressure" or the "cohesive energy density." Since the vaporization of a material represents complete separation of the molecules as a gas phase, it is a measure of the amount of energy which has to be put into one cc of liquid to overcome all of the intermolecular forces holding the molecules together. The term cohesive energy density is, therefore, highly appropriate because $\Delta E/V$ measures the concentration of forces that cause the molecules to cohere.

The heat of mixing per cc at a given concentration is equal to the square of the difference between the square roots of the cohesive energy densities of the components. The square root of the cohesive energy density is obviously an important quantity in determining heat effects. It is, therefore, convenient to assign to this quantity the symbol δ. Expressed mathematically $\delta = (\Delta E/V)^{1/2}$. If we place δ's in the right-hand side of the rearranged equation we can easily see that the unit heat of mixing of two substances is dependent on $(\delta_1 - \delta_2)^2$. If the heat of mixing is not to be so large as to prevent mixing, then $(\delta_1 - \delta_2)^2$ must be relatively small. In fact, if $(\delta_1 - \delta_2)^2 = 0$, solution is assured by the entropy factor. As the value approaches zero, $\delta_1 \rightarrow \delta_2$. This is mathematically equivalent to saying that if the δ values of two substances are nearly equal, the substances will be miscible. For this reason, Hildebrand has termed δ the solubility parameter.

In deriving the solubility parameter, no assumptions were made about polarity, solvation, association or any such mysterious quantities. Keep in mind, however, that solubility parameter governs only the heat of mixing of liquids or amorphous polymers. The heat fusion of crystals must be considered as an entirely separate factor. A noncrystalline polymer will, therefore, dissolve in a solvent of similar δ without the necessity of solvation, chemical similarity, association or any specially directed intermolecular force. As we have seen, the high entropy change possible with polymers is reason enough for solution to occur.

The solubility parameter of a solvent, δ, is a readily calculable quantity. The following section will detail a way of ascertaining or estimating the numerical value. Determining δ_p, the solubility parameter of a polymer (or for any nonvolatile substance) cannot be done directly because most polymers cannot be vaporized without decomposition. δ_p is therefore defined as the same as that of a solvent in which the polymer will mix (a) in all proportions, (b) without heat effect, (c) without volume change, and (d) without reaction or any special association.

Calculation of Solubility Parameters

It can be shown that $\Delta E = \Delta H - RT$, where ΔH = latent heat of vaporization at temperature T (°K) and R = Gas Constant = 1.986, so that $\Delta E_{25°} = \Delta H_{25°} - 600$.

As a specific example, consider the following data for carbon tetrachloride:

$$\text{Molecular weight} = 153.8$$
$$\text{Density, } 20°C = 1.595 \text{ g/cc}$$
$$\Delta H_{20°} = 7790 \text{ cal/mol}$$

$$\delta = \left(\frac{\Delta H - RT}{V}\right)^{1/2} = \left(\frac{7790 - 580}{153.8/1.595}\right)^{1/2} = 8.6$$

For most solvents, direct measurement of the heat of vaporization at the desired temperature have not been made or cannot be found in the literature. In such cases we must resort to one of the various known methods for estimating ΔH; for example, the Clausius-Clapeyron equation. Perhaps the most convenient of the estimations is Hildebrand's equation:

$$\Delta H_{25°C} = 23.7 T_b + 0.020 T_b^2 - 2950$$

where T_b is the boiling point in °K. Figure 28 is an adaptation of Hildebrand's curve in which RT has already been subtracted from ΔH so that ΔE may be read directly from the boiling point in °C at 760 mm. In each of these cases,

the data are reasonably accurate only for liquids that are not hydrogen bonded. They do not yield accurate data for esters, ketones, alcohols, etc. It has been found, however, that a final correction has been applied to the δ calculated from ΔE read from Figure 27, so that the solubility parameter estimate is sufficiently close for practical applications. These corrections are:

- For alcohols, add 1.4 to calculated δ.
- For esters, add 0.6 to calculated δ.
- For ketones, add 0.5 to calculated δ if the boiling point is under 100°C. Otherwise add nothing.

The use of Figure 27 is illustrated, again with carbon tetrachloride:

$$\text{Molecular weight} = 153.8$$
$$\text{Density} = 1.595$$
$$\text{Boiling point} = 76°C$$
$$\Delta E \text{ (from Figure 27)} = 7200 \text{ cal/mol}$$

$$\delta = \left(\frac{\Delta E}{V}\right)^{1/2} = \left(\frac{7200}{154/1.60}\right)^{1/2} = 8.6$$

Based on these concepts, solvents could be arranged by chemical types and solubility parameter (δ) as shown in Table 18. The solubility parameters of polymers could also be determined and arranged in groups of chemical families, as shown in Table 19. The great practical contribution of the Hildebrand concept was the prediction that any given polymer should be soluble in a specific solvent so long as their individual solubility parameters were $\delta \pm 2$ units. Beyond this limit, the solvent became a swelling agent, and further beyond, the polymer was totally insoluble in that specific solvent.

Table 20 has been compiled from manufacturer's bulletins and arranged so that the solvents are listed in order of increasing solubility parameter. It may be seen that chlorinated rubber is soluble in solvents within the range of δ 8.5 to 9.9 and insoluble outside that range so that here the theory seems to hold well. Ethyl cellulose seems to be soluble from δ 8.5 to 14.5, but two exceptions may be seen. For cellulose acetate and nitrocellulose the correlation is not nearly so good and many exceptions in the solubility series were noted. Apparently, the relationship in some cases was very good, but it still did not predict all observable phenomena. If some additional qualifying condition could be found, perhaps a more universal rule could be devised. As we shall see, this additional qualifying condition involved a second solubility parameter.

The Search for a Second Parameter

Following publication of the solubility parameter concept, the effect of various intermolecular forces on solu-

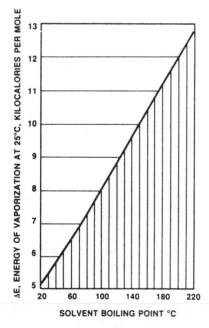

Figure 28. Graph used for the easy determination of ΔE from the boiling point of solvents. In turn, the Hildebrand solubility parameter δ can be calculated from δ = (ΔE/V)$^{1/2}$, where V = mol wt/density.

TABLE 18. Solubility Parameters of Selected Solvents Arranged by Chemical Types

Aliphatic Hydrocarbons	δ		Esters	δ
isobutylene	6.7		butyl acetate	8.5
low odor mineral spirits	6.9		Cellosolve acetate	8.7
pentane	7.0		propyl acetate	8.8
hexane	7.3		butyl Cellosolve	8.9
heptane	7.4		ethyl acetate	9.1
octane	7.6		propyl formate	9.2
VM&P	7.6		dibutyl phthalate	9.4
methylcyclohexane	7.8		methyl acetate	9.6
turpentine	8.1		ethyl lactate	10.0
cyclohexane	8.2		butyronitrile	10.5
dipentene	8.5		acetonitrile	11.9
			propylene carbonate	13.3
Aromatic Hydrocarbons	**δ**		ethylene carbonate	14.7
Solvesso #150	8.5			
Solvesso #100	8.6		**Ketones**	**δ**
ethylbenzene	8.8		diisobutyl	7.8
xylene	8.8		diisopropyl	8.0
toluene	8.9		methyl isobutyl	8.4
benzene	9.2		methyl amyl	8.5
tetralin	9.5		methyl propyl	8.7
			diethyl	8.8
Chlorinated	**δ**		isophorone	9.1
2,2 dichloropropane	8.2		diacetone alcohol	9.2
carbon tetrachloride	8.6		methyl cyclohexanone	9.3
1,2 dichloropropane	9.0		methyl ethyl	9.3
chloroform	9.3		cyclohexanone	9.9
trichlorethylene	9.3		acetone	10.0
tetrachlorethylene	9.4		cyclopentanone	10.4
chlorobenzene	9.5		cyclobutandione	11.0
methylene chloride	9.7			
ethylene dichloride	9.8		**Alcohols**	**δ**
o-dichlorbenzene	10.0		Butyl Carbitol	8.9
			Butyl Cellosolve	8.9
Ethers	**δ**		diethylene glycol	9.1
diethyl	7.4		2-ethylene glycol	9.1
dimethyl	8.8		Carbitol	9.6
dichloroethyl	9.8		Cellosolve	9.9
dioxan	9.9		methyl isobutyl carbinol	10.0
Cellosolve	9.9		n-octanol	10.3
			2-ethylbutanol	10.5
Esters	**δ**		n-hexanol	10.7
isobutyl n-butyrate	7.8		sec. butanol	10.8
isopropyl isobutyrate	7.9		n-pentanol	10.9
methyl amyl acetate	8.0		n-butanol	11.4
butyl butyrate	8.1		cyclohexanol	11.4
sec. butyl acetate	8.2		isopropanol	11.5
sec. amyl acetate	8.3		n-propanol	11.9
isobutyl acetate	8.3		ethanol	12.7
isopropyl acetate	8.4		ethylene glycol	14.2
amyl acetate	8.5		methanol	14.5
			glycerol	16.5

bility became apparent. The approach of Hansen [32,33], which utilized a hydrogen bonding component (δ_H), a polar component (δ_p), and a nonpolar component (δ_D) became particularly useful. In mathematic terms, the Hansen solubility parameter could be expressed as:

$$\delta^2 = \delta_D^2 + \delta_p^2 + \delta_n^2$$

In the Hansen method, the solubility of any given polymer is determined by examining the polymer behavior in a variety of solvents that cover all levels of the parameters concerned. From the plot of the resulting data, the polymer "envelope" is defined by those solvents which dissolved the polymer.

Using the Hansen solubility parameter system, the plot is three-dimensional; however, for practical purposes, the solubility parameter (δ) versus hydrogen bonding is sufficiently accurate. Thus, the hydrogen bonding index of solvents is the "second parameter" needed to predict most polymer/solvent behavior phenomena.

Thus, the basic principle involved in the application of solubility parameters is a simple one—when the value for a solvent falls within the parameter range of a polymer, the polymer will be soluble in that solvent. Additionally, in applying the solubility parameter concept, the hydrogen bonding strength of the solvent must be considered. As a first step, solvents are divided into three basic classes, depending on the relative energy of the hydrogen bridges, as follows:

Class I   *Poorly Hydrogen-Bonded.*
          Aliphatic, aromatic, chlorinated and nitrohydrocarbon solvents

Class II   *Moderately Hydrogen-Bonded.*
          Esters, ethers, ketones and glycol monoethers

Class III   *Strongly Hydrogen-Bonded.*
          Alcohols, amines, acids, amides and aldehydes

Table 21 provides the solvent spectrum of several solvents in terms of hydrogen-bonding activity. Table 22

TABLE 19. Solubility Parameters of Polymers

Polymer	δ
Alkyd, medium oil length	9.4
Amine type	
Beetle 227-8	10.1
Uformite MX61	9.6
Cellulose Derivatives	
Cellulose dinitrate	10.6
Cellulose nitrate, ½ sec.	11.5
Cellulose diacetate	10.9
Cellulose, ethyl (N22)	10.3
"Epon" 1004	10.9
Ester gum	9.0
Nylon 66	13.6
Nylon Type 8	12.7
Phenolic, BR17620	11.5
Polyacrylonitrile	15.4
Polyethylene	7.9
Polyglycol terephthalate	10.7
Polymethacrylonitrile	10.7
Polymethyl chloroacrylate	10.1
Polymethyl methacrylate	9.5
Polyvinyl acetate	9.4
Polyvinyl bromide	9.6
Polyvinyl chloride	9.7
Polyvinylidene chloride	12.2
Polyvinyl chloride acetate	10.4
Polystyrene	9.1
Rubbers	
Buna N	9.4
Chlorinated	9.4
GRS	8.1
Natural	8.3
Neoprene GN	9.2
Polybutadiene	8.6
Polyisobutylene	8.1
Thiokol F & FA	9.4
Thiokol RD	9.0
Silicone, polydimethyl	7.3
Teflon	6.2

presents data comparing solubility parameters, hydrogen bonding index, with corresponding molecular weights and densities, which are the parameters used to compute the Hildebrand solubility parameter. Figure 29 visually represents the parameter locations for major solvent groups.

Solubility Parameters of Biomaterials and Blood Components

As discussed in the previous paragraphs, the Hildebrand solubility parameter/hydrogen bonding index is a measure of the total forces holding the molecules of a solid as a liquid together.

Every polymer and solvent is characterized by a specific solubility parameter/hydrogen bonding index; polymer and solvents having approximately the same values are mutually miscible (soluble). Those with very different values are mutually immiscible (insoluble).

Table 23 presents calculated solubility parameters of several important biomaterials and blood components. This table explains many experimental observations described in the literature. For example, heart valves made of silicone rubbers were found to change dimensions significantly; this dimensional change eventually discouraged the use of silicone in heart valves. With a solubility parameter in the 7.3 to 7.6 range, it can readily be predicted that cholesterol, cholesterol esters and triglyceride with a solubility parameter in the 8.0 to 8.5 range would display some "miscibility" with the silicone rubber.

TABLE 20. Test of Hildebrand Solubility Parameter

Solvent	δ	Chlorinated Rubber	Ethyl Cellulose	Cellulose Acetate	½ sec. Nitrocellulose
Hexane	7.3	I	I	I	I
Ethyl ether	7.4	P	S	I	P
VM&P Naphtha	7.6	I	I	I	I
Turpentine	8.1	I	P	I	I
Dipentene	8.5	P	S	I	I
Butyl acetate	8.5	S	S	I	S
Carbon tetrachloride	8.6	S	S	I	I
Cellosolve acetate	8.7	-	S	I	S
Xylene	8.8	S	S	I	I
Toluene	8.9	S	S	I	I
Ethyl acetate	9.1	S	S	S	S
Diacetone alcohol	9.2	S	P	S	S
Methyl cellosolve acetate	9.2	-	S	S	S
Benzene	9.2	-	S	I	I
Methyl ethyl ketone	9.3	S	S	S	S
Chloroform	9.3	-	S	I	I
Butyl lactate	9.4	-	S	I	S
Pentachloroethane	9.4	-	S	I	I
Methyl acetate	9.6	S	S	S	S
Methylene chloride	9.7	-	S	I	I
Ethylene dichloride	9.8	S	S	I	I
Cyclohexanone	9.9	-	S	S	S
Cellosolve	9.9	S	S	I	S
Dioxane	9.9	-	S	S	S
Ethyl lactate	10.0	-	S	S	S
Acetone	10.0	P	S	S	S
Methyl cellosolve	10.8	-	S	S	S
Cyclohexanol	11.4	-	S	I	I
Butanol	11.4	I	S	I	I
Ethanol	12.7	I	S	I	I
Methanol	14.5	I	S	I	I

S = Soluble
I = Insoluble
P = Swollen

TABLE 21. Solvent Spectrum

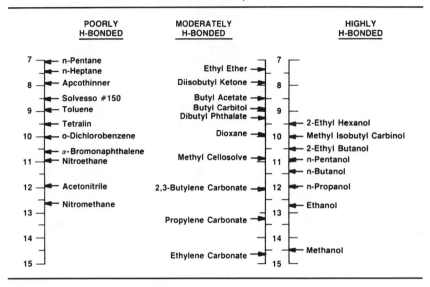

TABLE 22. Characteristic Parameters for Some Solvents at 25°C

Solvent	Solubility Parameter, Hildebrands, $(cal/cm^3)^{\frac{1}{2}}$	Hydrogen Bonding Index	Molecular Weight	Density, g/cm^3
Acetone	10.0	5.7	58.08	0.792
Acetonitrile	11.9	4.5	41.05	0.786
Acrylonitrile	10.5	4.3	53.06	0.806
n-Amyl alcohol	8.5	8.9	88.15	0.817
Aniline	11.8	8.7	93.13	1.022
Benzene	9.2	2.2	78.11	0.879
n-Butanol	11.4	8.9	74.12	0.806
tert-Butyl alcohol	10.5	8.9	74.12	0.789
Carbon disulfide	10.0	2.2	76.14	1.266
Carbon tetrachloride	8.6	2.2	153.82	1.594
Chlorobenzene	9.5	2.7	112.56	1.106
Chloroform	9.3	2.2	119.38	1.492
Cyclohexane	8.2	2.2	84.16	0.774
Cyclohexanone	9.9	6.4	98.15	0.951
n-Decane	6.6	2.2	142.27	0.726
Diethyl carbonate	8.8	4.0	118.13	0.969
Diethylene glycol (DEG)	14.2	8.5	106.12	1.116
DEG, monobutyl ether	8.9	6.9	162.23	0.955
DEG, monoethyl ether	9.6	6.9	134.18	0.988
Diethyl ether	7.4	6.9	74.12	0.714
N,N'-Diformylpiperazine	15.4	9.4	142.16	---
Diisopropyl ether	6.9	6.6	102.18	0.725
N,N'-Dimethylacetamide	10.8	6.6	87.12	0.937
N,N'-Dimethylformamide	12.1	6.4	73.10	0.944
Dimethyl sulfoxide	13.0	5.0	78.13	1.096
1,4-Dioxane	9.9	5.7	88.11	1.028
Ethyl acetate	9.1	5.2	88.11	0.901
Ethanol	12.8	8.9	46.07	0.785
Ethylbenzene	8.8	2.7	106.17	0.863
Ethylene carbonate	14.7	4.0	88.06	1.321
Ethylene dichloride (or 1,2-dichloroethane)	9.8	2.7	98.96	1.246
Ethylene glycol (EG)	14.6	9.6	62.07	1.113
EG, monobutyl ether (or 2-butoxyethanol)	8.9	6.9	118.18	0.901
EG, monoethyl ether (or 2-ethoxyethanol)	9.9	6.9	90.12	0.925
Ethylene oxide	11.1	5.8	44.05	0.887
2-Ethylhexanol	9.5	8.9	130.23	0.829
Formamide	19.2	16.2	45.04	1.133
Furfural	11.2	4.7	96.09	1.160
Glycerol	16.5	8.5	92.10	1.261
n-Heptane	7.4	2.2	100.21	0.680
n-Hexane	7.3	2.2	86.18	0.655
Isophorone	9.4	7.0	138.21	0.923
Isopropyl acetate	8.4	5.3	102.14	0.872
Isopropyl alcohol	11.5	8.9	60.10	0.800
Kerosene (typical)	7.2	2.2	---	0.800
Methyl chloride	9.7	2.7	84.93	1.315
Methyl ethyl ketone	9.3	5.0	72.11	0.800

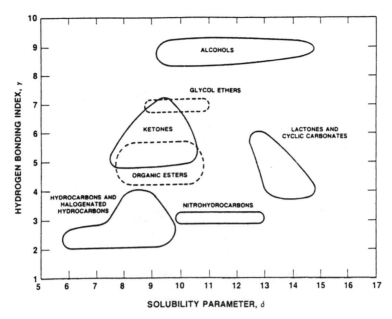

Figure 29. *Parameter locations for major solvent groups.*

Indeed, the reason for the dimensional change was finally traced to lipid absorption by the rubber.

Polyurethanes, such as Biomer and Mitrathane with solubility parameters higher than silicone rubbers can be predicted to be less susceptible to lipid absorption, but still capable of being penetrated and plasticized by cholesterol, cholesterol esters, and lipids. On the other hand, phospholipids should only be surface adsorbed rather than matrix absorbed as predicted by this concept.

Solvency, Swelling and Surface Fissuring

The "power," "activity" or "goodness" of solvents can be judged by many different criteria such as ability to reduce viscosity, ability to dissolve large quantities of polymer, and ease of solution at room temperature with minimal stirring. Although it is rather difficult to generalize, most solvents capable of dissolving polyurethane elastomers share solubility parameters in the range of 10 to 13, and

Table 23. Calculated Solubility Parameters of Biomaterials and Blood Components

Polymer or Blood Component	Solubility Parameter δ $(cal/cm^3)^{\frac{1}{2}}$
Segmented Polyetherurethane (Biomer)	
Soft segment	10.5
Hard segment	13.0
Aliphatic Polyurethane	
Soft grades (80A–85A)	9.0 - 12.0
Hard grades (60D–72D)	10.0 - 13.0
PTMEG	8.0 - 9.5
Silicone Oil	6.2
Polydimethylsiloxane (Silicone rubber)	7.3 - 7.6
Poly(ethylene terephthalate)	9.7 - 10.7
Glutaraldehyde-treated tissue valves (Unused)	12.0 - 13.0
Glutaraldehyde-treated protein surfaces ("Biolized" materials)	10.0 - 12.0
Cholesterol and esters	8.4 - 8.9
Triglycerides	8.0 - 8.3
Lipid-soluble vitamins	8.6 - 10.9
Phospholipids	> 16
Proteins (Non-denatured)	> 18
Water	23.2

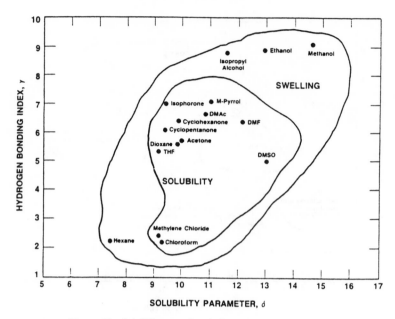

Figure 30. Solubility map for aliphatic polyurethane resin.

display either poor or moderate hydrogen bonding indexes.

Solvents close to the periphery of these values swell the polymers significantly, and may contribute to eventual surface fissuring by inducing residual stresses. Solvents far away from these values can be safely used for surface cleaning of polyurethane prostheses.

Based on these considerations, we can construct a solubility map for the aliphatic family shown in Figure 30. As shown, aliphatic resins are dissolved by solvents possessing solubility parameters in the 9 to 13 range, and either poor or moderate hydrogen bonding indexes. It should be noted that softer grades behave differently than harder grades, since the polyether segment molecular weight, the percent soft segment, and the end groups are different, as listed below:

Shore Hardness	PTMEG Molecular Weight	Percent Hard Segment	Nominal End Group
80A	2000	27	Isocyanate
85A	2000	36	Hydroxyl
93A	1000	51	Hydroxyl
100A	1000	57	Hydroxyl
60D	1000	59	Isocyanate
65D	1000	63	Hydroxyl
72D	1000	70	Hydroxyl

In our laboratories we use a variety of solvents for the processing and assembly of aliphatic-based medical prostheses. These prostheses include catheters, wound dressings, medicated wound dressings, skin buttons, and transcutaneous energy transmission systems. Solvents and non-solvents are listed in Tables 24 and 25 in alphabetical order, with special characteristics noted relating to the aliphatic polyurethanes.

By the judicious application of the solubility parameter concept as presented in this section, the astute technology will have a rational and reliable scientific method for the selection of the most appropriate solvent, swelling agent or non-solvent for use with aliphatic resins.

BIOSTABILITY OF POLYURETHANE ELASTOMERS

Permanent polyurethane leads were first implanted in humans in 1975 (neurologic) and in 1977 (cardiac). In 1981, a relatively short-term cardiac implant was discovered with insulation failure due to a previously undiscovered cracking mechanism. As of October 1987, many pacing leads distributed have been returned with similar insulation failures. The primary failure mechanism has been determined to be environmental stress cracking (ESC), although secondary mechanisms have been identified.

Prior to the introduction of polyurethane pacemaker lead insulation, the materials of choice were silicone rubber, or polyethylene. Silicone rubber performed well, but required the use of a thick wall because of its inferior mechanical properties.

Controversy has arisen about the use of Pellethane 2363-80A polyurethane because of biodegradation in the form of shallow surface fissures. This was the first clinical manifestation of polyurethane biodegradation. Certain models have demonstrated excellent biostability, while others have experienced unacceptably high degrees of biodegradation.

Table 24. Effects of Solvents on Aliphatic Medical-Grade Thermoplastic Polyurethane Elastomers

Name	Solubility Parameter	Hydrogen Bonding	Comments
Acetone BP = 55.1°C	10.0	5.7	Will solvate resins at low solids. Causes surface tackiness and initiates cracking and splitting of fabricated parts.
Chloroform BP = 61.2°C	9.3	2.2	Used primarily as a fast evaporating solvent for grades below EG-60D. Difficult to control viscosity because of rapid evaporation.
Cyclohexanone BP = 155.6°C	9.9	6.4	A slow evaporating solvent, used extensively for bonding tubing to fittings. Best for Tecoflex EG-80A and EG-85A at low solid contents.
Cyclopentanone BP = 130.5°C	9.4	6.2	Similar to cyclohexanone, but a slightly faster evaporating solvent, more advantageous in processes utilizing oven drying.
Dimethyl Acetamide BP = 165.5°C	10.8	6.6	A preferred solvent for all grades of Tecoflex. Recommended solids between 10 to 17 percent, with a viscosity of 1000 cps at 60°C.
Dimethyl Formamide BP = 153°C	12.1	6.4	A powerful solvent for the harder grades of Tecoflex. High solids solutions can be obtained when heated to 65°C.
Dimethyl Sulfoxide BP = 189°C	13.0	5.0	A marginal solvent for the harder grades of Tecoflex.
Dioxane BP = 9.9°C	9.9	5.7	A low-cost alternative to tetrahydrofuran.
Isophorone BP = 215.4°C	9.4	7.0	Stable, colorless solvent for the softer grades of Tecoflex. Mild odor.
Methylene Chloride BP = 39.8°C	9.2	2.4	Good solvent for EG-80A and EG-85A. Highly volatile clear solvent with an ethereal odor. Nonflammable.
M-Pyrrol BP = 202°C	11.0	7.1	Good solvent for harder grades of Tecoflex. Clear liquid with a mild amine-like odor.
Tetrahydrofuran BP = 66°C	9.1	5.3	An excellent solvent for all grades of Tecoflex. A fast evaporating solvent, with a rate of evaporation between acetone and methyl ethyl ketone. Tecoflex coatings for PVC.

Table 25. Effects of Nonsolvents and Swelling Agents on Tecoflex

Name	Solubility Parameter	Hydrogen Bonding	Comments
Ethanol BP = 78.3°C	12.8	8.9	A swelling agent for softer grades. Surface tackiness develops by leaching of lubricant.
Hexane BP = 68°C	7.4	2.2	A swelling agent if Tecoflex is exposed for prolonged periods. Good surface cleaning solvent.
Isopropyl Alcohol BP = 82°C	11.5	8.9	A swelling agent for softer Tecoflex grades. Will leach lubricant, leaving a tacky surface.
Methanol BP = 64.7°C	14.6	9.1	Swells Tecoflex EG-80A and 85A. Leaches lubricant leaving a tacky surface.
Methyl Ethyl Ketone BP = 79.6°C	9.3	5.0	Powerful swelling agent for softer grades. Leaches lubricant. Does not affect EG-60D, EG-65D or EG-72D.
Toluene BP = 108°C	9.1	3.1	Preferred swelling agent for all grades, with softer grades displaying greatest swelling. Examples after 90 minutes: ID x OD — Exposed — ID x OD EG-80A Tubing 0.110" x 0.160" 0.208" x 0.290" EG-60D Tubing 0.110" x 0.160" 0.130" x 0.192"
Freon TF (Trichloro Trifluoroethane) BP = 47.6°C	Not Applicable	Not Applicable	Exceptional surface cleaning agent for all grades. Recommended for vapor degreasing. Swelling of 5 to 6 percent may occur with EG-80A if left exposed to this agent for extended periods of time.

In 1981, Parins of Cardiac Pacemakers Inc. [34] alerted the biomaterials community to the *in vivo* degradation of polyurethane pacemaker leads. This initial report was soon followed by Guerrant [35] of Intermedics Inc., and McArthur of Pacesetter Systems [36].

In November 1983, a French physician reported the failure of 10 Medtronic 6991-U leads, and in January 1984 the Lancaster General Hospital noted a 20% failure rate with Medtronic 6972 pacemaker leads [37]. As a result, 27,000 Model 6972 bipolar leads, manufactured between December 1975 and February 1982 were involved in an FDA Class II recall [38].

This section discusses the known and hypothesized factors involved in the biostability/biodegradation of polyurethanes. For our purposes, we will define biodegradation as the "structural or chemical changes in a biomaterial that are initiated or accelerated by the vital activity of the biological environment." Thus, biodegradation is not merely the *in vitro* degradation of the biomaterial, since that does not involve any vital activity of the host organism.

Cardiac Pacemaker Leads

Cardiac pacing systems are utilized for patients with some impairment of the heart's natural electrical system that limits the heart's ability to pump blood throughout the body at a rate suitable to fulfill the body's needs. Under normal circumstances, the rhythmic contractions of the heart are stimulated by small electrical signals emitted by the sinus node, the heart's natural pacemaker. These signals are conducted downward along nerve fibers to the four chambers of the heart, first to the two upper chambers or atria, which serve to prime the two lower chambers or ventricles, which in turn perform the principal pumping function of the heart.

When the heart's natural pacing mechanism is impaired, a pacemaker may be used to remedy the problem by electrically stimulating the heart to restore its regular rhythmic muscular contractions. Pacemakers are generally implanted and connected to the heart by means of insulated wire leads and electrodes called lead/electrodes. Since the right and left sides of the heart contract in unison, it is necessary to pace only one side, and only the right side is commonly paced. Most modern pacemakers are hermetically sealed, usually in titanium metal cases containing a long-life lithium-based battery and appropriate electronic circuitry to generate pulses and control their characteristics. Pacemakers currently on the market range from approximately 35 to 100 grams (one and one-quarter to three and one-half ounces) in weight and from approximately 15 to 50 cc in volume. The useful lives of these pacemakers typically range from 5 to 10 years.

The cardiac pacing industry began in the 1960s with the development of relatively simple, single-chamber pacing devices providing a continuous stream of electrical pulses at a fixed rate, generally to the right ventricle of the heart. By the early 1970s the industry had almost entirely converted to more advanced single chamber "demand" pacemakers capable of sensing or monitoring the heart's natural rhythm and providing stimulation only when the natural rhythm was inadequate.

In the mid-1970s programmable pacemakers came into increasing use, offering the ability to modify without surgery several operating parameters of the pacemaker, including pulse rate and pulse energy, simply by activating a programming unit communications head held against the skin over the implanted pacemaker. The ability to adjust certain operating parameters enabled the physician to regulate the pacemaker to best meet the patient's needs, to extend the expected life of the pacemaker under certain conditions, and to eliminate the need for surgical replacements in some cases where the physiological condition of the patient's heart had changed. Later in the 1970s, such external control was extended in multiprogrammable pacemakers enabling the physician to program additional operating parameters.

Another important development during the late 1970s was the creation of pacing systems that enabled bidirectional telemetry between the implanted unit and an external programmer. This improvement enabled the physician for the first time to interrogate the implanted unit and to receive back information confirming that the pacemaker had received, and responded correctly to, the programming signals and to ascertain the operating characteristics of the implanted pacemaker. Such telemetry systems also permitted transmission of important physiologic and operating data on how the heart and pacemaker function together.

The next advance in pacing systems was the development of dual-chamber devices, the first practical versions of which were released commercially in 1981. Unlike single-chamber systems, which stimulate only the right ventricle of the heart through a single lead/electrode, dual chamber systems are capable of synchronized stimulation of both the right atrium and right ventricle through two separate lead/electrodes. This synchronized stimulation can increase blood flow with less strain on the heart. As a result, physicians are recommending the use of dual chamber systems for increasing numbers of patients.

Recently, more advanced dual chamber systems have been developed. These devices not only provide synchronized stimulation of both chambers, but are also capable of sensing and tracking in both chambers as well. When a dual-chamber pacemaker senses that there is a regular natural atrial rhythm, it will assure that the ventricles track this rhythm in synchrony. When a regular atrial rhythm is not present, an atrial pulse is delivered by the system followed by a synchronized ventricular pulse.

Because dual-chamber systems more closely simulate the heart's actual physiological rhythm, thereby more effectively meeting the individual physiological needs of each patient, these pacemakers are expected to increase from 20 percent in 1984 to 50 percent of all implanted pacemakers by 1990.

Advances in cardiac pacemakers are allowing more patients to play tennis, swim, even jog. And that is important, since almost 100,000 patients receive pacemakers in the U.S.—a quarter of them between the ages of 25 and 45.

The FDA has just approved a new pacemaker, Activitrax, which adjusts heart rhythm by sensing vibrations that indicate activity. Another pacemaker, the Kelvin 500, regulates the heart beat by sensing slight excursions in body temperature after exercise or other physiological activity. Through it all, the newer devices are not only more sophisticated than their predecessors, they are also small enough to fit inside a tablespoon. A recent review in the *Annals of Internal Medicine* foresees dual-chambered pacemakers that monitor blood oxygen and pH levels, a device particularly important for patients with pulmonary disease.

Compared to standard silicone rubbers, polyurethane elastomers offer several advantages including higher tensile strengths, significantly higher tear resistance, and excellent abrasion resistance. In the manufacture of cardiac pacing leads, these advantages have resulted in the introduction of polyurethane leads with significantly reduced wall thicknesses. These thinner-wall leads have resulted in easier surgical insertion, less traumatic introduction of multiple leads when inserted into single veins (for dual-chamber pacing), and greater elasticity for the implanted lead.

Vascular Grafts

Vascular disease, such as atherosclerosis, is usually progressive. A fatty streak in the vessel can develop rapidly into fibrous plaque deposits and ultimately to a complex material that impedes blood flow. Some patients eventually need vascular grafts to bypass severely obstructed arteries. Vascular disease resulting in an arterial aneurysm, a balloon-like dilation of an artery, may also require a graft replacement.

To date, no organization is marketing arterial grafts suitable for the replacement of the coronary arteries. Each year, there are 320,000 coronary bypass surgeries. Surgeons still harvest saphenous vein grafts from the patient and are interested in a viable off-the-shelf arterial substitute. Thus, a major new market opportunity exists in the development of an improved small-diameter (4 mm or less) vascular prosthesis. If that product could be used for both peripheral and coronary applications, the vascular graft market could grow to $500 million annually.

Two biomaterials currently dominate the vascular graft market: dacron and PTFE (polytetrafluoroethylene). Dacron (polyethylene terephthalate) monofilaments are woven into various intricate designs to form the grafts; these grafts are generally used in the large diameter category (12 to 22 mm diameter). Blown PTFE grafts are generally used in the intermediate diameter category (6 to 12 mm diameter).

PTFE is a full fluorinated polymer with the structural formula $(-CF_2-CF_2)_n$. It was discovered accidentally in 1938 by DuPont researcher R. J. Plunkett. PTFE, with an unusually high crystalline melting point of 342°C and a melt viscosity of 10^{11} P at 380°C, rendered the polymer intractable to conventional processing.

In 1963, Shinsaburo Oslinge of Sumitomo Industries in Japan discovered a process for expanding PTFE during extrusion. This opened the way for the production of expanded PTFE vascular grafts as we know them today. These expanded grafts consist of nodes and fiber; nodes are open channels perpendicular to the graft axis, while fibers are open channels parallel to the graft axis.

The porosity of these PTFE grafts encourages the formation of a biological lining on the lumenal surface, variously known as a neointimal or pseudointimal lining. A strict biological definition classifies a neointimal lining as a cellular lining, whereas a pseudintimal lining refers to a mostly acellular lining, composed of various fibrous proteins, such as fibrin and/or collagen. In humans, the linings seen in PTFE grafts are pseuodointimal linings since they are essentially acellular.

Dacron and PTFE grafts are clinically acceptable for peripheral vascular surgery, arteriovenous shunts, and aneurysm repairs where the internal diameter exceeds 6 mm. For diameters smaller than 6 mm, studies indicate that anastomic hyperplasia, thickened fibrin linings and kinking all contribute to poor *in vivo* performance. Occlusive thrombus at both anastomic ends results in postoperative failures, with reported 50 to 75 percent patency rates at 12 weeks.

Polyurethane grafts with improved compliance matching to the native vessels are, at present, the best alternative. However, with the specter of surface fissuring (and subsequent fiber breakdown) overhanging the polyurethanes, we must await the solution to bioinstability before a successful small-bore, polyurethane-based vascular graft becomes a clinical reality.

Artificial Hearts

Cardiovascular disease is the most significant medical problem in the United States. Cardiovascular disease is still the leading cause of death, responsible for almost as many deaths as all other causes combined. Consequently, its diagnosis, monitoring, and treatment is a national concern. According to American Heart Association estimates, Americans will spend over $50 billion this year for drugs, physician and nursing services, and hospital and nursing home services, to diagnose, monitor and treat cardiovascular disease.

While the number of deaths from coronary artery and cardiovascular disease is decreasing in the U.S., the prevalence of CHF is increasing. Congestive heart failure accounts for almost 400,000 deaths each year in the U.S. alone. Approximately half of these deaths are sudden, and presumably related to the particularly high incidence of ventricular arrhythmias in patients with congestive heart failure. In 1971, the Framingham study found that, for those who have acquired CHF, the probability of dying within five years was 62 percent for men and 42 percent for women. The investigators stated, "despite early recognition and increasingly sophisticated and potent treatment of CHF, its clinical cause and prognosis remains surprisingly grim and not much better than those for cancer in general." Unfortunately, this statement remains true 16 years later.

Congestive heart failure is a condition in which the heart pumping function is inadequate to supply the metabolic need of the body; in other words, CHF is present when the heart fails in its function as a pump. When cardiac pumping is inadequate, congestion (or pooling of blood) is observed in the lungs, legs, and stomach, depending upon which side of the heart is affected.

The heart's prime mechanical function is to generate sufficient force to propel blood throughout the peripheral vasculature. Within its ventricular chambers the normal heart generates enough driving pressure to perfuse downstream components of the vasculature where the blood pressure is lower. One fundamental measure of mechanical function is cardiac output, which is a clinical expression of the heart's performance as a pump. Whenever cardiac output is inadequate on a chronic basis, we say the patient suffers from CHF.

The clinician treating cardiogenic failure patients has little hope of saving these desperately ill patients. Drug therapy is the only choice available at this time other than a biologic heart transplant. Drug therapy is effective initially, but limited in many ways because the disease state progresses to a point where the natural heart cannot provide the necessary energy level to maintain life. At that point, biologic heart transplant is the only other choice. Significant progress has been made on this front, although the lack of sufficient donor hearts has greatly limited this activity. It is estimated that between 1500 and 2000 donor hearts are available yearly while there are approximately 40,000 patients a year in CHF who need them. Obviously, there is a significant clinical need to provide an alternative for those patients in CHF who require cardiac support.

At present, the only hope for patients with CHF is twofold: biological heart transplants or artificial hearts. Since only a maximum of 2000 donor hearts become available per year, the only logical alternative is the development and widespread clinical availability of artificial hearts. Artificial hearts are best utilized in those patients who have developed cardiogenic shock, a condition resulting from sudden decline in cardiac output secondary to CHF, usually a myocardial infarction.

The societal need for artificial hearts is large. We estimate that of 400,000 deaths caused by CHF, approximately 84,000 occur as a result of cardiogenic shock. This is the primary patient population that could benefit from either biologic heart transplants or artificial hearts. We further subdivide artificial hearts into total heart (where the natural heart is surgically excised) and ventricular assist devices (where the natural heart remains in place, and the assist device is surgically connected in parallal between the left ventricle and the aorta).

With few exceptions, polyurethane is used for the flexing diaphragms of permanently implantable artificial hearts. The goal of artificial hearts is to implant these devices in patients for periods of ten years. Again, the biostability of polyurethane-based diaphragms is a matter of concern in artificial hearts, since breakage of the diaphragm would be a medical emergency. Solving the puzzle of polyurethane surface fissuring is a high priority in the biomaterials community.

The Magnitude of the Problem

From the preceding sections, it is clear that polyurethanes are crucial in pacemaker leads, small-bore vascular grafts and artificial hearts. These are all chronic implants that depend on the long-term biostability of the polyurethane for their ultimate performance.

In pacemakers, the unit provides the energy output, while the lead provides the pathway into the heart. The lead insulation may be the most simple-looking part of the device, but it is one of the most critical components. While we accept several potential pacemaker/unit exchanges during the life of the implant, the lead is expected to remain unchanged, and provide absolute reliability for a period of 10 to 15 years!

Based on estimates from industry analysts, the worldwide pacemaker utilization reached 250,000 units in 1986, representing a billion dollar market of which approximately 55 percent were implanted in the U.S., as shown in Table 26.

Polyurethane vascular grafts could be utilized for shunts, peripheral vascular surgery and coronary artery grafts, with current usage presented in Table 27. The selling price of biostable polyurethane grafts are expected to be: $300 for shunts, $600 for peripheral vascular surgery, and $1000 for coronary artery grafts. Thus, the potential worldwide market for successful polyurethane vascular grafts is nearly one billion dollars.

Table 26. Pacemaker Market Projections

	1986	1990 (E)
Units		
U.S.	110,000	135,000
Overseas	140,000	180,000
Totals	250,000	315,000
Sales (millions)		
U.S.	$ 550	$ 825
Overseas	450	675
Totals	$ 1,000	$ 1,500

The Artificial Heart represents another great opportunity for polyurethanes. Although not generally appreciated, the term "artificial heart" encompasses both Total Artificial Hearts (TAH), as well as Ventricular Assist Systems (VAS). In either case, the artificial heart discussed here is intended to provide *permanent* support for patients in chronic cardiogenic shock, or with progressive cardiomyopathies.

The National Heart Lung and Blood Institute (NHLBI) convened a committee of experts in the aftermath of the revolutionary Barney Clark implant to review the overall purpose of the national artificial heart program, and make recommendations regarding the advisability of the program. In May 1985, the committee issued its final report which contained a sweeping endorsement of the overall concept and purpose, and recommended greatly expanded federal research efforts [39]. The committee estimated that each implant will eventually cost about $150,000, recipients will survive an average of 54 months, and 17,000 to 35,000 Americans below the age of 70 could benefit from this treatment annually. The report notes that if these projections are accurate, the annual budget for artificial hearts in the U.S. will be in the range of $2.5 to 5.0 billion dollars.

Pacemakers, vascular grafts and artificial hearts may be the most visible devices requiring biostable polyurethanes, but other long-term implants, such as skin buttons, vascular access, implantable infusion pumps, and peritoneal dialysis, also deserve attention.

Because of its importance, the biomaterial community is committed to elucidate the mechanisms underlying the susceptibility of polyurethane to biodegradation, to correlate molecular changes with observed failures and, finally, to provide an appropriate answer to this vexing problem.

MOLECULAR CORRELATIONS TO SURFACE FISSURING

In 1983, Szycher and McArthur [40] first proposed that polyether-based polyurethanes were susceptible to *in vivo* oxidation of the polyether chain. Our studies showed that, in this chain, the most susceptible groups is the $-CH_2$ group in the alpha position to the ether oxygen, which undergoes oxidation and eventually chain cleavage, leading to significant reductions in molecular weight *at the surface*, and eventual surface fissuring.

Based on these preliminary results, we hypothesized that progressive surface degradation is caused, in part, by stress-induced oxidation of the polyether macroglycol used in the synthesis of polyurethane elastomers. Our hypothesis has been reinforced by experimental evidence that surface cracking can be significantly reduced, if not eliminated, by using higher-durometer polyurethanes, because these polymers contain fewer polyether macroglycol chains in the molecular backbone that comprises the soft segment.

It was our contention that surface fissuring could be traced to molecular degradation of the soft segment. The molecular degradation was caused by chain cleavage occurring principally at areas of: (1) residual stress from improper draw-down ratio during extrusion, utilization of inappropriate solvents during assembly, and (2) induced stresses from dynamic bending and vein ligation sites.

We suggested three possible ways to reduce surface fissuring of polyurethane-based pacemaker leads: (1) utilize higher durometer polyurethanes, since they are inherently less susceptible to stress-induced oxidation at the soft segments, (2) lower the ligature stress at the ligation

Table 27. Usage of Vascular Grafts by Procedure

	Peripheral	Shunts	Coronary Artery Bypass
Dacron	30,000	---	---
PTFE	80,000	75,000	---
Biograft	7,000	1,000	---
Saphenous Vein	233,000	---	320,000
Other	---	74,000	---
Total	350,000	150,000	320,000

site by the use of a silicone anchoring sleeve which spreads the stresses over a larger area and, finally, (3) control the manufacturing process to minimize the drawdown ratio of the tubing. We should add: (4) use of an appropriate swelling solvent during manufacture that does not cause excessive residual stress at the surface after drying.

Stress and Surface Fissuring

As presented during the ASTM Symposium on Corrosion and Degradation of Implant Materials in 1983, we utilized two polyurethane elastomers for our study.

Polyurethane leads made of Pellethane 2363-80A and aliphatic polyurethane 60D were implanted in the right heart of experimental animals (dogs) for varying periods of time. Following explantation, the leads were cleaned with pepsin, a proteolytic enzyme, by digestion at 37°C with pH controlled at 1.0 for several hours to remove biologic deposits. The efficacy of the pepsin digestion was experimentally demonstrated by totally removing known biologic debris after soaking for only 30 minutes. The specimens were subsequently dried and readied for Scanning Electron Microscopy (SEM).

Experimental leads were ultrastructurally compared with returned clinical leads made of Pellethane 2363-80A. These leads were explanted from patients, and the surfaces were enzymatically cleaned with pepsin and Tergazyme prior to SEM evaluation.

Finally, stressed and unstressed Tecoflex EG-60D specimens were implanted subcutaneously in swine for three months. After pepsin treatment, the surfaces were chemically analyzed by Attenuated Total Reflectance Infrared (ATR-IR) spectroscopy, and compared to unimplanted controls which provided baseline spectral data.

Our results indicated that most surface fissuring of the polyurethanes identified in this study appeared to be related to the combination of manufacturing induced and environmentally induced stresses. Much of the observed surface fissuring occurred at the vein ligation site, probably because of excessive pressure of a suture on the lead. Even shallow surface fissuring (not at ligation sites) seems to initiate at points of environmentally induced chronic stress (although extrusion stress probably contributes) such as the section immediately adjacent to the connector where the lead is looped in the pocket or near the electrode end where dynamic flexure is greatest in the heart.

The relationship between surface cracking and stress is dramatically illustrated in Figure 31. Figure 31(a) shows the surface of a molded Tecoflex EG-60D specimen implanted subcutaneously (unstressed) in a swine for three months. Figure 31(b) shows the surface of another molded Tecoflex EG-60D specimen implanted subcutaneously in the same animal, for an identical period of time; this sample shows unmistakable and characteristic surface fissuring, since it was deliberately implanted in a highly

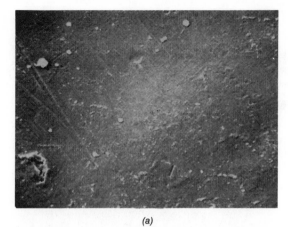

(a)

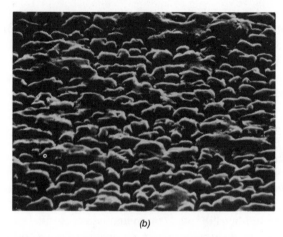

(b)

Figure 31. Relationship between surface cracking and stress. (a) Surface of molded Tecoflex EG-60D implanted subcutaneously in swine for three months. This specimen was implanted in an unstressed manner (1000×). (b) Surface of molded Tecoflex EG-60D in the same animal, for an identical period of time. This specimen was deliberately implanted in a highly stressed configuration, and shows characteristic surface fissuring (1000×).

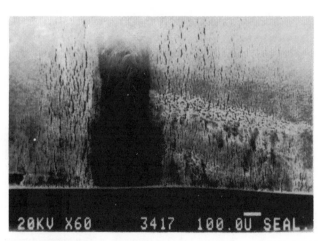

Figure 32. Pellethane 2363-80A lead explanted from patient after 9 months at site of vein ligation showing extent and morphology of surface fissuring (60×).

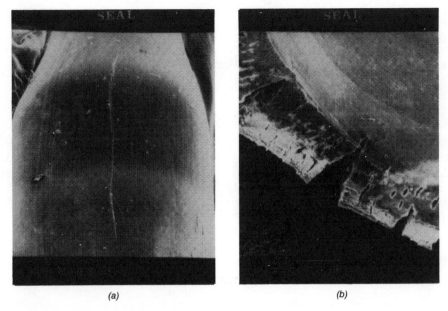

(a)   (b)

Figure 33. *Effect of constant stress on surface fissuring. (a) Pellethane 2363-80A lead explanted from patient after 7 months at section of tube expanded over electrode ($\approx 60\%$ stress) showing cracking in expanded area, none in relaxed area ($30\times$). (b) Enlargement at $180\times$ of cracked section of expanded Pellethane 2363-80A tube.*

stressed configuration. We must conclude that even the hardest grades of Tecoflex are susceptible to microcracking.

The relationship between surface cracking and excessive stress is further illustrated in Figures 32 and 33. These scanning micrographs of implanted leads show surface fissures confined exclusively to the ligature site, or at the section of Pellethane 2363-80A polyurethane tube stretched over the electrode [Figures 33(a) and 33(b)],

where the polyurethane is under constant stress. The micrographs clearly depict surface cracking at the sites of stress with a rapid decrease in surface cracking with distance from the site of highest stress. Furthermore, at relaxed areas, no surface cracking is visible.

A comparison of the effects on harder (Tecoflex EG-60D) vs. softer (Pellethane 2363-80A) polyurethanes is shown in Figures 34 and 35. Leads constructed from the two materials were implanted in dogs without silicone

Table 28. Changes in Spectral Features of Explants Compared with Unimplanted Control

Mode	Sample	Urethane	Urea	Polyether	Presence of Mobile Component	Evidence of Oxidation
Unimplanted Control	Control				Yes	No
	Mobile film on control	1700 band reduced	Similar	Significantly reduced		No
	Control after extraction with ethanol	Similar	Decreased	Increased	No	
Explants	Unstressed explant	Possible increase in H- bonded urethane	Bands at 5310, 1640, 1560 absent	Similar	No	No
	Stressed explant	Similar	Similar	Similar	Yes	Some indication of -OH and -NH bands at 3500
	Mobile film on stressed explant	Similar to mobile film from control				Small CO band at 1700

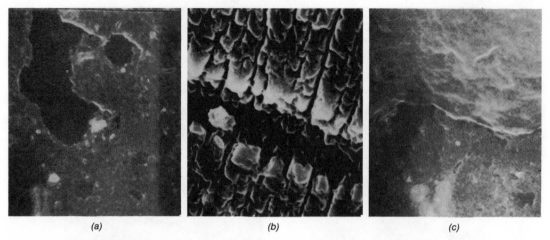

Figure 34. *3-month dog implant leads, Tecoflex EG-60D. (a) Lead body section near connector, showing no cracking (5000×). (b) At site of vein ligation, view showing slight cracking (2000×). (c) Lead body section near electrode, view showing no cracking (5000×).*

support sleeves at the ligature sites. At varying implant times, leads were explanted and analyzed by SEM for cracking. Samples were taken from the ligature site of the lead body near the connector end, and the lead body near the electrode end. On two leads implanted for 90 days, Figure 34(b) shows significantly less deep or severe cracking on the harder Tecoflex EG-60D lead at the ligature site, compared to the equivalent Pellethane 2363-80A section, shown in Figure 35(b). Similarly, Figure 35(a) shows slight cracking in the lead body near the connector on the softer Pellethane 2363-80A sample, while none was seen in Figure 34(a), the corresponding section on the harder Tecoflex EG-60D lead.

No cracking was seen near the electrode in either lead at 90 days. Thus, it appeared that surface fissuring was significantly reduced in the harder Tecoflex polyurethane lead, compared to the softer Pellethane lead in the same environment. Unfortunately, microcracking cannot be totally eliminated in these elastomers.

Chemical analysis by ATR-IR spectroscopy showed significant differences among stressed (cracked) and unstressed (not cracked) implanted specimens and the unimplanted control. These differences are shown in Figures 36 and 37, and are summarized in Table 28. In this study, a mobile film was found on both the control and stressed samples. The films transferred to the IR crystal and their spectra were found to be similar and, in both, the relative amounts of polyether and polyurethane contributions were reduced. As would be expected when this film was removed by extraction from the control, the extracted control showed an increased polyether contribution. The mobile film from the stressed sample did show a small

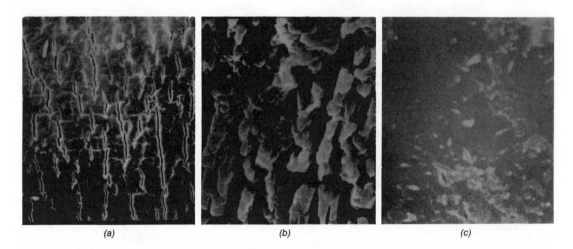

Figure 35. *3-month dog implant leads, Pellethane 2363-80A. (a) Lead body section near connector end, view showing slight cracking (1000×). (b) At site of vein ligation, view showing significant cracking (2000×). (c) Lead body section near electrode, showing no cracking (5000×).*

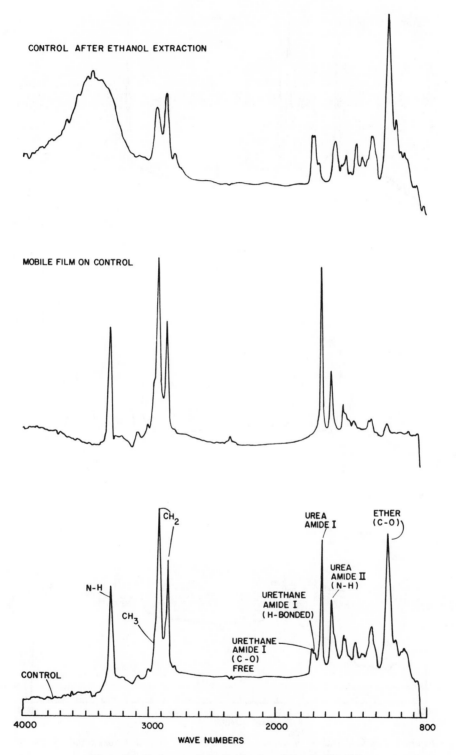

Figure 36. *Surface analysis of unimplanted Tecoflex EG-60D.*

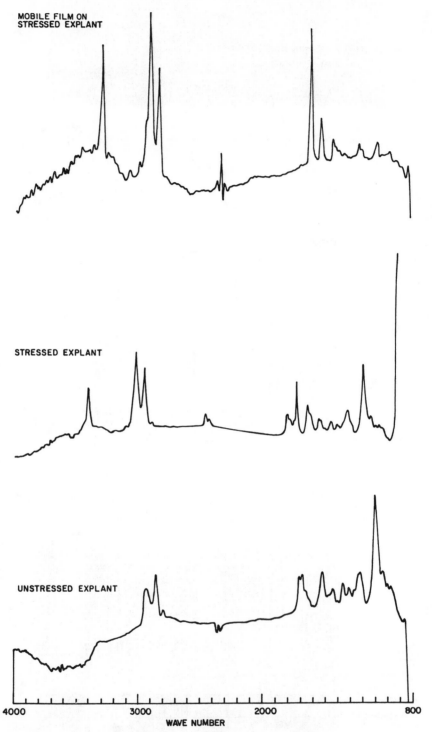

MOBILE FILM ON
STRESSED EXPLANT

STRESSED EXPLANT

UNSTRESSED EXPLANT

WAVE NUMBER

Figure 37. *Surface analysis of cracked Tecoflex EG-60D explanted from swine after three months.*

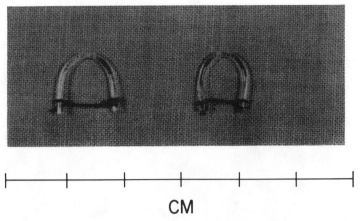

CM

Figure 38. Tecoflex® rods (1 mm dia.) after 3 months subcutaneous implantation in rabbits.

carbonyl peak which could be indicative of oxidation. The unstressed implant did not have the mobile phase, but did show a decrease in urea bands. Possible oxidation was seen in the stressed sample by the presence of −NH and −OH bands and 3500 cm⁻¹.

A tentative explanation suggested by these results is that polyether-based polyurethanes are susceptible to *in vivo* oxidation of the soft segment particularly when the polymer is under chronic stress. In the polyether chain, the most susceptible group is the −CH₂ group in the alpha position to the ether oxygen, which undergoes peroxidation, free radical dissociation and eventual chain cleavage.

Our hypothesis has been reinforced by experimental evidence that surface fissuring can be significantly reduced with the use of higher durometer polyurethanes, since these polymers inherently contain fewer polyether macroglycol chains in the molecular architecture. Pande

[41] compared the long-term *in vivo* stability of a soft polyurethane (Shore 80A) to a harder one (Shore 55D). At intervals of up to one year, samples were explanted and observed under SEM. No evidence of surface fissuring was observed in the harder polyurethane. However, similar tests on the softer polyurethane, conducted for comparison purposes, did show some evidence of surface fissuring.

Further Evidence of Stress-Induced Fissuring

In 1984, during the Second World Congress on Biomaterials, Society for Biomaterials held in Washington D.C. we presented further evidence of the crucial effect of stress on surface fissuring [42].

Our experiment consisted of extruding Tecoflex EG-

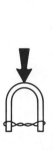

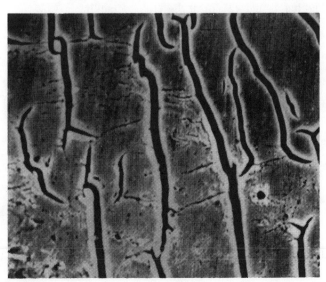

Figure 39. Surface cracking at top of Tecoflex rod (1000×).

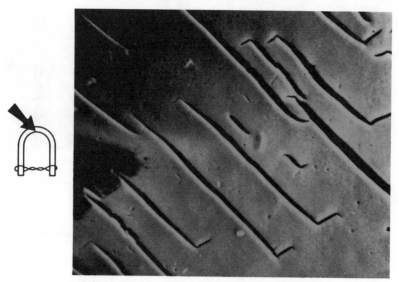

Figure 40. Surface cracking at side of Tecoflex rod (1000×).

80A (a susceptible grade of Tecoflex), bending the 1-mm-diameter solid rod 90 degrees, ligating both ends with suture material and, finally, annealing the best rods at 110°C for 6 hours. The rods were subsequently implanted subcutaneously for a period of 3 months, as shown in Figure 38.

After retrieval, the rods were incubated in 0.01 percent pepsin solution acidified to pH = 1.0 overnight at 38°C, followed by a final cleaning with 0.15 percent Tergazyme solution buffered to pH = 7.0 overnight at 50°C, to remove any biological material from the surface. The rods were then scanned in the electron microscope for any evidence of surface fissuring.

As expected, surface fissuring occurred in those locations where the rod was subjected to tensile stress (top, Figure 39), compressive stress (at bottom of U, Figure 40), at the ligature site (Figures 41 and 42), or at the U

(Figure 43). By contrast, no fissuring was observed anywhere else in the rods, as exemplified in Figure 44, at the center post of the rod, at an area where no stresses were present.

These results led us to conclude that low durometer polyurethanes could be made less susceptible to surface fissuring *if properly annealed*, but any stresses would result in oxidation of the soft segments, leading to fissuring caused by Biologically-Induced Environmental Stress Cracking (BI-ESC).

These results also led us to the conclusion that BI-ESC can be reduced by choosing higher durometer polyurethanes, since these polymers inherently contain fewer soft segments. Our recommendation was corroborated by Stokes, who reported at the 1984 ANTEC that harder aromatic polyurethanes are indeed more resistant to stress cracking.

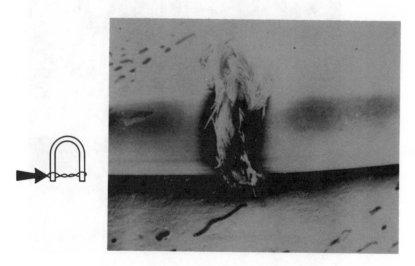

Figure 41. Surface cracking at ligature site (50×).

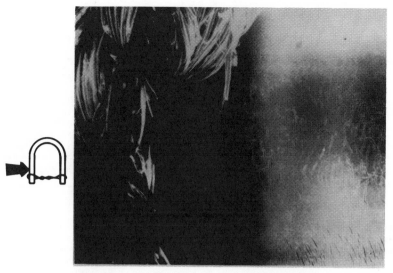

Figure 42. *Detail of fissuring at ligature site (250×).*

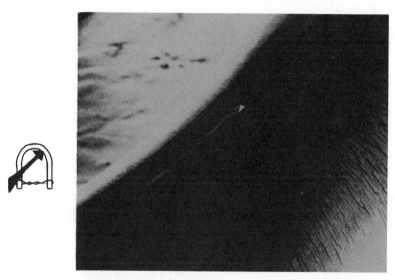

Figure 43. *Low-power panoramic view of fissuring which occurred at the U (50×).*

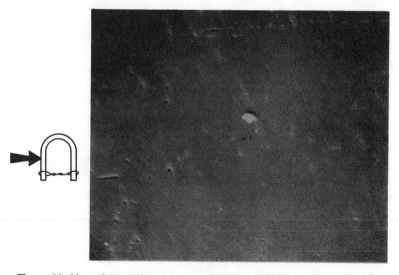

Figure 44. *No surface cracking at center of rod where no stresses occur (1000×).*

Table 29. Polyurethane Degradation Mechanisms*

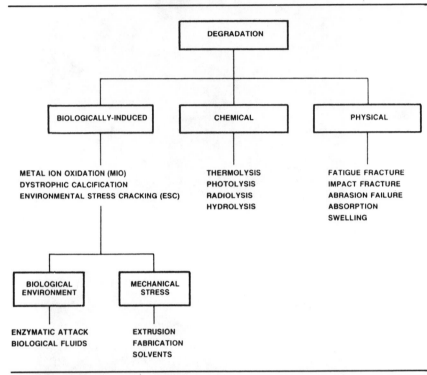

*Although we are focusing on the polyurethanes, most polymers undergo similar degradation mechanisms.

In this important study, extruded tubing 2.0 × 2.2-mm in diameter was placed over a mandrel and strained to elongations ranging from 0 to 500 percent in increments of 100 percent, with firm ligatures placed over the tubing at each end of the mandrels to fix the strain. Specimens were implanted subcutaneously in rabbits, and explanted weekly for 12 weeks. Results are summarized in the following table.

Polymer	Induction Time Before Failure (weeks)	Strain Threshold Before Failure ($\%E$)
Pellethane 80A	4	>214
Pellethane 80A (annealed)	>12	>300
Pellethane 55D	None	None
Tecoflex 80A	1–2	<200
Tecoflex 60D	9	>400

We must conclude that only Pellethane 55D does not microcrack, but this material has recently been withdrawn from the market for chronic implantation.

Biologically Induced Environmental Stress Cracking

It is well known that all polymers undergo some degradation. Typically, we think of polyurethane degra-

dation in terms of physical, or chemical terms. Now we must add biologically induced degradation to the list, as presented in Table 29.

At present, we recognize two main mechanisms responsible for surface fissuring: Environmental Stress Cracking (ESC) and Metal Ion Oxidation (MIO). Stress cracking requires both stress (strain) in excess of a threshold level and a reactive chemical media, such as the biological environment. Metal Ion Oxidation of polyurethanes, particularly in contact with molybdenum, chromium, or cobalt greatly accelerates polyurethane degradation and fissuring, but is confined to degradation observed only with pacemaker leads, since these ions are not freely circulating in blood. To better appreciate the important differences between these two degradation mechanisms, refer to Table 30.

Beyond surface fissuring, polyurethanes undergo a variety of other degradation mechanisms. Unlike metallic and ceramic surfaces, polyurethane surfaces are mobile, and the distribution of hard/soft segments can be rearranged in response to the biological environment in an effort to minimize free energy. Polyurethanes exposed to blood and extracellular fluids function like the stationary phase in partition liquid chromatography; that is, lipids and protein are not only absorbed on the surface, but are absorbed or solubilized into the bulk of the polymer. This leads to plasticization, swelling and loss of mechanical properties.

An important degradation mechanism is the loss of averaged molecular weight by the polyurethanes when ex-

Table 30. Comparison of In Vivo Stress Cracking and Autooxidation Mechanisms Affecting Implanted Polyether Polyurethanes

Stress Cracking (ESC)	Autooxidation (MIO)
Requires direct tissue contact.	Does not require direct tissue contact (occurs within device).
Crazed cracks, with rough spiculated crack walls.	Smooth crack walls.
Cracks to failure always occur at locations normal to stress vectors - not at coil contact points (unless severely stressed at those points).	Stress on the polymer is not necessary but does provide a slight accelerating effect. MIO usually initiates from coil-tubing contact points.
Cracked areas may appear whitish due to light dispersion, but true polymer color unchanged.	Polymer is brittle and amber or soft and gummy without color development.
No change in bulk tensile strength and elongation of polymer.	Severe loss of mechanical properties.
Mechanism dependent upon molecular morphology - can be exacerbated or eliminated by thermal processes.	Mechanism negligibly affected by molecular morphology - dependent on presence of oxidants with electrode potentials > 0.7 V.
Cannot (so far) be duplicated in vitro. Does not occur in 3% H_2O_2 even in the presence of metal ions.	Can be duplicated in vitro in 3% H_2O_2 in presence of certain metals.
Can be accelerated in vivo in the presence of stress (strain) and in the absence of metals. The time to failure is dependent on the amount of stress (strain) in excess of a critical value.	Have been so far unable to accelerate mechanism in vivo. The time to failure is dependent on the corrosion rate of certain metals or concentration of certain metal ions.
No change in bulk infrared spectrum.	Bulk infrared spectra show loss of PTMO ether and other changes.
Bulk tubing may contain no more metals than unimplanted tubing.	Bulk tubing always contains relatively large concentrations of transition metals.

posed to the biological environment. Since most mechanical properties are directly related to molecular weight, reductions in the *bulk* molecular weight of the polymer have profound effects on the long-term suitability of polyurethane-based prostheses.

Molecular Weights and Biodegradation

A brief discussion of polymerization and molecular weight distributions is in order. Polymers may be synthesized by two main mechanisms: addition chain polymerization and condensation step polymerization, presented in Table 31. Polyurethane elastomers are synthesized via a condensation polymerization reaction.

Polyurethanes are composed of long chains of covalently bonded repeat units. The length of the polymer chain is specified by the number of repeat units in the chain, and this number is referred to as the degree of polymerization (DP). Typically, polyamides (nylons) begin to have adequate mechanical properties at a DP of about 40, cellulosics at 60, and vinyl polymers at 100 or more. Polymers with network structure or significant secondary interactions (like the nylons and the polyurethanes) usually require much lower DP values for useful properties than simple linear polymers like polystyrene. At an average molecular weight of 40,000, inefficient property development has occurred. This M_n is obtained with polyurethanes at ratios of 0.98 and higher.

Table 31. Distinguishing Features of Chain- and Step-Polymerization Mechanisms

Addition Chain Polymerization	Condensation Step Polymerization
Only growth reaction adds repeating units one at a time to the chain.	Any two molecular species present can react.
Monomer concentration decreases steadily throughout reaction.	Monomer disappears early in reaction: at DP* 10, less than 1% monomer remains.
High polymer is formed at once; polymer molecular weight changes little throughout reaction.	Polymer molecular weight rises steadily throughout reaction.
Long reaction times give high yields but affect molecular weight little.	Long reaction times are essential to obtain high molecular weights.
Reaction mixture contains only monomer, high polymer, and about 10^{-8} part of growing chains.	At any stage all molecular species are present in a calculable distribution.

* Degree of polymerization

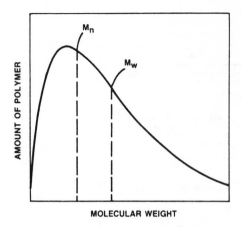

Figure 45. *Distribution of molecular weights in a typical polymer.*

In normal polymer synthesis a polymer is produced with a distribution of chain lengths, or molecular weights. When distinguishing between different samples of the same polymer, it is useful to define an average molecular weight. Several different averages which have a statistical basis are important. The number average molecular weight (M_n) is the first moment of the molecular weight distribution and is an average over the number of molecules. The weight average molecular weight (M_w) is the second moment of the molecular weight distribution which averages over the weight of each polymer chain. These averages are defined by the equations below:

The number average molecular weight M_n

$$\overline{M}_n = \frac{w}{\sum\limits_{i=1}^{\infty} N_i} = \frac{\sum\limits_{i=1}^{\infty} M_i N_i}{\sum\limits_{i=1}^{\infty} N_i}$$

simply divides the total weight of material present by the number of molecules in the material, and is particularly useful for properties that depend primarily on the smaller

molecules. The weight average molecular weight (designated M_w) in the equation

$$\overline{M}_w = \frac{\sum\limits_{i=1}^{\infty} w_i M_i}{w} = \frac{\sum\limits_{i=1}^{\infty} N_i M_i^2}{\sum\limits_{i=1}^{\infty} N_i M_i}$$

considers the weight of material of each size rather than the number of molecules of each size, and thus places greater emphasis upon the higher-molecular-weight fractions and upon properties that depend primarily upon the larger molecules. The weight average molecular weight is thus always greater than the number average molecular weight. In a homogeneous polymer of narrow molecular weight distribution, this difference may not be very great and the ratio M_w/M_n may be only 1.5 to 2.0; whereas, in a polymer of very broad molecular weight distribution, the difference may be very large and the ratio may be as high as 20 to 50. Thus this ratio may be used as a simple expression of the broadness or poly-dispersity of the molecular weight distribution.

Figure 45 typifies the molecular weight distribution and average weights for a polymer. Typical linear polyurethane elastomers have number average molecular weights in the range 25,000 to 100,000 and weight average molecular weights from 50,000 to 300,000. It should be noted that the higher the molecular weight, the more difficult it is to melt process a polymer. In general, the physical properties of polymers generally increase with molecular weight, though in the case of the polyurethanes and other highly polar condensation polymers, the most rapid increase in properties occurs before about 20,000 number average molecular weight [43].

As far back as 1980, Lemm et al. [44] showed that the average molecular weight of Biomer decreases more than 50 percent after exposure to urease enzyme, and by approximately 20 percent after 6 months' subcutaneous im-

Table 32. Biodegradation of Biomaterials In Vivo [44] Test Materials

Material	Chemical Composition	Original Molecular Weight
Plathuran UM 8300	Polyesterurethane	175,000
Pellethane 2363-80A	Polyetherurethane	230,000
PU - X	Polyetherurethane	120,000
Avcothane 51	PEU-PDMS-Block-Copolymer	110,000
Biomer	Polyetherurethane	125,000
PEO/PET	Polyester (60/40)	40,000
Kraton 2104	Synthetic Rubber	135,000

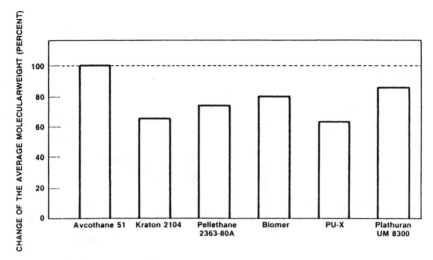

Figure 46. *Reduced molecular weight of some biomaterials after six months subcutaneous implantation (from Reference 45).*

plantation. Since that molecular weight distribution influences the mechanical characteristics of all polymers, significant reductions in this distribution can be expected to adversely affect the durability and biostability of the polyurethanes used in long-term implanted devices.

Lemm and colleagues followed their initial work [45] with a study where several polyether/polyester-based polyurethanes and Kraton were tested *in vivo*. Table 32 and Figure 46 present their data, which show all polymers (except Avcothane, a cross-linked polymer) to have undergone significant reductions in average molecular weight. The authors further observed "a serious destruction of the surface was found on Pellethane 2363-80A and PU-X after nine months of implantation" by SEM analysis, perhaps the first reported observation of surface fissuring.

Similar results were published by Williams [46] who implanted Avcothane, Pellethane, Biomer, Estane, Lycra, PU-X and Plathuran in rats for periods of up to nine months. All implanted polyurethanes (with the exception of Avcothane) showed more or less severe surface ruptures and cracks, which started preferentially at surface defects such as microbubbles, although the loss in molecular weight did not materially influence the mechanical strength. Figure 47 is a copy of the original figure.

At this point we must emphasize the difference between *bulk* molecular weight and molecular weight at the biological *interface*. Since oxidation of the ether linkages naturally occurs at the surface, we would expect a smaller molecular weight reduction in the bulk, and a larger reduction of molecular weight at the surface. Since the mechanical properties of the polymer are related to bulk molecular weight, the mechanical strength of even surface-degraded polyurethanes would remain largely unchanged; only after the degradation has progressed inward into the bulk of the polymer can the mechanical properties be expected to deteriorate significantly.

The difference between bulk and surface molecular weight is convincingly demonstrated in Stokes' data pre-

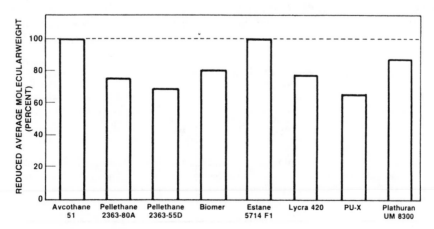

Figure 47. *Reduced average molecular weight of some polyurethanes after six months subcutaneous implantation (after Reference 46).*

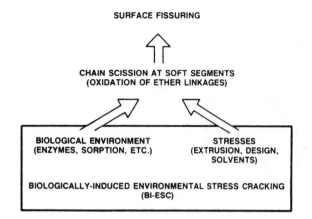

Figure 48. *Hypothesized sequence of events leading to surface fissuring.*

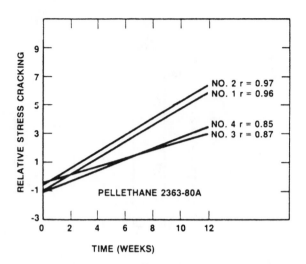

Figure 49. *Effect of antioxidant on stress cracking. Sample No. 1 = extracted material. Sample No. 2 = extracted material plus processing wax. Sample No. 3 = extracted material plus antioxidant. Sample No. 4 = extracted material plus antioxidant plus processing wax (from Reference 48).*

sented in this issue. After 24 months implant, Pellethane and Tecoflex exhibited the following characteristics:

Property	Pellethane 80A	Pellethane 55D	Tecoflex 80A	Tecoflex 60D
M_w	−4% (bulk)	−1.6% (bulk)	−40% (surface)	−20% (surface)
M_n	+1% (bulk)	+3.1% (bulk)	−40% (surface)	−16% (surface)

As can be expected, the molecular weight of the polyurethane is reduced in proportion to implant time. This is because oxidation is initiated within the soft segments, and in the segmented polyurethane elastomers there is a significant excess of polyether soft segments at the surface, compared to the average bulk composition. Ratner [47] elegantly demonstrated by x-ray photoelectron spectroscopy that a surface excess of soft segment domains are commonly present within 20 Å of the surface, with the nitrogen-containing hard segment domains being largely excluded from this region. Once oxidation starts at the polyurethane/biological interphase, a progressive wave of degradation proceeds unimpeded as demonstrated in Table 33.

Additional evidence of chain scission is provided by Phillips (in this issue) who reports the M_w of explanted clinical pacemaker leads with a control $M_w = 187,000$ dalton, $M_w = 69,000$ at the area of surface fissuring, and a $M_w = 167,000$ only two inches away from the fissured area. Equally significant, at the area of fissuring, the percentage of hard segments increases, again pointing to the soft segment as the area of maximum biological vulnerability.

Based on this evidence, we conclude that most of the observed surface fissuring is caused by biologically induced, stress-related oxidation of the polyether macroglycol which composes the soft segments of polyurethane elastomers. Pictorially, we can summarize our hypothesis as shown in Figure 48.

Effect of Antioxidants

First, the good news: antioxidants protect polyurethanes from oxidative stress-cracking mechanisms. And

Table 33. Molecular Weight of Tecoflex Polyether Polyurethane Surface Material as a Function of Implant Time

Implant Time (Months)	Tecoflex EG80A x 10³ $\bar{M}w$	Tecoflex EG80A x 10³ $\bar{M}n$	d	Tecoflex EG60D x 10³ $\bar{M}w$	Tecoflex EG60D x 10³ $\bar{M}n$	d
0	181	156	1.16	120	103	1.13
3	149	141	1.05	120	89	1.35
6	147	141	1.04	98	63	1.55
12	138	129	1.07	94	61	1.64
18	107	94	1.14	95	87	1.09

After Stokes, K. B., "Polyether Polyurethanes: Biostable or Not?," this issue of the *Journal of Biomaterials Applications*, pp. 228–259.

now for the bad news: antioxidants are sacrificial, and compromise biocompatibility if used in large concentrations.

Davis reported a significant reduction of stress cracking in Pellethane 2363-80A reformulated with antioxidant [48]. Pellethane was extracted in chloroform for 48 hours; four tubing compositions were extruded: (1) extracted material, (2) extracted material plus processing wax, (3) extracted material plus antioxidant, and (4) extracted material plus antioxidant, plus processing wax. Results, shown in Figure 49, show that materials 3 and 4 had less severe damage than materials 1 and 2.

Antioxidants are organic compounds that extend and maintain the useful service life of polymers by inhibiting or retarding oxidative degradation. They protect polymers during processing, storage, and end use. A variety of in-

trinsic, as well as external, agents can initiate such degradation in polymers. These can include impurities; peroxide or hydroperoxide; metal contamination, oxygen (O_2); other gases, H_2S, chlorine, oxides of nitrogen, SO_2, etc.; heat; light (weathering); ozone; shear (processing); water (humidity); high pH; and radiation (gamma, cobalt, or electron beams).

Polymers undergo degradation through a sequence of chemical reactions resulting in radical formation and peroxide oxidation. The consequences of polymer degradation are discoloration, loss of tensile strength, loss of elongation, loss of impact strength, loss of gloss and clarity, change in molecular weight, and change in molecular weight distribution. Chain scission and cross-linking reactions (depending upon the nature of the polymer) broaden molecular weight distribution of the polymer,

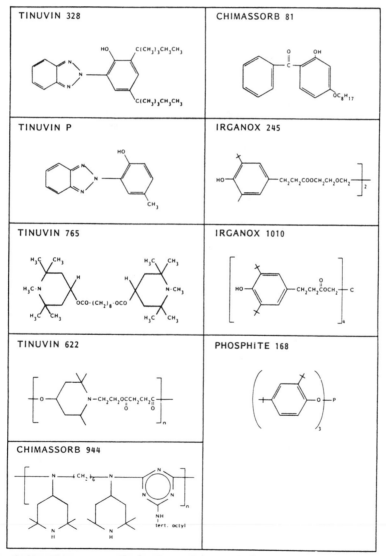

Figure 50. *Chemical structures of common UV absorbers, antioxidants, and phosphate stabilizers.*

Table 34. Major Reactions—Polymer Oxidation, Inhibition, Chain Scission, and Crosslinking

Initiation

$$ROOH \xrightarrow{\text{Heat}} RO\cdot + HO\cdot$$

$$2\,ROOH \longrightarrow RO\cdot + ROO + H_2O$$

$$R'H \xrightarrow{\text{Heat/Light}} R'\cdot + H\cdot$$

$$R'\cdot + O_2 \longrightarrow R'OO\cdot$$

$$RO\cdot + R'H \longrightarrow ROH + R'\cdot$$

Propagation

$$ROO\cdot + R'H \longrightarrow ROOH + R'\cdot$$

$$RO\cdot + R'H \longrightarrow ROH + R'\cdot$$

$$HO\cdot + R'H \longrightarrow H_2O + R'\cdot$$

$$R'\cdot + O_2 \longrightarrow R'OO\cdot$$

$$R'OO\cdot + R'H \longrightarrow R'\cdot + R'OH$$

Termination and crosslinking

$$R'\cdot + R'\cdot \longrightarrow R'\text{-}R'$$

$$R'O\cdot + R'\cdot \longrightarrow R'OR'$$

$$R'OO\cdot + R'\cdot \longrightarrow R'OOR'$$

$$R'OO\cdot + R'O\cdot \longrightarrow \left. \right\} \text{Non-radical}$$

$$R'OO\cdot + R'OO\cdot \longrightarrow \left. \right\} \text{products}$$

Chain scission

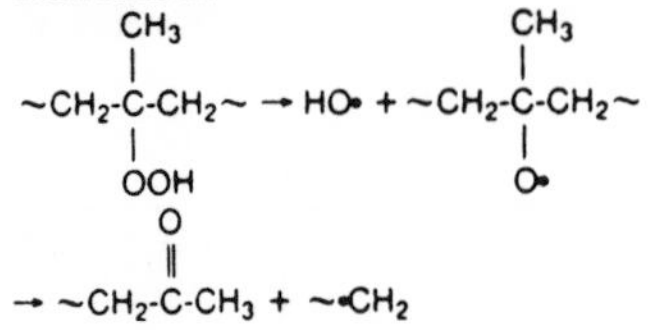

$$ROOH = \text{Peroxide (impurities)}$$
$$R'H = \text{Polymer}$$

Table 35. Inhibition Reactions by Antioxidant

$$
\begin{aligned}
R'OO\cdot \\
R'O\cdot \\
HO\cdot \\
R'\cdot
\end{aligned}
\left. \right\} + AH \longrightarrow
\begin{aligned}
R'OOH + A\cdot \\
R'OH + A\cdot \\
H_2O + A\cdot \\
R'H + A\cdot
\end{aligned}
$$

$$A\cdot + R'OO \rightarrow R'OOA$$

AH = Antioxidant
A• = Stable antioxidant radical

Efficiency of antioxidant on trapping radicals

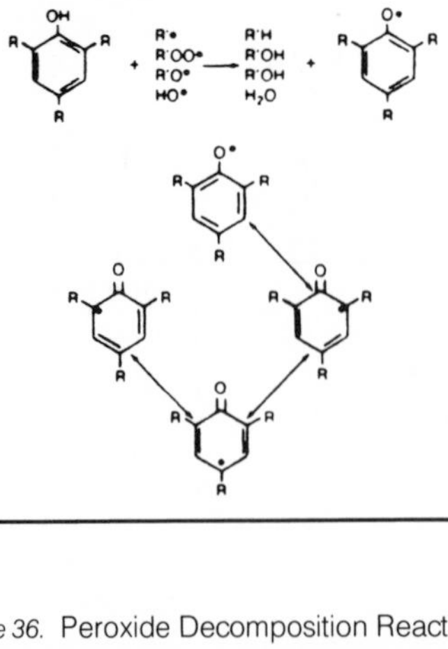

Table 36. Peroxide Decomposition Reactions

$$ROOH + \text{peroxide decomposer} \longrightarrow \text{Stable, non-radical products}$$

$$ROOH + (R_1O)_3P \longrightarrow ROH + (R_1O)_3P{=}O$$

$$ROOH + R_1SR_2 \longrightarrow ROH + R_1\text{-}\overset{O}{\underset{O}{S}}\text{-}R_2$$

Table 37. Antioxidants Believed to Be Used in Medical-Grade Polyurethane Elastomers

Polymer	Chemical Name	Chemical Structure
Biomer	4,4' Butylidene bis (6-tert-butyl-m-cresol) (Santowhite)	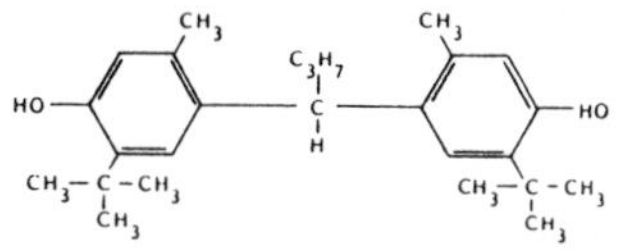
Pellethane	Octadecyl 3,5-di-tert-butyl 4 Hydroxyhycinnamate (Irganox 1076)	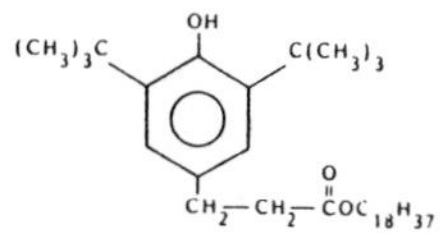
Tecoflex	Tetrakis [methylene (3,5-di-tert-4 hydroxyhydrocinnamate) methane]	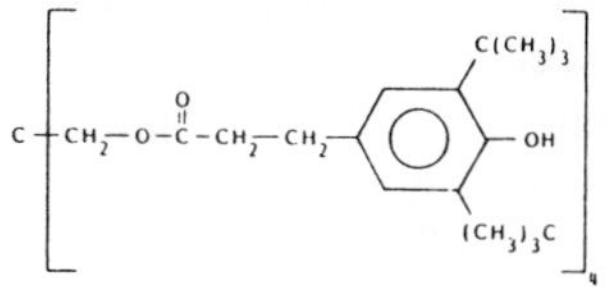

and large quantities of oxygen in the form of hydroxyl, carbonyl, ester, and acid groups are introduced. Oxidation also may result in significant deterioration of the polymer—formation of polar groups and color producing unsaturated sequences—with little change in the size of the polymer chains and the molecular weight.

The reactions of radical chain oxidation of hydrocarbon polymers are detailed in Table 34.

Agents in polymer degradation can initiate the degradation in polymers via free radical formation and peroxide oxidation. The radicals react with oxygen and yield a peroxy radical. This peroxy radical abstracts a labile hydrogen to yield hydroperoxide and another free radical that propagates the cycle, eventually degrading the polymer. The hydroperoxide, however, is itself unstable. It decomposes into two new radicals—an alkoxy and a hydroxyl. These radicals initiate new degradation cycles. The cycle ends when the radicals themselves combine to form stable products. At that point, deterioration is significant.

There are two major types of antioxidants, so classified by their inhibition mechanisms, radical chain terminators, and peroxide decomposers, as shown below:

I	Primary, radical chain terminators, free/radical scavengers	Hindered phenols Hindered amines
II	Peroxide decomposer	Phosphates Sulfur compounds

Primary, or free radical scavenging antioxidants, inhibit oxidation via chain-propagating radicals. They have reactive OH or NH functional groups, such as hindered phe-

nolic or secondary aryl amines. They transfer hydrogen to free radical $R'\cdot$ or, principally $R'OO\cdot$, peroxy radicals. In general, the phenolic antioxidants are nonstaining, nondiscoloring, and are available in a wide range of molecular weights and efficiencies.

Amine antioxidants are very effective antioxidants. However, they tend to discolor and stain and to interfere with peroxide cross-linking. They can only be used where the color addition can be masked or tolerated. The inhibition reactions by antioxidant are shown in Table 35.

Another class of antioxidants, secondary or peroxide decomposing stabilizers, decompose peroxides and hydroperoxides into nonradical and stable products (Table 36). This class includes phosphorus- or sulfur-containing compounds, particularly phosphites and thioesters.

Phosphites reduce hydroperoxide to alcohols as they are oxidized to phosphate. They are nondiscoloring and are highly effective processing stabilizers for various polymers.

Thioester antioxidants also are nondiscoloring and often exhibit synergism with primary antioxidants for long-term heat stability.

The use of two or more antioxidants can provide enhanced protection against this type of degradation. Combinations of antioxidants and UV-absorbers are equally synergistic for polyurethanes, especially the aromatic types. Figure 50 presents some common antioxidants, UV-absorbers and phosphite stabilizers.

All medical-grade polyurethanes contain antioxidants at different concentrations. In general, the lower the concentration the greater the biocompatibility, and vice versa. Being fully aware of this circumstance, most manufacturers attempt to optimize the concentration of antioxidant for the best protection against surface fissuring and the best biocompatibility. Table 37 presents, to the best of our knowledge, the type of antioxidant used in medical-grade polyurethane elastomer.

Effect of Annealing

Again this is a good news/bad news topic. The good news is that a properly annealed polyurethane will be more resistant to biologically-induced environmental stress cracking (BI-ESC). The bad news is that "proper annealing," per se, cannot totally prevent BI-ESC.

Annealing can be summarized as slow crystallization by heat treatment without large-scale melting. Annealing improves the properties of segmented polyurethanes that normally would be associated with crystallinity, and it also reduces (or eliminates) stresses on the polymer induced by manufacturing or design features.

To reduce BI-ESC in Tecoflex polymers, we recommend annealing at 110°C for a minimum of one hour under a nitrogen blanket to prevent surface thermoxidation.

FUTURE TRENDS

The recognition that polyurethanes can be susceptible to *in vivo* degradation under certain conditions has forced the biomaterials community to focus on this problem.

We are beginning to understand some of the mechanisms underlying this phenomenon; at present, BI-ESC and MIO are leading hypotheses.

As we have seen, the soft segments of the polyether-based polyurethanes are implicated by most investigators. Therefore, it appears likely that future trends to solve surface fissuring will focus on: (1) changing the basic structure of the soft segments, (2) protecting the susceptible polyether linkages, (3) using antioxidants, (4) removing residual stresses by annealing, better designs and improved manufacturing techniques, and (5) developing surface coatings.

REFERENCES

1 RINKE, H., H. Schild and W. Siefken. U.S. Patent No. 2,511,544 (1938).

2 LANGERAK, E. O., L. J. Prucino and W. R. Remington. U.S. Patent No. 2,692,893 (to DuPont) (1954).

3 SCHOLLENBERGER, C. S. U.S. Patent No. 2,871,218 (to BF Goodrich) (1955).

4 NYILAS, E. "Polysiloxane – Polyurethane Block Copolymers," U.S. Patent No. 3,562,352 (to Avco Corp.) (1971).

5 BORETOS, J. W. *J. Biomed. Mater. Res.*, 6:473–476 (1972).

6 COLAVOS, G. C., H. W. Bonk and H. Ulrich. "Thermoplastic Polyurethane: An Alternative to PVC for Food and Medical Applications," SPE National Technical Conference, Nov. 8 to 10, 1977, Denver, Colorado.

7 SZYCHER, M., V. L. Poirier and D. Dempsey. "Synthesis and Fabrication of Polyurethane Elastomers for Cardiac Assist Systems," *Proc. SPE 35th Annual Technical Conference*, 35:743 (1977).

8 SZYCHER, M. "Extrudable Polyurethane for Prosthetic Devices Prepared from a Diisocyanate, an Ether Glycol and 1,4 Butane Diol," U.S. Patent No. 4,447,590 (May, 1984).

9 SZYCHER, M. and V. L. Poirier. "Synthetic Polymers in Artificial Hearts: A Progress Report," *Industrial Chemistry Engineering*, 22(4):588 (1983).

10 PENTZ, W. J. and R. G. Krawiec. "Hydrolytic Stability of Polyurethane Elastomers," *Rubber Age*, 107(2):39–43 (1975).

11 GAHIMER, F. H. and F. W. Nieske. "Hydrolytic Stability of Urethanes and Polyacrylate Elastomers in a Human Environment," *J. Elast. Plast.*, 1:266 (1969).

12 OSSEFORT, Z. T. and F. B. Testtroet. "Hydrolytic Stability of Urethane Elastomers," *Rubber Chem. and Tech.*, 39(4) (1966).

13 POIRIER, V. L. "Fabrication and Testing of Flocked Blood Pump Bladders," in *Synthetic Biomedical Polymers*. M. Szycher and W. Robinson, eds. Lancaster, PA:Technomic Publishing Co., p. 106 (1980).

14 DARBY, T. D., H. J. Johnson and S. J. Northrup. "An Evaluation of a Polyurethane for Use as a Medical-Grade Plastic," *Toxicol. Appl. Pharmacol.*, 46:449 (1978).

15 STEINHOFF, D. and E. Grundmann. "Zur Cancerogenen Wirkung Von 3-3′-dicholoro-4,4′-diaminodiphenylmethan Bei Ratten," *Naturwissenschaften*, 58:578 (1971).

16 National Toxicology Program Technical Report on the Carcinogenesis Bioassay of 4,4′-Methylene-dianiline Dihydrochloride, NTP-81-143, NIH Publication No. 82-2504, National Institutes of Health, Bethesda, Maryland (1982).

17 SHIMIZUR, H. and N. Takemura. "Mutagenicity of Some Aromatic Amino Compounds, and Its Relation to Carcinogenicity," *Sangyo Igaku*, 18:138 (1976).

18 MCLAUGHLIN, J., JR., P. P. Marliac, M. J. Verrett, M. K. Mutchler and J. G. Fitzhugh. "The Injection of Chemicals Into the Yolk Sac of Fertile Eggs Prior to Incubation as a Toxicity Test," *Toxicol. Appl. Pharmacol.*, 5:760 (1963).

19 CASARETT, L. J. "Toxicologic Evaluation," in *Toxicology: The Basic Science of Poisons*. L. H. Casarett and J. Daull, eds. New York:Macmillan, p. 24 (1976).

20 SZYCHER, M., V. L. Poirier and D. J. Dempsey. "Development of an Aliphatic Biomedical-Grade Polyurethane Elastomer," *J. Elast. Plast.*, 15:81 (1983).

21 ULRICH, H. and H. W. Bonk. "Emerging Biomedical Applications of Polyurethane Elastomers," *Proc. SPI 27th Annu. Conf., Bal Harbor, Florida*, p. 143 (1982).

22 SZYCHER, M., V. Poirier, D. Dempsey and W. Robinson. "Development and Testing of Melt-Processable Aliphatic Polyurethane Elastomers," *Trans. Soc. Biomater.*, 6:49 (1983).

23 SZYCHER, M. and V. L. Poirier. "Polyurethanes in Implantable Devices," *MDDI*, 6:5, 46 (1984).

24 "Clinical Applications of Biomaterials," presented at the Consensus Development Conference, National Institutes of Health, Bethesda, Maryland, Nov. 1–3, 1982.

25 ZDRAHALA, R. J., D. E. Spielvogel and M. A. Strand. "Softening of Thermoplastic Polyurethanes: A Structure/Property Study," *J. Biomat. Appl.*, 4(2):544 (1988).

26 LYMAN, D. J., F. J. Fazzio, H. Voorhees, G. Robinson and D. Albo, Jr. *J. of Biomat. Res.*, 12:337 (1978).

27 MARTZ, H., R. Paynter, J. C. Forest, A. Downs and R. Guidoin. *Biomaterials*, 8:3 (1987).

28 STENQUIST, O., I. D. Linder and B. Gustavsson. *Acta. Anaesthesiol. Scand.*, 27:153 (1983).

29 ZDRAHALA, R. J., D. D. Solomon, D. J. Lentz and C. W. McGary, Jr. *Polyurethanes in Biomedical Engineering, II*. H. Planck et al., eds. Elsevier Science Publishing Co., p. 1 (1987).

30 DRAHALA, R. J. and C. W. McGary, Jr. *Mat. Res. Society Symposium Proc.*, 55:407 (1986).

31 HILDEBRAND, J. *Chem. Rev.*, 44:37–45 (1949).

32 HANSEN, C. M. *J. Paint Tech.*, 39(505):104–117 (1967).

33 HANSEN, C. M. and A. Beerbower. In *Kirk-Othmer Encyclopedia of Chemical Technology. Suppl Vol. 2nd Ed.* A. Standen, ed., pp. 889–910 (1971).

34 PARINS, D. J., K. D. McCoy and N. J. Horvath. "*In vivo* Degradation of a Polyurethane," Cardiac Pacemakers, Inc., St. Paul, Minnesota (1981).

35 GUERRANT, K. "Biostability of a Polyurethane," Intermedics, Inc., Freeport, Texas (1981).

36 MCARTHUR, W. A. "Long-Term Implant Effects on Three Polyurethane Leads in Humans," Pacesetter Systems, Inc., Sylmar, California (April, 1982).

37 *MD&DI Reports*, 10(12), Chevy Chase, Maryland (March, 1984).

38 *Changing Medical Markets*, Issue 65 (May, 1984).

39 ALTMAN, L. K. "U.S. Panel Strongly Endorses Artificial Heart," *The New York Times*, Sec. A, p. 1, col. 3 (May 24, 1985).

40 SZYCHER, M. and W. A. McArthur. "Surface Fissuring of Polyurethanes Following *in vivo* Exposure," in *Corrosion and Degradation of Implant Materials*. Fraker and Griffin, eds. Second Symposium, ASTM, STP, 859, Philadelphia, Pennsylvania, pp. 308–321 (1985).

41 PANDE, G. S. "Polyurethane Insulation for Cordis Permanent Pacing Leads," Technical Memorandum 35 (April, 1982).

42 SZYCHER, M., D. Dempsey and V. L. Poirier. "Surface Fissuring of Polyurethane-Based Pacemaker Leads," *Second World Congress on Biomaterials, Tenth Annual Meeting of the Society for Biomaterials, Washington, DC*, p. 24 (1984).

43 LELAH, M. D. and S. L. Cooper. *Polyurethanes in Medicine, 6.* CRC Press (1986).

44 LEMM, W., L. Pirling and E. S. Bucherl. "Biodegradation of Some Biomaterials *in vitro*," *Proc. Europ. Soc. Artif. Organs*, 7:86–90 (1980).

45 LEMM, W., T. Krukenberg and G. Regier, et al. "Biodegradation of Some Biomaterials After Subcutaneous Implantation," *Proc. Europ. Soc. Artif. Organs*, 8:71–75 (1981).

46 WILLIAMS, D. F. "The Biodegradation of Surgical Polymers," in *Polyurethanes in Biomedical Engineering*. Planck, ed. Elsevier Science Publishing Co. (1984).

47 RATNER, B. D., R. W. Paynter and H. R. Thomas. "Polyurethane Surfaces—An XPS Study," *Trans. 9th Annual Meeting, Society for Biomaterials, Birmingham, Alabama*, p. 21 (1983).

48 DAVIS, M. W. and K. B. Stokes. "*In vivo* Oxidative Stress Cracking of Polyether Polyurethanes," *Trans. 11th Annual Meeting, Society for Biomaterials*, p. 54 (1985).

CHAPTER 5

Sterilization of Medical Devices

MICHAEL SZYCHER, Ph.D.[1]

INTRODUCTION

The effective use of proper disinfectants and sterilization procedures constitutes a significant factor in preventing nosocomial infections. Physical agents such as moist or dry heat play the dominant role in sterilization procedures in hospitals, and chemical germicides are used primarily for disinfection and antisepsis.

On the other hand, ethylene oxide (EtO) or, more recently, gamma sterilization, plays the dominant role in sterilization procedures by medical device manufacturers.

As used in this paper, the term "medical devices" includes instruments, equipment, and medical devices, the use of which involves significant risk of transmitting infection to patients or hospital personnel. Consequently, these items should be either sterilized or disinfected to prevent cross-contamination and infection.

The nature of instrument and equipment disinfection can be understood more readily if medical devices, equipment, and surgical materials are divided into three general categories based on the risk of infection involved in their use. These categories were first suggested by Spaulding [1,2]. Although one risks oversimplification in dividing medical devices into such categories, we have elected to retain Dr. Spaulding's classification system because it is fairly straightforward and logical and has been used for years by epidemiologists and microbiologists when discussing or planning strategies for disinfection and sterilization.

Spaulding believed that strategies for sterilization and disinfection could be better understood and implemented if equipment and items for patient care were categorized by the degree of infection risk involved in their use. He described three categories of such items: critical, semicritical, and noncritical.

Critical items, the first category, are so called because the risk of acquiring infection is great if such an item is contaminated. These are instruments or objects that are introduced directly into the human body—either into the blood or into normally sterile areas of the body. Examples are scalpels, transfer forceps, cardiac catheters, implants, pertinent components of the heart-lung oxygenator, and the blood side of artificial kidneys. The requirement for these items prior to use is sterility; consequently, one of several accepted sterilization procedures should be chosen.

Items in the second category are classified as semicritical in terms of the degree of risk of infection; examples are flexible fiberoptics, endotracheal and aspirator tubes, bronchoscopes, respiratory therapy equipment, cystoscopes, and urinary catheters. Although these items come in contact with intact mucous membranes, they do not ordinarily penetrate body surfaces. Sterilization of many of these items, although desirable and often more cost-effective if steam autoclaves can be used, is not absolutely essential. Semicritical items should be subjected, at a minimum, to a procedure that can be expected to destroy ordinary vegetative bacteria, most fungal spores, the tubercle bacilli, and small nonlipid viruses. In most cases, meticulous physical cleaning, followed by an appropriate high-level disinfection treatment, gives a reasonable degree of assurance that the items are free of pathogenic microorganisms.

A third category is noncritical items. These do not ordinarily contact the patient directly or, if they do, they contact only unbroken skin. Such items include face masks, humidifiers, rebreathing bags, x-ray machines, and a variety of accessory medical and surgical items. Use of these items carries relatively little risk of transmitting

[1]Chairman, Chief Technical Officer, PolyMedica Industries, Inc. Burlington, Massachusetts 01803, U.S.A.

infection. Consequently, depending on the particular piece of equipment or item, cleansing with a good detergent in hot water may be sufficient, but with some, the added assurance of chemical disinfection with a low-level disinfectant may be appropriate.

If all medical and surgical materials could be sterilized by steam autoclaving, there would be no need to establish these categories. In reality, however, many such medical devices and articles in everyday use cannot be sterilized by steam autoclaving or irradiation, and chemical germicides must be used. In this context, one must then consider the differences between chemical sterilization and chemical disinfection.

Definition of Terms

Sterilization

Sterilization is defined as the use of a physical or chemical procedure to destroy all microbial life, including highly resistant bacterial endospores. In the hospital, this pertains particularly to those microorganisms that may exist on inanimate objects. Moist heat by steam autoclave, EtO gas, and dry heat are the major sterilizing agents used in hospitals. As will be seen, however, there are a variety of chemical germicides that have been used for purposes of sterilization and that appear to be effective when used appropriately. These germicides, used in a different manner, actually may be a part of a disinfection process. Unfortunately, some health professionals refer to "disinfection" as "sterilization," which leads to a degree of confusion that often becomes magnified with routine use.

A good example of this is the use of 2% glutaraldehyde germicides for the disinfection of certain flexible fiberoptic endoscopes. Some practitioners refer to this as "sterilization" of endoscopes. A 2% glutaraldehyde solution is capable of sterilization, but only after extended contact time in the absence of extraneous organic material. Unfortunately, flexible fiberoptic endoscopes are not physically capable of withstanding immersion in fluid for 6 to 10 hours—in fact, most manufacturers recommend that immersion times not exceed 10 minutes. Thus, the procedure the endoscopes are subjected to is one of disinfection and not sterilization, in spite of the fact that colloquially it is referred to in the hospital as "sterilization."

Disinfection

Disinfection is generally a less lethal process than sterilization. It eliminates virtually all recognized pathogenic microorganisms, but not necessarily all microbial forms (e.g., bacterial endospores) on inanimate objects. As can be seen by this definition, disinfection does not ensure an "overkill," and disinfection processes lack the margin of safety achieved by sterilization procedures. The effec-

tiveness of a disinfection procedure is controlled significantly by a number of factors, each of which may have a pronounced effect on the end results. Among these are the nature and number of contaminating microorganisms (especially the presence of bacterial endospores), the concentration of and length of exposure to the germicide, the amount of organic matter (soil, feces, blood) present, the type and condition of the medical and surgical materials to be disinfected, and the temperature.

Disinfection then, is a procedure that reduces the level of microbial contamination. But, there is a broad range of activity extending from sterility at one extreme to a minimal reduction in the number of microbial contaminants at the other. It is emphasized that the acceptance of such distinctions is consistent with the ability of a nonsporicidal disinfectant solution to completely destroy microbial contamination on medical and surgical materials. Indeed, this probably happens often when spores are absent. Nevertheless, it should not be called sterilization; one would expect that microbiologic assays would be negative only when the item was free of bacterial spores, because of the way it was either used or cleaned or both. This is an important achievement and, consequently, there is a need for a term to distinguish between sterilization and the destruction of microbial contamination that is free of bacterial endospores. *Decontamination* is the most appropriate term to be used in this sense, and it implies that items and devices treated as such are rendered safe to handle.

By definition, chemical disinfection differs from sterilization by its lack of sporicidal power. This is an oversimplification of the actual situation, because a few chemical germicides in fact do kill spores, although they may require a high concentration and several hours to do so.

Nonsporicidal disinfectants may differ in their capacity to produce decontamination. Some germicides kill rapidly only the ordinary vegetative forms of bacteria such as staphylococci and streptococci, and some forms of fungi and lipid-containing viruses, whereas others are effective against such relatively resistant organisms as the tubercle bacillus, mycobacterium tuberculosis, other fungi and nonlipid viruses. The latter group, therefore, represents a level of activity between that of sporicides and many commonly used germicides. Furthermore, absolute sterility is difficult to prove and, as a result, sterility is commonly defined in terms of the probability that a contaminating organism will survive treatment. For example, sterilizing processes are challenged usually with a high number (10^6 to 10^7) of dried bacterial endospores, and sterilization is defined as the state in which the probability of any one spore surviving is 10^{-6} or lower. This rationale has been used to establish cycles for steam autoclaves and EtO gas sterilizers, and it produces a great degree of overkill as well as a quantitative assurance of true sterilization. It is virtually impossible to evaluate liquid chemical disinfection processes by using these criteria, and disinfection

TABLE 1. Levels of Germicidal Action

| | Bacteria | | | | Viruses | |
	Vegetative	Tubercle Bacillus	Spores	Fungi*	Lipid and Medium-Size	Nonlipid and Small
High	+**	+	+	+	+	+
Intermediate	+	+	−	+	+	+
Low	+	−	−	±	+	−

*Includes usual asexual "spores," but not necessarily chlamydospores and sexual spores.
**Plus signs indicate that a microbial effect can be expected when the normally used concentrations of disinfectants are properly employed.

procedures cannot be assumed to have the same reliability as sterilization procedures.

Antiseptic

An antiseptic is defined as a germicide that is used on skin or living tissue for the purpose of inhibiting or destroying microorganisms. It should be realized that the distinction between an antiseptic and a disinfectant often is not made. As defined, a disinfectant is a germicide that is used solely to destroy microorganisms on inanimate objects; an antiseptic germicide, however, is one that is used on or in living tissue. Although some specific germicides may be used for both purposes (e.g., alcohols), the adequacy for one purpose does not ensure adequacy for the other. Consequently, it is not good practice to use an antiseptic for the purposes of disinfection and vice versa, because manufacturers specifically formulate germicides for their intended use.

Levels of Disinfection

As mentioned previously, Spaulding categorized medical and surgical materials into critical, semicritical, and noncritical items. He also proposed three levels of germicidal action to be recognized for properly carrying out strategies for disinfection in hospitals. The terms "high," "intermediate," and "low" will be used to designate these levels of germicidal action.

High-Level Disinfection

A number of critical items are damaged by high temperatures, cannot be heat sterilized, and must be disinfected with chemical germicides. As can be seen from Table 1, an essential property of a high-level disinfectant is effectiveness against bacterial endospores; usually, if the contact time is long enough, this type of germicide can be used as a sterilant. High-level disinfectants are used often to treat medical and surgical materials; in the absence of bacterial spores, they are rapidly effective. The absence of spores usually cannot be ensured, although it has been shown that the number of spores on items subjected to such treatments is generally low.

The sporicidal activity of the high-level disinfectant depends on both the specific chemical agent and the manner in which it is used. Table 2 shows several disinfectants categorized as having high-level activity. These include aqueous 2% glutaraldehyde, 8% formaldehyde solution in 70% alcohol, 6 to 10% stabilized hydrogen peroxide, and EtO gas.

In addition, a number of germicides are available commercially that have been approved by the U.S. Environmental Protection Agency (EPA) as sterilants and sporicides. As will be pointed out later, the Association of Official Analytical Chemists (AOAC) sporicidal test is highly stringent, so that chemical germicides designated as sporicides or sterilants by the AOAC are most likely effective. Some of these products combine various chemicals, such as glutaraldehyde with formaldehyde and glutaraldehyde with phenol and phenate. Peracetic acid in liquid and vapor has been described in the past as a high-level disinfectant, but its application presents major difficulties [3,4], especially with medical and surgical items.

Germicides classified as sporicides have been shown to kill large numbers of resistant bacterial endospores under stringent test conditions. However, these may require 24 hours of contact time [5]. Although this type of germicide may qualify technically as a cold sterilant because of the time involved, it may receive little use. In addition, most medical devices in actual practice are not contaminated with extraordinarily high levels of bacterial endospores, so that if a small number of spores comprised the initial population, sterilization may occur much more quickly than 24 hours [6]. In other words, given the circumstances of relatively few bacterial spores present, sterilization can be achieved by a weaker germicide. Since medical devices and items are not routinely monitored microbiologically, however, one cannot consistently ensure the absence of bacterial spores, so that with certain critical types of medical devices, it may be good practice to rely on those germicides that have been documented in the scientific literature to produce a sporicidal effect in a given amount of time and/or approved by the EPA as sporicides or sterilants.

There is no way to verify microbiologically the sterility of medical devices and items that are sterilized without

TABLE 2. Activity Levels of Selected Germicides

Class	Use-Concentration of Active Ingredient	Activity Level
GAS		
Ethylene Oxide	450 to 500 mg/L*	High
LIQUID		
Glutaraldehyde, Aqueous**	2%	High
Formaldehyde + Alcohol	8% + 70%	High
Stabilized Hydrogen Peroxide	6 to 10%	High
Formaldehyde, Aqueous	3 to 8%	High to intermediate
Iodophors	30 to 50 mg/L free iodine/ 70 to 150 mg/L available iodine	Intermediate
Iodine + Alcohol	0.5% + 70%	Intermediate
Chlorine Compounds	0.1 to 0.5% free chlorine	Intermediate
Phenolic Compounds, Aqueous	0.5 to 3%	Intermediate to low
Quaternary Ammonium Compounds	0.1 to 0.2% aqueous	Low
Mercurial Compounds	0.1 to 0.2%	Low

*In autoclave-type equipment at 55° to 60°C.
**There are several proprietary formulations on the U.S. market, i.e., 4% glutaraldehyde and 3% formaldehyde; glutaraldehyde 2% and 7% buffered phenol; and glutaraldehyde 2%, low pH and normal and raised temperatures.

sampling the item itself. The usual procedure is to verify that the germicide can inactivate 10^6 to 10^7 spores of Bacillus subtilis or Clostridium sporogenes. This can be determined in a laboratory, but variation caused by human error cannot be measured, so that the existence of an established set of procedures associated with the sterilization procedure and the germicide used takes on critical importance. A good example of this is the use of 2% glutaraldehyde germicides, which are capable of sterilization, but only after extended contact time and in the absence of extraneous organic material. Unfortunately, some materials are not physically able to withstand immersion in these fluids for 6 to 10 hours. Even if prolonged contact were possible, the treated materials would have to be rinsed thoroughly with sterile water, dried in a special cabinet with sterile air, and stored in a sterile container to ensure that the materials remain sterile.

Intermediate-Level Disinfection

Intermediate-level disinfectants do not necessarily kill large numbers of bacterial endospores in a relatively short time, i.e., 6 to 12 hours, but they do inactivate the tubercle bacillus, which is significantly more resistant to aqueous germicides than are ordinary vegetative bacteria. These disinfectants are also effective against fungi (asexual spores but not necessarily dried chlamydospores or sexual spores) as well as lipid and nonlipid medium-size and small viruses. Examples of intermediate-level disinfectants (Table 2) include 0.5% iodine, 70 to 90% ethanol and isopropanol, chlorine compounds (free chlorine, i.e., hypochlorous acid as derived from sodium hypochlorite, calcium hypochlorite or gaseous chlorine) at 500 mg/L

and some phenolic and iodophor-based disinfectants, depending on formulation.

Although intermediate-level disinfectants are considered effective against viruses, there appear to be some exceptions. Klein and Deforest (1963) have shown that the resistance of viruses to chemical disinfectants varies significantly. They reported that small nonlipid viruses were significantly more resistant to chemical germicides than medium-size viruses with lipid in their protein coats. Some of the most widely used liquid germicides failed to destroy picornaviruses, which include the enterovirus group and the rhinoviruses of the common cold. The point here is that simply because a germicide has good tuberculocidal activity, it cannot be assumed categorically that these germicides are effective against all viruses.

Moreover, there are a number of viruses for which tissue culture systems are not yet available and for which documented laboratory testing with various germicides has not yet been accomplished. For example, the human hepatitis viruses (B, and non A/non B) have been difficult to study because they have not yet been cultured in the laboratory. There is no evidence, however, that any of these viruses are unusually resistant to physical or chemical agents [7]. It has been proposed that the resistance level of the hepatitis B virus, for example, is between that of the tubercle bacillus and the bacterial spores, but nearer that of the former [8]. Since there is a doubt, the most conservative approach would be to use high-level disinfectants for decontamination and disinfection when hepatitis B virus contamination is known or suspected.

Some chemical germicides with good tuberculocidal activity can destroy small nonlipid viruses. As shown by Klein and Deforest [9], both 70% ethanol and isopropanol are rapidly tuberculocidal [10], whereas only the former was found by Klein and Deforest to destroy the small nonlipid viruses they studied. On the other hand, Wright [11] reported that ethanol failed to kill a test virus that, on the basis of Klein and Deforest's study, would be expected to be quite susceptible. At best, an intermediate-level tuberculocide may not necessarily be an intermediate-level virucide.

The germicidal resistance of fungi in general is probably similar to that of gram-positive vegetative bacteria [12,13]. Bacteriostasis may not have been eliminated in many of these reports, however, and there is now reason to believe that some forms of pathogenic fungi may be considerably more resistant than most vegetative bacteria. Since it is likely that germicidal chemicals that kill the more resistant fungi may not also be tuberculocidal and virucidal, intermediate-level microbicidal capabilities should be examined with separate classes of microorganisms and referred to specifically.

Low-Level Disinfection

Low-level disinfectants are those that cannot be relied upon to destroy, within a practical period of time, bacterial endospores, the tubercle bacilli, or small nonlipid viruses. These disinfectants may be useful in actual practice because they can kill rapidly vegetative forms of bacteria and fungi as well as medium-size, lipid-containing viruses. Examples of low-level disinfectants are quaternary ammonium compounds and mercurials. In addition, the germicidal activity is flexible, depending on the concentration of the active ingredient. Disinfection levels of iodophors and phenolic compounds may be classified as intermediate or low depending on concentrations of the germicide. All germicidal chemicals do not have this capacity. For example, even a 5 to 10% concentration of a quaternary ammonium compound may fail to meet the tuberculocidal or virucidal criterion of intermediate-level disinfection. An appraisal of commonly used disinfectants is shown in Table 3.

Efficacy of Germicides

Microorganisms vary widely in their responses to physical and chemical stresses. Those most resistant to such stresses are bacterial endospores; few, if any, other microorganisms approach the broad resistance of endospores. A number of factors, some of which are associated with

TABLE 3. Relative Efficacy of Commonly Used Disinfectants

	Disinfectant*	Comment
GAS		
Ethylene Oxide	9–10	Sporicidal, toxic; good penetration. Requires relative humidity of 30 percent or more. Microbicidal activity varies with apparatus used. Absorbed by porous material. Dry spores highly resistant. Moisture must be present; presoaking most desirable.
LIQUID		
Glutaraldehyde, Aqueous	6–8	Sporicidal, toxic. Active solution unstable.
Stabilized Hydrogen Peroxide	6–8	Sporicidal. Use-solution stable up to 6 weeks. Toxic orally and to eyes; mildly toxic to skin. Little inactivation by organic matter.
Formaldehyde + Alcohol	6–8	Sporicidal, toxic, volatile; noxious fumes.
Formaldehyde, Aqueous	2–6	Sporicidal, toxic; noxious fumes.
Phenolic Compounds	6–8	Stable, corrosive; irritates skin. Little inactivation by organic matter.
Chlorine Compounds	4–6	Fast action; inactivation by organic matter. Corrosive; irritates skin.
Alcohol	2–3	Rapidly microbicidal except for bacterial spores and some viruses. Volatile, flammable. Dries and irritates skin.
Iodine + Alcohol	1–2	Corrosive, rapidly microbicidal, flammable. Causes staining, irritates skin.
Iodophors	2–4	Somewhat unstable, relatively bland, corrosive. Staining temporary.
Quaternary Ammonium Compounds	2–4	Bland; inactivated by soap and anionics; absorbed by fabrics. Old or dilute solution can support growth of gram-negative bacteria.
Mercurial Compounds	1–2	Bland; much inactivated by organic matter; weakly bactericidal.

*Rating = Maximal usefulness is indicated by 10; little or no practical usefulness by 1.

the microorganisms themselves and others with the surrounding physical and chemical environment, influence the antimicrobial efficacy of chemical germicides. Some factors are more important than others, but all of them should be considered when planning strategy for the chemical disinfection of medical and surgical materials.

Nature of the Medical Device

The easiest surface to disinfect chemically is one that is smooth, nonporous, and cleanable, such as a scalpel blade. Crevices, joints, and pores constitute barriers to the penetration of liquid germicides and require prolonged contact times to accomplish disinfection; in fact, it is possible for a disinfection procedure to fail under these circumstances. This is also true of EtO gas, which has a high degree of penetrability. If microorganisms are entrapped in impervious spaces or within organic materials, the EtO sterilization procedure may fail, especially when the level of contaminating microorganisms is high and composed of bacterial spores. In the last 10 to 15 years, a number of devices have been made of heat-labile materials that require chemical germicides for sterilization or high-level disinfection. If sterilization is the objective of a treatment, contact times of 6 to 10 hours are required, and this is often detrimental to the material in the devices.

For example, flexible fiberoptic endoscopes cannot be subjected to long contact times in liquid germicides without risking the eventual degradation of lenses and other components. It is for this reason that, if sterilization is to be accomplished, EtO sterilization is the only feasible treatment. Since these instruments are expensive and frequently used, some practitioners have elected to practice high-level disinfection rather than sterilization of these instruments.

The size of a medical device also limits the types of germicides that can be used and governs whether sterilization or high-level disinfection will be the intended treatment. If an instrument is too large to be conveniently immersed in solutions or placed in any EtO chamber, disinfection may be accomplished by wiping with a liquid. This would include primarily semicritical or noncritical devices.

Thus, the nature and use of a medical device or item may dictate the type and use of a chemical germicide. Practitioners should be aware of this, and when purchasing medical devices, at least one criterion should be the ease with which the device can be cleaned, sterilized, or disinfected.

Bioburden

Under a given set of circumstances, the higher the level of microbial contamination, the longer must be the exposure to the chemical germicide before the entire microbial population is killed. This factor does not stand alone,

because the amount of time necessary to inactivate 100 bacterial spores would be significantly longer than the time required to inactivate 100 cells of Staphylococcus aureus or most other ordinary vegetative bacteria. When considering a natural microbial population composed of various types of microorganisms that have different degrees of resistance to physical or chemical stress, the survivor curve with all factors controlled would be parabolic and not straight (as it might be if a pure culture of a particular microorganism were used). Furthermore, the most resistant microbial subpopulation, even though it may be present in a fairly lower concentration than the entire microbial population, tends to control sterilization or disinfection time.

Resistance to Chemical Germicides

Microorganisms vary widely in their resistance to chemical germicides and, thus, the types that are present on medical items or surgical materials may have a significant effect on the time as well as the concentration of germicides needed for sterilization or disinfection. The most resistant types of microorganisms are bacterial spores, some of which are significantly more resistant to both chemical and physical stresses. In a broad descending order of relative resistance, considerably below that of bacterial endospores are the tubercle bacilli, fungal spores, small or nonlipid viruses, vegetative fungi, medium-size or lipid viruses, and vegetative bacterial cells. Obviously, the biggest differences in resistance are between bacterial spores and vegetative cells. Smaller, but important, differences exist between the tubercle bacillus and nonacid-fast bacteria and among viruses and fungi. The human hepatitis viruses (B and non A/non B) are difficult to place in this order; it has been estimated [14] that their resistance levels are intermediate between bacterial spores and the tubercle bacilli, but more probably toward the latter.

The differences in chemical resistance exhibited by various vegetative bacteria are relatively minor, except for the tubercle bacilli and other nontubercular but acid-fast mycobacteria [15], which, presumably because of their hydrophobic cell surfaces, are comparatively resistant to a variety of disinfectants, especially those in the low-level category. Among the ordinary vegetative bacteria, staphylococci and enterococci are somewhat more resistant than most other gram-positive bacteria. It is interesting to note that antibiotic-resistant "hospital" strains of staphylococci do not appear to be more resistant to chemical germicides than ordinary isolates. A number of gram-negative bacteria, such as pseudomonas, klebsiella, enterobacter, and serratia, also may show somewhat greater resistance to some disinfectants than other gram-negative bacteria. This may be significant, because many of these gram-negative bacteria are known to often be responsible for outbreaks of hospital infections, especially in compromised hosts.

Gram-negative water bacteria that have the ability to grow well and achieve levels of 10^3 to 10^7/ml in distilled, deionized, or reverse-osmosis water have been shown to be significantly more resistant to a variety of disinfectants in their "naturally occurring" state (i.e., isolated and grown in pure culture in water without subculturing on laboratory media) as compared to bacterial cells subcultured in the normal fashion.

These differences in resistance, although minor, become important when low-level disinfectants are used, particularly at marginal or dilute concentrations, or when disinfectants having greater germicidal properties are used inappropriately (e.g., ingredients used to prepare them are not fresh or significant organic loads are allowed to develop). The resistance of naturally occurring microorganisms also extends to bacterial spores, and it has been shown by Bond [16] that naturally occurring bacterial spores in soil are significantly more resistant to dry heat than those that are subcultured, as shown in Figure 1.

Chemical Sterilization by EtO

Ethylene oxide (EtO) is an effective bacteriocide, active at temperatures as low as 60°C. For this reason, many products are currently sterilized with EtO, including those that cannot be sterilized by other means. However, new, tougher standards for occupational exposure of workers involved in EtO sterilization, and stricter standards for re-sidual EtO in sterilized devices, may restrict the future use of EtO sterilization.

Steam sterilization (which will be discussed in subsequent sections) can only be used for heat-stable items such as metal surgical instruments, packs of linen, and gloves. However, thermoplastics, such as PVC and PU's, can deform under steam pressure and temperature; therefore, not all medical devices can be safely steam sterilized.

Radiation is an efficient method of sterilization, but the equipment can be prohibitively expensive. In addition, high radiation doses may crosslink or alter the chemical composition of synthetic polymers, and should be used only after thorough analysis of its possible effects.

These discussions are designed to help the reader decide the question: Which should be used, steam, EtO, or radiation, to sterilize medical devices? There is no universal answer to the question. The answer will depend on the complexity of the product, the desired degree of sterility assurance, the permanency of the required sterility package, the consequences of nonsterility, the effect of each process on the medical device and the cost of sterilization.

Principles of EtO Sterilization

We begin this section with an overview of the principles of EtO sterilization, and a detailed discussion of the most important operating parameters necessary to fully understand this widely used sterilization method.

The use of EtO as a sterilant in the reduction or elimina-

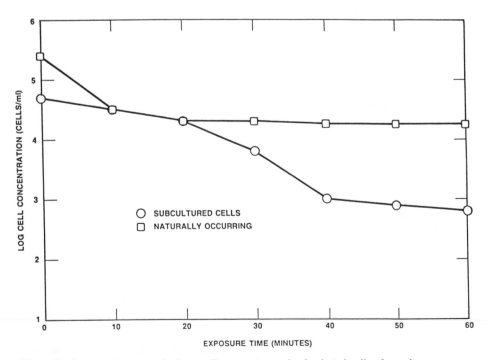

Figure 1. *Comparative survival of naturally occurring and subcultured cells of pseudomonas aeruginosa exposed dry heat.*

tion of bacteria, mold, spores and fungus is accepted worldwide. Because EtO is highly diffusive and can permeate many materials, it is possible to sterilize heat- or moisture-sensitive materials through sealed plastic wrapping films, shipping cartons and containers.

The growing use of sophisticated heat- and moisture-sensitive medical prostheses requiring sterilization has produced an increasing need for dependable gas sterilizers. Hospitals that deliver advanced levels of health care use gas systems to sterilize instruments such as anesthesia circuits, respirators, endoscopes or special equipment used in operative cases, such as operating microscopes.

The technique protects instruments, such as those used in ophthalmic surgery, from the deterioration that occurs with repeated autoclaving. Use of gas sterilization may also enable hospitals to reuse certain expensive plastic items, such as cardiac catheters and embolectomy catheters. To meet these needs for dependable, nondamaging sterilization of heat- and moisture-sensitive items, many manufacturers also find EtO sterilization acceptable.

Initial investigations of the EtO sterilization process focused on the crucial parameters that determine efficacy. Experimental results emphasized the important interaction of EtO concentration, duration of exposure, and temperature [17]. Using a standardized challenge of 10^6 bacillus subtilis spores, it was demonstrated that an exponential relationship exists between spore death rate and the concentration of EtO exposure, expressed as mg/liter. For example, at 75°F, sterilization was achieved using EtO concentrations of 44 mg/liter for 24 hours. At elevated temperatures, fewer mg/liter-hours of EtO exposure are necessary to achieve sterilization. For example, at 98°F, exposure to an EtO concentration of 44 mg/liter sterilized the spore challenge in 6 hours. In order to attain those results, however, additional requirements of the EtO sterilization process must be met.

Subsequent experiments demonstrated the importance of the state of humidification of organisms at the time of their exposure to EtO [18–21]. Desiccation of the spores prior to EtO exposure produces a small but significant percentage of organisms which are highly resistant to the sterilization process. Similar resistance to destruction by EtO occurs in desiccated staphylococcus aureus. Rehumidification of such organisms can require prolonged exposure to an atmosphere having a 50 to 90 percent relative humidity. Wetting of desiccated organisms, however, either by brief immersion in water or by spraying with water, instantaneously reverses EtO resistance.

Moisture has been found to be a critical factor in achieving sterility with gaseous EtO. No gas sterilizer can effectively kill desiccated spores.

Spore formers have the unique ability to transform reversibly from a vegetative form to an encapsulated form. In the encapsulated form, they are usually incapable of reproduction, but can exist without nutrients and are completely impervious to a hostile environment. The spore is a result of condensation of essential cell substance with the subsequent development of the highly resistant capsule.

The influence that moisture has on EtO sterilization has been studied in detail. The conclusions drawn from these studies are:

- The atmosphere surrounding the product and bacteria should contain moisture.
- Unsterile products should not be in a state of extreme desiccation.
- The moisture content or relative humidity of the atmosphere in those areas where product packaging is conducted should not be less than 30 percent, preferably close to 50 percent, to avoid unintentional dehydration.

The other vital prerequisite of EtO sterilization processes is penetration. Ethylene oxide must be able to reach a microorganism in order to destroy it. Barriers to penetration, such as coatings of salts, or the proteinaceous material present in blood or pus, can prevent sterilization. Similarly, EtO cannot penetrate glass or metal. Therefore, instruments must be disassembled prior to EtO exposure. Stylets, plungers or plugs must be removed in order to permit free access of EtO. Wrapping materials must allow EtO diffusion (e.g., paper, cloth, some plastic films).

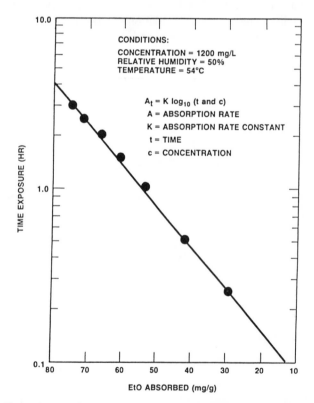

CONDITIONS:
CONCENTRATION = 1200 mg/L
RELATIVE HUMIDITY = 50%
TEMPERATURE = 54°C

$A_t = K \log_{10} (t \text{ and } c)$
A = ABSORPTION RATE
K = ABSORPTION RATE CONSTANT
t = TIME
c = CONCENTRATION

Figure 2. EtO absorbed on polyvinyl chloride (PVC) as a function of time [from Bruch, C. W. "FDA Activities in EtO Residuals," Proceedings, HIMA, Report 77-7, p. 12 (November 1977)].

TABLE 4. Summary of Acute Response of Animals to Inhalation Exposure to Ethylene Oxide OHEW (NIOSH) Publication No. 77-200

ppm by Volume in Air	Exposure Time (hr)	Animal	Results
250–280	8	Guinea pig	Slight respiratory changes; no deaths
	48	Guinea pig	An occasional death
560–600	7	Guinea pig, cat and dog	No deaths
	8	Guinea pig	An occasional death
	22	Guinea pig and cat	Death during (or following) exposure
	22	Rabbit and dog	No deaths
710	4	Dog	0/3 died in 14 days
1,100	5	Rat, guinea pig, and rabbit	Moderate injury, no deaths
	8	Guinea pig, dog, and rabbit	Slight injury, no deaths
	8	Rat and cat	Death within 24 hours
1,300–1,400	8	Guinea pig	Majority died in 1 to 8 days
	4	Dog	3/3 died first day
2,200	1.5	Cat	Injurious, no deaths
	3	Cat	Death within 24 hours
	4	Guinea pig	Injurious, few deaths
	4	Rabbit	Injurious, no deaths
	4	Dog	Death within 24 hours
3,000	1	Guinea pig	No deaths
	3	Guinea pig	Death of majority within 1 to 8 days
	8	Guinea pig	Death of majority within 24 hours
4,000	4	Rat	No deaths (of 6)
7,000	20 min	Guinea pig	No evidence of injury
	1	Guinea pig	Death of majority within 1 to 8 days
	2.5	Guinea pig	Death within 24 hours
8,000	4	Rat	6/6 died
14,000	10 min	Guinea pig	No evidence of injury
	20 min	Guinea pig	Majority died in 1 to 8 days
	1	Guinea pig	Death within 24 hours
51,000–64,000	5 min	Guinea pig	Majority died in 1 to 8 days
	10 min	Guinea pig	Death in 24 hours

Following the sterilization cycle, attention must be given to the requirement for aeration. Ethylene oxide, a small, highly reactive molecule, actually dissolves in porous materials. The amount of EtO retained in an item and the rate of EtO elution depends on a number of variables. These include the composition and surface area of the item, the packaging material, the presence or absence of a soluble diluent gas like Freon, and the temperature at which aeration occurs.

Polymers sterilized with EtO gas absorb and retain varying amounts of EtO [22]. Residual EtO in sterilized plastic tubing has been reported to cause hemolysis of blood in heart-lung surgery [23,24]. Other publications reported the effects of gas sterilization in 14 different plastic devices, and concluded that adverse hemolytic reac-

tions were caused when blood was exposed to the plastics that retained significant quantities of residual EtO [25,26].

Toxicity of EtO

To knowledgeable scientists in the biomedical field, it comes as no surprise that EtO possesses toxic properties, which are listed in Table 4. Toxicity is, after all, an unavoidable requirement for any effective sterilant. It has been known for over 20 years that EtO is a highly reactive alkylating agent and a radiomimetic agent [27]. A substance is considered radiomimetic if the effects of its reaction in biological systems mimic the effects of radiation.

To illustrate, Figure 2 shows the amount of EtO ab-

TABLE 5. Extent of Ethylene Oxide Absorption by Plastic and Rubber Materials during a Standard Gaseous Sterilization Cycle

Material	Residue Level (ppm)
PVC	10,000–30,000
Polystyrene	15,000–25,000
Polyethylene	5,000–10,000
Polypropylene	15,000
Natural Rubber	20,000–35,000
Synthetic Rubber	20,000
Silicone Rubber	15,000–20,000

(From Ernst, R. R. and Whitbourne, J. E., "Study of the Requirements, Preliminary Concepts, and Feasibility of a New System to Process Medical/Surgical Supplies in the Field," pp. 46–57, Appendix, Contract No. DADA 17-70-C-0072, U.S. Army Medical R&D Command, Washington, D.C.)

sorbed by polyvinyl chloride (PVC) as a function of time when exposed to a concentration of EtO of 1200 mg/liter at 50-percent relative humidity and 54°C. Researchers studied EtO residual levels for various materials upon removal from the sterilizer (after having been exposed to 650 mg/liter at 54°C for 4 hours) and concluded that all levels are acutely toxic. Table 5 summarizes these findings.

These results show conclusively that insuring removal of EtO residuals from sterilized polymers is a desirable goal. Normally, the rate at which sorbed gases dissipate from exposed prostheses is dependent upon the nature of the polymer and the conditions under which the prostheses are stored following exposure. Removal of residual gases could be conducted by placing specimens in a well-ventilated area at room temperature. Unfortunately, dissipation of residual EtO is not a rapid process at room temperature. Many manufacturers of EtO sterilizer equipment routinely recommend at least three, and preferably five days' aeration for EtO sterilization plastic tubing intended for use in heart-lung surgery.

Of utmost importance is the time required for adequate aeration of the type of material sterilized. Highly porous materials such as paper, cloth, and natural rubber lose EtO very rapidly. No significant EtO remains in such materials after 1 to 2 hours aeration at 120°F. Items composed of filled synthetic rubber, such as black anesthesia masks or red rubber endotracheal tubes, lose EtO more slowly. A red rubber endotracheal tube, for example, requires several hours aeration at 120°F to reduce the EtO level below 250 ppm. Of all the materials currently EtO sterilized, the one that retains the most EtO and requires the longest aeration is vinyl, otherwise known as polyvinyl chloride or PVC. For example, a PVC intestinal tube generally requires about 8 hours aeration at 120°F to reach EtO levels under 250 ppm. The form of the material, particularly the ratio of the surface area to the volume, significantly affects the rate of EtO elution.

Materials used in wrapping also influence the rate of EtO absorption and the time required for aeration. Ethylene oxide rapidly penetrates traditional paper or cloth wrappers, which do not constitute a significant gas barrier. Plastic packaging materials, however, may reduce the speed of EtO absorption, and also prolong the rate of EtO

TABLE 6. Properties of Ethylene Oxide Mixtures

	Carbon Dioxide Mixtures			Fluorocarbon Mixture
Ethylene Oxide				
% by Weight	10	20	30	12
% by Gas Volume	10	20	30	27
Carbon Dioxide				
% by Weight	90	80	70	—
% by Gas Volume	90	80	70	—
Fluorocarbon 12				
% by Weight	—	—	—	88
% by Gas Volume	—	—	—	73
Vapor Pressure (full cylinder) at 21°C (70°F), psig	750	675	600	60
Ethylene Oxide, mg/L at 54°C (130°F)	470 (29.4 psig)	1020 (33.0 psig)	1167 (22.0 psig)	600 (7.3 psig)
Flammability	Nonflammable	16.5 to 43.5% in air with spark ignition at atmospheric pressure	Approximately the same flammability range as the 80/20 mixture	Nonflammable in storage and shipment and in concentration used in practice in ordinary rooms or vaults or in suitable vacuum fumigation vaults

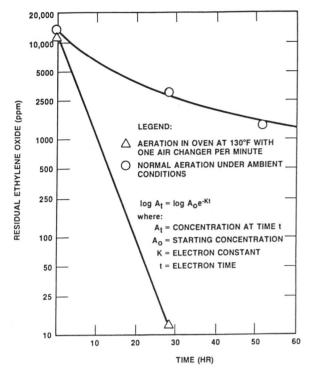

Figure 3. *Effect of aeration on EtO content of PVC endotracheal tubes packaged in 3-mil polyethylene film.*

elution. A number of packaging substances are so impermeable to EtO that they must not be used in gas sterilization processes. These include Nylon®, cellophane, and metallic films such as aluminum foil.

The temperature at which aeration occurs greatly influences the rate of EtO elution: the lower the temperature, the slower the aeration process. Elevated temperature aerators significantly accelerate EtO elution. Temperatures above 140°F may damage heat-sensitive medical devices. Therefore, most aerators operate at temperatures between 120° and 140°F.

When the requirements for humidification and penetration have been met, and an adequate number of mg/liter-hours of EtO exposure are provided at an appropriate temperature, reliable sterilization of large numbers of resistant organisms can be achieved. Following the sterilization cycle, porous materials that retain EtO must dwell in a controlled temperature environment for sufficient time to assure adequate elution of EtO residues. At the completion of those processes, the user can have a high level of assurance that fragile instruments are sterile, and are undamaged by the procedure; sealed in a protective package, they will have a prolonged shelf life.

Since elution time is directly related to temperature, an increase in temperature results in a faster elution rate. Figure 3 graphically demonstrates the linear release of residual EtO under forced aeration at 54°C versus the rather exponential degassing rate under ambient conditions. In

these experiments, PVC endotracheal tubes were wrapped in 3-mil polyethylene.

Regarding commercially available sterilant gases, a number of mixtures of EtO are frequently used as shown in Table 6. In most cases, carbon dioxide and Freon are utilized, since 100 percent EtO gas can form explosive mixtures. The most frequently used mixtures are the 10-90 and 20-80 EtO/CO_2 systems, as well as the 12-88 EtO/Freon system.

Bactericidal Action

The mode of action of EtO can be considered first as a general reaction, as shown in Figure 4, part A, and then the postulated mode of action of EtO with bacterial walls, shown in part B.

EtO is a chemical compound that has a molecular weight of 44 Daltons, a boiling point of 10.4°C at atmospheric pressure, and a vapor pressure of 1095 mmHg (gauge) at 20°C (properties are summarized in Table 7). Ethylene oxide is the simplest member of the alkylene ox-

TABLE 7. Physical Properties of Ethylene Oxide*

LIQUID	
Molecular Weight	44.05
Apparent Specific Gravity at 20/20°C (68/68°F)	0.8711
Δ Sp. gr./Δt at 20° to 30°C (68° to 86°F)	0.00140
Coefficient of Expansion at 20°C (68°F)	0.00161
Water Solubility	Complete
Heat of Vaporization at 1 atm	6.1 kcal/g-mole
Surface Tension	28.0 dynes per cm
Viscosity at 10°C (50°F)	0.28 cps
Vapor Pressure at 20°C (68°F)	1095 mmHg
Boiling Point at 760 mm	10.4°C (50.7°F)
at 300 mm	−11.0°C (−12.2°F)
at 10 mm	−66°C (−86.8°F)
ΔBP/ΔP at 740 to 760 mmHg	0.033°C per mm
Freezing Point	−112.6°C (−170.7°F)
Refractive Index, n_D at 7°C (44.6°F)	1.3597
Heat of Fusion	1.236 kcal/g-mole
Specific Heat at 20°C (68°F)	0.44 cal per g per °C
Explosive Limits in Air at 760 mmHg—Upper	100% by volume
—Lower	3% by volume
Flash Point, Tag Open Cup (ASTM Method D 1310)	< −18°C (<0°F)
VAPOR	
Critical Temperature	196.0°C (384.8°F)
Critical Pressure	1043 psia
Autoignition Temperature in Air at 1 atm	429°C (804°F)
Decomposition Temperature of Pure Vapor at 1 atm	560°C (1040°F)
Heat of Combustion of Gas, Gross	312.15 kcal/g-mole
Heat of Formation	12.2 kcal/g-mole

*Data from Union Carbide Corp., New York.

ides, or epoxides, basically consisting of two carbon atoms and an oxygen atom, linked together in an unstable, three-membered ring. Under proper conditions, the three-membered ring opens, and enters into an alkylation reaction through attachment to a molecule via its positively charged carbon atom.

Alkylating agents react with a variety of biologically important cellular compounds, which are vital to normal metabolism and reproduction. Some of these compounds include constituents of nucleic acids, such as adenine and guanine. Alkylating agents also react with proteins. Susceptible reaction sites are sulfhydryl, amino, carboxyl and hydroxyl groups of the proteins. Because of such alkylating reactions, it is thought that critical molecular sites can be blocked, seriously impairing normal bacterial metabolic processes.

Many investigators have demonstrated the lethal effect of EtO on microorganisms including bacteria, viruses and fungi. It is theorized that EtO exerts its primary effect by alkylation of susceptible molecules. The term alkylation refers to the replacement of a hydrogen atom in a molecule by an alkyl group.

Although it is not known whether nucleic acids or proteins are preferentially attacked, it has been shown that the nucleic acids have a high affinity for alkylating agents. In this connection, it is widely accepted that one need look no further than the inactivation of DNA for an explanation of the lethal effect of EtO [28]. The present state of knowledge, however, does not rule out the possibility that some of the end effects of alkylating agents could be due to other causes, such as inactivation of sensitive enzyme systems. Enzymes are proteins that act as biological catalysts.

The rate at which the destruction of organisms occurs, is partially related to the rate of diffusion of the gas through the cell wall, amount of gas present, availability or accessibility of chemical groups to react with EtO and other relevant factors such as humidity, temperature, exposure time and deaeration.

Typical Sterilizing Cycles

Figure 5(a) shows a typical EtO process cycle in which the chamber is initially evacuated to remove air; steam is admitted to raise the humidity, which conditions the surface of the materials to be sterilized. The humidity is held for an adjustable period. The sterilant is injected to the proper concentration; exposure takes place for a variable period, generally 2 to 4 hours. After exposure, the chamber is re-evacuated to remove the sterilant. Finally, filtered air is admitted to bring the system back to atmospheric pressure. The cycle is now complete.

Figure 5(b) presents a typical 12-88 process cycle; this means 12 percent EtO, 88 percent Freon. Note that, in this case, the exposure time is 4 to 5 hours long, and two air washes are utilized.

One final word about EtO sterilization. Assurance of an effective EtO sterilization process requires administrative control (operator training programs, equipment maintenance, especially dedicated clean areas), it requires process control (thermocouples, pressure gauges, chemical indicators), and it requires biological control (biological indicator challenges, product cultures).

- Chemical indicators are used to monitor gas concentrations. Chemical ink indicators consist of chemochromic inks printed on paper. When exposed to EtO, the ink undergoes a chemical reaction, which results in color change.

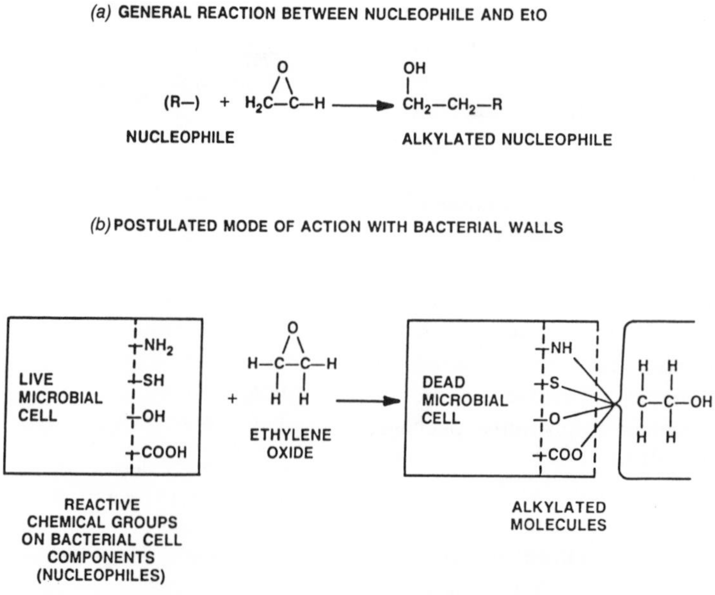

(a) GENERAL REACTION BETWEEN NUCLEOPHILE AND EtO

(b) POSTULATED MODE OF ACTION WITH BACTERIAL WALLS

Figure 4. Bactericidal action of ethylene oxide.

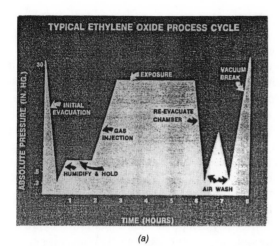

(a)

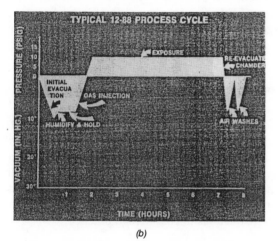

(b)

Figure 5. *Typical EtO process cycles.*

- Indicators are placed within each product package. Proper color change is a precondition for release.
- Biological indicators are used to assure sterility. These indicators consist of a standardized preparation of *Bacillus subtilis* var. *globigii* as monitors of sterilization.
- *Bacillus subtilis* var. *globigii* spores are among the most resistant to EtO. These bacteria are more resistant to EtO than the anticipated product contamination, thus providing a rigorous challenge to the sterilization process.
- Five biological monitors are generally used in each sterilizer load, and are placed on those areas most difficult to sterilize, such as the geometric center and the upper and lower regions of both front and rear sterilizer load.

Items to be sterilized by EtO gas are customarily packaged in special wrapping materials to maintain sterility following a sterilization. The ideal packaging mate-rial for products to be sterilized by EtO should have the following characteristics:

- ready availability
- permeability to EtO
- permeability to water vapor
- permeability to air (important for sterilizers with vacuum cycles)
- permeability to microbes to maintain sterility during storage

Although no plastic films meet all the above requirements, some data are available that allow for intelligent choices among competing films.

Polyethylene, for example, meets almost all the requirements for an ideal wrapping material and is especially desirable because of its transparency. This film is readily permeable to EtO and moisture from 1.0 to 4.0 mils. There are three grades of polyethylene: low, medium, and high density. For gaseous sterilization, the low-density film is recommended because it has a higher permeability rate to EtO and moisture than either of the other grades. It is also most suitable for heat sealing, due to its lower melting point.

Occupational Exposure to EtO

Ethylene oxide is used extensively within health care facilities for sterilization of equipment and supplies which are heat sensitive. It is unique for this purpose. Alternative chemicals or processes have, in themselves, serious limitations or health hazards. The National Institute for Occupational Safety and Health (NIOSH) recognizes, therefore, that the continued use of EtO as a gaseous sterilant is highly desirable in many situations. Recent results of tests for mutagenesis have increased the concern for potential health hazards associated with exposure to EtO. In order to assess the potential for exposure and associated hazards, NIOSH has undertaken this Special Occupational Hazard Review. An assessment is made of the evidence for toxic effects of EtO, especially with respect to mutagenic, teratogenic, and carcinogenic potentials. Additionally, a limited field survey was conducted by NIOSH to document the use, problems, and potential for human exposure in medical facilities. The results of this survey were in agreement with data made available by the American Hospital Association, the U.S. Army, other federal agencies, and industrial and professional organizations. Based on this review, measures for control of occupational exposure are recommended.

The acute toxic effects of EtO in man and animals include acute respiratory and eye irritation, skin sensitization, vomiting, and diarrhea. Known chronic effects consist of respiratory irritation and secondary respiratory infection, anemia, and altered behavior.

The observations of: (a) heritable alterations in at least 13 different lower biological species following exposure to EtO, (b) alterations in the structure of the genetic material in somatic cells of the rat, and (c) covalent chemical bonding between EtO and DNA support the conclusion that continuous occupational exposure to significant concentrations of EtO may induce an increase in the frequency of mutations in human populations. At present, however, a substantive basis for quantitative evaluation of the genetic risk to exposed human populations does not exist.

No definitive epidemiological studies, and no standard long-term carcinogenesis assays, are available with which to assess carcinogenic potential. Limited tests by skin application or subcutaneous injections in mice did not reveal carcinogenicity. However, the alkylating and mutagenic properties of EtO are sufficient bases for concern about its potential carcinogenicity. Neither animal nor human data are available on which to assess the potential teratogenicity of EtO.

NIOSH recommends that EtO be considered as mutagenic and potentially carcinogenic to humans, and that occupational exposure to it be minimized by eliminating all unnecessary and improper uses of EtO in medical facilities. Whenever alternative sterilization processes are available that do not present similar or more serious hazards to the employee, they should be substituted for EtO sterilization processes whenever possible. Although this review is limited to EtO, concern is also expressed for hazards from such hydration and reaction products of EtO as ethylene glycol and ethylene chlorohydrin, the latter a teratogen to some lower biological species.

In his report, Glaser [29] includes a summary of the airborne EtO concentrations measured within health care facilities as part of the field survey. NIOSH estimates that there are in excess of 10,000 EtO sterilizers in use in U.S. health care facilities, and that approximately 75,000 workers are potentially exposed to EtO in those facilities. Reasons for the unnecessary exposure of personnel were found to include: improper or inadequate ventilation of sterilizers, aerators, and working spaces; improper handling and/or storage of sterilized items; untrained workers operating some sterilization equipment; improper operating techniques leading to mishandling of some EtO sterilizing equipment; poor design of the sterilization facility; and design limitations of the sterilization equipment.

NIOSH recommends, based on the recent results of tests for mutagenesis, that exposure to EtO be controlled so that workers are not exposed to a concentration greater than 135 mg/m³ (75 ppm) determined during a 15-minute sampling period, as a ceiling occupational exposure limit and, in addition, that the provision that the time-weighted average (TWA) concentration limit of 90 mg/m³ (50 ppm) for a workday not be exceeded. As additional information on the toxic effects of EtO becomes available, this recommended level for exposures of short duration may be altered. The adequacy of the current U.S. EtO standard, which was based on the data available at the time of promulgation, has not been addressed in this report. NIOSH strongly recommends that control strategies such as those described in this document, or others considered to be more applicable to particular local situations, be implemented to assure maximum protection of the health of employees. Good work practices will help to assure their safety.

Where the use of EtO is to be continued, improved techniques of exhausting the gas from the sterilizer, the aerator, and the sterilized items need to be implemented. Gas sterilization should be supervised, and the areas into which EtO may escape should be monitored to prevent all unnecessary exposure of personnel. When proper control measures are instituted, the escape of EtO into the environment will be greatly reduced. Under such control, the use of EtO as a gaseous sterilant in medical facilities can be continued with considerably less risk to the health of occupationally exposed employees.

PHYSICAL METHODS OF STERILIZATION

As we have seen, sterilization is an absolute term, meaning the destruction of all microorganisms. Sterilization is a radical process, which may alter or damage the polymer(s) that comprise the medical device. Sterilizing methods have traditionally been classified as "physical" or "chemical" as depicted on Table 8, although there are no sharp distinctions in commercial practice.

Steam Sterilization

The oldest and most recognized agent of destruction is heat. From early recorded history, due consideration was

TABLE 8. Traditional Classification of Sterilization Methods

	a. Chlorine Compounds (Hypochlorites, Chloramines)
	b. Iodine Compounds (Betadine, Iodophors)
	c. Phenolic Compounds (Bisphenol, Nitrophenol)
	d. Alcohols
	e. Hydrogen Peroxide
	f. Nitrogen Compounds (Dowicil, Vancide)
1. Chemical	g. Surfactants
	h. Mercurials (Thimerosal, Mercurochrome)
	i. Silver Compounds (Sulfadiazine)
	j. Heavy Metals (Ni, Zn, Pb)
	k. Aldehydes (Glutaraldehyde, Formaldehyde)
	l. Ethylene Oxide
2. Physical	a. Steam
	b. Ultraviolet Irradiation
	c. Ionizing Radiation ——— Electron Beam / Gamma Rays

TABLE 9. Times Required for Lethal Effect on Bacterial Spores by Thermal Exposure

Organisms	Moist Heat Time (min)			Dry Heat Time (min)		
	100°C	110°C	121°C	120°C	140°C	170°C
B. anthracis	5–15	—	—	—	180	—
C. botulinum	330	90	10	120	60	15
C. welchii	5–10	—	—	50	5	—
C. tetani	5–15	—	—	—	15	—
Soil bacilli	>1020	120	6	—	—	15

Source: Avis, K. E. "Sterilization," in *The Theory and Practice of Industrial Pharmacy, 2nd Edition*. Lachman, Lieberman and Kanig, eds. Philadelphia:Lea and Febiger, pp. 567–585 (1976).

given to dangers associated with the inception and transmission of disease. The use of fire and water as purifying agents was incorporated in the Mosaic Law. Moist and dry heat are classic sterilizing media. Moist heat includes either saturated steam or boiling water. Although boiling water at ambient pressures is not a good sterilizing agent because of its relatively low temperature, its principal advantage is its availability. Steam under pressure is inexpensive and sterilizes penetrable materials and exposed surfaces rapidly.

Dry heat, on the other hand, is relatively slow, requiring higher temperatures of application. However, dry heat will penetrate all kinds of materials, such as oils, petrolatum, and closed containers, that are not permeable to steam.

Down through the years, steam sterilization has been an important process. Today, pre-vacuum, high-temperature steam sterilizers are considered to be the safest, most practical means of sterilizing the majority of surgical instruments, surgical dressings, fluids, fabrics and other absorbent materials.

In the process of steam sterilization, although the death of each single organism might be considered as an independent incident, the process of destroying a great number of bacteria closely parallels many ordinary chemical reactions. Both involve a definite relationship between *time* and *temperature*.

Even though, in steam sterilization, some organisms may die during the first few minutes of exposure, a definite time period is necessary to kill *all* microbiological life as presented in Table 9. The basic time-temperature requirements for accomplishing sterilization in saturated steam is based on a logarithmic thermal death curve with allowance for a proper "margin of safety." No pathologic organism has been found that will survive more than 3 minutes at 250°F; however, the total time of steam sterilization cycles depends on many variables such as type of material, the way it is loaded, and the system design.

Microbial Resistance

One of the most important requirements for sterilization is the determination of microbial resistance to any sterili-

zation technique. Sterilization process parameters are developed from this determination. Due to its importance, certain principles of microbial resistance are of interest, such as: (a) the mathematical expression of microbial death, (b) the definition of microbial death, and (c) the mechanism of microbial death [30].

Mathematically, microbial death appears to follow a first-order, logarithmic rate. Such a phenomenon allows expression of microbial death in mathematical terms. It also becomes a basis for describing sterilization effectiveness of different processes.

In general, a logarithmic order of death is described by a straight line, when the logarithm of the number of bacterial survivors following exposure to a sterilizing agent is plotted versus increments of time. There are some exceptions to this phenomenon. For example, some spore populations upon initial exposure to sterilizing agents, such as steam, may actually increase in number due to a phenomenon called activation. Other populations may contain a few extremely resistant cells, causing tailing of the curve.

The definition of microbial death is, for all practical purposes, the inability of microorganisms to reproduce. This definition does not necessarily mean that the microorganisms are actually dead; certain metabolic reactions and growth characteristics may continue to persist even though microorganisms may not be capable of reproducing. The definition is very important because it reflects the technological state of the art, applied to sterilization in a practical sense. It is also important to recognize that a "sterile" product is one that has been confirmed as such within the framework of this definition. Additionally, it is noteworthy that when certain microorganisms are "dead," chemical substances may still persist (in the form of endotoxins), which could cause a pyrogenic response.

Although the phenomenon of the logarithmic order of death is not yet fully clear, the mechanism of death is often considered to be a severe interaction of the sterilizing agent with critical protein or nucleic acid in the cell; for example, (a) with ultraviolet light, death appears to be due to the formation of thymine dimers on the same DNA strand; (b) with heat, it is proposed that hydrogen bonds are broken in DNA; and (c) in EtO, alkylation of amine groups on nucleic acids may be responsible for death [31].

Heat resistance varies among proteins, among microbial species, and among bacterial spores. Many of the bacterial spores are the forms of life most resistant to most chemical and physical killing agents, and particularly to heat. There is a notable difference between thermal resistance to moist heat and to dry heat. A species of bacterial spore highly resistant to moist heat is not necessarily highly resistant to dry heat and vice versa. A case in point is the comparison of spores of the thermophile *B. stearothermophilus* with spores of the mesophile *B. subtilis* var. *niger*. These are the spores most often used to monitor sterilization processes for moist and dry heat, respectively. To inactivate 100,000 spores of *B. stearothermophilus* in saturated steam at 121°C requires 12 minutes of exposure, but 1,000,000 spores of *B. subtilis* are inactivated in less than 1 minute at the same temperature. However, *B. subtilis* var. *niger* is much more resistant to dry heat than *B. stearothermophilus* when both are subjected to the same high temperature.

Other factors can enhance or lower the heat resistance of spores. An innate thermoresistance appears to be associated with certain spores of bacteria that have a greater resistance to heat than other spores. Beyond this, however, environmental influences such as pH, ion concentrations, and constituents of growth and sporulating media enhance the thermoresistance of spores.

The D Value

The rate at which microorganisms are killed may be expressed kinetically. Kinetic death rates, when plotted on logarithmic paper, permit their expression in terms of D values (the time required to destroy 90 percent of the bacterial cells or spore population under a given set of conditions). The D value is generally noted according to the specific sterilizing conditions; for example, D_{121} is the time required to reduce a population of cells (vegetative or spores) by 90% (one log) when exposed to a moist heat temperature of 121°C. D values are frequently used in describing the effectiveness of a sterilization process, such as the number of D values achieving a desired reduction of a microbial population in a sterilization process. For example, the notation 12D* indicates the reduction of a microbial population by 12 logs or a theoretical kill of 10^{12} microorganisms. Figure 6 shows the D values obtained from test data. The general equation of the straight line survivor curve is:

$$D \text{ value} = \frac{T_u - T_o}{\log N_o - \log N_u}$$

*12D has traditionally been applied to canning processes in the food industry. The designated D value of *Clostridium botulinum* is used as the standard.

where

N = microbial population
N_o = initial number
N_u = surviving population

The Steam Sterilization Cycle

A steam sterilizing cycle is divided into three phases: (1) the heating phase or time necessary to bring the chamber up to temperature, before timing begins, (2) the sterilizing phase, or period in which bacteria are exposed to killing temperatures, and (3) the venting, cooling and drying phase. A pre-vacuum, steam pulsing sterilizing cycle is presented in Figure 7.

In the heating phase, for loads other than liquids, it is absolutely essential that as much air as possible be removed from the chamber and product, because any air present in the load will inhibit the penetration of steam, and lower the temperature. A pre-vacuum high-temperature cycle improves the efficiency of the steam sterilization process. Regardless of the fact that the sterilizer might be incorrectly loaded or overloaded, the pre-vacuum cycle will ensure full heating of the load, and will shorten the overall cycle to make possible the use of fast killing high temperatures, with a less deleterious effect on the load.

High-speed resterilization of surgical instruments is an absolute requirement in today's busy hospital operating suites. The most effective and quickest method of resteril-

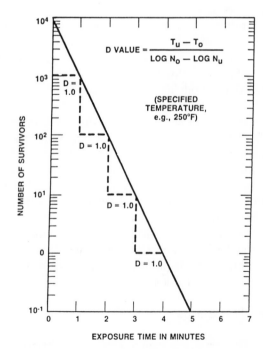

Figure 6. Thermal death kinetics D value.

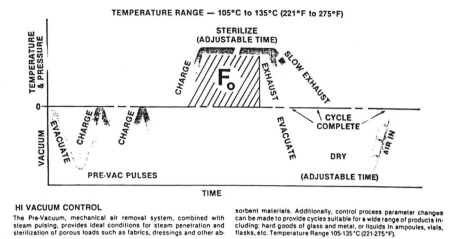

HI VACUUM CONTROL

The Pre-Vacuum, mechanical air removal system, combined with steam pulsing, provides ideal conditions for steam penetration and sterilization of porous loads such as fabrics, dressings and other absorbent materials. Additionally, control process parameter changes can be made to provide cycles suitable for a wide range of products including: hard goods of glass and metal, or liquids in ampoules, vials, flasks, etc. Temperature Range 105-135°C (221-275°F).

Figure 7. A typical pre-vacuum, steam pulsing sterilizing cycle.

ization of undegradable operative equipment has been shown to be steam sterilization [32]. Steam under pressure is inexpensive and sterilizes penetrable materials and exposed surfaces rapidly. Steam sterilization is effective only if used properly. Moisture penetration and air removal are essential for effective sterilization. The use of steam sterilization requires knowledge of its use, some of its thermodynamic properties, correct selection of materials, and the proper setting in the sterilizer.

In summary, steam sterilization—the oldest of the sterilization techniques—provides ideal conditions for penetration and sterilization of porous materials such as fabrics, dressings and other absorbent materials. Additionally, steam sterilization is also widely used in the sterilization of ampules, vials and liquids.

Ultraviolet Sterilization

The practical applications of ultraviolet (UV) irradiation depend on the killing action of the radiation on agents such as yeasts, molds, bacteria, rickettsiae, mycoplasma, and viruses. Some of the other effects of UV include increases in the rate of mutation, chromosomal aberration, and changes in cellular viscosity. UV affects such vital processes as respiration, excitability, and growth.

There is a delicate balance in living things between the deterioration of cellular components after exposure to UV and their biochemical repair. If the amount of damage exceeds the cell's capacity to repair this damage, the cell will die. The reversal of injurious effects of UV by visible light, i.e., photoreactivation, was recognized as a general phenomenon following its rediscovery by Kelner [33] in bacteria and by Dulbecco [34,35] in bacteriophage. Fungus spores, bacteria, animal and plant cells, viruses, and nucleic acids inactivated by UV are photoreactivated by treatment with visible light or near UV, in the vicinity of about 330 to 480 nm.

Viruses, mycoplasma, bacteria, and fungi may be destroyed by UV, whether they are suspended in air or in liquids or deposited on surfaces. Because UV will not penetrate most substances, foods and fabrics, for example, cannot be sterilized by this radiation. The more important applications of UV are directed at: (1) destruction of airborne organisms, establishing by this action satisfactory air hygiene; (2) inactivation of microorganisms located on surfaces or suspended in liquids, but accessible to UV; and (3) protection and disinfection of many products of unstable composition that cannot be treated by conventional methods. Bacterial spores are more resistant than vegetative bacteria, and there is quite a wide difference in resistance between species.

Mercury Vapor Germicidal Lamps

The most practical method of generating UV radiation is by passage of electric discharge through low-pressure mercury vapor enclosed in special glass tubes, known commercially as germicidal lamps. The principle of all germicidal lamps is the same, that of electron flow between electrodes through ionized mercury vapor. The arc in a fluorescent lamp operates on the same basic principle and produces the same type of UV energy. The difference between the two is that the bulb of the fluorescent lamp is coated with a phosphor compound that converts UV to visible light. The glass used in ordinary fluorescent lamps filters out all germicidal UV. The germicidal lamp is not coated with phosphor and is made of special glass that transmits the UV generated by the mercury in addition to visible light. About 95 percent of the UV is in wavelengths of 253.7 nm. These lamps have germicidal efficiency of 5 to 10 times that of high-pressure quartz mercury arcs (400 to 60,000 mmHg or 0.5 to 75 atm).

Operational efficiency of germicidal lamps depends on the surrounding temperature and movement of air. Commercial lamps are generally designed to operate most efficiently at an ambient temperature of 27°C. Cooling the lamp below 27°C by passing air currents over it or by submerging it in liquid lowers its output. Special lamps that operate efficiently under otherwise undesirable conditions are available commercially [36].

In addition to transmission of 253.7 nm, the glass used in low-pressure mercury lamps will transmit a certain amount of 184.9 nm. Energy of this wavelength forms ozone by breaking the bonds of the oxygen molecule. The amount of ozone produced is controlled entirely by the transmission of the glass tubes and decreases more rapidly than emission of 253.7 nm with the age of the lamp. The concentration of ozone in a given area is measured in parts of ozone per million parts of air. The amount of ozone will vary with temperature, humidity, and air movement. The limit of permissible concentration specified by the Council on Physical Medicine of the American Medical Association is one part per 10 million in a conventionally occupied environment. Special germicidal lamps are made with glass envelopes allowing transmission of high concentration of 184.9 nm along with the germicidal 253.7 nm.

Bacterial tubes depreciate rapidly during the first 100 hours of operation; consequently, commercial tubes are rated initially as though they had already operated for 100 hours. Meters are available to monitor the output of a particular lamp, as well as to measure the intensities of germicidal energy at various locations in the room and reflectance of germicidal energy by walls and ceilings [37,38].

Various germicidal tubes are available, operating at different current ratings. The maximum intensity of a tube is provided at its own surface. Absorption of UV by air is negligible. However, distance from the source of radiation imposes certain restrictions in calculation of intensity. An inverse relationship exists between distance from the source and intensity of radiation out to about one half of the effective length of the source, and between the square of the distance at greater than this length from the source. Slim-line germicidal lamps start instantly and use a coil filament on each end that operates hot. Lamp life is governed by the electrode life and frequency of starts. These lamps are used when high UV intensity is desired, as in treatment of water or air or of products on conveyer belts. Cold cathode bactericidal lamps also start instantly but are not affected by number of starts. Their useful life is determined entirely by the transmission of the bulb. They have a longer life than other lamps and perform well at cold temperatures. Because of their long life and moderate intensity, they are often used in occupied areas and when frequent starting is desirable. Most bactericidal lamps operate best in still air at room temperature, and UV output is measured at an ambient temperature of 77°F. Higher or lower temperatures decrease the output of the lamp.

The lamps should be cleaned periodically by wiping with a cloth dampened in alcohol or ammonia and water to maintain maximum output of UV. No oils or waxes should be used for moistening the wiping cloth. When a lamp drops to about 60 percent of its 100-hour rating, or after it has been used for three fourths of its rating time, it should be replaced.

Installation of UV lamps in an enclosed space has become an exacting procedure that should be handled by a lighting engineer. Preliminary ideas regarding certain aspects of installation may be gathered from pamphlets and handbooks put out by the manufacturers of these lamps [39].

Applications in Hospitals and Pharmaceuticals

Numerous and extensive experiments were conducted to determine the efficacy of UV light for protection against infections in hospitals and for reduction of the incidence of respiratory infections in populations routinely sharing a common environment, as exemplified by wards, schools, and barracks.

The first successful application of UV air disinfection in the hospital was pioneered by Hart [40], followed by Overholt and Betts [41]. Hart installed unshielded UV lamps a short distance above the operating team in a surgical amphitheater, allowing the intensity of radiation to be 18 to 30 μW/cm² at the level of the operating table. Prior to the use of UV, postoperative mortality from overwhelming infection after clean operations was 1.12% (19 deaths after 1782 operations). Twenty-nine years after the installation of UV lights [42], no deaths occurred following 2600 operations, including thoracoplasties and neurosurgery. During the same period, wound infection rates dropped from 11.6% (207 out of 1782 operations) to 0.25% (6 out of 2460 operations) in clean primary incisions. According to Hart, contamination with staphylococci did not present a problem because continuous use of UV during and between operations controls the spread of bacteria by air. He considers the air route of spread to be the greatest factor in seeding of clean operative wounds and exposed sterile supplies with pathogenic bacteria. Hart emphasized the use of adequate precautions for the patient and the surgical team, as well as the necessity of installing the proper equipment.

In spite of these results, the use of direct UV did not achieve wide popularity and had only limited acceptance. In 1962, only about 15 hospitals were using this procedure in the United States. Although alarm over epidemic of infections due to *Staphylococcus aureus* in supposedly clean wounds became evident, the medical profession as a whole has not become convinced of the practicability of using UV. This attitude could be attributed primarily to the following factors: The intensity of UV was considered to be insufficient; there was a lack of control of relative humidity in the operating rooms; dirty tubes precluded penetration of UV; and the installation was expensive and difficult because the decrease in UV intensity is inversely proportional to the square of the distance from the source.

A Linde–Robbins UV aseptic air system was installed in the entire operating suite, obstetric room, nursery, and emergency room of a new 60-bed hospital. Careful hospital design allowed this air system to counteract the negative factors just mentioned and to function at above 99 percent efficiency in killing airborne pseudomonas, *Bacillus subtilis*, and *Staphylococcus aureus*. Of 3971 operations performed by 90 surgeons over 22 months, no bacteria were recovered in sampling air with petri dishes. The infection rate in this hospital was 0.002 percent. In another hospital using the same system only in surgery, a 0.0019 percent infection rate was recorded over two years. This is compared with a 1.3 percent rate in two hospitals without the Linde-Robbins UV system. The authors pointed out that surgical infection rates usually vary from 0.96 percent to 13.6 percent. It is interesting to note that the results of a survey carried out by the authors revealed that 20 U.S. and Canadian hospitals in the planning or building stages were incorporating the aseptic air units as a part of the design.

Using a similar apparatus and Anderson's air sampler [43] obtained an inactivation rate of greater than 99 percent for adenovirus type 2, Coxsackie B_1, influenza A, Sindbis, and vaccinia viruses.

Infection represents a major problem in dialysis treatment, and the dialyzing room should be as free of microbial agents as possible. Inamoto et al. [44] installed one 15-watt bare UV lamp for 13.5 m² of the ceiling and used them after working hours. Bacteria were killed even in the area of low UV intensity, possibly by reflected rays and ozone. Easy application and low cost would make this method more advantageous than other procedures used in room disinfection.

Application of localized high-intensity radiation over production lines is used by the pharmaceutical industry [45,46,47] in sterile transfer rooms and hoods, in filling and capping rooms, in air-duct systems to provide sterile air to working areas, and in any locations or situations where microbial contamination may be a problem. While no claims are made for complete removal of microorganisms, it is indicated that better sanitation is brought about as a result of UV radiation. In addition, certain chemicals and plastics were sterilized by UV without producing untoward changes [48,49]. Finally, we must not omit from this discussion the use of UV in many research procedures requiring the use of certain filter membranes, special plastic-coated instruments, and similar apparatus that cannot be subjected to conventional microbial decontamination.

Electron Beam Sterilization

Sterilization of plastic medical devices and supplies by ionizing radiation is increasingly being employed as an alternative to gaseous EtO sterilization. Ethylene oxide is toxic, is readily absorbed by many polymers, and is not always easily or readily desorbed or eliminated. Many plastic materials cannot be sterilized by techniques that require heat (dry heat or steam), nor is treatment with cold (aqueous) sterilants satisfactory in many instances. Ionizing radiation, therefore, is assuming an increasingly important role in the sterilization of many medical products and is becoming a well-established industrial process. Although this technique is not limited to the sterilization of polymeric materials, it is probably the most applicable method for many of these materials.

The various types of ionizing radiation in the electromagnetic spectrum produce bactericidal effects by transferring the energy of a photon into characteristic ionizations in or near a biologic target. In addition to creating pairs of positive and negative electrons, ions can also produce free radicals and activated molecules. These effects, which are produced without any appreciable rise in temperature, have been termed "cold sterilization" when applied to the destruction of microorganisms.

Radiation sterilization by the electron beam (EB) method is of increasing interest since the advent of EB machines of true industrial reliability. These new accelerators have two distinct applications areas in the sterilization field: in-line sterilization of individual devices or intermediate packages at about 1 to 4 MV as part of the manufacturing process, and terminal sterilization shipping cases at 4 to 12 MeV.

Commercial sterilization with electron beams is both very old and fairly new as shown in Table 10. The first EB sterilization application was at Ethicon beginning in 1957. However, Ethicon gave up EB and went to cobalt in the early 1960's, for reasons related to the reliability of their first-generation EB machines. So, EB fell into disuse in sterilization; cobalt sources are the dominant method of industrial radiation sterilization. Meanwhile, modern EB machines have shown on-stream reliabilities fully comparable with other industrial equipment. These accel-

---

TABLE 10. Abbreviated History of Radiation Sterilization

1895—X-Rays discovered by Roentgen
1896—X-Rays shown to kill microorganisms
1930—Exponential relationship demonstrated between dose and kill
1956—Ethicon pioneers EB sterilization for sutures
1960—Demonstration gamma facility operational at Wantagh, UK
1960—First commercial gamma plant built in Australia for sterilizing goat hair
1964—Ethicon establishes commercial gamma sterilization facility in Edinburgh, Scotland
1975—World's largest EB service facility (7 million Curie Co⁶⁰ equivalent) for medical product sterilization on Long Island

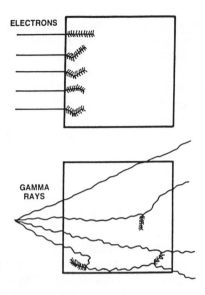

Figure 8. High-energy electrons display some penetrability into matter, but much less than gamma rays.

erators are in use for crosslinking wire and cable insulation, partial vulcanization of rubber tire components, and manufacture of heat-shrink food wrap film, among other applications.

Particle Radiation Biology

The particles usually considered in radiation biology are the α, β, neutron, meson, positron, and neutrino. The only particle that currently is applicable to sterilization is the β particle or electron. Alpha particles, although capable of causing dense ionizations, have limited penetrating ability; neutrons, which are uncharged, have great penetrating power into matter but induce radioactivity.

Mesons and protons are produced only by expensive, high-energy machines, and therefore are not commercially important.

Beta radiation, arising from radioactive disintegrations, consists of electrons with a single negative charge and a low mass. Beta radiation from an isotopic source cannot penetrate materials deeply, but electrons (cathode rays) produced in manmade machines can be accelerated to high energies with a subsequent improvement in penetrating ability as shown in Figure 8. The penetration of electrons into matter is expressed by the Feather equation:

$$R_{max} = \frac{0.542E - 0.133}{\varrho}$$

where R_{max} is the maximum range (g/cm³) for cathode rays in matter of density ϱ, and E is the voltage (MeV) by which the electrons have been accelerated. The penetrating abilities of the various radiations are compared in Table 11.

Penetration Characteristics

Penetration characteristics are not a constant as with cobalt, but vary with voltage or energy. Also, the variation of ionization (or dose) as the radiation penetrates matter is of a special form. Figure 9 illustrates this, comparing penetration characteristics of 12 MeV electrons in plastic with cobalt radiation. The radiation effect of the electrons actually increases as the beam penetrates, then decreases steadily until the maximum range of the electrons is reached. The useful range of this beam extends to the point on the descending side of the curve at which the radiation effect or dose is the same as at the surface. If the thickness of the object has this value or less, every portion

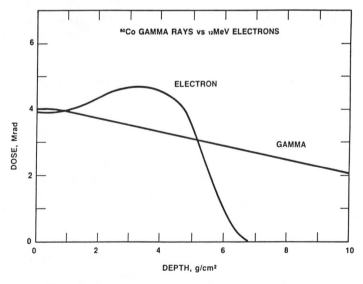

Figure 9. Comparative penetration, gamma rays vs electrons.

TABLE 11. Useful Penetrations Achieved with Different Ionizing Radiations Using Typical Irradiation Sources*

		Useful Penetration (cm)	
		Irradiating from One Side	Irradiating from Both Sides
γ Rays	Co⁶⁰	10.2	40.6
X-Rays	50 KeV	<0.1	~0.5
	10 MeV	12.7	61.0
Cathode Rays	1 MeV	~0.3	~0.8
	5 MeV	1.8	4.3
	10 MeV	3.8	8.6
β Rays	Sr⁹⁰	<0.1	~0.3

*The dose received at any one point will exceed 60% of that at points of maximum intensity.

Source: Hannan, R. S., M. J. Thornley. "Radiation Processing of Foods," Food Mfg. (Oct–Dec 1957).

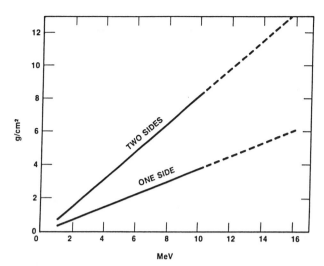

Figure 10. *Practical EB sterilization thickness vs electron energy.*

will receive at least the entrance dose. However, if we irradiate from two opposite sides, the corresponding maximum thickness is not simply twice the "one-side" thickness, but twice the thickness at which the dose on this curve is only 50 percent of the entrance dose. Thus in opposed irradiation, the tails of the two penetration curves can add up when the thickness is correct. The plots of these "one-side" and "two-side" thicknesses vs voltage are shown in Figure 10. The graphs are extrapolated above 10 MeV, but data points at 10 and 12 MeV indicate that the values are either reasonable or conservative. Note also that the ordinate values correspond to centimeters of water. Since packages of medical disposable items are generally considerably less dense than water, correspondingly greater thicknesses may be penetrated. Practically all medical disposables in existing packaging designs can be penetrated by 10 to 12 MeV electrons, at least by taking advantage of the two-side penetration method.

In conclusion, although the use of EB systems for radiation processing is now an established industrial process, the limited penetrability of electrons precludes its use in densely packaged products. As a consequence, radiation sterilization of most medical devices is accomplished using the more penetrating gamma rays from Large Co⁶⁰ radioisotope sources. Nonetheless, EB sterilization systems compete in some cases with gamma sterilization, since there are two major disadvantages to the use of large Co⁶⁰ sources for radiation sterilization: first is the hazard associated with the transportation, handling and storage of large quantities of radioactive material, and second is the limited source of supply of Co⁶⁰.

Gamma Sterilization

In both gamma and electron radiation, the lower energy electrons produce chemical changes in the medium and lead to the destruction of microorganisms. The degree of sterilization achieved in any device is directly related to the amount of radiation absorbed. The radiation absorbed dose is normally measured in rads. Rad is defined as 100 ergs of absorbed energy per gram of material irradiated (shown in Table 12). In the case of gamma radiation, sterilization or destruction of live bacteria and other microorganisms is conveniently carried out by exposing the material to the ionizing radiation emitted from radioactive materials. Sources of radioactive material are gamma rays generated from isotopes such as Co⁶⁰ or Ce¹³⁷. Cesium 137, although having a much longer shelf life, requires a greater quantity to obtain the same radiation level; for this reason the universal choice of radioactive source is Co⁶⁰.

When applied to a packaged product, Co⁶⁰ gamma rays effectively penetrate the packaging (regardless of configuration or density) and sterilize the product by killing all contaminating microorganisms. Similar to x-rays but more powerful, gamma rays cannot cause anything to become radioactive.

In comparison to other methods (heat, EtO), gamma radiation is a much simpler process involving only one variable. As detailed in Table 13, it is necessary with other processes to maintain close control over packaging and product configuration, vacuum, pressure, temperature,

TABLE 12. Units and Conversion Factors in Radiation Chemistry

1 roentgen (r)	= 2.58 × 10⁻⁴ coulombs/kg (standard conditions)
1 rad	= 100 erg/g
	= 10⁻² joules/kg
	= 6.29 × 10¹³ eV/g
	= 2.4 × 10⁻⁶ cal/g
1 gray* (Gy)	= 100 rad
1 Megarad (Mrad)	= 10⁶ rad
G value	= molecules of a product/100 eV absorbed

*The gray is the International System unit for absorbed dose, and is being used with increasing frequency. It is equal to the energy imparted by ionizing radiation to mass corresponding to one joule/kg. Sterilization doses are expressed in megarads (10 kgy = 1 Mrad).

TABLE 13. Comparison of Sterilization Methods

Consideration	Steam	Ethylene Oxide	Gamma Radiation
1. Product Design	No sealed cavity	No sealed cavity	No restrictions
2. Materials of Construction	Most materials satisfactory except for those which are heat or moisture sensitive	Most materials satisfactory	Most materials
3. Product Packaging	Permeable material or second sealing process	Permeable material or second sealing process	No restrictions
	Provision for expansion of packaging during vacuum	Provision for expansion of packaging during vacuum	No restrictions
	Seals must withstand vacuum stress	Seals must withstand vacuum stress	No restrictions
4. Parameters to be Controlled during Sterilization	Vacuum Pressure Temperature Relative humidity Time	ETO concentration Vacuum Pressure Temperature Relative humidity Time	Time
5. Reliability of Sterilizing Process	Good	Good	Excellent
6. Post Sterilization Microbiological Testing	Desirable	Required	Can be eliminated
7. Quarantine Period	7 to 14 days	7 to 14 days	Can be eliminated
8. Post Sterilization Treatment	Dry product	Aerate to remove toxic residues	None
9. Quantitative Process Monitoring Possible	No	No	Yes
10. Economics	Good on low and high volumes	Good on low and high volumes	Good on high volumes

Source: Isomedix Inc., Whippany, N.J.

humidity and time. Post-sterilization treatment is also required to dry the product, or aerate and remove toxic residues.

With gamma radiation there are no residuals, no post-sterilization treatment, and no seasonal sterilization problems (caused by varying moisture content factors). The only variable with gamma sterilization is exposure time.

Fundamental Principles

Any discussion of gamma sterilization requires a knowledge of radiation principles. Radiation is energy that travels through space, and is generally divided into two forms: (1) electromagnetic waves, such as gamma rays, and (2) fast moving particles, such as alpha and beta particles.

Figure 11 shows the energy levels and wavelengths of the different types of nonparticulate (or electromagnetic) radiation. Gamma rays resemble hard (short-wavelength) x-rays, and are emitted at one or two fixed wavelengths by Co^{60} (half-life = 5.3 years), a byproduct of atomic fission reactions.

An understanding of radiation begins with the basic building block of all matter: the atom. An atom contains:

(1) a central nucleus containing two kinds of subatomic particles, protons and neutrons, and (2) a series of shells containing electrons of different energy levels. Isotopes are atoms with the same number of protons, but a different number of neutrons in the nucleus; the total number of neutrons and protons in the nucleus is called the mass number.

Isotopes are generally identified by the name of the element, followed by the mass number, as shown below:

Co^{59} (Stable)	Co^{60} (Unstable)
27 electrons	27 electrons
27 protons	27 protons
32 neutrons	33 neutrons

A neutron consists of a proton and an electron. After ejecting the electron (β particle), the neutron becomes a proton, depicted below:

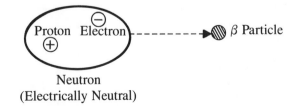

Neutron
(Electrically Neutral)

and so,

$$Co_{27}^{60} \longrightarrow Ni_{28}^{60} + \beta_{-1}^{0} + \gamma \text{ rays}$$

The source of gamma rays is intranuclear. Gamma rays are products of nuclear energy transitions, where unstable Co^{60} decays to Ni^{60} emitting both beta and gamma radiation. The emission of an x-ray from an atom occurs when there is a transition of an electron from an outer shell to a vacancy further within an inner shell, and is produced commercially by bombarding a heavy metal target with fast electrons in a man-made accelerator; by contrast, gamma radiation is the result of a transition of an atomic nucleus from an excited (unstable) state to a ground (stable) state.

Mode of Action

Radiation's effect on organisms, especially microorganisms, was first investigated soon after x-rays were discovered by Roentgen in 1895. These early investigators realized also that ionizing radiation had the ability to penetrate bringing a lethal effect to even the most inaccessible contaminating cell. It was not until 1930 that work was done to correlate a kill/dose–response ratio.

In 1964, the first commercial irradiator was built at Ethicon in Somerville, NJ and used to irradiate sutures. In the late 1950's, when disposable medical products began to become an important segment of the health care industry, a method of sterilization that was effective, and yet would not adversely effect the products, was necessary. Gamma sterilization was pioneered in Europe and has rapidly spread to the U.S. in the last decade. It has become a preferred radiation–sterilization method for an increasing number of medical devices throughout the world.

In contrast to heat, radiation injury does not cause denaturation of protein but induces ionization of vital cell components, particularly the deoxyribonucleic acid (DNA) of the nucleus. The extent of ionization of the irradiated molecules depends on the energy level of the radiation used. High energy radiations above 5 MeV may induce radioactivity in the irradiated material and are, therefore, unsuitable for sterilization of medical equipment or foods.

Two theories have been proposed to explain the lethal action of ionizing radiation. The first is the target (direct action) theory in which it is suggested that ionization of DNA is directly induced. This is supported by the exponential relationship between dose and effect. The diffusion (indirect action) theory postulates primary ionization of water molecules in the cell, thereby producing free hydrogen and hydroxyl radicals which, in turn, initiate secondary reactions in DNA molecules. Both theories may be reconciled with one another by postulating that the target molecules are surrounded by a water film [50].

In addition, many other chemical changes may also be induced and these often result in the development of undesirable food flavors [51], discoloration of glass and fabrics, loss of fiber strength and the release of chlorine from plastics such as polyvinyl chloride. The effects of radiation on medical plastics will be discussed separately.

A typical gamma site shown in Figure 12 is composed of a central gamma cell source around which the product to be sterilized is transported. The product is generally placed in metal trays and exposed to the radiation source in a continuous operation, until the required dose level has been obtained. By this procedure, both batch and continuous operations are possible. When not in use, the radioisotope source, Co^{60}, is generally immersed 20 feet below the surface of a pool of water. A blue fluorescent effect develops, known as the "Cerenkov Effect," which is the consequence of an excited state in the water molecule, produced from ionizing radiation.

Disposal of waste or spent Co^{60} has been a prevalent problem. However, methods are now being developed in the U.S. and Europe to reactivate such material. These wastes are also finding use where low level radiation is required in medical applications.

Dosimetric methods are used to control the radiation process. Two systems widely used are: dyed acrylic–

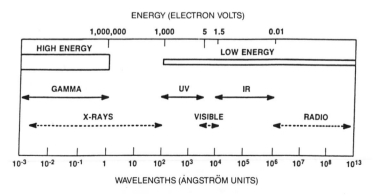

Figure 11. *Wavelengths and energy levels of different types of electromagnetic radiations.*

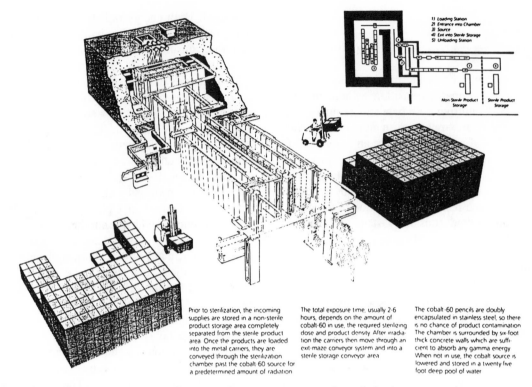

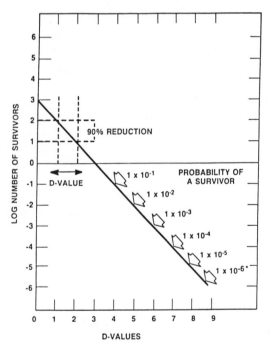

Prior to sterilization, the incoming supplies are stored in a non-sterile product storage area completely separated from the sterile product area. Once the products are loaded into the metal carriers, they are conveyed through the sterilization chamber past the cobalt 60 source for a predetermined amount of radiation

The total exposure time, usually 2-6 hours, depends on the amount of cobalt-60 in use, the required sterilizing dose and product density. After irradiation the carriers then move through an exit-maze conveyor system and into a sterile storage conveyor area

The cobalt-60 pencils are doubly encapsulated in stainless steel, so there is no chance of product contamination. The chamber is surrounded by six-foot thick concrete walls which are sufficient to absorb any gamma energy. When not in use, the cobalt source is lowered and stored in a twenty-five foot deep pool of water

Figure 12. Sterilization process (courtesy: Isomedix Inc.).

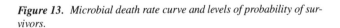

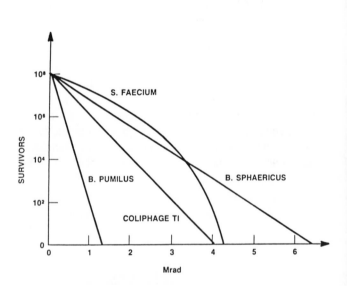

Figure 14. Inactivation curves for various microorganisms.

*One chance in million of contamination is the commonly accepted value of probability for sterile medical implants.

Figure 13. Microbial death rate curve and levels of probability of survivors.

TABLE 14. Sterilizing Doses for Ionizing Radiation

Group	Organisms	Dose Range Mrad
Sensitive	Vegetative Bacteria* Animal Viruses (>75 mμ)	0.05–0.5
Moderately Resistant	*Bacillus Anthracis* (Spores) *Clostridium Sp.* (Spores) Moulds and Yeasts Animal Viruses (20–75 mμ)	0.5–2.0
Resistant	*Bacillus Pumilus* (Spores) *Micrococcus Radiodurans* Animal Viruses (<20 mμ) Bacterial Viruses	2.0–4.0

*Including acid-fast bacilli.

Source: Rubbo, S. D. and J. F. Gardner. *A Review of Sterilization and Disinfection, Year Book.* Chicago:Medical Publishers (1965).

plastic chip, and radiochromic film dosimeters. Generally, measurements are made of the optical density changes that take place in proportion to the absorbed dosage. The radiochromic-type dosimeters are quite small and can conveniently be placed at almost any point within a carrier in a radiation system. In Europe, the general radiation level used is 2.5 Mrad. In the United States, interest has been shown in the possibility of using radiation sterilization doses that are lower than 2.5 Mrad, provided that the product bioburden is sufficiently low. As a result of this approach, levels of 1.5 Mrad or lower are possible for adequately sterilizing medical devices. Some generalizations obtained from recent preliminary field data has shown control of bacteria at 0.5 Mrad, spores at 2.0 Mrad and most resistant spores at 2 to 6 Mrad, as shown in Table 14.

All of which brings us to the concept of bioburden. In this context, the bioburden is the number of microorganisms on a device prior to sterilization. Every manufacturer strives to assemble devices with the lowest possible bioburden; for example, to reach a level of probability of survivors of 10^{-6} (for medical implants), as shown in Figure 13.

The biological effect of ionizing radiation involves special characteristics which need to be known before the optimum conditions of sterilization of a product can be defined. When a microbial culture is submitted to the effect of a radiation, one notices an exponential reduction in the number of germs that survive with respect to the dose received (Figure 14). If we designate by D_{10} the dose which causes the reduction of the microbial population to 1/10 of its initial value, this dose generally depends on the initial contamination.

The exponential reduction of the number of germs makes it impossible to define a dose for absolute sterilization. It is only possible to say that a determined dose brings about a determined reduction for a certain microorganism. Moreover, it is impossible to state that no germ

has survived the treatment; it can be said only that the probability of finding a surviving germ, under controlled conditions, is, for example: 10^{-3} or 10^{-6} (see Table 15). Therefore we are led to the notion of the probability of sterility which can sometimes appear surprising. It must be noted, however, that it is not possible to be sure of sterility. When sterility tests are made on samples, one does not determine whether the batch is sterile or not, but rather a certain probability of sterility for this batch.

If gamma sterilization offers only a certain probability of sterility, it is essential to know if this probability is sufficient, taking into account the intended use of the product, especially if it is comparable with the guarantees offered by other methods. Therefore, it is conceivable that the dose necessary to ensure a satisfactory sterility varies, on the one hand, with the initial contamination and, on the other, with the final use of the product. This is of special interest for the radiosterilization of pharmaceutical products which, at the beginning, are almost germless and to which it is often impossible to give large doses.

As for disposable articles, systematic tests for contamination before sterilization have been carried out in different countries. Satisfactory doses of sterilization determined by bacteriologists vary from 2.5 to 4.0 Mrad. It seems difficult to make an industrial installation of gamma irradiation operate so that the dose distributed varies with the products treated. Most installations in service in the world have been set up so that the minimum dose received by the product is 2.5 Mrad.

Gamma Sterilization of Plastic Medical Devices

Sterilization of plastic medical devices and supplies by ionizing radiation is increasingly being employed as an alternative to EtO sterilization. Ethylene oxide is extremely toxic, is readily absorbed by many polymers and is not always easily or readily desorbed or eliminated.

TABLE 15. Estimates of Probability of Survivors for Sterilized Items

Item	Probability of Survivor/Unit
Canned Chicken Soup[a]	10^{-11}
Large Volume Parenteral Fluid	10^{-9}
Intravenous Catheter and Delivery Set[a]	10^{-6}
Syringe and Needle[a]	10^{-6}
Urinary Catheters[a]	10^{-3}
Surgical Drape Kit[a]	10^{-3}
Small Volume Parenteral Drug (Sterile Fill)	10^{-3}
Laparoscopic Instruments (processed with Liquid Chemical Sterilants)[b]	10^{-2}

[a]Dosimetric Release: No sterility test.
[b]Limits of USP Sterility Test: $10^{-1.3}$ (with 95% confidence).

Source: Bruch, C. W. "Process-Control Release of Terminally Sterilized Medical Devices," in *Sterilization of Medical Products.* E. R. L. Gaughran and R. F. Morrissey, eds. New Brunswick, NJ:Johnson & Johnson, p. 104 (1981).

TABLE 16. Effects of Radiation on Selected Thermoplastic Polymers

Polymer	Radiation Stability	Radiation Dose to Produce Significant Damage (Mrads)	Number of Potential Sterilizations*
ABS (Acrylonitrile–Butadiene–Styrene)	Good	100	M
Acetals	Poor	1–2	0
Acrylics		5	
PMMA (Polymethylmethacrylate)	Fair	5	1
Others	Fair	10	1–2
Amides (Nylons)			
Aliphatic	Fair	50–100	1–2
Aromatic	Excellent	1000	M
Cellulosics	Fair	20	1–2
Fluoropolymers			
PTFE (Polytetrafluoroethylene)	Poor	1	0
PCTFE (Polychlorotrifluoroethylene)	Fair	10–20	1–2
FEP (Fluorinated Ethylene Propylene)	Fair	20	M
PVF, PVF₂, PETFE, PECTFE	Good	100	M
(Polyvinylfluoride), (Polyvinylidine Fluoride),			
(Polyethylene–Tetrafluoroethylene),			
(Polyethylene–Chlorotrifluoroethylene)			
Polycarbonate	Good	100 +	M
Polyesters (Aromatic)	Good	100	M
Polyolefins			
Polyethylene	Good	100	M
Polypropylene	Fair	10	M
Polymethylpentene	Good	30–50	M
Copolymers	Good	50	M
Polystyrene	Excellent	1000	M
Copolymer	Good	100–500	M
Polysulfones	Excellent	1000	M
Polyvinyls			
PVC (Polyvinyl Chloride)	Good	50–100	M
Copolymers	Fair	10–40	1–2

*Sterilization potential of polymers divided into four categories:
    0—nonsterilizable
    1—one procedure
  1–2—somewhat more than one
    M—multiple sterilization possible
This potential is based primarily on the mechanical properties of the polymers and for other reasons, such as optical clarity or gas evolution, the material may not be suitable for the noted number of sterilizations.

Many plastic materials cannot be sterilized by techniques that require heat. Ionizing radiation, therefore, is assuming an increasingly important role in the sterilization of many medical products and, indeed, at this time is becoming a well-established industrial process. Although this technique is not limited to the sterilization of polymeric materials, it is probably the most applicable method for many of these materials.

Polymers discussed in this application are organic materials made up of specific monomers bonded together in multiple repeat units to form a high molecular weight material.

The arrangement of molecules in macromolecules may be very regular or completely random, thus providing zones of potentially high crystallinity or those with little or no apparent crystallinity. The degree of crystallinity is highly dependent, not only on the molecular makeup, but also upon the processing conditions used to form the material.

In addition to the macromolecules themselves, commercial polymer products frequently contain varying amounts of other components to aid in processing, to stabilize the polymer, or to provide particular desirable properties to the product. These additives are generally small molecules which function in the polymer matrix as antioxidants, UV light stabilizers, plasticizers, inert fillers, and processing aids, usually in low concentrations, although some additives acting as fillers or reinforcing agents may be used in quantities from 10 to 70 percent.

The effects of the interaction of ionizing radiation with polymers vary greatly with the basic chemical structure of the polymer. Thus, the dose necessary to produce similar significant effects in two different polymers may vary from values as low as about 4×10^4 rads in polytetrafluorethylene to 4×10^9 rads or more in styrene or polyimides. These interactions, even at low doses, can significantly affect the mechanical and physical properties of the polymer. For instance, in a typical polyethylene with an average molecular weight of about 100,000 and readily soluble in a solvent such as decalin, only one crosslink per 14,000 monomer units can cause gelatin. Radiation effects on the properties of a polymer are often difficult to predict. Certain additives have very distinct protective action in preventing radiation damage to plastics. These compounds are frequently termed "antirads" and usually are materials that also act as antioxidants. The action of these additives can be either that of a reactant which combines readily with radiation-generated free radicals in the polymers, or that of a primary energy absorber, preventing radiation's interaction with the polymer itself.

Radiation generally interacts with polymers in two basic manners, both resulting from excitation or ionization of atoms in the polymer by the high energy source. Alterations in molecular structure of the polymer as a result of these interactions appear as changes in the chemical and physical properties. The two major mechanisms of degradation, or change, occurring as polymers are irradiated are: (1) chain scission, occurring as a random rupturing of bonds which reduce the molecular weight of the polymer and (2) crosslinking of polymer molecules, which results in the formation of large three-dimensional networks. Usually, both of these mechanisms occur as polymeric materials are subjected to ionizing radiation, but frequently one mechanism predominates with a specific polymer. As a result of chain scission, very low molecular weight fragments, gas evolution, and unsaturated bonds may appear. Crosslinking generally results in an initial increase in tensile strength, while impact strength decreases, and the polymer becomes more brittle with increased dose.

For polymers with carbon–carbon chains (backbones) it is observed that crosslinking generally will occur if the carbons have one or more hydrogens attached to them, whereas scission occurs at tetrasubstituted carbons. Polymers containing aromatic molecules generally are much more resistant to radiation degradation than aliphatic polymers. This is true, whether the aromatic group is directly in the chain backbone or not. Thus, both polystyrene (with a pendant aromatic group) and polyimides (with an aromatic group directly in the polymer backbone) are relatively resistant to high doses. From a product/use viewpoint, the loss of mechanical properties is the most important characteristic affected by irradiation of polymers. These properties include tensile strength, elastic modulus, impact strength and shear strength and

also elongation. Embrittlement may occur even as irradiated polymers decrease in hardness. Crystallinity and, therefore, density characteristics, may also change as chain scission continues.

Another consideration resulting from irradiation of polymers is the development of color. This is usually an undesirable development, whether the change results in only yellowing or in complete opacity. These changes, which usually occur at widely differing doses in various polymers, are often influenced by the presence of oxygen and may either diminish or develop with storage after irradiation.

A great deal of the information available from government reports, industrial literature, and scientific publications concerning radiation effects on polymers, deals with their properties after exposure to extremely high doses, and frequently little data are available concerning biomedical polymers in the exposure range of sterilization.

Radiation dose conditions used for sterilization, although varying significantly from process to process or device to device, generally appear to be in the 1 to 5 Mrad range. It is assumed that the effects of radiation on polymers are cumulative with each subsequent exposure.

The conditions of irradiation can significantly affect the properties of the material. The presence of oxygen or air may alter the results of the interaction of radiation with polymers. Free radicals produced in polymers by irradiation in air are often rapidly converted into peroxidic radicals. The fate of these radicals is dependent on both the nature of the irradiated polymer and the presence of additives, and also on other parameters such as temperature, total dose, dose rate and sample size. Conditions may also change the interaction of radiation with polymer additives resulting in gas evolution and formation of other degradation products from these small molecules, with the possibility of producing irritants or other undesirable products.

We will discuss in detail, the effects of radiation on selected thermoplastic polymers listed in Table 16. We begin with ABS (acrylonitrile–butadiene–styrene).

Although ABS materials are less radiation-resistant than styrene or styrene–acrylonitrile polymers, they will withstand one or more radiation sterilization procedures of up to 5 Mrads dose with no observable effect on properties.

POLYACETALS

Homopolymers and copolymers making up the polyacetals are derived from formaldehyde as the primary monomer. Both the copolymers and homopolymers are relatively sensitive to radiation. Radiation doses exceeding 1.0 Mrad appear to cause undesirable changes in these materials and, although they have many desirable properties as structural plastics, they should be used with caution where they may be expected to receive radiation doses in excess of 1 Mrad. The radiation damage threshold is estimated at 0.5 Mrad with 25 percent damage at 1.1 Mrad.

POLYACRYLICS

This important group of materials consists of a number of commercially available polymers and copolymers with a wide range of uses and properties. The most commonly used acrylic polymer, polymethyl methacrylate (PMMA), has relatively poor ionizing radiation resistance. It is certainly capable of withstanding at least one sterilizing radiation procedure in most of its finished product forms without noticeable effect; however, multiple doses in the Mrad range can be expected to affect its mechanical properties significantly. A dose in the 10^7 rad range degrades this polymer to produce an unacceptably brittle product. Perhaps more important, one of PMMA's most desirable properties, optical clarity, is considerably affected. Discoloration may occur at doses as low as 0.5 Mrad, and light transmission can decrease by more than 50 percent after a 5-Mrad exposure. Some recovery of transmission occurs during storage in oil, and certain additives help protect the polymer against radiation damage.

Other acrylic polymers such as polyacrylonitrile, polyacrylates, polyhydroxyacrylates and polycyanoacrylates appear to have somewhat better resistance to radiation than PMMA, but none of these materials should be sterilized by radiation many times.

POLYAMIDES

These polymers, referred to as nylons (in some cases aramids), are among the most commonly used for many applications. The aliphatic polyamides, nylons 6, 66, 6/10, 12, etc., show little difference in their stability to radiation. Nylons of this type generally crosslink under the influence of radiation and initially show increases in tensile strength and hardness, with corresponding decreases in elongation and impact strength. Thus, these materials can readily withstand single radiation sterilization; however, the advisability of multiple sterilizations should be questioned, depending upon the use and the particular polymer.

The aromatic family of polyamides called aramids, although most frequently appearing in fiber form, have very excellent radiation (10^9 rads) and thermal stability and can be expected to retain all their properties after multiple sterilizations by radiation or other techniques.

Most recently some new transparent (amorphous) polyamides have been made available and may be very useful in some applications, but may be expected to be sensitive to multiple sterilizations.

CELLULOSICS

The cellulosic polymers considered in biomedical applications are primarily the cellulose esters (including mixed esters) and cellulose ethers, particularly ethyl cellulose. They exhibit fair radiation resistance and, although their resistance varies considerably from material to material, an average dose value at which significant (~ 25 percent) degradation takes place is, for example, in cellulose acetate, about 20 Mrad. Thus, these materials appear to be able to withstand a limited number of sterilizations without significant effect on their properties.

FLUOROPOLYMERS

Fluorinated polymers, particularly polytetrafluoroethylene (PTFE), are renowned for their chemical stability and their high temperature use characteristics. However, some of these materials are extremely sensitive to radiation and are among the poorest known polymers in terms of radiation stability. PTFE, perhaps the best known and most used of the group, shows significant radiation damage at exposures as low as 0.04 Mrad and is, thus, unsuitable for radiation sterilization. PTFE does not crosslink on irradiation, but instead liberates fluorine atoms which, in turn, react to break carbon–carbon bonds in the polymer, causing severe degradation at low doses.

Other fluoropolymers have somewhat better resistance to radiation. Polychlorotrifluoroethylene (PCTFE) reportedly shows threshold radiation damage at about 1 Mrad and 25 percent damage at 20 Mrad. FEP (copolymer of hexafluoropropene and tetrafluoroethylene) polymer is considerably more radiation resistant than PTFE and can be sterilized satisfactorily. Other fluoropolymers containing carbons with hydrogen, as well as fluorine bonds such as polyvinyl fluoride, polyvinylidene fluoride, and copolymers of ethylene and tetrafluoroethylene (PETFE), show much less sensitivity to radiation (100 Mrad), tend to crosslink on exposure, and are capable of multiple sterilizations by radiation.

POLYCARBONATE

The commercial polycarbonate polymers contain aromatic rings in their main chain structure and, as might be predicted, show quite good resistance to radiation. Their strength is retained well after exposures up to 800 Mrad.

POLYESTERS (AROMATIC)

Aromatic thermoplastic polyesters have been used extensively in structural and biomedical applications in recent years. The most common type of polyester is poly (ethyleneglycolterephthalate) which shows fairly good radiation resistance (25 percent damage at 90 Mrad). Recently, these materials have appeared in a variety of filled and unfilled as well as transparent (amorphous) products that should find many applications in medical devices and packaging. These materials, of course, can withstand radiation sterilizations without significant degradation.

POLYOLEFINS

These materials are among the most widely used and the most economical thermoplastic materials. They are widely used in biomedical applications and packaging. They are divided into broad groups, and one of the most important of the groups, polypropylene, is discussed in detail especially in connection to its response to radiation.

POLYETHYLENE

Polyethylene is produced in differing types known as low density, high density, linear low density and ultrahigh molecular weight varieties by modifying the processes by which the monomer ethylene is polymerized. All forms are reasonably resistant to radiation and can generally withstand doses up to 100 Mrad without a significant change in properties. Polyethylene reacts primarily with ionizing radiation to crosslink the polymer. Recent experiments have measured a value of 0.3 for the ratio of chain scission to crosslinking in irradiated polyethylene, thus indicating that although crosslinking predominates as a mechanism, considerable carbon–carbon bond cleavage also occurs. With irradiation, the average molecular weight increases and the degree of crystallinity decreases. Some mechanical properties such as tensile strength do show change, with slight increases up to about 10 Mrad followed by a gradual decrease. The modulus of elasticity reacts oppositely, first falling, and then increasing, while the impact strength falls continuously after about 50 to 80 Mrad.

POLYPROPYLENE

Polypropylene is a very important polymeric material used in a wide range of biomedical and medical disposables applications. Both chain scission and crosslinking are observed to occur in irradiated polypropylene at about equal levels. This might perhaps be predicted since it has a structure intermediate between polyethylene, which primarily crosslinks, and polyisobutylene (quaternary carbon atom), which degrades largely by scission upon irradiation. Radiation doses, which cause only minor (25 percent or less) degradation to polyethylene, may render polypropylene useless. Even a single sterilization of polypropylene may result in problems that may not develop for a period of time after irradiation.

Because of the potential utility and importance of this polymer in medical applications and because it has been thoroughly studied, the following description is given, detailing the effects of radiation of polypropylene. This account illustrates problems that may result from the interaction of polymers with radiation, although polypropylene is perhaps an extreme example.

In recent years, radiation sterilization of polypropylene has become increasingly important for industrial purposes due to both economic factors and ease of processability. Polypropylene, which is widely used in numerous biomedical products, degrades very readily with irradiation and suffers more than many other thermoplastic materials. Basically, there are two main degradation problems that arise with irradiated polypropylene. First, polypropylene articles will often discolor during irradiation, giving the product an undesirable color tint. The second and more severe problem is the polymer's embrittlement, which begins during irradiation. More importantly, the physical properties continue to deteriorate with time following irradiation, often leaving a product highly embrittled after a few months of normal aging.

Discoloration. It has been found that pure polypropylene does not discolor upon irradiation. However, the stabilizers that are added to improve the polymers thermal and irradiation stability can and often do discolor upon irradiation. In general, irradiation imparts a "yellowish" color to the polymer which is essentially permanent, although there is a slight reduction in intensity with time. The discoloration becomes even more pronounced with dose. This coloration problem is best resolved by avoiding the use of any additives which discolor at sterilizing doses of radiation. However, the more severe problem of polymer degradation during irradiation is not as easily resolved.

Physical Properties. Examination of a polypropylene specimen before and after irradiation indicates that the irradiation sterilization cycle embrittles the substrate. When normal molding-grade polypropylene formulations are used to fabricate syringe barrels or related biomedical products, several additional practical problems emerge which are related to the fundamental irradiation embrittlement of the polymer: flange breakage, luer cracking, and tip breakage. All three classes of mechanical failure after irradiation can be characterized physically by stating that the polymer no longer possesses the elongation characteristics needed to accommodate the normal strains encountered in practice. Consequently, items such as syringe barrels, which will be subjected to considerable stress loads in practice, must also fall within product strength specifications after radiation sterilization.

In summary, the degradation of the polypropylene chain is mainly an auto-oxidative scheme. It is apparent that, if the radical population can be minimized, the possibility of main-chain oxidation occurring can be reduced. Several variables in polypropylene fabrication influence the ultimate free-radical population, and the net effect of these variables on radical stability can be measured by electron spin resonance. The effects of polymer morphology—especially crystallinity—has a very pronounced influence on the radical population and, consequently, the long-term stability of the polypropylene. Although it is not the intent of the current discussion to resolve the irradiation degradation problem, it is important to recognize that potential embrittlement begins with molding techniques and is further magnified by irradiation conditions.

POLYMETHYLPENTENE

This transparent polyolefin material has a number of desirable properties and, although not a great deal of information is known concerning its radiation behavior, it is expected to have stability between that of polyethylene and polypropylene. Information from its manufacturer states, "polymer is stable against electron and gamma radiation, and can be subjected to such radiation, as required by sterilization procedures, without discoloration or embrittlement even on prolonged exposure."

COPOLYMERS

Polyallomers are copolymers of ethylene and propylene and, in some cases, a third monomer. They are relatively crystalline block copolymers which exhibit many of the same properties as polyethylene and polypropylene and, indeed, show some of the best properties of both, such as stress–crack resistance, low brittleness temperature and ease of processing. These copolymers have good radiation resistance with the primary effect being crosslinking and may be multiply sterilized by radiation. Poly(ethylene–vinyl acetate) and poly (ethylene–acrylate) are ethylene copolymers normally containing relatively large ratios of ethylene. Because they are quite stable to radiation (similar to polyethylene), they are suitable for multiple sterilization procedures. Some of these materials, being almost elastomeric in nature, widen the selection of properties available in polyolefin-type polymers.

POLYSTYRENE

This well-known polymer is the most radiation stable of the common and inexpensive molding and extrusion materials. Its properties remain unaffected and gas evolution is insignificant to a higher radiation dose than any other plastic in its class. Its stability is believed to be due to the protective action of the pendant aromatic rings. Crosslinking of styrene occurs almost to the total exclusion of chain scission, and a radiation dose of about 4000 Mrad is necessary to cause significant damage.

Poly(Styrene Acrylonitrile) (SAN). Copolymers of styrene, although not exhibiting the same degree of radiation stability as polystyrene itself, nevertheless have reasonably good resistance and may be expected to withstand multiple sterilizations without damage.

POLYSULFONES

This is a relatively new group of sulfur-containing, aromatic-backbone polymers which, in general, have very promising thermal and radiation resistance properties. There are at least three commercial products available (polysulfone, polyethersulfone and polyphenylsulfone), all of which reportedly can withstand radiation doses of greater than 1000 Mrad without significant damage.

Another similar macromolecule of interest, polyphenylene sulfide, although not a sulfone, is a high-performance sulfur-containing polymer displaying outstanding radiation stability. Technical representatives of the manufacturer report little change in tensile strength and flexural modulus of this material after exposure to 5000 Mrad.

POLYVINYLS

Polyvinyl chloride (PVC) is the most widely used vinyl polymer in medical products and finds application both as a plasticized (flexible) and an unplasticized (rigid) material. PVC is found to crosslink to a considerable extent

TABLE 17. Radiation Sensitivity of Selected Elastomers

Material (Rubbers)	Radiation Threshold Damage Mrads	Dosage 25% Damage Mrads
Polyacrylic	2–4	10–15
Butyl	2–3	10
Chlorosulfonated Polyethylene	—	30
EPDM (Ethylene-Propylene-Diene)	10	100+
Fluoro-	5	50–70
Natural	10	100–200
Nitrile	—	100
Polychloroprene (Neoprene)	6	50
Silicones	—	50–100
Styrene-Butadiene	6–8	100+
Urethane	20	600–800

under irradiation. Its stability to radiation is reported to be very similar to polyethylene—at about 100 Mrad significant damage begins to appear. Plasticizers have some effect on PVC's radiation sensitivity and small amounts of HCL are produced as a result of irradiation. PVC is certainly suitable for single and, in most instances, multiple radiation sterilizations. However, radiation may cause undesirable color changes in some PVC products.

Other Vinyl Polymers. Copolymers of VC, such as vinyl chloride–vinyl acetate, as well as other vinyls, such as polyvinylidene chloride, polyvinylformal and polyvinylbutyral, all appear to be more sensitive to radiation than PVC. Damage with these polymers begins in the range of 1 to 4 Mrad, and 25 percent damage is observed at about 10 to 40 Mrad. Therefore, it is probable that these materials can be used in single sterilization, but may not be suitable for multiple procedures.

There are many additional thermoplastic polymers that have not been mentioned in this review. An attempt was made to include the major families of thermoplastics and the most commonly used polymers in these groups. There are certainly many other potentially useful materials which might be applicable for specific purposes. The radiation sensitivity of polymers not mentioned specifically in this review may be roughly forecast based on the rules set forth earlier in this course and on comparisons of their structures with those of polymers whose irradiation response is known. However, once a specific material is selected for an application, its radiation sensitivity should be determined on prototypes.

So far we have discussed the thermoplastic polymers. Thermosets can be sterilized by gamma radiation without difficulty, so we will not treat them in detail. Just for completeness, thermosets such as phenols, urea formaldehyde, epoxies, unsaturated polyesters and polyimides are highly resistant to gamma radiation, and may be multiply sterilized if desired.

Elastomers (rubbers) represent a large group of polymeric products which have some unique properties quite distinct from those of the thermoplastic and thermoset materials. They have a variety of applications in the area of medical products. Their resistance to radiation varies over a considerable range, although generally not as greatly as with the thermoplastic polymers. Table 17 lists a selected group of elastomers and compares the average radiation resistance of one of each of these types of rubbers. It suggests radiation doses at which threshold damage occurs (at least one physical property begins to change) and values at which about 25 percent damage occurs (represented by a 25 percent change in one property). Although this gives only a brief insight into the radiation stability of these materials, it does permit some selectivity for their use in applications where radiation sterilization may be used.

The values given are only meant to represent averages;

it must be pointed out that fillers and plasticizers used in the formulation of the elastomers can have a very substantial influence on radiation stability. For instance, the addition of aromatic plasticizers to neoprene compositions make these rubbers much more stable to radiation. The partial substitution of phenyl groups for methyl groups in silicone rubbers increases the radiation stability considerably. Most of the elastomers listed, with the possible exception of the first two (polyacrylic and butyl), are certainly capable of being radiation sterilized one or more times.

PACKAGING OF STERILE MEDICAL DEVICES

The prime function of a package containing a presterilized medical item is to ensure that the sterility of the contents is maintained up to the time the package is intentionally opened and that provision is made for the contents to be removed without contamination. Failure to achieve this aim negates the efforts of technologists to control sterilization methods and the standards of sterility that have been set. The recommendation that any sterilization procedure should achieve a statistical probability of not more than one nonsterile article occurring in one million articles processed, loses its practical significance if the package fails to achieve a similar standard. In order to achieve such standards, many factors involved in the design and manufacture of a package must be carefully considered and the major ones are listed as follows:

- suitability of packaging material for the sterilization method
- resistance of the material to bacteria
- strength of package
- type of package
- testing of the package
- type of opening

Although this list of the factors involved is not complete, it probably includes the major ones encountered. These factors have not been listed in any order of importance as this would be extremely difficult. Many of these items are interdependent and, in many instances, failure to overcome one problem will negate the whole package function.

Suitability of Packaging to Sterilization

Although materials suitable for all methods of sterilization are available, care must be taken in selecting the correct material for the sterilization method to be used since each process imposes certain limitations.

The steam process demands adequate air and moisture permeability of material and, because of the high temperatures involved, many thermoplastic materials cannot be used. Nevertheless, certain thermoplastics such as high-density polyethylene, polypropylene, and nylon are suitable. Medical-grade paper is the most widely used material for steam sterilization and is often used in conjunction with heat-resistant plastic materials.

The gas process does not restrict the use of thermoplastic materials because it is carried out at low temperatures, but the permeability of the packaging material is a very important factor. This limitation is often not due to gas penetration but rather air permeability; most gas processes involve vacuum cycles which can impart considerable physical stresses on the package if entrapped air in the package is not easily removed. Because there is no standard gas process in use, it is essential that the packaging material be selected and tested in the cycle for which it is intended.

Radiation sterilization offers the widest choice of packaging materials; high temperatures are not involved so that many thermoplastic materials can be used and, since radiation penetrates all common packaging materials, the permeability factors associated with the steam and gas processes are not relevant. Some materials can be affected, however, such as polypropylene, which can lose strength and discolor, and polyvinylchloride which tends to discolor and yield free hydrochloric acid. Nevertheless, radiation-resistant grades of these polymers are available.

Since no packaging material is a single chemical entity, many materials are available commercially in different chemical forms, although they may be classified as a single product. For example, a common thermoplastic material can contain different plasticizers, stabilizers, and slip additives in various proportions. These small variations may result in different end results when the materials are sterilized. This is further complicated when packaging converters combine basic raw materials in different ways using various adhesives, etc. It is most important, therefore, that guidance be obtained from the packaging manufacturer; preferably the packaging material should be subjected to the sterilization process and thoroughly tested before it is regularly used.

Bacterial Permeabilities of Packaging Materials

A detailed examination of the bacterial permeabilities of packaging materials has not been carried out, probably because of the difficulties of measuring this property under practical conditions. The most important factor affecting bacterial permeability is the frequency and size of pinholes in the packaging material. Ideally, the package material chosen for an application should be completely free of pinholes. Pinholes are frequently found in single-ply materials which should be employed only in thicknesses where the occurrence of pinholes is very remote. Coatings will often effectively fill in pinholes that occur in a base material, and when two plies of material are laminated together, not only will the laminant tend to fill in pinholes but it is also unlikely that pinholes in one ply will occur directly opposite those in another ply to produce a continuous hole.

In theory, only pinholes that are smaller than the smallest known bacterial cell can be tolerated, but in practice this standard may be unnecessary. An investigation [52] using a sizegrading, split-sampler technique of the size distribution of airborne particles carrying various species of bacteria and fungi found in hospital and office premises has shown that most organisms associated with human disease were usually found on particles in the range 4–20 μ equivalent diameter. Many fungi, however, appeared to be present in the air as single spores. There must also be a force to drive organisms through pinholes in a package to render the contents nonsterile. It is well known that paper packages held in humid storage conditions or in direct contact with water stand considerable risk of contamination by bacteria growing through the paper. The use of waterproof packaging materials is, therefore, always to be preferred, and sterile packages should, wherever possible, be stored in dry and good storage conditions, particularly if they are made in any part from uncoated paper. Water is not, however, the only driving force that can promote the passage of bacteria through pinholes in a package. Pressure differences between the inside and outside of a package can cause ingress of airborne bacteria. These pressure differences can be caused by temperature changes, the opening of cupboards and drawers, impact during transport, or simply by handling so that a "bellows effect" is produced.

Therefore, although no standards exist which control the frequency or size of pinholes that can be tolerated in packaging materials, it is important to develop and use techniques for determining pinholes. Also, it is necessary to measure pinholes in packaging materials that have been flexed, abraded, and creased, since these actions can cause pinholes in materials that are pinhole-free when examined in sheet form.

Package Opening and Contents Removal

The weakest link in the sterility chain—from manufacturer to patient—is almost certainly the opening of the package and removal of the contents. It is difficult to assess the degree of contamination that occurs when this exercise is carried out, but reference to some published work can indicate the minimum level that can be expected.

During a series of bacteriological experiments designed to evaluate various wrapping materials and containers for packaging surgical dressings [53], the bacteriological efficiency of the packaging materials was measured by the degree to which its contamination rate exceeded a "blank" or "zero" figure. The "zero" figure was measured by using test swabs contained in tins that had been sterilized in hot air; 518 control swabs were tested and 20 gave positive cultures so that a "zero" contamination rate of 3.8% was obtained for these experiments. A further series of experiments, carried out by three industrial laboratories on the radiation–sterilization of disposable syringes, utilized syringes treated at 10 Mrad for determining the "zero" contamination levels of the laboratories. These "zero" levels were found to be <0.1% in two laboratories and <0.6% in the third, but the authors pointed out that these low figures were achieved by the aid of laminar airflow cabinets and using double packaging of the syringes.

These experiments, since they were carried out by trained bacteriologists, would indicate that in practice it is reasonable to expect that contamination levels in the order of 1–5% can be expected when a singly wrapped product is removed from its package. If this order of contamination is experienced, then the sterilization standard of one in a million, previously mentioned, is largely negated; it is essential, then, that packages be designed with opening devices that enable the product to be removed with the least possible chance of contamination.

For many years it was considered essential by several investigators [54,55] that a sterile article should not be drawn over a nonsterile edge so that cutting or tearing were not methods of opening a flexible package that should be encouraged. Nevertheless, determinations [56,57] indicate that cutting open a package, even with unsterile scissors, offers slight risk in contaminating the sterile products when it is withdrawn. Unfortunately, statistical data to show if the unsterile edge of a cut package is of practical significance are not available. However, if a package is to be cut open, then either sterile or nonsterile scissors must be provided. The provision of sterile scissors for opening every package does not appear to be practical considering the very large number of prepackaged sterile items that are in current use, and it is inconceivable to suggest to a nurse that she may use nonsterile scissors to start a sterile procedure.

Probably the easiest way of opening a flexible package is to provide a method of tearing and this technique has been widely used, particularly for packaged syringes. This method may require the introduction of starting aids such as a notch, but an essential feature for this type of opening to be successful is that the material should have a low degree of stretch on tearing. A tear tape or string incorporated into a package might be considered as a further tearing aid, but such a method inevitably increases the risk of imperfect sealing. An alternative approach is to break the package open by pressing the object through the wall of the package.

Packaging is, therefore, of the same order of importance as the method that is used to sterilize the product. Unfortunately, there is no such thing as a perfect package into which a range of products can be contained. The package requirements for each item must be independently assessed. Many of the problems encountered in selecting and testing a sterile package have been considered in this paper, but it must be recognized that even a perfect package will probably not satisfy the standards that bacteriologists would like to achieve.

Packaging manufacturers can provide a very wide range of materials and package designs suitable for pre-sterilized disposable products. However, the greater assistance of bacteriologists, particularly in the area of opening the package, would help packaging manufacturers ensure that they fully contribute to the main objective of the hospital services and the manufacturers of presterilized medical products—to provide acceptable products which can be used with the highest degree of confidence to the benefit of the patient.

POSTSCRIPT: WHICH SHOULD I USE— RADIATION OR GAS?

Having reviewed the options available to device manufacturers, we must now ask ourselves the $64,000 question: Which should I use? In this section we attempt to summarize some of the key points.

- Gas is basically a surface sterilant. Radiation is basically a volume sterilant; that is, it sterilizes through the item, the inside as well as the outside. This becomes especially important where bacterial migration to the surface may occur, where material may abrade, or where material is punctured.
- Gas depends on the proper environment, especially moisture being present, at the bacterial site. This limits packaging materials to those that will allow air to pass out and gas and moisture to pass in, while maintaining a bacterial barrier. This also limits the complexity of the device which must have all open paths without sealed spaces, plugs or caps.

Radiation requires only that the material be placed in the radiation field for the appropriate length of time. Since the radiation penetrates completely, the product can be packaged in as many barriers as desired and sealed in the final shipping carton. Radiation is insensitive to environment, working well in air or vacuum, dry or moist conditions.

- Resistant strains: gas kills those strains sensitive to its effects and leaves a population of resistant organisms (generally dry spores). This is partly because of technique and partly because of using washed spore strips to monitor unwashed spore kill effects.

Radiation kills all organisms in a measured, predictable

manner. While various strains have differing radio-sensitivity, their lethal dose (LD-90) can be readily and accurately measured. A large number of organisms have already been cataloged by their LD-90.

- Degree of sterility awareness: It is no longer adequate to define sterility as "the absence of microorganisms." In the food industry, with many products coming from the soil, it was quite common to encounter very high bacterial populations (10^6 to 10^8). When these were treated with heat, bacterial reduction of 10^8 or 8-decades (8-D) were common. Reductions of 12-D were sought and were possible, but generally resulted in food being overcooked. Gas "sterilization" of dry products (especially spices) could achieve high D-value reductions, but was often "sterile" only in the relative sense of "less than 1000" survivors. It killed large populations of sensitive organisms, but left a residual of resistant organisms. A typical case of EtO treatment of black pepper with a mixed population starting count of 4×10^7 gives a 5-D reduction to 400 counts. A radiation exposure of 750 kilorads achieves the same effect. But continued radiation further reduces the count while continued gas exposure does not.

With the advent of disposable medical devices, the U.S. used existing gas sterilizers to do the job (while the rest of the industrial world used radiation). But, the cases were different. Medical devices do not have the high initial contamination of food products. In fact, most plastics are initially almost sterile, handled by people in a "peopled" atmosphere. There is no effective way of determining the difference between a "near sterile" item versus a "just past sterile" item. Sterility testing was adopted—applying a statistical basis and sampling techniques to the items tested. Under ideal conditions, this can give a 99 percent confidence level that no more than 1 in 1000 not tested is "nonsterile" or a sterility assurance of 10^3. In actual practice, "sterility testing" generally gives a 95-percent confidence level that no more than 5 percent of a lot is nonsterile.

Since it is not possible to monitor the gas process at the point of bacterial concentration or "the most difficult point," biological indicators became a necessity, but they must challenge the process. With radiation, it is technically only necessary to know the D value of the most resistant strain encountered in the product, and the maximum pre-sterilization concentration. The proper amount of radiation can then be delivered to give any required degree of sterility assurance. The 2.5 megarad exposure often cited, is a 15-D reduction of an indicator species generally recognized as more radiation resistant than any organism encountered in practice. People-related bacteria are generally quite sensitive to radiation. For example, a 2.5 Mrad exposure would achieve a 750-D (10^{750}) reduction in Pseudomonas aeruginosa or a 125-D (10^{125}) reduction in E. coli. Since the radiation process can be monitored and predicted, neither biological indicators nor sterility testing have any value in a real or technical sense. It is because of this facet of irradiation that sterility testing of irradiated devices has been eliminated in other countries.

- Reactions with the product: EtO is a highly reactive gas. It will react with water to form a toxic compound and, since moisture must be present for EtO to kill bacteria, toxic compounds will be formed.

Radiation is not very reactive in the chemical sense. It does produce ionization, which allows reactions to take place. In solids, with a high dielectric constant, or powders, the "ionization" forms charge centers, or "F" centers, which produce an optical color change.

Therefore, *any* product subjected to *any* sterilization procedure should be checked for effect. Any form of primary energy addition (heat, light or radiation) can cause a change of physical properties, and any chemical reaction (EtO) can cause changes in chemical, physical and toxicological properties. It is prudent for every manufacturer to be aware of the effect of all sterilization techniques on his products.

REFERENCES

1 SPAULDING, E. H. "Chemical Disinfection and Antisepsis in the Hospital," *J. Hosp. Res.*, 9:5–31 (1972).
2 SPAULDING, E. H., K. R. Cundy and F. J. Turner. "Chemical Disinfection of Medical and Surgical Materials," In *Disinfection, Sterilization, and Preservation, 1st Edition.* C. A. Lawrence and S. S. Block, eds. Philadelphia:Lea & Febiger, pp. 654–684 (1977).
3 PORTNER, D. W. and R. K. Hoffman. "Sporicidal Effect of Peracetic Acid Vapor," *Appl. Microbiol.*, 16:1782–1785 (1968).
4 HOFFMAN, R. K. and B. Warshowsky. "Beta-Propiolactone Vapor as Disinfectant," *Appl. Microbiol.*, 6:358–362 (1958).
5 ORTENZIO, L. F. "Collaborative Study of Improved Sporicidal Test," *J. Assoc. Off. Anal. Chem.*, 49:721–726 (1966).
6 SPAULDING, E. H. "Principles and Application of Chemical Disinfection," *AORN J.*, 1:36–46 (1963).
7 MINER, N. A. "Viral Hepatitis: Prevention and Control," *Postgrad. Med.*, 60:19–22 (1978).
8 BOND, W. W., N. J. Peterson and M. S. Favero. "Viral Hepatitis B: Aspects of Environmental Control," *Health Lab. Sci.*, 14:235–252 (1977).
9 KLEIN, M. and A. Deforest. "Antiviral Action of Germicides," *Soap Chem. Spec.*, 39:70–72, 95–97 (1963).
10 HEISTER, D., C. H. Shaffer, Jr., M. Hill and L. F. Ortenzio.

"Studies on the A.O.A.C. Tuberculocidal Test," *J. Assoc. Off. Anal. Chem.*, 51:3–6 (1968).

11 WRIGHT, H. S. "Test Method for Determining the Virucidal Activity of Disinfectants Against Vesicular Stomatitis Virus," *Appl. Microbiol.*, 19:92–95 (1970).

12 PRINDLE, R. F. and E. S. Wright. "Phenolic Compounds," In *Disinfection, Sterilization, and Preservation, 1st Edition*. C. A. Larence and S. S. Block, eds. Philadelphia:Lea & Febiger, pp. 401–429 (1968).

13 LAWRENCE, C. A., "Quaternary Ammonium Surface-Active Disinfectants," in *Disinfection, Sterilization, and Preservation, 1st Edition*. C. A. Lawrence and S. S. Block, eds. Philadelphia:Lea & Febiger, pp. 430–452 (1968).

14 BOND, W. W. and M. S. Favero. "*Bacillus Xerothermodurans* Sp. Nov., A Species Forming Endospores Extremely Resistant to Dry Heat," *Int. J. Syst. Bacteriol.*, 27:157–160 (1977).

15 CARSON, L. A., N. J. Petersen, M. S. Favero and S. M. Aguero. "Growth Characteristics of Atypical Mycobacteria in Water and Their Comparative Resistance to Disinfectants," *Appl. Environ. Microbiol.*, 36:839–846 (1978).

16 BOND, W. W., M. S. Favero, N. J. Petersen and J. H. Marshall. "Dry-Heat Inactivation Kinetics of Naturally Occurring Spore Populations," *Appl. Microbiol.*, 20:573–578 (1970).

17 KERELUKK, K. and R. S. Lloyd. "Ethylene Oxide Sterilization," *J. Hosp. Res., American Sterilizer Company*, Erie, Penn. (1969).

18 KAYE, S. and C. R. Phillips. "The Sterilizing Action of Gaseous Ethylene Oxide: IV—The Effect of Moisture," *Am. J. Hygiene*, 50:296, 306 (1949).

19 KAYE, S. "Synergistic Effect of Ethylene Oxide and Other Agents," Symposium on Sterilization Techniques for Instruments and Materials as Applied to Space Research, London:COSPAR (1967).

20 GILBERT, G. L., V. M. Gambill, D. R. Spiner, R. K. Hoffman and C. R. Phillips. "Effect of Moisture on Ethylene Oxide Sterilization," *Appl. Microbiology*, 12(6):496–503 (1964).

21 OPFELL, J. B., J. P. Hohmann and A. B. Latham. "Ethylene Oxide Sterilization of Spores in Hygroscopic Environments," *Science Education, J. Am. Pharm. Assoc.*, 48:617–19 (1959).

22 FREEMAN, M. A. R. and C. F. Barwell. "Ethylene Oxide Sterilization in Hospital Practice," *J. Hyg. (Cambridge)*, 58(3):337–45 (September 1960).

23 CLARKE, C. P., W. L. Davidson and J. B. Johnston. "Hemolysis of Blood Following Exposure to an Australian-Manufactured Plastic Tubing Sterilized by Means of EtO Gas," *Austral. & New Zealand J. Surg.*, 36:53 (August 1966).

24 CUNLIFFE, A. C., F. C. Path and F. Wesley. "Hazards from Plastics Sterilized by Ethylene Oxide," *Brit. Med. Jour.*, (5551):575 (May 1967).

25 O'LEARY, R. K. and W. L. Guess. "Toxicological Studies on Certain Medical-Grade Plastics Sterilized by Ethylene Oxide," *J. Pharm. Sci.*, 57(1):12–17 (January 1968).

26 O'LEARY, R. K., W. D. Watkins and W. L. Guess. "Comparative Chemical and Toxicological Evaluation of Residual Ethylene Oxide in Sterilized Plastics," *J. Am. Pharm. Assoc.*, NS8(4):180 (April 1968).

27 EHRENBERG, L., K. D. Hiesche, S. Osterman-Goldar and I. Wennberg. "Evaluation of Genetic Risks of Alkylating Agents: Tissue Doses in the Mouse from Air Contaminated with EtO," *Mutuation Res.*, 24:83–103 (1974).

28 ROSS, W. C. J. "Chemistry of Cytotoxic Alkylating Agents: IV—1,2-Epoxides," in *Advances in Cancer Research*, by J. P.

Greenstein and A. E. Haddow. N.Y.:Acad. Press, Inc., 1(4):429–35 (1953).

29 GLASER, Z. R. "Ethylene Oxide: Toxicology Review and Field Study Results of Hospital Use," *J. Environ. Pathol. and Toxic.*, 2:173–208 (1979).

30 *Parenteral Solutions Handbook*, Berkeley, Calif.:Cutter Laboratories (1978).

31 *Hospital Supply Index*, Product Analysis 1B:1743, Ambler, Penn.:IMS America, (1983).

32 ERNST, R. R. "Sterilization by Heat," in *Disinfection, Sterilization, and Preservation, 2nd Edition*. H. Block, ed. Philadelphia, Penn.:Lea & Febiger Press, pp. 494–510 (1977).

33 KELNER, A. "Effect of Visible Light on the Recovery of *Streptomyces Griseus Conidia* from Ultraviolet Irradiation Injury, *Proc. Natl. Acad. Sci.*, 35:73–79 (1949).

34 DULBECCO, R. "Photoreactivation," in *Radiation Biology, Volume II*. A. Hollaender, ed. New York:McGraw-Hill, pp. 455–486 (1955).

35 DULBECCO, R. "Experiments on Photoreactivation of Bacteriophages Inactivated with Ultraviolet Radiation," *J. Bacteriol.*, 59:329–347 (1950).

36 KAUFMAN, JOHN E. (ed) "Miscellaneous Applications of Radiant Energy," in *IES Lighting Handbook*. New York:Illuminating Engineering Society, pp. 1–24 (1972).

37 JAGGER, A. "A Small and Inexpensive Ultraviolet Dose-Rate Meter Useful in Biological Experiments," *Radiol. Res.*, 14:394–403 (1961).

38 MPELKAS, C. C. "Germicidal and Short-Wave Ultraviolet Radiation," *Engineering Bull.*, 0-342. Danvers, Mass.:Sylvania Lighting Center (1970).

39 General Electric Company, "Germicidal Lamps," *Bulletin TP-122*, Cleveland (1970).

40 HART, D. "Sterilization of the Air in the Operating Room with Bacterial Radiation," *J. Thorac. Surg.*, 7:525–535 (1938).

41 OVERHOLT, R. H. and Betts, R. H. "Comparative Report on Infection of Thoracoplasty Wounds: Experiences with Ultraviolet Irradiation of Operating Room Air," *J. Thorac. Surg.*, 9:520–529 (1940).

42 HART, D. "Bactericidal Ultraviolet Radiation in the Operating Room. Twenty-Nine-Year Study of Control of Infection," *IAMA*, 172:1019–1027 (1960).

43 ANDERSON, A. A. "New Sampler of Collecting, Sizing and Enumeration of Viable Airborne Particles," *J. Bacteriol.*, 76:471–488 (1958).

44 INAMOTO, H, et al. "Dialyzing Room Disinfection with Ultraviolet Irradiation," *J. Dial.*, 3:191–205 (1979).

45 MATELSKY, I. "Germicidal Lamps in the Pharmaceutical Industry," *Pharm. Int.*, 21:147 (1951).

46 HOSLER, W. W. "Germicidal Ultraviolet Tubes Kept Strong-Cobb Packing Pure," Elec. Prod. Mag., 24:115 (1951).

47 PHILLIPS, G. B. and Novak, F. E. "Application of Germicidal Ultraviolet in Infectious Disease Laboratories: II—Ultraviolet Pass-Through Chamber for Disinfecting Single Sheets of Paper," *Applications in Microbiology*, 4:95–96 (1956).

48 SALALYKIN, V. I., S. A. Lebedeva and D. T. Ostromogolskii. "Sterilization of Urea by Means of Ultraviolet Rays," *Vopr. Neirokhir*, 1:10–11 (1963).

49 HENNICKE, A. "On the Sterilization of Medical Plastic Substances by Ultraviolet Rays," *Strahlentherapie*, 111:626–631 (1960).

50 HUTCHINSON, F. "Molecular Basis for Action of Ionizing Radiation Injury," *Science*, 134:533 (1961).

51 HORNE, T. and B. A. Bridges. "Radiation Microbiology as Applied to Foods," *Int. J. Appl. Radiol.*, 6:100 (1959).

52 NOBLE, W. C., O. M. Lidwell and D. Kingston. *J. Hygiene, Camb.*, 61:385–391 (1963).

53 ALDER, V. G. and F. I. Alder. *J. Clin. Pathol.*, 14:76–79 (1961).

54 HARE, R. P., P. J. Helliwell and R. A. Shocter. *Lancet*, i:774 (1961).

55 CUNLIFFE, A. C. et al. *Lancet*, ii:582–583 (1963).

56 DARMANDY, E. M. et al. "Packaging for Radiosterilization," *Proc. Symp.* UK Panel for Gamma and Electron Irradiation, London (1961).

57 CHRISTENSEN, E. A. J. *J. Danish Hospitals*, 10:107–109 (1970).

CHAPTER 6

Polyvinyl Alcohol as a Biomaterial

A. J. ALEYAMMA[1] and
CHANDRA P. SHARMA, Ph.D.[1]

ABSTRACT: Polyvinyl alcohol (PVA), due to its good biocompatibility and versatility, has found a major position in the hydrogel category of biomaterials. The use of PVA in a variety of biomedical applications, such as blood prosthetic devices, artificial skin and hemodialysis membranes is discussed. From our preliminary studies, it seems that polyelectrolyte modified PVA is a suitable candidate for a hemodialysis membrane, and polyethylene glycol modified PVA is a suitable candidate for an artificial skin.

KEY WORDS: Polyvinyl alcohol, blood prosthetic devices, artificial skin, hemodialysis.

INTRODUCTION

Polyvinyl alcohol is one of the most important hydrogels that has been extensively used in the biomedical field. Hydrogels are polymeric networks (crosslinked structures) which exhibit the ability to swell in water or biological fluids and retain a significant fraction of water within its structure without dissolving. The biocompatibility of hydrogels is attributed to their ability to simulate the natural tissue due to their high water content and their special surface properties. Their low interfacial tension, high permeability to small molecules, and soft and rubbery nature, make hydrogels well-suited candidates for biomaterials. Their major disadvantage is their relatively low mechanical strength. This can be overcome either by cross-linking, by formation of interpenetrating networks, or by crystallization that induces crystallite formation and drastic reinforcement of the hydrogel structure.

PVA is a film-forming, highly hydrophilic water soluble polymer with outstanding chemical stability [1]. For medical purposes, most commonly, it is crosslinked with formaldehyde or glutaraldehyde, rendering insoluble, but water swellable, PVA networks (PVA hydrogels). In recent years, PVA hydrogels have had a wide variety of applications in the biomedical field. Here we give a brief review of some of these applications in biomedical field, including blood contact applications, artificial skin and wound covering, and controlled release devices.

PVA IN BLOOD CONTACT APPLICATIONS

PVA hydrogels, both in their native form and as heparinized materials, have been studied extensively as potential biomaterial for contact with blood. Contact of blood by any surface [2] other than healthy vascular endothelium results in fibrin formation and platelet aggregation. Heparin is the standard anticoagulant used during extracorporeal circulation to prevent thrombosis, but it does allow platelet adhesion to foreign surfaces. In addition, heparin anticoagulates the patient as well as the extra corporeal device and therefore produces a serious risk of hemorrhage.

Ikada et al. [3] observed low protein adsorbability and good blood compatibility with nonannealed PVA. Peppas et al. [4,5] examined the physical and surface properties of PVA hydrogels used in blood compatible applications and studied the importance of surface hydroxyl groups in the heparinization reactions. Although many approaches have been used to prepare blood compatible materials [6], heparinization—ionic or covalent immobilization of heparin to artificial surfaces—has been one of the successful methods. A heparin–PVA hydrogel appears to be the most extensively studied biomaterial. This is useful

[1]Division of Biosurface Technology, Biomedical Technology Wing, Sree Chitra Tirunal Institute for Medical Sciences and Technology, Poojapura, Trivandrum–695012, India

for short-term applications, e.g., AV shunts during surgery. However, exchange occurs between ionically bound heparin and blood components [7–9], making this approach unsuitable for long term implants. Covalent coupling [10,11], while increasing the stability of the heparin, has typically resulted in inactivation of the heparin, producing materials with very limited thromboresistance. Improved blood compatibility has been reported for materials prepared by the covalent coupling of heparin to polyvinyl alcohol through an acetal bridge [12–15].

A heparin–PVA coating procedure has been devised, using a modified form of the acetal bridge technique of Merril and Wong [12,13], to produce thromboresistant materials. In vitro studies show that the immobilized heparin is effective in imparting thromboresistance to the PVA hydrogel (prolonged partial thromboplastin, thrombin, and plasma recalcification times) by accelerating the formation of a surface-bound thrombin-antithrombin III inactive complex in the absence of a significant release of heparin, and by accelerating the creation of a heparin microenvironment [16,17].

Ex vivo studies are also performed with experimental materials [18]. Tubing (1.7 mm i.d.) made from a styrene–butadine–styrene elastomer (SBS) is surface hydroxylated, coated with the heparin–PVA hydrogel and implanted as an acute carotid–jugular arteriovenous (AV) shunt in pigs [18]. However, the patency of these shunts at the relatively high shear rates ($\sim 1000/s$) associated with blood flow is found to be the same as that of identical shunts coated with PVA but without heparin [14]. Fong et al. [19] found that the patency of heparin–PVA coated polyethylene tubing is significantly longer than control tubes (PVA, no heparin) at low flow rates in dogs using a novel parallel flow AV shunt, designed to avoid surgical artifacts.

In a series of publications, Sefton and his associates [20–22] made a detailed study of heparinized PVA and elucidated the mechanisms of cross-linking and heparinization. Protein or platelet adsorption on these materials has also been reported [23–25].

Recent studies have demonstrated that a PVA hydrogel prepared by glutaraldehyde cross-linking (with or without heparin) is reactive towards platelets in a chronic canine arteriovenous shunt, when blood flows for extended periods of time [25]. Several approaches have been taken toward solving this problem. In one attempt, Sefton et al. [27] immobilized a monoaldehyde terminated PEG-6000 onto PVA, but observed little effect on protein adsorption and platelet consumption. Llanos et al. [28] initiated a pilot study on the incorporation of antiplatelet agents, e.g., prostaglandin, onto the PVA hydrogel. They demonstrated the feasibility of immobilizing compounds other than heparin to the PVA hydrogel. However, they neither demonstrated that the immobilized prostaglandin retained its biological activity nor that there is a beneficial effect toward platelets [29].

In an attempt to increase the blood compatibility of PVA, we have developed [29] a blend of polyvinyl alcohol and a heparinoid polyelectrolyte. In vitro evaluation of this membrane by platelet adhesion studies demonstrated a reduction in the number of adhered platelets [29].

Modifications leading to antithrombogenicity of PVA are in progress. We have developed a polyvinyl alcohol–polyethylene glycol blend (PVA–PEG) making use of the nonthrombogenic character of PEG (unpublished work). Further studies are being planned to evaluate the blood compatibility aspects of this blended membrane.

PVA in Hemodialysis Devices

A number of efforts to use PVA membranes in artificial kidneys have been presented, but cellulosic membranes continue to be the material of choice in dialysis. Limited studies of the use of PVA in hemodialyzers have been reported by M. Luttinger et al. [30]. These studies demonstrated that the dialyzing characteristics of the commercial PVA films are promising with respect to urea and uric acid, but somewhat slower than the cellulosics with respect to creatinine.

We have developed [29] a dialysis membrane from PVA using paraformaldehyde as cross-linking agent, curing at room temperature for 48 hours. Mechanical properties are satisfactory that a dry membrane experiences a tensile modulus (at a relative humidity of 90% at room temperature) of 488 kg/cm^2, along with its high elastic nature (288% elongation at break). The permeabilities of various solutes (e.g., urea, creatinine, uric acid, inulin and albumin) through these membranes were evaluated using a mixture of the above, prepared in phosphate buffer of pH = 7.4. Superior permeability characteristics, in comparison to cellulosic materials currently being used, were obtained with PVA membrane (Table 1). Plasma proteins such as albumin were almost excluded from the gel matrix indicating that the gel was fairly cross-linked [29].

PVA–Polyelectrolyte Blended Membrane

Beugeling et al. [31] observed good anticoagulant activity with a synthetic polyelectrolyte (PE) having sulfamate and carboxylate groups, which can be used as a substitute for heparin. Recent studies show that this polyelectrolyte derived from natural rubber is very effective in modifying polymeric substrates [31–33]. We have developed [29] a PVA–PE blended membrane without affecting its permeability and mechanical properties significantly. This membrane has demonstrated a reduced platelet surface attachment. A PVA–PE blend in the ratio 100:10 is selected as the more suitable formulation (least platelet adhesion). A PVA membrane surface modified with polyelectrolyte via Co^{60} γ-irradiation is also found to be an effective membrane [29].

The effect of sterilization on these membranes was stud-

TABLE 1. Permeability (%) of Various Molecules through Modified and Bare PVA Membranes

Molecule	Membrane[a]	% Passed[b]			
		1 hr	2 hrs	4 hrs	6 hrs
Urea	1.	32.9 ± 2.2	43.1 ± 3.1	49 ± 2.8	58.1 ± 3.5
	2.	34.7 ± 1.5	42.8 ± 1.1	47.7 ± 2.9	56.3 ± 2.6
	3.	34.5 ± 3.8	44.4 ± 1.7	48.1 ± 3.8	56.6 ± 2.6
	4.	36.5 ± 1.9	42.4 ± 4.7	51.4 ± 0.5	53.9 ± 1.7
	5.	21.7 ± 0	32.8 ± 0.8	46.2 ± 0.9	53.2 ± 2.5
Creatinine	1.	27.6 ± 1.6	36.2 ± 2.5	44.2 ± 2.2	49.2 ± 2.8
	2.	26.7 ± 1.8	36.7 ± 1.4	44.3 ± 1.2	43.2 ± 1.5
	3.	27.0 ± 2.2	34.3 ± 1.6	41.5 ± 2.4	47.4 ± 0.7
	4.	28.4 ± 1.9	42.1 ± 2.6	45.6 ± 2.3	50.0 ± 0.53
	5.	16.9 ± 0.6	19.8 ± 0.7	31.5 ± 1.5	43.5 ± 0.7
Uric Acid	1.	14.0 ± 1.2	27.4 ± 2.0	35.1 ± 1.5	42.2 ± 2.5
	2.	14.9 ± 1.9	28.5 ± 1.7	39.6 ± 0.5	40.9 ± 1.3
	3.	15.2 ± 1.1	26.9 ± 0.8	36.1 ± 3.3	40.5 ± 2.2
	4.	21.3 ± 3.3	31.7 ± 1.3	37.4 ± 1.3	40.5 ± 1.5
	5.	5.3 ± 1.1	12.3 ± 1.2	21.2 ± 1.2	33.5 ± 0.5
Albumin	1.	0	0	1.4 ± 0.4	2.8 ± 0.6
	2.	0	2.5 ± 0.2	0	0.65
	3.	0	0	0	0
	4.	0	0.36 ± 0.5	2.0 ± 1.1	3.2 ± 0.48
	5.	0.79 ± 0	0	1.40 ± 0.1	2.6 ± 0.5

[a]1. Bare PVA [29].
2. PVA–polyelectrolyte blend (in the ratio 100:10 [29]).
3. Surface modified PVA [29].
4. PVA–PEG
5. Standard cellulose acetate [29].
[b]Values expressed as mean ± standard deviation.

ied, and Co^{60} γ-irradiation seems to be the best method [29]. Glutaraldehyde treatment is also effective. However, greater attention is needed to remove any traces of glutaraldehyde before use.

PVA–PEG Blended Membrane

In recent years several research groups have found that polyethylene glycol (PEG) in different forms is relatively inert toward biological species. These forms include PEG in free homogeneous solution, adsorbed onto substrate, grafted onto polymer surface and formed into networks. George [34] reported that platelets did not adhere to glass surface treated with PEG when suspended in plasma or serum. Wasiewski et al. [35] observed reduced thrombin adsorption on PEG surface. PEG has been used as a concentrator of plasma proteins in blood [36], suggesting it is inert toward plasma proteins. Several studies involving networks, thus hydrogels, containing PEG have been reported [37,38]. On the basis of these studies, it appears that the use of PEG and PEG-containing materials for blood interfacing applications is a promising approach toward reducing the adhesion of blood components. PVA modified with a PEG-6000 exhibits permeability characteristics which are not altered significantly from those of bare PVA. A slight reduction in mechanical properties is observed. However, the resulting properties are quite satisfactory (tensile modulus = 422 kg/cm² ± 37.5 and

percentage elongation at break = 217 ± 23.2). Here, also, Co^{60} γ-irradiation seems to be the best method of sterilization.

POLYVINYL ALCOHOL SPONGE (IVALON)

A polyvinyl alcohol sponge known as Ivalon was developed in 1949 [39] as a plombage after pneumonectomy in dogs. Since then, it has been extensively utilized by surgeons for a variety of applications. A review of this material was presented by Boretos [40]. Ivalon is white, odorless and porous, with pore size of 0.1–4 mm. The moistened foam is supple, hygroscopic, can be compressed up to ratios of about 16:1 and has a high tensile strength. This was investigated for a wide variety of tissue reconstructions.

Ivalon was used in cardiac surgery to bridge septal defects and to support incompetent valves. Benjamin et al. [41] repaired congenital septal defects in animals using Ivalon and combinations of Ivalon–nylon and Ivalon–Teflon. PVA sponge [42,43] was used to repair the heart valve cusps and supports for sutures to draw the valves into close approximation. The use of Ivalon sponges as minor components or linings of the mechanical heart systems were studied by Harrison [44]. Evaluation of this material from the toxicity point of view has led to inconclusive results [45].

In vascular surgery, PVA sponge has been used as a venous prothesis to revascularize the tissue by providing channels for collaterial circulation [46]. Crowford et al. [47] used the sponge for arterial prothesis but found that it rapidly became brittle.

Ivalon was extensively studied as an artificial skin [48–54]. Chardack et al. reported the use of microporous sponge for preparing a fresh granulated wound bed for autografting [50–52] (see section on PVA as an Artificial Skin also). Initial studies were favorable, but further clinical studies [53,54] limit the use of Ivalon for this purpose, and Ivalon currently is not used as artificial skin. When used as a short-term temporary skin dressing [55], regularly removed PVA sponge cleanses wounds, stimulates granulation tissue and reduces bacterial colonization of the wound. This is due to high fluid absorption and strong adherence to the wound surface, especially in infected wounds. Furthermore, PVA sponge can be soaked with antiseptic solutions, facilitating the treatment of granulating surfaces, infected wounds and infected open fractures.

In plastic surgery, Ivalon has been used for various types of subcutaneous implants. The use of PVA sponge [56] in the repair of complete anorectal prolapse is well established and widespread. The investigation of Ivalon as a surgically implanted breast prothesis was not at all successful. There was evidence of tissue infiltration, loss of resilience [57], unavoidable infection [58], and excessive shrinkage with time.

PVA sponge was successful as a tantalum mesh for the repair of hernias [59–61]. Dailey et al. [62] used PVA sponge as a filler for pulmonary post-resection spaces with over five years of successful implant experience recorded. Taking advantage of the natural growth of adhesions around PVA sponge, a treatment was developed for ascites of the liver secondary to cirrhosis [63]. Bergan et al. [64] attempted to develop a bile duct replacement by epithelialization of the synthetic tube. Unfortunately, their expectations were short–lived. Middle ear tympanoplasty to restore conductive hearing loss was evaluated using PVA sponge [65], but there was greater foreign body reaction to the PVA sponge than to other materials tried.

In orthopedic surgery, PVA sponge has been investigated as a synthetic scaffold [66] for new bone growth. However, encapsulation by scar tissue limits the possible ingrowth of bone [66]. The sponge has also been reported to aid in the reconstruction of knee joints and can be used as an interposition membrane to prevent adhesions [67,68].

Extensive clinical experience has revealed many negative properties such as loss of tensile strength and a tendency to become brittle in vivo [69]. For example, invascular grafts this led to early rupture and later to aneurysms. Uncompressed sheets of PVA showed a tendency towards fragmentation and dissolution, and therefore had little value as supporting prostheses. PVA implants were not tolerated in the presence of infection. Further, progressive calcification occurred over a 7½ month study, with extensive fibrous tissue ingrowth. Finally, too little effort was made to control the fabrication and storage of PVA. As a result of these factors, Blumberg et al. [69] stated that PVA was far from ideal as a prosthetic material, and in the 1960's, clinical use of Ivalon material in human cases was largely abandoned. However, because of the early work with PVA sponge, valuable knowledge and experience in the quest for satisfactory surgical implants had been gained.

PVA AS AN ARTIFICIAL SKIN

Special dressing and artificial skin have long been of interest to hospitals searching for a means to overcome the development of scar tissue and loss of body fluids in cases of severe and extensive burns and wounds [70]. In the early sixties, Chardack reported extensively [49–53] on the use of the Ivalon sponge. Clinical experience initially suggested success in terms of preparing a fresh granulating wound bed for autografting. By virtue of its hydrophilic character, water loss could be maintained at a satisfactory level. However, it was discovered from further clinical studies that autograft-taking was poor in the majority of cases. Biopsies of the underlying tissue immediately after removal of the Ivalon sheets showed embedded fragments of Ivalon impurities. Another factor mitigating against the use of Ivalon is that it is rigid when dry. Therefore, Ivalon has fallen from favor and currently finds no use in autografting.

Mutschler et al. [54] used a PVA–formaldehyde foam as a skin cover for burns and infected wounds in pigs. Macroscopic, histological and bacteriological examination over a period of 18 days after application of PVA showed better wound cleansing, significantly reduced bacterial flora, and more rapid growth of the epithelium than do other materials used as skin covers.

Collagen has been used by various workers for the development of artificial skin, due to its cell binding characteristics and fast wound healing properties [70,71]. Albuminated substrates have been found to encourage normal tissue growth [72]. We have used a combination of albumin and collagen onto PVA for developing artificial skin [73]. The biological inertness of polyethylene glycol (PEG) is well known [33–35] and has been demonstrated by many investigators. Considering this evidence, we have tried a PVA–protein coated and PVA–PEG blend with protein coatings on rabbits and guinea pigs, respectively [73]. These were used to treat excised wound beds of animals by grafting them on full thickness wound beds of 1.5 cm × 3 cm area.

The experimental results [73] with rabbits were not satisfactory. Neither protein coated PVA nor bare PVA showed any effect on the enhancement of wound healing. Furthermore, infection could not be controlled properly. This is probably due to the use of gluteraldehyde for sterilization, because the hydrophilic PVA can absorb excess glutaraldehyde. PVA–PEG samples (γ-irradiation sterilized, with and without protein modification) tested on guinea pigs demonstrated quite promising results. Fast wound healing was achieved and no infection was observed [73].

The period of time taken for complete closure of the wound when treated with a PVA–PEG blend is given in Table 2.

PVA AS A CONTROLLED-RELEASE SYSTEM

Controlled release systems represent a relatively new development that evolved out of a continuing need for prolonged and better-controlled drug administration. Each drug has a therapeutic range above which it is toxic and below which it is ineffective. Maintaining the appropriate plasma drug concentration in any patient at a particular time depends on the patient's compliance with the prescribed routine. This is particularly problematic if the toxic and minimum effective levels are close together. The goal of a controlled-release system is to ensure that the drug concentration remains in the therapeutic range for a prolonged time using a single dosage form.

PVA hydrogel was one of the materials studied for potential controlled-release applications [15,16,74]. Swellable, controlled-release systems may be prepared by a variety of techniques. Details of these experimental techniques have been presented by Korsmeyer et al. [75,76] and Gander et al. [77].

Colombo et al. [78] used PVA based systems which were coated with a thin layer of PVA cross-linked by UV irradiation.

Korsmeyer et al. [75,79] reported PVA based controlled-release devices, using theophylline as a model drug. These devices were prepared by forming a 10% aqueous solution of PVA and adding a cross-linking agent such as glutaraldehyde. The cross-linking reaction was performed on flat surfaces at room temperature for 48 hours. Slabs of $2 \times 2 \times 0.2$ cm were cut and tested for swelling kinetics. Theophylline was incorporated either during the

TABLE 2. Wound Healing Pattern of Modified PVA When Implanted in Guinea Pigs

Sample	Sterilization method	Time taken for complete wound closure, days[a]
1. PVA. PEG blend [A]	γ-irradiation	57.24 ± 9
2. [A] + Collegen + Albumin	γ-irradiation	48.3 ± 5.9

[a]Each value expressed as mean ± standard deviation of 3 animals (6 wounds).

crosslinking process or after preparation of the cross-linked polymers by soaking the slabs in a concentrated aqueous solution of theophylline. Typical release rates showed that the initial drying process and crosslinking affect the mechanism and amount of drug released.

Langer and Folkman [80] reported a PVA system that can release macromolecules such as polypeptides, e.g., soyabean trypsin inhibitor with molecular weight 21,000. These systems show release times from a few days to a week, and have proved useful in releasing a variety of different polypeptide growth factors and in greatly facilitating a variety of biological studies.

PVA matrixes have been used in neuroscience studies. Mayberg and coworkers [81] developed a method to actually coat PVA containing the histochemical agent, horseradish peroxidase, onto blood vessels. The enzyme was continuously and directly released into brain blood vessels for at least one day. Moskowitz [82] and coworkers then used this technique to trace the prevascular meningeal projections from trigeminal ganglia. This led to an understanding of how headaches occur.

In an effort to render the employed preparative techniques to current pharmaceutical technology, Korsmeyer et al. [83,84] attempted to prepare blends of hemopolymers by compression of granular polymers. Compressed systems of PVA, polyvinyl pyrrolidone, polyethylene glycol, and their mixtures were prepared and KCl, phenyl propanolamine, and bovine serum albumin were used as model drugs of widely varying molecular size. Zero-order release was achieved with a compressed PVA controlled-release system over a period of 15 hr. Similarly, Gander et al. [75] attempted to shift this technology toward the formation of swelling controlled-release microparticles, using cross-linked PVA. By studying the release behavior of proxyphylline from these systems, they showed that the method of incorporation of the drug may, in some situations, make a significant difference in the mechanism and level of release.

OTHER BIOMEDICAL APPLICATIONS OF PVA

Replacement of Articular Cartilage

The articular cartilage of the synovial joint is a 1–2 mm thick covering of the opposed bony faces of the joint. This cartilage aids in absorbing force and reducing friction between the surfaces of the bones [85]. The cartilage contains 70 to 80% synovial fluid. The dry weight contains collagen (45 to 60%) and chondroitin sulfate (15 to 25%). The cartilage has a low water permeability, and the pore structure has an average radius of 62 Å. It is a rather hard material with a tensile modulus of 0.58 Mpa. Semicrystalline PVA hydrogel has been used as one of the "natural" materials for articular cartilage replacement [86].

Bray and Merril [86] used amorphous PVA networks of varying degrees of cross-linking, produced by electron beam irradiation of aqueous PVA solutions, to prepare semicrystalline hydrogels upon heat treatment (crystallization) at 90°C. The tensile moduli of these materials varied from 0.19 to 4.68 Mpa. These hydrogels were further grafted with the reagents to obtain material with surface charge densities of 1 meq/g PVA. Peppes [85] used a modified technique to obtain pseudocomposite PVA hydrogels. These materials were made by crystallization of relatively thick hydrogel films at 160 to 200°C for 15 minutes to 1 hour. During this process only the outer layers of the hydrogels crystallized (with degrees of crystallinity up to 29% on a swollen basis), whereas the center of the films remained predominantly amorphous (crystallinity lower than 5%). Thus, improved tensile moduli were determined (as high as 62 Pa), whereas the high water content in the center provided the weeping lubrication characteristics necessary in cartilage use.

Artificial Pancreas Applications

Exogenous administration of insulin in patients suffering from diabetes mellitus is possible by a variety of devices. Hydrogels have been used as membranes in insulin pumps or as carriers for β-cells [87]. A. M. Sun et al. [87] developed a bioartificial pancreas consisting of living pancreatic islets of Langerhans cultured on the outside surface of semipermeable tubular membranes. A major drawback to practical application of the device has been the necessity of preventing blood coagulation inside the fiber by a high dosage of circulating anti-coagulants. This problem was lessened, although not eliminated, by coating the inner surface of the semipermeable fiber with a thromboresistant heparin–PVA film. Devices with heparinized, 0.5 mm inner diameter fibers remained patent for 2, 3, 5 or 6 days in pancreatectomized monkeys before thrombosis at the anastomosis caused occlusion of the hollow fiber.

PVA Membranes for Plasmapheresis

Plasmapheresis is a technique of separation of plasma from whole blood, which has become quite popular in clinical applications in recent years. PVA membranes [88,89] were found to have significantly higher hydraulic permeability and almost double the plasma flux of other membranes.

PVA–Contact Lens Applications

A number of uses of PVA as a contact lens material have been reported [90,91], although PVA hydrogels have not been as successful as PHEMA because of their high water content (when amorphous) or their poor optical properties (when semicrystalline). However, copolymers of PVA containing HEMA have been better candidates for contact lens applications [92].

PVA in Reconstruction of Vocal Cords

Injection of polymer solutions or suspensions onto vocal cords has been used as a method to correct certain vocal cord impairments [93]. Peppas et al. [94,95] developed a method of intracordal injection of aqueous PVA solutions and in situ gelation using stoichiometric quantities of glutaraldehyde as a cross linking agent. The material of choice is a PVA hydrogel with average molecular weight = 7426, cross-linked in situ within 17 minutes and exhibiting a modulus of approximately 0.04 MPa, an ultimate tensile strength of 0.035 MPa and an elongation at break of 125%. This material does not exhibit the undesirable effects and tissue reactions that have been reported [96] for PVA sponge implants.

CONCLUSION

It seems that PVA is a highly competitive material in the biomedical field. As discussed above, most reports concerning the short-term bio-compatibility of PVA implants mention a relatively mild foreign-body reaction. Further modifications of this material are required to exploit it for a wide range of long-term applications in the biomaterial field.

ACKNOWLEDGEMENTS

We appreciate the help received from Mr. K. Rathinam and Mrs. R. S. Jayasree for artificial skin evaluation. This work was funded by DST and ICMR, India. We are also thankful to Dr. Thomas Chandy for his assistance during the preparation of this paper.

REFERENCES

1 PETER, S., N. Hese and R. Stefan. *Desalination*, 19:161 (1976).
2 MARMUR, A. and S. L. Cooper. *J. of Colloid and Inter. Sci.*, 89:458–465 (1982).
3 IKADA, Y., H. Iwata, F. Horri, et al. "Blood Compatibility of Hydrophilic Polymers," *J. Biomed. Mater. Res.*, 15:697–718 (1981).
4 PEPPAS, N. A. and E. W. Merrill. "Development of Semicrystalline PVA Networks for Biomedical Applications," *J. Biomed. Mater. Res.*, 11:423 (1977).
5 PEPPAS, N. A. and T. W. B. Gehr. "New Hydrophilic Copolymers for Biomedical Applications," *Trans. Am. Soc. Artif. Intern. Organs*, 24:404 (1978).
6 RUCKENSTEIN, E. and R. Srinivasan. "The Origin of Platelet Deposition—Is It Kinetic or Thermodynamic," *J. Biomed. Mater. Res.*, 16:169–172 (1982).

7 BAIER, R. E. "Cell Adhesion to Biomaterials Surfaces: Conflicts and Concerns," *J. Biomed. Mater. Res.*, 16:173–175 (1982).

8 NEUMAN, A. W., O. S. Hum, D. W. Francis, W. Zingg and C. J. Van Oss. "Kinetic and Thermodynamic Aspects of Platelet Adhesion from Suspension to Various Substrates," *J. Biomed. Mater. Res.*, 14:499–509 (1980).

9 RUCKENSTEIN, E., A. Marmur and S. R. Rakower. "Sedimentation and Adhesion of Platelets onto a Horizontal Glass Surface," *Thromb. Haemostas.*, (Stuttgart) 36:334–342 (1976).

10 SRINIVASAN, R. and E. Ruckenstein. "Kinetically Caused Saturation in the Deposition of Particles or Cells," *J. Colloid Interface Sci.*, 79:390–398 (1981).

11 ABSOLOM, D. R., C. J. Van Oss and A. W. Neumann. "Elution of Human Granulocytes from Nylon Fibres by Means of Repulsive Van der Waals Forces," *Transfusion*, 21:663–674 (1982).

12 VAN OSS, C. J., R. D. Absolom and A. W. Neumann. "Repulsive Van der Waals Forces II. The Mechanism of Hydrophobic Chromatography," *Sep. Sci. Technol.*, 14:305–317 (1979).

13 VAN OSS, C. J., D. R. Absolom, A. L. Grossberg and A. W. Neumann. "Repulsive Van der Waals Forces I. Complete Dissociation of Antigen-Antibody Complexes," *Immunol. Commun.*, 8:11–29 (1979).

14 HAVANEC, D. L., D. R. Absolom, C. J. Van Oss and E. A. Gorzynski, "The Relationship to Coagulation of Immunoglobin Class Dissociated from Escherichia Coli-Antibody Complexes," *J. Clin. Microbiol.*, 12:608–609 (1980).

15 VAN OSS, C. J., D. Beckers, C. P. Engelfriet, D. R. Absolom and A. W. Neumann. "Elution of Blood Group Antibodies. I Red Cell Antibodies," *Vox Sang*, 40:367–371 (1981).

16 GOOSEN, M. F. A., M. V. Sefton. "Properties of a Heparin–Poly (vinyl Alcohol) Hydrogel Coating," *J. Biomed. Mater. Res.*, 17:359–373 (1983).

17 BASMADJIAN, D. and M. V. Sefton. "Relationship Between Release Rate and Surface Concentration for Heparinized Materials," *J. Biomed. Mater. Res.*, 17:509–518 (1983).

18 SEFTON, M. V. and W. Zingg. "Patency of Heparinized SBS Shunts at High Shear Rates," *Biomat. Med. Dev. Artif. Org.*, 9:127–142 (1981).

19 WAN FONG, I. P., Walter Zingg and M. V. Sefton. "Parallel Flow Arteriovenous Shunt for the Ex Vivo Evaluation of Heparinized Materials," *J. Biomed. Mater. Res.*, 19:161–178 (1985).

20 GOOSEN, M. F. A., M. V. Sefton and M. W. C. Hatton. "Inactivation of Thrombin by Antithrombin III on a Heparinized Biomaterial," *Thromb. Res.*, 20:543 (1980).

21 GOOSEN, M. F. A. and M. V. Sefton. "The Fate of Surface Bound Heparin," in *Biomaterials: Interfacial Phenomena and Applications, Vol. 199*, S. L. Cooper, N. A. Peppas, A. S. Hoffman and B. D. Ratner, eds. *Advances in Chemistry Series*, Washington, D.C.:ACS, p. 147 (1982).

22 SEFTON, M. V. et al. "The Thromboresistance of a Heparin-PVA Hydrogel," *Chem. Eng. Commun.*, 30:141 (1984).

23 HATTON, M. W. C., G. Rollason and M. V. Sefton. *Thromb. Hemost.*, 50:873 (1983).

24 ZUCKER, M. B. "Heparin and Platelet Function," *Fed. Proc. Fed. Am. Soc. Exp. Biol.*, 36:47 (1977).

25 LINDON, J. et al. "Interaction of Human Platelets with Heparinized Gel," *J. Lab. Clin. Med.*, 91:47 (1978).

26 CHOLAKIS, C. H. Ph.D. Thesis, University of Toronto (1987).

27 SEFTON, M. V. and G. Llanos. "Immobilization of Polyethylene Glycol onto a Poly Vinyl Alcohol Hydrogel for Reduced Platelet Reactivity," *Trans. Society. Biomaterial*, 11:21–25 (April 1988).

28 LLNOS, G. and M. V. Sefton. "Immobilization of Prostaglandin PGF$_{2\alpha}$ on Poly Vinyl Alcohol," *Biomaterials*, 9:429 (1988).

29 ALEYAMMA, A. J. and C. P. Sharma. "Poly Vinyl Alcohol-Polyelectrolyte Blended Membranes: Blood Compatibility and Permeability Properties," submitted to *Progress in Biomedical Polymers*, Charles G. Gebelein, ed. ACS Symposium Series (1988).

30 LUTTINGER, M. and C. W. Cooper. "Improved Hemodialysis Membranes for the Artificial Kidney," *J. Biomed. Mater. Res.*, 1:67 (1967).

31 BEUGELING, T., L. Van der Does, A. Bantjes and W. L. Sederel. *J. Biomed. Mater. Res.*, 8:375 (1974).

32 LUNDELL, E. O., G. T. Kwiatkowski, J. S. Byck, F. D. Osterholtz, W. S. Creasy and D. O. Stewart. in *Hydrogels for Medical and Related Application*, Joseph and Andrade, eds. ACS Symp., 31:305 (1976).

33 SHARMA, C. P. and K. Ajanta. *Trans. Soc. Biomaterials*, 10:100 (1988).

34 GEORGE, J. N. *Blood*, 40:862 (1972).

35 WASIEWSKI, W., M. J. Rasco, M. B. Martin, J. C. Detwiler and J. W. Fenton. "Thrombin Adsorption to Surfaces and Prevention with Poly Ethylene Glycol 6000," *Thromb. Res.*, 8:881 (1976).

36 FRIED, M., and P. W. Chun. in *Methods in Enzymology*, New York:Academic Press, 22:238 (1971).

37 LYMAN, D., B. Loo and R. Crawford. "New Synthetic Membranes for Dialysis I. A Copolymer–Ester Membrane System," *Biochemistry*, 3:985 (1964).

38 LYMAN, D. "New Synthetic Membranes for Extracorporeal Hemodialysis," *Ann. N.Y. Acad. Sci.*, 146(1):113 (1968).

39 SORENSEN, W. R. in *Encyclopedia of Mate. Sci. and Engg.*, Michael B. Bever, ed. 5:3809 (1986).

40 BORETOS, JOHN W. "Cellular Polymers for Medical Use. The Vital Role of Porosity and Permeability," *Cellular Polymers*, 3:345–358 (1984).

41 BENJAMIN, R. W. et al. "The Gradual Closure of Interfacial Defects," *J. Thorac. Surg.*, 34:679 (1967).

42 LILLEHEI, C. W. et al. "Surgical Correction of Pure Mitral Insufficiency by Annulo Plasty Under Direct Vision," *Lancet*, 77:446 (1957).

43 BARNARD, C. W. et al. "Ivalon Baffle for Posterir Leaflet Replacement in the Treatment of Mitral Insufficiency: A Follow-up Study," *Surgery*, p. 727 (1968).

44 HARRISON, J. H. *Am. J. Surg.*, 95:3 (1958).

45 AKUTSU, T. and A. Kantrowifz. "Problems of Materials in Mechanical Heart Systems," *J. Biomed. Mater. Res.*, 1:33 (1967).

46 PIFARRE, R. et al. "Experimental Evaluation Epicardiectomy and Ivalon Sponge Operation for the Treatment of Coronary Artery Disease," *J. Thorac. Cardiovas. Surg.*, 48:465 (1964).

47 CRAWFORD, E. S. et al. "Clinical Use of Synthetic Substitutes in 317 Patients," Arch. Surg., 76:261 (1958).

48 CHARDACK, W. M., C. E. Day, G. Fazekas, N. Minsley, *J. Trauma.*, 1:54 (1961).

49 CHARDACK, W. M., D. A. Brueske, A. P. Santomauro, G. Fazekas. *Ann. Surg.*, 155:127 (1962).

50 CHARDACK, W. M. *Milt. Med.*, 127:335 (1962).

51 CHARDACK, W. M., M. M. Martin, T. C. Jewett and B. E. Boyer. *Plast. Reconstr. Surg.*, 30:554 (1962).

52 JEWETT, T. C. and W. M. Chardack. *Amer. J. Surg.*, 106:24 (1963).

53 MARTIN, M. M. and B. E. Boyer. *J. Trauma*, 3:87 (1963).

54 TAYLOR, P. H., J. A. Moncrief, W. E. Switzer, L. R. Rose and L. Q. Pugsley. *Arch. Surg.*, 86:250 (1963).

55 MUTSCHLER, W., E. Burri, L. Claes, R. Frankenhauser and E. Plank. "A Comparative Study of Temporary Skin Covers in Contaminated Wounds and Burns," in *Advances in Biomaterials*, G. D. Winter, D. F. Gibbons, H. Plank, eds. New York:Wiley, 3:41–48 (1980).

56 MORGAN, C. N., N. H. Porter and D. J. Kluyman. "Ivalon Sponge in the Repair of Complete Rectal Prolapse," *Br. J. Surg.*, 59(19):84–86 (1972).

57 BROWN, J. B. et al. "Investigation and Use of Dimethyl Siloxanes, Halogenated Carbons and Poly Vinyl Alcohol as Subcutaceous Prostheses," *Ann. Surg.*, 152:534–547 (1960).

58 PERRAS, C. "The Prevention and Treatment of Infections Following Breast Implants," *Plast. Reconstr. Surg.*, 35:649–656 (1965).

59 SWAITZ, A. W. et al. "Experimental Study of Poly Vinyl-Formal (Ivalon) Sponge as a Substitute for Tissue," *Plast. Reconstr. Surg.*, 23:1–14 (1960).

60 SCHOFIELD, T. L. "Poly Vinyl Alcohol Sponge, An Inert Plastic for Use as a Prosthesis in the Repair of Large Hernias." *Brit. J. Surg.*, 42:618–621 (1955).

61 HAUPT, G. J. et al. "Poly Vinyl Formalinized (Ivalon) Sponge in the Repair of Diaphramatic Defects," *Arch. Surg.*, 80:613 (1960).

62 DAILEY, J. E. et al. "Ivalon Sponge Prosthesis with Pulmonary Resections Over Five Years Experience," *Dis. Chest*, 38:604–615 (1960).

63 GAGE, A. A. "Control of Experimental Ascites by Hepatopexy," *JAMA*, 192:377–381.

64 BERGAN, J. J. et al. "Vascularized Poly Vinyl Sponge Prothesis," *Arch. Surg.*, 8:301–305 (1962).

65 JOHNSON, F. "Polyvinyl in Tympanic Membrane Perforations," *Arch. Otolaryng*, 86:152–155 (1967).

66 FREIDENBERG, Z. B. and R. Lawrence. "Bone Growth in Poly Vinyl Sponge," *Surg. Gynec. Obstet.*, 109:291 (1959).

67 FRIEDENBERG, L. B. "Poly Vinyl Sponge in Osteochrondral Joint Defects," *Surg. Gynec. Obstet.*, 110:719–722 (1960).

68 COBEY, M. C. "Arthroplastics Using Compressed Ivalon Sponge Long Term Follow Up Studies in 109 Cases," *Clin. Orthop.*, 54:139–144 (1967).

69 BLUMBERG, J. B. et al. "The Effect of Specific Compression on Soft-Tissue Responses to Formalized Poly Vinyl Alcohol (Ivalon) Sponge: A Critical Evaluation," *Ann. Surg.*, 151:409–418 (1980).

70 YANNAS, I. V., J. F. Burke, C. Huang and P. L. Gordon. "Correlation of In Vivo Collagen Degradation Rate with In Vitro Measurements," *J. Biomed. Mater. Res.*, 9:623–628 (1975).

71 QUINN, K. J., J. M. Courtney, J. H. Evans, J. D. S. Gaylor and W. H. Reid. "Principles of Burn Dressings," *Biomaterials*, 6:369–377 (1985).

72 COOPER, S. L., ed. *Biomaterials: Interfacial Phenomena and Application*, Washington:ACS Publications (1982).

73 SHARMA, C. P. et al. "Surface Modification: Tissue Compatibility Towards the Development of Artificial Skin," *ICMR Project Report* (1989).

74 YAMAUCHI, A., Y. Matsuzawa, Y. Hara, M. Saishin, K. Nishioka, S. Nakao and S. Kamiya. "The Use of (Poly Vinyl Alcohol) Hydrogels as Drug Carriers," *Polymer Prepr.* 20(1):575 (1979).

75 KORSMEYER, R. W. and N. A. Peppas. "Effect of the Morphology of Hydrophilic Polymeric Matrices on the Diffusion and Release of Water Soluble Drug," *J. Membr. Sci.*, 9:211 (1981).

76 REINHART, C. T., R. W. Korsmeyer and N. A. Peppas. "Macromolecular Network Structure and Its Effects on Drug and Protein Diffusion," *Int. J. Pharm. Technol.*, 2(2):9 (1981).

77 GANDER, B., R. Gurny, E. Doelker and N. A. Peppas. "Cross-linked PVA Micromatrices for Swelling-Controlled Drug Release," *Proc. Int. Symp. Controlled Release Pharm.*, 5 (1983).

78 COLOMBO, P., C. Caramella, U. Conte and A. Gazzaniga. "Surface Crosslinking of Compressed Polymeric Mini-matrices for Drug Release Control," *Proc. Int. Symp. Controlled Release Bioact. Mater.*, 11:123 (1984).

79 KORSMEYER, R. W. and N. A. Peppas. "Swelling-Controlled Release from Hydrophilic Polymeric Networks," *Proc. Symp. Controlled Release Bioact. Mater.*, 8:85 (1981).

80 LANGER, R. and J. Folkman. "Polymers for the Substained Release of Proteins and Other Macromolecules," *Nature*, London, 263:797 (1976).

81 MAYBERG, M., R. Langer, N. Zervas and M. Moskowitz. "Perivascular Meningeal Projections from Cat Trigeminal Ganglia: Possible Pathway for Vascular Headaches in Man," *Science*, 213:228 (1981).

82 MOSKOWITZ, M., M. Mayberg and R. Langer. "Controlled Release of Horseradish Peroxidase from Polymers: A Method to Improve Histochemical Localization and Sensitivity," *Brain Res.*, 212:460 (1981).

83 KORSMEYER, R. W., R. Gurny, E. Doelker, P. Buri and N. A. Peppas. "Mechanisms of Solute Release from Porous Hydrophilic Polymers," *Int. J. Pharm.*, 15:25 (1983).

84 GURNY, R., E. Doelker, P. Buri, R. W. Korsmeyer and N. A. Peppas. *Proc. Congr. Int. Pharmac. Technol. APGI*, 3:97 (1983).

85 PEPPAS, N. A. "Characterization of Homogeneous and Pseudocomposite Homocopolymers and Copolymers for Articular Cartilage Replacement," *Biomater. Med. Devices Artif. Organs*, 7:421 (1979).

86 BRAY, J. C. and E. W. Merril. "PVA Hydrogels for Synthetic Articular Cartilage Material," *J. Biomed. Mater. Res.*, 7:431 (1973).

87 SUN, A. M., G. M. O'Shea and M. F. A. Goosen. "Development and In Vivo Testing of an Artificial Endocrine Pancreas," in *Biocompatible Polymers, Metals and Composites*, M. Szycher, ed. Lancaster, PA:Technomic Publishing Co., Inc., pp. 929 (1983).

88 MALEHESKY, P. S., J. Wojcicki and Y. Nose. "Membrane Effects in Plasma Separation," in *Progress in Artificial Organs 1983*, K. Atsumi, M. Mackawa and K. Ota, eds. Cleveland:ISAO Press, p. 649 (1984).

89 RANDERSON, D. H. and J. A. Taylor. "Protein Adsorption and Flux Decay on Membrane Plasma Separators," in *Plasmapheresis*, Y. Nose, P. S. Malchesky and J. W. Smith, eds. Cleveland:ISAO Press, p. 69 (1983).

90 YANG, W. H., V. F. Smolen and N. A. Peppas, "Oxygen Permeability Coefficients of Polymers for Hard and Soft Contact Lens Applications," *J. Membr. Sci.*, 9:53 (1981).

91 PEPPAS, N. A. and W. H. Yang. "Polymer Structural Effects on the Oxygen Permeation of Soft Contact Lens Materials," *Proc. IUPAC*, 27(4):28 (1980).

92 REFOJO, M. F. "Contact Lenses," in *Encyclopedia of Chemical Technology*, New York:John Wiley and Sons, 6:720 (1979).

93 ARNOLD, G. E. "Vocal Rehabilitation of Paralytic Dysphonia IX. Technique of Intracordal Injection," *Arch. Otolaryngol*, 76:358 (1962).

94 PEPPAS, N. A. and R. E. Benner, Jr. "Proposed Method of Intracordal Injection and Gelation of PVA Solution in Vocal Cords," *Biomaterials*, 1:58 (1980).

95 PEPPAS, N. A. and R. E. Benner, Jr. "Hydrophilic Polymeric Materials for Reconstruction of Vocal Cords," *Proc. IUPAC*, 26:1539 (1979).

96 CHEN, R. W., A. W. Musser and R. Postlethwait. "Alterations of and Tissue Reaction to PVA Sponge Implants," *Surgery*, 66:899 (1969).

CHAPTER 7

Biocompatibility and Toxicological Screening of Materials

THOMAS CHANDY, Ph.D.[1] and
CHANDRA P. SHARMA, Ph.D.[1]

ABSTRACT: Medical devices such as catheters, haemodialysers, oxygenators, heart valves and blood vessel prostheses are frequently used in humans as a consequence of natural and accidental deterioration of the body. In this paper, a broad outline of the materials being used in medical applications, and their limitations, is discussed. Possible ways of anchoring tissue interfaces, and current evaluation procedures for blood compatibility and toxicity protocols are also reviewed. Finally, the need for awareness of moral and ethical issues and the development of a code of ethics for the engineers, scientists and physicians working in the field of biomaterials are discussed.

As we get older, our vital organs and tissues deteriorate because of many factors. Though the processes involved are not clearly understood, the consequences are quite clear: painful teeth, arthritic joints, fragile bones which may break, circulatory system blockages due to thrombus formation, loss of control of the heart's vital pumping rhythm, calcification of the heart's valves, and diminished powers of hearing and vision. Accidents may also enhance the processes of bodily deterioration, including disfigurement. The emerging need for the replacement of living tissues has stimulated scientists, engineers and doctors to explore the development of body implants having good interfacial compatibility.

USE OF MATERIALS FOR BIOMEDICAL APPLICATIONS

The materials used for developing body implants or interfaces are commonly called biomaterials. A biomaterial may be defined as a material that is used in the treatment of patients and which, at some stage, interfaces with living tissue for a significant length of time. Therefore, the interaction between the tissue and the material is an important factor in the treatment [1]. The emphasis of the definition is on the time of contact between the material and the tissue of the patient. It is this time period that distinguishes a biomaterial from other materials used only transiently by a surgeon or physician, such as the steel used for a scalpel blade or the tungsten carbide used in a dental bur. In effect, the definition excludes all materials that contact tissues for a short period of time, but includes all those that interface with tissues for durations of more than a few hours. The definition, therefore, embraces all those nonvital materials that are used medically in, on and about the body, and that are in contact with tissues other than the epidermis [1].

According to the Clemson Advisory Board for Biomaterials, "a biomaterial is a systemically, pharmacologically inert substance designed for implantation within or incorporation with a living system," a definition adopted at the Sixth Annual International Biomaterials Symposium, April 20–24, 1974 [2]. Recently, Black has stated: "A Biomaterial is any pharmacologically inert material, viable or non–viable, natural product or man-made, that is a part of or is capable of interacting in a beneficial way with a living organism" [3]. Thus, the term "biomaterials" encompasses all materials used for medical applications that are interfaced with living systems or other systems developed for extracorporeal uses [4]. The biomaterials include metals, ceramics, natural polymers (biopolymers), synthetic polymers of simple or complex chemical and/or physical structure. A list of some of the devices and their functions is given in Table 1 [5].

Control over the biomaterials–tissue interface is the paramount problem in this field of biomaterial science [6]. Thus, the relative success or failure of a biomaterial reflects the scientific and engineering judgement used in solving this problem. The interaction of many complex

[1]Division of Biosurface Technology, Biomedical Technology Wing, Sree Chitra Tirunal Institute for Medical Sciences and Technology, Poojapura, Trivandrum-695012, India

TABLE 1. Implant Devices Currently in Use or Being Tested

Device	Function	Biomaterials
SENSORY AND NEURAL SYSTEMS		
1. Artificial vitreous humor	Fill the vitreous cavity of the eye	Silicone Teflon sponge; polyglyceryl methacrylate (PGMA)
2. Corneal prosthesis, intraocular lens	Provide an optical pathway to the retina; correct problems caused by cataracts	Polymethylmethacrylate (PMMA)
3. Electrical control of epileptic seizure	Conduct electrical signals to brain	Pt and Pt–Ir wires and electrodes; stainless steel; silicone rubber; PMMA
HEART & CARDIOVASCULAR SYSTEM		
4. Heart pacer	Maintain heart rhythm	Stainless steel; Ti cans; silicone rubber; wax epoxy encapsulants; Pt or Pt–Ir alloy electrodes
5. Chronic shunts and catheters	Assist haemodialysis	Polyethylene, hydrophilic coatings
6. Arterial and vascular prostheses, heart assist device	Replace diseased arteries; replace the diseased heart portions	Segmented polyurethanes; silicone rubber; HEMA coated polymers; Dacron velours; Teflon
7. Cardiac heart valves	Replace diseased valves	Co–Cr alloy; low temperature isotropic carbon; porcine grafts; Ti alloy with silastic or pyrolytic carbon disks or balls
SKELETAL AND DENTAL		
8. Artificial total hip, knee, shoulder, elbow, etc.	Reconstruct arthritic or fractured joints	Stems; 316L stainless steel; Co–Cr alloys; high density polyethylene; metal bioglass coating; porous Teflon; Ti and Ti alloys
9. Spinal fusion	Immobilize vertebrae to protect spinal cord	Bioglass; stainless steel
10. Tooth replacement implants	Replace diseased, damaged, loosened teeth	Co–Cr–Mo alloys; Al_2O_3 Bioglass; PMMA; porous calcium aluminate
MISCELLANEOUS SOFT TISSUE		
11. Artificial skin	Treat severe burns	Processed collagen; ultrathin silicone membrane; polycaprolactone foam, collagen grafted polyurethane

physical, biological, clinical and technological factors must be considered.

THE BASIC CRITERIA FOR BIOMATERIALS

The basic criteria for developing biomedical devices from materials are very rigid [7,8]:

(a) They should be nontoxic. The material should not produce any undesirable inflammation and/or clinically significant changes in the tissues or the fluids of the body.

(b) They should be easily fabricable. The methods must be available to fabricate the implant, possibly on a mass production basis, with accurate dimensions. Such methods must be reproducible and capable of yielding good quality products with improved mechanical properties.

(c) They must be sterilizable. The sterilization of these materials is essential; they must be kept free from bacteria or any other micro-organisms, and must be stable and safe during sterilization by any of the recognized methods.

(d) They must be stable during implantation. Any

changes that occur in mechanical, physical or chemical properties during the period of implantation must not cause the implant to lose its efficiency. The mechanical properties should match the nature of the prosthesis that substitutes for the body parts.

(e) They should not corrode or degrade to liberated products that may induce local or systemic harmful effects.

(f) They should not be carcinogenic. The biomaterial, once in the body, should not induce mitogenic properties in the tissue as a result of its degradation product, leaching components or corroded materials.

In addition to these criteria, the cost of the finished product should be as low as possible.

The selection of materials for a device depends mainly upon the end application of the device, i.e., the design characteristics, duration of usage and the basic nature of the application.

BIOCOMPATIBILITY

In the past 20 years, the development of artificial organs and devices to maintain life functions has stimulated research into the biocompatibility of materials. "Biocompatibility" describes the ability of a biomaterial to exist within a living body without adversely and significantly affecting the body, and without the material itself suffering any adverse and significant effects [1]. These two broad aspects of biocompatibility, the effects on the material and the effects on the tissue, are very much interrelated. An adverse effect on a material by the physiological fluids may lead to the release of particulate or soluble matter from the material, which results in an adverse response from the tissues. So, biocompatibility mainly involves the chemical interactions that take place between the materials and the bodily fluids, and the physiological responses to these reactions [1].

Broadly speaking, biocompatible materials are those which are acceptable to the living physiological environment. However, in the exact sense, it is very difficult to define this term, since it may also have some correlation within the narrow confines of a specific material prepared for a specific purpose. Hence, a material used as a blood interface is called blood-compatible, but the same material, if it is used as a tissue interface, is called tissue-compatible.

Blood–Material Interface

Blood compatibility may be defined as the inability of an artificial surface to activate the intrinsic blood coagulation system or to attract or alter platelets or leucocytes [9]. All artificial materials known until now induce the coagu-

lation of blood and/or the adhesion and aggregation of blood platelets, eventually leading to the formation of thrombus on the material surface [9,10]. There is a wide range of thrombogenic effects, varying from complete occlusion to a degree of consumption of the blood clotting factors, or formed elements. Despite many recent advances by biomedical scientists, the ideal blood-compatible surface of endothelium has not been matched in its nonthrombogenic properties by any artificial material [11].

Current research has shown that, upon exposure of synthetic surfaces to whole, flowing blood, most materials become rapidly coated with a layer of blood proteins, in parallel with the adhesion of platelets, leading to thrombus formation [11,12]. To overcome such problems, research has been directed toward several areas: production of materials that prevent thrombosis; modification of material substrates to improve blood compatibility; use of therapeutic substances that prevent deposition of fibrin and formed elements of blood–surface interactions; and possible surface modifications to enhance the blood compatibility of substrates. These aspects have been reviewed earlier [8,13].

Tissue–Material Interface

There are many possible causes of tissue changes adjacent to implants. Although most of these causes are a direct or indirect consequence of implant insertion, they are not all due to the chemical nature of foreign material. The reactions exhibited between an implant material and the environment of the body control the ability of the implant to maintain functionality throughout its period of use [6]. This, indeed, is of utmost importance; it is the environmental compatibility between the implant and the body tissues or fluids that is most important in determining the usefulness of any implant. Now it is known that the chemical and geometrical nature of the surface of the prosthetic material itself dictates the compatibility between an implant surface and the tissues. This compatibility is certainly controlled by the cellular activity at the interface.

When the material can be considered chemically and physically inert, the response of the tissues to the implant may be only slightly different from normal postoperative healing. The material provokes only the formation of a thin, fibrous capsule around it. This capsule is most suitable clinically, because the material is then virtually extracorporeal and is effectively ignored thereafter by the body.

On the other hand, if the material is less inert or more "irritant," then the foreign body giant cells are produced. This is a clinically undesirable feature, indicating basic tissue instability. Healing is delayed when these cells are present, and the eventual scar or fibrous tissue layer is usually much thicker than in their absence. The fibrous layer is due to a nonspecific response by the tissue to the physical presence of the implant as a solid foreign body. However, this physical explanation for the reactive fibrosis, does not rule out the possibility that the cellular response at the tissue–implant interface may be mediated or modified by protein adsorbed onto the metal or polymer surface at the time of its insertion [14]. Thus, it appears that achieving the necessary match, or gradient, in physical properties across the interface between living and nonliving matter is a formidable scientific challenge.

GENERAL METHODS OF CONTROLLING TISSUE–MATERIAL INTERFACES

The interfacing of living tissue with man-made materials is, by definition, associated with placing prosthetic devices in the human body [5]. Interactions at the tissue–material interface may determine whether a material is tissue compatible and can coexist with the physiological environment. Currently, biomaterial research is exploring the use of porous metals and ceramics as a class of high-strength materials that are compatible with living tissue and are capable of anchoring or attaching a prosthetic device to living tissue within the body [5,15]. It is conceivable that the tissue can grow into the pores, or surface depressions if the pores are big enough, and maintain a vascular supply and tissue vitality [5].

It has been suggested that the porous biomaterials can be resistant to corrosion and deterioration in the body due to the large interfacial area they can provide to tissue and tissue fluids [16]. Bioceramics, especially aluminum oxide and a few metals such as titanium and cobalt–chromium alloys, have potential for microstructural control of the interface. These materials may exhibit sufficient corrosion resistance to be considered for use in porous implants [17]. It appears that the soft connective tissue may grow into pores of greater than 50 micrometers in diameter and remain healthy over periods of at least several years; on the other hand, bigger pores, having greater than 100 μm size are required for bone growth [5]. Therefore, the optimization of pore size and density may provide for control of tissue interfaces.

A second method of controlling the biomaterials–tissue interface is chemical breakdown via the resorption of the material, where the foreign material may be replaced by regenerating tissues [5,18]. Polymer systems based on poly(glycolic acid), poly(lactic acid) and their copolymer systems decompose in the tissue interfaces and are used clinically as resorbable sutures and implantable drug delivery systems [19]. However, the strength of these absorbable biomaterials decreases as resorption occurs, leaving the materials too weak to be used as replacements for bones and joints.

The third approach to control of the interface is to use biomaterials with controlled surface reactivity. In this case, the biomaterial is designed to react chemically with the physiological system, producing a strong bond between the tissues and the implant surface [16]. This interface stabilization prevents further deterioration, makes the implant passive, and produces more flexibility in device design and fabrication. Four major categories of surface active biomaterials have been developed: dense hydroxyl apatite ceramics, bioactive glasses, bioactive glass-ceramics, and bioactive composites. These materials have found suitable orthopaedic and dental applications. However, the ultimate safety and performance of materials as tissue interface depend on the physical performance, reliability and compatibility with the biological environment of its end use.

TESTS TO EVALUATE THROMBOGENESIS ON ARTIFICIAL SURFACES

Tests to evaluate the thrombogenic potential and the haemostatic defects induced by artificial surface exposure are now available for selecting suitable blood-compatible substrates for implantation [9,13]. Most evaluations necessitate both in vitro and in vivo studies. A few in vitro test methods adopted for evaluating blood compatibility of materials are suggested in the following sections.

Coagulation Time Test

The coagulation is initiated by two processes: the intrinsic system (via the activation of factor XII), and the extrinsic pathway (via tissue factor). Exposure of blood to a foreign material can initiate the activation of the intrinsic coagulation by conversion of the zymogen factor XII (Hageman factor) into activated factor, XIIa. This conversion takes place after the adsorption of factor XII to the material surface and requires the participation of the complex of high molecular weight kininogen–prekallikrein-factor XI. Activated factor XII converts prekallikrein into kallikrein, which in turn activates surface bound factor XII, resulting in a burst of activated factor XII. Factor XIIa converts factor XI into XIa, which in turn activates factor IX. Activated factor IX combines with factor VIIIa, phospholipids and Ca^{++} ions to form a complex which is able to convert factor X into Xa. Next, factor Xa combines with factor Va, phospholipids and Ca^{++} ions to form a complex, which converts prothrombin into thrombin. Thrombin in turn converts fibrinogen molecules into fibrin monomers, which are stabilized by factor XIIIa to fibrin gel. The extrinsic pathway is activated by the tissue factor and factor VII, which directly activates factor X. Thereafter a well-known pathway for fibrin formation [8,10,13] is followed.

The material to be tested is coated inside a test tube and

the time required for the formation of a firm clot is determined. Usually, an enhanced coagulation time compared to an uncoated glass substrate is proposed to be nonthrombogenic.

Recalcification Time Test

Citrated plasma is recalcified and clotting takes place via the intrinsic pathway, being initiated by the surface activity of the clotting tube. Plasma recalcification time is measured by adding 0.025 M CaCl$_2$ to citrated plasma.

Thrombin Time Test

A known concentration of human thrombin and calcium is added to the test plasma. The clotting time is a direct measure of the amount of fibrinogen present, the function of the fibrinogen and the presence of antithrombins, e.g., heparin. Therefore, a prolonged thrombin time is usually considered to be due to either a decrease in fibrinogen, or the presence of heparin or high concentrations of fibrin–fibrinogen degradation products, which prevent the formation of the fibrin clot.

Activated Partial Thromboplastin Time (APTT) Test

Platelet substitute, in the form of a partial-thromboplastin, usually prepared from rabbit brain, is incubated with a contacting agent to provide optimal activation of the intrinsic coagulation factors. The clotting time is determined after the addition of excess calcium.

Stypven (Russell's Viper Venom) Clotting Time Test

In the presence of calcium ions and phospholipid, a potent coagulant substance in the venom of Russell's viper accelerates plasma coagulation. Stypven activates factor X directly, without the need for other coagulation factors. Stypven/phospholipid reagent is incubated with plasma for 30 seconds. Then, a known amount of CaCl$_2$ is added and the clotting time recorded.

Antithrombin III Binding Studies

Antithrombin III neutralizes thrombin in physiological milieu to reduce the thrombus formation. Hence, substrates having antithrombin III binding capacities cause a reduction in the activity in the plasma.

The defibrinated plasma is diluted in a buffered heparin solution, and a specific amount of thrombin is added to the diluted plasma. During a timed incubation, a portion of the added thrombin is neutralized by the antithrombin III present in the sample. An aliquot of the first stage is then mixed with a fibrinogen solution. The time required for clot formation is proportional to the amount of thrombin remaining after neutralization.

Whole blood clotting time and the assay of various clotting factors (e.g., II, V, VIII, XI and XII) are also performed for equating the thrombogenic potential of a material.

Platelet Function

Exposure of any synthetic substrate to whole blood, platelet-rich plasma or washed platelets results in the platelets adhering within seconds, depending on the nature of the surface, the flow conditions, the nature of the proteins adsorbed on the substrate and extent of platelet activation. The platelets adhering to the substrate can be quantitated and probably equated with thrombogenic character of the surface [20,21].

Platelet Adhesion

By centrifuging 0.38% citrated blood at $700 \times g$, a supernatant having platelet-rich plasma (PRP) is collected. This supernatant is further centrifuged at $1000 \times g$ to remove the white blood cells. The PRP is again centrifuged at $2000 \times g$ to get the platelets, which are washed with tyrode solution and suspended in the same solution. This platelet suspension is exposed to the polymer surface and rinsed with phosphate buffer. The adhered platelets are fixed with 2.5% glutaraldehyde and stained with Coomassie Blue G. The platelet density is measured using an optical microscope.

In Vitro Platelet Retention with Microbeads

In this test, materials prepared in the form of microbeads (0.2 to 0.5 mm in diameter) are exposed to whole human blood (heparinized and citrated) in a column under laminar flow condition at ~1 ml/min [22]. Blood is withdrawn in a polypropylene syringe having a silicone rubber plunger. After being heparinized and citrated, the blood is admitted through polypropylene tubing to the bottom of the column that is packed with the microbeads. The surface area of the beads is in excess of 1600 cm^2, whereas that of the tubing, syringe, and silicone rubber components is only 150 cm^2. The effluent blood is examined for evidence of blood–surface interactions, with particular attention to platelet retention and release of platelet constituents. The main limitations of this test are that materials must be prepared as beads, and that the blood comes in contact first with materials other than the test specimens.

Other platelet function studies include: (a) counting the platelets before and after exposing the material to the flowing blood; (b) evaluation of platelet aggregation in contact with material substrates in the presence of inducing agents such as ADP, Collagen, thrombin and epinephrine; and (c) quantitation of platelet release constituents such as PF$_4$, PF$_3$ and β-thromboglobulin using spectrophotometric methods.

Protein Adsorption Studies

It has been shown that the nature of the protein adsorbed onto the material surface is a factor in the adhesion of blood platelets, in the activation of the clotting mechanism, and, ultimately, in the thrombus formation [10,11]. It seems that platelets adhere less to albuminated surfaces [23]. But, on the other hand, γ-globulin and fibrinogen adsorbing substrates intensify the adhesion of platelets. This process has been detected by a number of physical and chemical methods including ellipsometry, radiolabelled proteins, electrophoretic techniques, ATR-IR, FTIR and immunological identification of adsorbed proteins [13,24,25].

The protein adsorption can vary with surface properties of the material. In general, proteins interact more strongly with hydrophobic surfaces than with hydrophilic ones, and hydrophilic surfaces seem to adsorb less protein than hydrophobic surfaces. The nature of the surface can be evaluated using contact angle techniques with a goniometer and pure solvents of known surface tension [13]. These measurements can provide information related to the hydrophilic or hydrophobic character of the surface and the changes in the surface. Accordingly, the interfacial energies at the solid–liquid interface can be correlated with blood compatibility.

Some of the methods commonly adopted to evaluate protein–surface binding are presented here. Adsorption-desorption experiments can be carried out using labelled proteins. Assuming that the labelled and unlabelled proteins adsorb to the same extent to a polymer substrate, the labelled protein acts as a tracer of the protein mixture [24]. Films of size 2×1.5 cm are dipped in buffer and shaken. Then the protein mixture, containing a known amount of one of the ^{125}I-labelled proteins, is added. This addition is carried out inside the medium to reduce the air–water interface. The films are removed at varying time intervals, shaken, rinsed and counted in a γ-counter to determine the surface protein concentration.

Polyacrylamide gel electrophoresis can be used to separate, identify and quantitate the adsorbed proteins [25] from a mixture of proteins, after desorbing them using Triton–X–100. The films are dipped in the protein mixture for 3 hours, taking care of the air–water interface. The unadsorbed proteins are removed by rinsing. The adsorbed proteins are removed using Triton–X–100 with repeated shaking. These proteins are then concentrated, and the polyacrylamide gel electrophoresis of the concentrate is carried out with 7% gels. The electrophoretogram can be scanned or photographed.

Ellipsometry is widely used for detecting the thickness and the refractive index of the adsorbed protein layer on the polymer substrate [4]. The thickness of the growing protein layer on the polymer surface can be measured in solution using a computer program that controls the stepping motors on the analyzer and polarizer. The substrate is measured ellipsometrically and pseudoconstants are found out using the program. These pseudoconstants are then used to obtain the thickness and refractive index of a film on this substrate, introducing very little error.

In Vivo Blood Compatibility Studies

Vena Cava Ring Test

Blood compatibility may be evaluated using the vena cava ring test, by implanting the material in contact with the flowing blood of animals [26]. Small rings (length 9.5 mm, O.D. 8.2 mm, I.D. 6.3 mm) are fabricated, with streamlined leading and trailing edges, from the test polymer. They are then implanted in the inferior vena cava of healthy dogs through a right thoracotomy during anaesthesia and secured in place with a ligature. The condition of the ring is assessed using a flow meter; the test may be allowed to continue for up to two weeks. The animals are then sacrificed and the rings are examined for thrombus formation.

Renal Embolus Test

A ring (length 8 mm, O.D. 8 mm, I.D. 6 mm) is implanted into the abdominal aorta of an anaesthetized dog immediately above the origin of the renal arteries. The procedure is accompanied by a subtotal constriction of the aorta below the origin of the renal arteries so that over 90% of the blood flowing through the ring must pass through the kidneys, as indicated by electromagnetic flow measurements. After 3 to 6 days of implantation, an autopsy is performed and the surface thrombosis is assessed by direct visual observation. The main limitation of these tests is the detachment of microemboli from the ring.

A Canine Ex Vivo Series Shunt for Evaluating Thrombus Deposition on Polymer Surfaces

This technique is used to examine the platelet and fibrinogen deposition on a series of up to ten different polymer surfaces in the same non-anticoagulated animal [27]. The test polymers may be in tubing form, extruded, or coated on the inner surface of 1/8 inch I.D. polyethylene tubing. The segments are joined together to form part of the shunt, which is then cannulated into the femoral vessels of a canine subject. Dynamic measurements of fibrinogen and platelet deposition on the polymer surfaces (over a 1/2- to 60-minutes blood contact period) are made, using labelled techniques and scanning electron microscopy. The series shunt allows for simultaneous testing of a number of polymers in the same animal and provides a method for direct comparison of these test substrates.

TOXICITY TESTS ON BIOMATERIALS

Toxicity testing is of primary importance in biomedical engineering applications. From "food grade" materials to materials for blood–tissue interfaces with the required properties, "end-use" considerations may necessitate the incorporation of additives or blends with other polymers. Once the functional properties of the material are matched to the application envisaged, biological safety and an appropriate toxicity testing protocol must be considered.

The test protocols published in 1965 in United States Pharmacopoeia (USP) and National Formulary (NF) became the official tests for evaluating materials that are to be in contact with parenteral drug solutions in the USA [28]. These biological tests have been the only guidelines available for the toxicologists, who have to evaluate materials for medical applications. Unfortunately, at present, there are no standards or internationally accepted battery of tests which can make a comprehensive protocol for the safety evaluation of raw materials and end products. However, there is a growing awareness amongst manufacturers, scientists, medical professionals and law enforcement agencies that a consensus on the formulation of acceptable standards is needed. Since the device manufacturing in this country is in its juvenile stages, the situation here is rather different.

Rationale of Testing

It may be worthwhile to clarify why biomaterials need a time-consuming testing protocol before their introduction to the human body [29]. The medical devices are made up of a variety of heterogeneous materials, such as metals, alloys, plastics and ceramics which are mostly man-made and are foreign objects to the living environment. When an artificial material is introduced into the body, it may give rise to various harmful effects.

Contact of a device with the skin, mucous membrane or blood, may cause ingredients to diffuse into the adjacent tissue, setting up a local response, e.g., inflammation or necrosis. On the other hand, if the ingredients get into the circulatory system, tissues and organs at remote sites can be affected, giving rise to varying degrees of systemic toxicity. In the case of material–blood interfaces, thrombus formation is the major unsolved problem. These harmful effects have to be reduced or eliminated to prevent the implant from being loosened, rejected and eventually failing. Therefore, it is of paramount importance that adequate and meaningful test protocols be evolved to ensure the safety of biomaterials.

Toxicity Test Protocol

Most evaluations necessitate both in vitro and in vivo studies. The USP, British Pharmacopoeia (BP) biological tests for toxicity evaluation of materials are summarized in Table 2 [29–32], and discussed in the following sections.

Acute and Chronic Toxicity Studies

In situ implantation—The objective of this test is to study the response of the rabbit muscle to the implanted test material over varying time intervals ranging from one week (acute) to two years (chronic). In this procedure, test materials are made into $1 \times 1 \times 10$ mm strips and implanted in the paravertebral muscles aseptically. The test animals are sacrificed at desired intervals of time and the tissues surrounding the implant site are subjected to macroscopic and histopathological examinations.

Tissue culture—Cell culture tests are usually ultrasensitive to a greater degree than the biological site tests. Thus, the absence of any pharmacological effect on cells adds to the degree of assurance from satisfactory in vivo results. Biomaterial strips or eluates are applied to cell monolayers in culture and then incubated. The toxicity of the biomaterial tested is determined by evaluating the sensitive parameters of cellular damage, such as neutral red uptake, trypan blue uptake, growth curve, plating efficiency and ^{51}Cr release.

Haemolysis test—The haemolytic potential of the test material is assessed by this test. Test material in the required quantity is exposed to oxalated rabbit blood and incubated for an hour at $35° \pm 1°C$, along with negative and positive controls. It is then centrifuged, and the absorbance of the supernatant is determined at 545 nm. The percentage of haemolysis is then calculated. If the haemolysis is 5% or less, the material can be considered to be nonhaemolytic.

Thrombogenic potential test—A quantitative, kinetic method is used for the determination of thrombogenic potential of medical devices. The evaluation is based on an in vitro comparison of the clot-forming property of the

TABLE 2. Toxicity Screening Protocol (General)

I. Acute Toxicity Tests	III. Sensitization
a. In situ implantation	IV. Carcinogenicity
b. Tissue culture	V. Mutagenicity
c. Haemolysis	VI. Special Tests
d. Thrombogenicity	a. Pyrogen test
e. Systemic Toxicity	b. Sterility test
f. Irritation test	c. In-use test
II. Chronic Toxicity studies	
a. In situ implantation	
b. Systemic Toxicity	
c. Irritation test	

test material to that of pyrex glass, which is one of the most thrombogenic materials.

Systemic toxicity—An extract of the test material is prepared as described in the USP XIX, 1975. Five mice are injected at a dose level of 50 ml/kg, through a specific route to suit the extracting medium. Five control mice are injected with the extracting medium alone. The animals are observed at various periods of time. Deaths and signs of toxicity are recorded over a period of seven days (acute toxicity). Chronic studies are performed on different species of animals via repeated injections of the extract.

Intracutaneous irritation test—0.2 ml of the extract of the material is injected intracutaneously at ten sites on the prepared dorsal side of the rabbit, while 0.2 ml of the extract of the medium alone are injected at ten sites on the contralateral side. The injection sites are critically observed at intervals of 24, 48, and 72 hours and scored to record erythema, oedema and necrosis to indicate the irritant potential of the test material.

Sensitization

Medical devices that are used for repeated or prolonged application need sensitization tests. The guinea pig maximization test may be appropriate as a standard procedure for revealing potent sensitizers. A biopsy of the lesion can help characterize the sensitization reaction.

Carcinogenicity

Testing for carcinogenicity, although time-consuming and tedious, is necessary because the possibility of chemical carcinogenesis is a reality. It appears that testing in several bacterial and insect systems coupled with a mammalian cell transformation system may be a reliable method to rule out chemical carcinogenesis in the field of medical devices.

Mutagenicity

The wider application of man-made materials such as implantable devices or extracorporeal circuits warrants the testing of these materials for mutagenicity. The widely used short-term in vitro assay for mutagenesis for which collaborative data with in vivo carcinogenicity exists is the Salmonella assay [31].

Special Tests

The special tests like the pyrogen test (for screening the presence of any pyrogenic material in situ, so as to limit the risks of a febrile reaction), the sterility test (to detect whether the material is free to viable forms of bacteria, fungi and yeasts) and the in-use test (to evaluate the efficiency of the products in their in-use condition before clinical trials) are also mandatory for medical devices.

ETHICS AND BIOMEDICAL RESEARCH

Biomaterials science has experienced a rapid growth phase during the last two decades, along with the rapid expansion in the whole field of biomedical engineering. The involvement of biologists, physical scientists, engineers and doctors in the development of body spares for improved life-style and patient care has made this field not only an interdisciplinary area, but also polydisciplinary [33]. The increasing complexity of a field so pertinent to the public health requires careful monitoring to control its direction and impact on society. Very little discussion has taken place on the need for developing ethical guidelines along with the technological advancement in biomaterials [34,35]. Thus, the rapid growth in the field of applied biomaterials poses new ethical problems in the design, manufacture, evaluation, and regulation of medical devices and implants.

Animal Research

Animals are being used as experimental models for many types of research work, including biomedical research. The welfare of animals is a very important subject, but one about which there is a great deal of confusion and muddled thinking. Today, a strong resurgence of concern over animal research is taking place. Hence, it is very important to determine the experimental protocols before experimenting on animals. This may help us alleviate their suffering. Responsibility for the humane care and use of animals involved in activities supported by grants or contracts from the Public Health Service (PHS) rests primarily with the institutions receiving the awards.

The biological and philosophical meaning of animal pain and suffering and the benefits of different types of knowledge gained from animal experimentation are being debated [36,37]. Therefore, a biomaterials specialist must not only consider the scientific criteria for animal experiments, but also the ethical issues involved. It is often suggested that animal experiment review committees assist in establishing a valuable dialogue between scientists and the lay public. Furthermore, these committees could provide the scientific community with the chance to reveal its own concern for the welfare of laboratory animals and their humane, non-profligate use. This would allay public disquiet, often fanned by inaccurate, emotional propaganda from extremist sources [38].

Human Experimentation

The ethical and legal issues involved in human experimentation are still more involved [39]. In 1973, the U. S. Department of Health, Education and Welfare (DHEW) proposed far-reaching regulations on human research, requiring organizational ethics committees to review such studies within individual organizations [36].

The Department of Health and Human Services (DHHS) succeeded DHEW and attempted to finalize regulations and reconcile them with the FDA. Currently, biomedical research involving humans is controlled by the DHHS and the FDA, and both require Institutional Review Boards to insure protection of human subjects [37]. The Institutional Review Boards ensure that the risks to the subject are minimized, that the risk–benefit ratio is reasonable, that selection of subjects is equitable, that documented informed consent is obtained from the subject or from a legal representative, that the course of the experiment is monitored to protect the safety of the subject, and that the confidentiality and privacy of the subject is respected [37,40].

Since biomaterials technology is growing at such a pace that large numbers of clinical trials using human beings will be needed for biomaterial research as a whole, the importance of ethical awareness of those working in this area becomes paramount. For this reason there are many governmental safeguards insuring that the patient is properly informed and supervised throughout the trial, and is able to withdraw at any time during the trial [37]. However, no matter how voluminous regulatory forms and procedures become, nothing can substitute for high moral standards among biomaterials scientists themselves.

Manufacturing and Evaluation of Biomaterials

Implants may fail due to many reasons (e.g., basic engineering defects, corrosion and other degradation of properties) and can become a factor in carcinogenic effects, metabolic effects, immunologic effects and bacteriologic effects [37,41]. Many of the mechanisms involved in the biological failure of biomaterials are not clearly understood. Thus, it is conceivable that even after adequate clinical trials for one type of the product, the implant may fail due to reuse or misuse. The reuse of certain materials not tested or designed specifically for reuse is of concern today. Some clinicians may reuse certain costly implants, e.g., pacemakers, to reduce the high cost of medical care.

In order to properly evaluate a product, all bias must be effectively reduced. Even the most honest investigator is not completely free of bias when making subjective clinical evaluations of the effectiveness of his own device. Recently, a "National Registry" has been instituted in the U. S. for the purpose of receiving reports of failures of implants and medical devices. This can help biomaterials scientists fulfill their ethical responsibility to confront the failure of implants and medical devices; valuable lessons can be learned from such cases and future failures can be minimized. Finally, the biomaterials scientists should strive for improvements in the investigative procedures so that the field of biomaterials science does not fall to discredit.

CONCLUSIONS

It has not been possible to explore in any great depth the various aspects which impinge upon the manufacture and use of biomaterials in medical applications, but it is hoped that we have pointed the way to a better awareness of the questions to be asked when confronting the problems that arise in this multidisciplinary field. As our understanding of the biochemical processes that regulate the growth and development of our tissues improves, we may see exciting developments in the interfacial problem, in which implants incorporate active ingredients that affect the healing and repair of damaged tissues. Finally, a code of ethics and new guidelines for professionals who design biomaterials and medical devices could help maintain high standards and improved health care.

REFERENCES

1 WILLIAMS, D. F. "Biomaterials and Biocompatibility," in *Fundamental Aspects of Biocompatibility*, D. F. Williams, ed. Florida: CRC Press, 1:1–10 (1981).

2 PARK, J. B. *Biomaterials Science and Engineering*, New York: Plenum Press, p. 1 (1984).

3 BLACK, J. "The Education of the Biomaterialist: Report of a Survey," *J. Biomed. Mater. Res.*, 16:159–167 (1982).

4 BAIER, R. E. and R. C. Dutton. "Initial Events in Interactions of Blood with a Foreign Surface," *J. Biomed. Mater. Res.*, 3:191–206 (1969).

5 HENCH, L. L. "Biomaterials," *Science*, 208:826–831 (1980).

6 WILLIAMS, D. F. *Implants in Surgery*, London:W. B. Saunders Comp. (1973).

7 LYMAN, D. J. "Polymers in Medicine and Surgery," in *Polymer Science and Technology*, R. L. Kronenthal, ed. New York:Plenum, 8:29–49 (1975).

8 SHARMA, C. P., V. K. Krishnan and M. S. Valiathan. "Perspectives and Problems of Blood-Compatible Polymers," *Polym. Plast. Technol. Eng.*, 18:233–244 (1982).

9 FORBES, C. D. and C. R. M. Prentice. "Thrombus Formation and Artificial Surfaces," *Brit. Med. Bull.*, 34:201–207 (1978).

10 VROMAN, L., A. L. Adams, M. Klings, G. C. Fischer, P. C. Munoz and R. Solensky. "Reactions of Formed Elements of Blood with Plasma Proteins at Interface," *Ann. N.Y. Acad. Sci.*, 283:65–76 (1977).

11 SALZMAN, E. W. "The Events That Lead to Thrombosis," *Bull. N.Y. Acad. Med.*, 48:225–231 (1972).

12 BAIER, R. E. "The Organization of Blood Components Near Interfaces," *Ann. N.Y. Acad. Sci.*, 283:17–36 (1977).

13 CHANDY, T. and C. P. Sharma. "Protein-Polymer Interaction— Changes with Plasma Components, Vitamins and Antiplatelet Drugs at the Interface," *Polym. Plast. Technol. Eng.*, 26:143–227 (1987).

14 WILLIAMS, D. F. and R. D. Bagnall. "Adsorption of Proteins on Polymers and Its Role in the Response of Soft Tissue," in *Fundamental Aspects of Biocompatibility*, D. F. Williams, ed. Florida:CRC Press, 2:113–128 (1981).

15 HIRSCHHORN, J. S., A. A. Mcbeath and M. R. Dustoor. "Porous Titanium Surgical Implant Materials," *J. Biomed. Mater. Res. Symp.*, 2:49–67 (1971).

16 HENCH, L. L. and J. Wilson. "Surface Active Biomaterials," *Science*, 226:630–636 (1984).

17 GARRINGTON, G. E. and P. M. Lightbody. "Bioceramics and Dentistry," *J. Biomed. Mat. Res.*, 2:333–343 (1972).

18 DE GROOT, K. "Bioceramics Consisting of Calcium Phosphate Salts," *Biomaterials*, 1:47–50 (1980).

19 HELLE, J. "γ, Controlled Release of Biologically Active Compounds from Bioerodible Polymers," *Biomaterials*, 1:51–57 (1980).

20 CHANDY, T. and C. P. Sharme. "Platelet Adhesion on Polycarbonate—Changes Due to L-Ascorbic Acid," *J. Colloid. Interface Sci.*, 92:102–104 (1983).

21 LEE, E. S. and S. W. Kim. "Adsorbed Glycoproteins in Platelet Adhesion on to Polymer Surfaces: Significance of Terminal Galactose Units," *Trans. Amer. Soc. Artif. Intern. Org.*, 25:124–131 (1979).

22 LINDON, J. N., R. Rodvien, D. Brier, R. Greenberg, E. Merrill and E. W. Salzman. "In Vitro Assessment of Interaction of Blood with Model Surfaces," *J. Lab. Clin. Med.*, 92:904–908 (1978).

23 PACKHAM, M. A., G. Evans, M. F. Glynn and J. P. Mustard. "The Effect of Plasma Proteins on the Interaction of Platelets with Glass Surfaces," *J. Lab. Clin. Med.*, 73:686–697 (1969).

24 UNIYAL, S. and J. L. Brash. "Patterns of Adsorption of Proteins from Human Plasma on to Foreign Surfaces," *Thromb. Haemostas*, 47:285–290 (1982).

25 CHIU, T. C., L. Craig, A. Metcalf and D. J. Lyman. "Electrophoretic Analysis of Protein Adsorbed on Polymer Surfaces," *J. Biomed. Mater. Res.*, 15:781–784 (1981).

26 BRUCK, S. D. "Current Activities and Future Directions in Biomaterials Research," *Ann. N.Y. Acad. Sci.*, 283:332–335 (1977).

27 LELAH, M. D., L. K. Lambrecht and S. L. Cooper. "A Canine Ex Vivo Series Shunt for Evaluating Thrombus Deposition on Polymer Surfaces," *J. Biomed. Mater. Res.*, 18:475–496 (1984).

28 The United States Pharmacopoeia, USP XVIII and The National Formulary, N. F. XIII (1965).

29 VINCENT, W. W. "Plastics in Medical Tubing Applications— Manufacturing Considerations," *Biomaterials*, 2:194–200 (1981).

30 VEDANARAYANAN, P. V., K. Rathinam and A. C. Fernandez. "Screening of Candidate Materials for the Fabrication of a Bubble Oxygenator—A Preliminary Report," *Bull. Mater. Sci.*, 5:97–102 (1983).

31 LOOMIS, T. A. *Essentials of Toxicology, 3rd edition*, Philadelphia:Lea and Febiger (1978).

32 WILLERT, H. G. "Proposed Guideline for the Biological Testing of Orthopaedic Implant," (Prepared by the working group on biomaterials of the German Society of Orthopaedics & Traumatology), *Biomaterials*, 1:179–182 (1980).

33 VON RECUM, A. F. *Handbook of Biomaterials Evaluation*, New York:Macmillan Publishing Company (1986).

34 SAHA, P. and S. Saha. "The Need of Biomedical Ethics Training in Bio-Engineering," *Biomedical Engineering I: Recent Developments*, S. Saha, ed. New York:Pergamon Press, pp. 369–373 (1982).

35 SAHA, S., S. Misra and P. Saha. "Bioengineers, Health-Care Technology and Bioethics," *J. of Med. Eng. Tech.*, 9:55–60 (1985).

36 ANTELYES, J. "Animal Rights in Perspective," *J. Am. Vet. Med. Assoc.*, 189:757–759 (1986).

37 SAHA, S. and P. Saha. "Bioethics and Applied Biomaterials," *J. Biomed. Mat. Res.*, 21:181–190 (1987).

38 BRITT, DAVID. "Ethics, Ethical Committees and Animal Experimentation," *Nature*, 311:503–506 (1984).

39 ENGELHARDT, H. T., Jr. and D. Callahan. *Science Ethics and Medicine*, New York:The Hastings Center, Hastings-on-Hudson (1976).

40 FLETCHER, J. C. "The Evolution of the Ethics of Informed Consent," *Research Ethics*, K. Berg and K. E. Tranoy, eds. New York:Alan. R. Liss, Inc., pp. 187–228 (1983).

41 BLACK, J. *Biological Performance of Materials*, New York & Basel:Marcel Dekker, Inc. (1981).

CHAPTER 8

Biomaterials for Blood Pumps

HELEN E. KAMBIC, Ph.D.[1] and
YUKIHIKO NOSE, Ph.D.[1]

ABSTRACT: In the United States, various forms of mechanical ventricular assist and total circulatory assist are now accepted means of therapy. This is the result of a directive initiated in 1964 by the National Heart, Lung and Blood Institute (NHLBI) with an overall program goal to develop a family of devices that could be used to rehabilitate patients with advanced heart disease [1]. Research during the decade of the 70's was oriented to the development of thrombus-free blood pumps and by almost "olympian" attempts to obtain the longest experimental animal survivors with pneumatically actuated blood pumps. The major goals for developing fully implantable devices of appropriate size, with adequate unloading of the ventricles, reliability and biological compatibility still remain, even after over 20 years of research on component reliability, energy conversion systems and biomaterials. The ultimate goal is the development of a totally implantable cardiac prosthesis that functions for a minimum of two years. The application of newly developed implantable actuation systems to cardiac prostheses offers many alternatives to the traditional pneumatic method. These methods should allow the patient to lead a nearly normal life. We summarize the recent work in the area of biomaterials and identify the relevant design features and problem areas associated with mechanical actuation for cardiac prostheses.

INTRODUCTION—DEFINITION OF BIOMATERIALS

Biomaterials are the basis for the construction of all artificial organs, whether they are constructed from totally synthetic materials or fabricated from specially treated natural tissues. During the Consensus Development Conference on the Clinical Applications of Biomaterials held at the National Institutes of Health in November 1982, the term "biomaterial" was defined as "any substance (other than a drug) or combination of substances, synthetic or natural in origin, which can be used for any period of time, as whole or part of a system which treats, augments, or replaces any tissue, organ, or function of the body" [2]. The requirements and use of biomaterials varies significantly depending on the intended duration of use, the intended method of application, and the function. In order to clarify these applications, the classification of biomaterials with respect to the above mentioned criteria is outlined in Table 1. The blood compatibility of materials is the most important consideration, even in transient applications. The medical need to replace or augment parts of the body has been met for several decades by substitution with natural tissue and selected synthetic materials. Since the beginning of this century, materials and devices were focused on life threatening situations. However, decades later "spare parts medicine," first made possible by materials developed for industrial purposes, has resulted in our present concepts of artificial organs and transplantation. The practical modifications of the composition, surface and bulk properties of both natural tissue and plastics has resulted in the development of the biomedical devices available today.

CARDIOVASCULAR MATERIALS

The development of cardiovascular materials has been hampered by the lack of satisfactory materials of sufficient durability and strength. Historically, blood clotting was the first biocompatibility problem recognized when blood comes into contact with a foreign material. The major research areas investigated were materials and their blood–surface interactions, particularly their potential for blood clot formation [3], pathological calcification [4,5], me-

[1]The Cleveland Clinic Foundation, Department of Artificial Organs, 9500 Euclid Avenue, Cleveland, Ohio 44106, U.S.A.

TABLE 1. Classification of Biomaterials

A. Intended period of use or application
    1. Permanent
    2. Long-term
    3. Transient

B. Intended method of application
    1. Reconstruction and augmentation of tissues and organs (spare parts, e.g., heart valves)
    2. Reconstruction and augmentation of physiological function, e.g., cardiac prosthesis, dialysis
    3. Therapeutic application, e.g., macromolecular modulation

C. Function
    1. Passive—structural components
    2. Active—moving structure

chanical failure [6], hemolysis, polymer degradation [7], and activation of coagulation factors [8,9]. The animal models and species-related differences for predicting clinical performance of materials for cardiovascular use were investigated by Bruck [10], Didisheim [11] and Dodds [12]. Compounding this problem in blood pumps are several parameters, including the flow, method of actuation, animal model, diaphragm movement, implant site, stroke volume, surface geometry and anticoagulant therapy (if required). The basic blood pump design considerations related to device development are outlined in Table 2.

Depending on the intended function, several types of cardiac protheses are available as outlined in Table 3.

Transient Cardiac Prostheses

This group of devices is used routinely in emergency situations and includes the intraaortic balloon pump, cardiopulmonary bypass, the temporary left ventricular

TABLE 2. Basic Blood Pump Design Considerations Related to Device Development

A. Blood–surface interactions	E. Placement
1. Cellular	1. Intrathoracical
2. Physicochemical	2. Parathoracical
3. Rheological	3. Extracorporeal
	4. Abdominal
B. Material durability	
1. Material selection	F. Size and weight
2. Design	
3. Fabrication	G. Mode of Pumping
4. Pump geometry	1. Nonpulsatile
5. Shelf life	a. Roller pump
6. Sterilization	b. Centrifugal pump
	2. Pulsatile
C. Actuation	a. Pusher-plate pump
1. Pneumatic	b. Sac type pump
2. Hydraulic	
3. Mechanical	
D. Power source	
1. Electric	
2. Thermal	

assist device (LVAD) and the biventricular bypass device. The failing natural heart would recover within several days to several weeks, after which the device would be removed so the patient's heart could resume its normal function.

Interim Cardiac Prostheses

This group of devices is used for transplant patients awaiting a suitable donor heart and includes the ventricular assist devices and the total artificial heart. A mechanical heart used in this way is called a "bridge" to transplant [13]. These devices could also be applied to heart transplant recipients during rejection crises of the transplanted heart. As temporary measures to save the dying patient, these prostheses need not be totally implantable since their use is intended for one month at most

Since the first mechanical heart was implanted by Denton Cooley in 1969 at the Texas Heart Institute in a 47 year old male patient as a bridge procedure to heart transplantation [16], there have been 116 total artificial hearts (TAH) implanted in 113 patients by 29 centers worldwide [14,15].

With the increased clinical application of mechanical circulatory support, not only is appropriate patient selection important, but the correct determination of whether the patient has right ventricular failure, left ventricular failure, or biventricular failure [17]. Devices capable of providing left ventricular support would be inadequate for patients with biventricular failure [18].

Early clinical trials and support with only an LVAD initiated the importance of the right heart [19]. Systems providing biventricular support may not be appropriate for patients with isolated left ventricular or right ventricular function, because of potentially increased device related complications [17,20].

Permanent Cardiac Prostheses

Development is still underway for this group of totally implantable mechanical devices geared to provide the potential for 2 years or longer of tether-free operation within the body. Electrically actuated left ventricular assist systems are now in the preclinical evaluation phase. The components include the blood pump, energy converter, variable volume compensation device, internal batteries, transcutaneous energy transmission systems, external batteries and diagnostic systems (Figure 1). In the U. S., at least 9 groups are involved in various stages of systems development (Table 4) with several of these devices available by the end of 1987.

Thermal engine ventricular assist systems are currently being pursued by 2 groups in the U. S. A. One such system, driven by a Stirling cycle engine, uses molten salt as a source of energy (Figure 2). The other alternative is the use of Plutonium 238 as a power source [21]. Although not

TABLE 3. Application of Cardiac Prosthesis

Type	Function	Device	Duration	Features
1. Transient	Temporary support of the failing heart	Intraaortic balloon pump (IABP) Cardiopulmonary bypass Temporary LVAD Biventricular bypass pump	Days-weeks (2)	Readily available and easily removed
2. Interim	Support patient awaiting transplantation	LVAD Biventricular bypass pump TAH	one month	Readily available and easily removed
3. Permanent	Total support of circulation	TAH, LVAD	2 years	Totally implantable

LVAD = left ventricular assist device, TAH = total artificial heart.

as advanced as the electrical systems, animal experiments are continuing to evaluate system performance using such alternate power sources.

BIOCOMPATIBILITY OF MATERIALS

The general requirements for blood pump materials must be divided into blood compatibility associated with the inner diaphragm surface and tissue compatibility of the outer housing surface. The blood-contacting inner surface of pumps includes the ventricular sac or pumping diaphragm, inflow and outflow valves and the ventricular housing. One important feature is the fatigue life of the diaphragm. A pump beating 100 times a minute would flex the diaphragm more than 50 million times a year. Therefore, materials are required with durability, ease of fabrication, nonreactivity towards blood and its constituents, and resistance to biodegradation.

For implantable pumps the ventricular housing must be durable, nonreactive to the surrounding tissue, and readily amenable for repairs or replacement. These components, for three types of blood pumps, are outlined in Figure 3.

Polymer Surfaces

Smooth surfaces were first used in the fabrication of blood pumps. Kolff and colleagues, using polyurethane, were able to implant a blood pump in a dog and keep him alive for up to 20 hours [22]. Material smoothness in early pumps was required to eliminate stagnant areas, seams and reduce clotting problems. However, the early prototypes were poorly designed. The availability of new synthetic polymers coincided with the emergence of improved blood pump design and actuation systems. The materials research emphasis was directed toward the specific blood–surface interactions involving plasma protein adsorption, platelet deposition leukocyte, erythrocyte adhesion, effects of flow, and shear rate [23]. The defini-

TABLE 4. Blood Pump Components and Energy Converters for LVAD and TAH Systems Under Development in the U.S.

Material	Blood Contacting Surface	Institution	Pump Configuration	Device	Actuation System
Angioflex	Smooth polyurethane	Abiomed, Danvers, Mass.	Sac type	LVAD	Electrohydraulic
Biomer	Smooth polyurethane trilaminar sac of butyl rubber sandwiched between 2 Biomer layers	Novacor Medical, Berkeley, Ca.	Diaphragm Dual pusher plate	LVAD	Electromechanical
Biomer	Textured microporous Urethane	Thoratec Inc., Berkeley, Ca.	Sac type	LVAD TAH	Pneumatic Pneumatic
Tecoflex	Polyester flock Titanium metal housing	Thermedics, Inc. Waltham, Mass.	Diaphragm type Pusher plate	LVAD	Electromechanical
Gelatin	Smooth aldehyde Treated gelatin Coated polyolefin Rubber, polyurethane housing	Cleveland Clinic Fdn. Cleveland, Ohio Nimbus, Inc. Rancho Cordova, Ca.	Pusher plate Diaphragm type	TAH LVAD LVAD LVAD	Pneumatic Electrohydraulic Thermal-pneumatic Pneumatic
Tecoflex	Polyester flock Diaphragm textured Powdered metal housing	Univ. of Wash. Whalen Biomedical, Inc. Cleveland Clinic	Pusher plate	LVAD	Thermal Hydraulic
Biomer	Smooth polyurethane graphite between Biomer layers	Symbion Salt Lake City, Utah	Sac type	TAH	Pneumatic

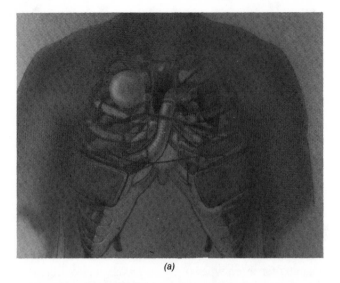

(a)

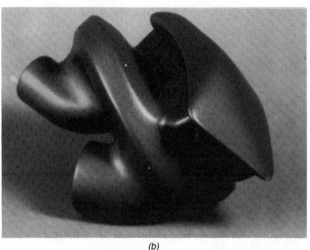

(b)

Figure 1. *(a) Completely implantable total artificial heart system proposed and developed by the Cleveland Clinic and Nimbus, Inc. The compliance chamber is located on the right. (b) Model of the integrated blood pump with attached electrohydraulic energy converter. Access to the modular energy system can be made without entering the thorax.*

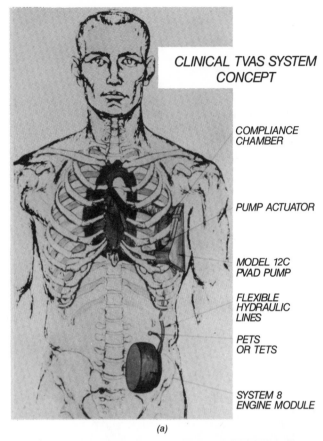

CLINICAL TVAS SYSTEM CONCEPT

COMPLIANCE CHAMBER

PUMP ACTUATOR

MODEL 12C PVAD PUMP

FLEXIBLE HYDRAULIC LINES

PETS OR TETS

SYSTEM 8 ENGINE MODULE

(a)

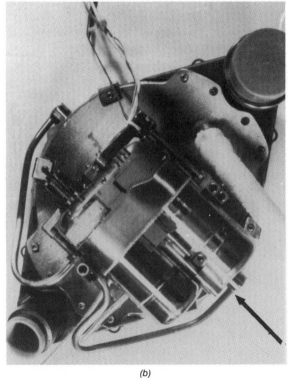

(b)

Figure 2. *(a) Locations of the pump actuator and engine module for the thermal ventricular assist system (TVAS). (b) The integrated thermal LVAD system couples a parathoracic ventricular device with a thermal energy converter (arrow) mounted directly onto the pump.*

tion of the laminary boundary layer with respect to blood flow, and the scale of roughness of a surface were new areas for study opened to evaluate and to define the blood–material contact phenomena occurring after immediate, short-term (<2 week) and long-term (years) time periods [24].

Although the bulk characteristics of a material and predictive tests concerning the mechanical properties are still considered important material parameters, the surface of the material which interacts with blood is the most crucial. Two approaches have since been directed to the development of surfaces that either (1) form blood linings (a pseudoneointima, PNI) or (2) minimize cellular or protein reactions. For short-term or interim use of the LVAD's, both approaches appear equally advantageous [25].

ARTIFICIAL HEART DESIGNS

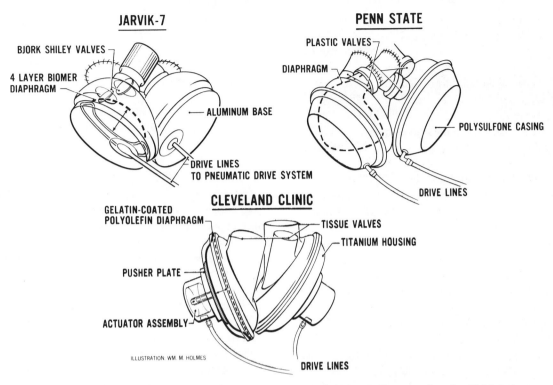

Figure 3. *Cross-section of the main components for three types of pneumatically actuated total artificial devices.*

One type of smooth "biolized" surface was developed at the Cleveland Clinic Foundation's Department of Artificial Organs [26]. Our group has initiated the development of mechanically actuated blood pump systems capable of coupling with either thermal or electrical actuation systems. One major objective of the LVAD for temporary use is the complete unloading of the left ventricle, with total capture of the cardiac output. The main blood-contacting components of the Cleveland Clinic blood pump include the housing, polyolefin rubber diaphragm and dura mater valves. The blood-contacting surface of the blood pump is a seamless glutaraldehyde-crosslinked gelatin layer coated on a textured polyolefin rubber (Hexsyn) diaphragm [27].

To mechanically anchor the biolized coating on both the pump housing and diaphragm, the surfaces must be textured. The diaphragm surface was integrally textured with the use of a salt casting technique after compression molding. The pump housing surface is coated with a textured layer of polyurethane (Avcomat 610), with the use of a similar technique. The resulting surface texture is nominally 100 μm thick, with open pores nominally 20 μm in diameter (Figure 4). After final assembly, biolization is done by dipping the entire pump into a gelatin solution, with the use of vacuum to fill the pores in the textured surfaces, and then crosslinking the gelatin coating in place with glutaraldehyde. By coating the pump after assembly,

the entire blood contact surface is seamless, with no discontinuities. With gelatin impregnated into the pores, additional coatings provide a smooth surface for blood contact. This biolized surface, combined with the natural tissue valves fabricated from human dura mater eliminates the need for anticoagulants.

Biolized surfaces provide a blood-compatible, hydrophilic, durable, and non-PNI generating surface. Clean,

SMOOTH GELATIN SURFACE

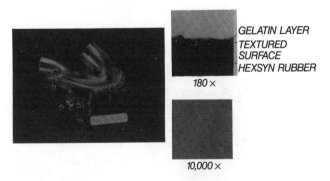

Figure 4. *(left) The biolized pusher plate LVAD. The salt texturization technique renders an integral porous surface on the polyolefin diaphragm, which is then coated with gelatin and glutaraldehyde crosslinked (top right). The smooth appearance of the gelatin surface applied to the diaphragm and inner housing of the pump (right bottom).*

thrombus-free blood pumps have been implanted in calves as total artificial hearts and left ventricular assist devices for over 10 months of implantation [28] (Figure 5).

The polyurethanes, initially prepared for industrial purposes, have found an increasing use in blood pump applications compared to that of the silicone elastomers and carbons. Equally good smooth surface properties can be developed with solvent cast and or thermoplastic polyurethane materials.

The segmented polyurethanes are a series of soluble non-crosslinked polyurethanes whose physical properties depend on the existence of soft and hard segments. Hard segments are formed by urethane and urea linkages while the soft segments are formed by polyether residues.

The most common polyether glycols used in the preparation of polyurethanes include polytetramethylenetherglycol (PYMEG), polytetrahydrofuran (THF) and polytetramethyleneoxide (PTMO). Diphenyl-methanediisocyanate (MDI) is the most commonly used diisocyanate. The MDI based polyurethane elastomers generally have physical and mechanical properties superior to otherwise identical polymers prepared from diisocyanates such as toluene diisocyanate (TDI), hexamethylene diisocyanate (HDI) and the hydrogenated analog of MDI called dicyclohexanediisocyanate (HMDI) [29].

As shown in the reactions forming the polyurethanes Biomer and Pellethane, the reaction of diisocyanate groups with low molecular weight reagents leads to chain extension and the formation of hard segments connecting the polyether (PTMEG) soft segments through urethane groups (Figure 6). In the formation of Pellethane (Figure 7) the diol chain extender is 1,4-butadiol, resulting in the repeating units connected by urethane groups. In the case of Biomer, the hard segment contains urea groups as a result of chain extension by ethylenediamine. Some biomedical polyurethanes available in the U. S. are listed in Table 5.

Several smooth surface synthetic polymers, including the silicone based elastomers, polyurethanes, pyrolytic carbons, polyethylene Biomer, Avcothane, and others have shown good blood compatibility. Certain types of smooth surfaces are believed not to activate the blood coagulation system. The use of smooth surfaces has the advantages of ease of fabrication, minimal thrombosis and fibrin deposition. Anticoagulation treatment may be required. A limited flex life may be due to undetected microscopic defects produced during fabrication; such surface imperfections can lead to degradation and calcification within the surface defects.

Fabrication processes to construct a device have a tremendous impact on thrombogenicity and calcification. Calcification on the surface of pumps and pannus forma-

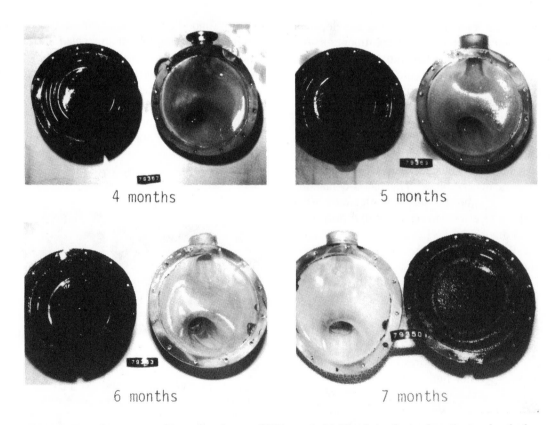

4 months   5 months

6 months   7 months

Figure 5. *Typical appearance of the pusher plate type LVAD coated with 5% gelatin after implantation in calves for four to seven months. The blood-contacting surface of both housing and diaphragm are clean without thrombus.*

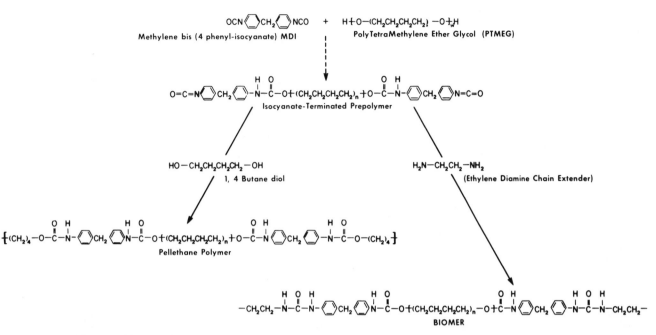

Figure 6. *Typical polymerization reactions leading to the formation of the polyurethanes Pellethane and Biomer.*

tion at the sutured orifice to valves and cannulae are typical examples [5,30]. Polyurethane elastomers for blood pump diaphragms have been used on the basis of their excellent mechanical properties (tensile strength and flex fatigue), which are based on their chemical structure. After contact in the biological environment, polyurethanes may change their original properties such as mechanical strength, average molecular weight or surface smoothness [7]. The surface chemistry of polyurethanes can vary significantly from the bulk chemistry. The molecular orientation at the surface and the preference of low molecular weight molecules to orient themselves to the surface has been supported by the extraction studies of Ratner et al. [31] to determine ESCA peak shifts of organic functional groups. Their analyses implicated polyether groups in platelet–surface reactions, with little

reactivity of the hard segment (carbamate and nitrogen groups) towards blood. Similar studies were done by Merril and Salzman [32], using ESCA (electron microscopy for chemical analyses) to analyze platelet–surface reactivity. The leaching out of low molecular weight compounds from polyurethanes may result in changes in surface structures and surface morphology that may be related to the surface morphology observed in polyurethanes after implantation.

Rough Surfaces

Rough surfaces generate a pseudoneointima (PNI). Typical examples are textured materials such as the woven Dacrons, polytetrafluoroethylene (PTFE), knitted velours, and sintered metal surfaces. A strongly adherent bi-

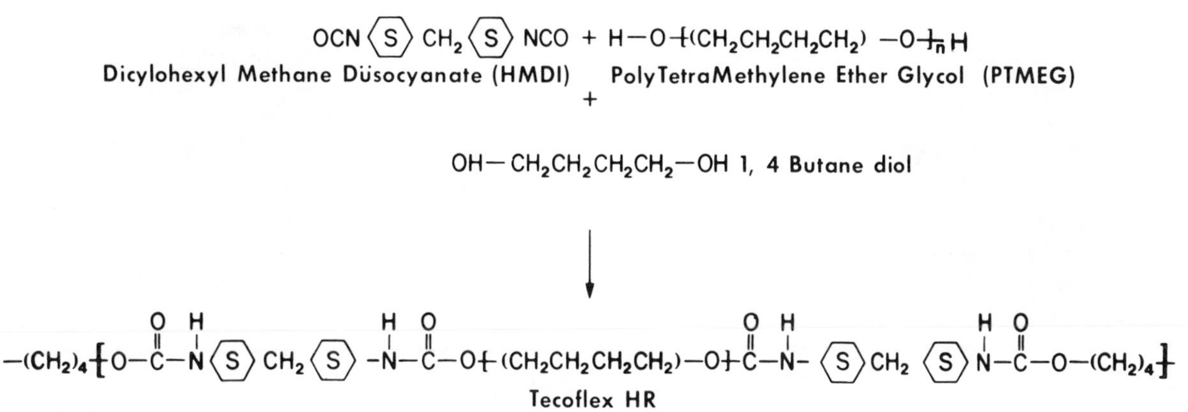

OCN ⟨S⟩ CH₂ ⟨S⟩ NCO + H—O—(CH₂CH₂CH₂CH₂) —O—ₙ H

Dicylohexyl Methane Düsocyanate (HMDI)   PolyTetraMethylene Ether Glycol (PTMEG)

+

OH— CH₂CH₂CH₂CH₂—OH 1, 4 Butane diol

—(CH₂)₄—O—C—N ⟨S⟩ CH₂ ⟨S⟩ —N—C—O—(CH₂CH₂CH₂CH₂)—O—C—N— ⟨S⟩ CH₂ ⟨S⟩ N—C—O—(CH₂)₄—

Tecoflex HR

Figure 7. *Typical polymerization reactions to yield the polyurethane Tecoflex.*

TABLE 5. Selected Polyurethanes Available in the U.S.

Generic Trade Name	Manufacturer	Preparation	Polyether Based Polyurethane
Cardiomat 610 Cardiothane 51 Cardiomat 40	Kontron Medical Everett, Mass	15% by weight solution contains 10% silicone 5% by weight	Medical grade Block copolymer of Polyurethane and Polyorganosiloxane Polymer silicone system
Biomer/ (Lycra, Spandex)	Ethicon, Inc. Somerville, N.J.	Solvent cast 30% solution	Medical grade Aromatic Segmented polyurethane
Pellethane 2363	Dow Corning Corp. La Porte, Texas	Resin form Thermoplastic	Aromatic Segmented polyurethane
Tecoflex	Thermedics Waltham, Mass	Solvent Cast	Medical grade Alphatic Linear segmented polyurethane
Mitrathane M2007	Mitral Medical International Inc. Wheat Ridge, Co.	Solvent cast 25% by weight	
Q-thane	K.J. Quinn, Co., Inc. Malden, Mass	Resins	Polyether/polester Alphatic
Surethane	Cardiac Control Systems Palm Coast, Florida	20% solution	
REN:C:O-thane RP 6403	Ciba-Giegy Corp. East Lansing, Mich		2 component polyurethane Casting elastomer
Polathane XPE Systems	Polaroid Corp. Assonet, Mass		2 component Ether linked polyurethane Elastomer

ological PNI lining is produced, which requires anticoagulation to control layer thickness. The PNI linings on blood pump bladders perform as stable biological linings derived first from the deposition of circulating blood elements and result in the formation of an organized fibrin matrix. With time, cellular proliferation occurs and in situ collagen may be observed [33]. The disadvantages in their use is the possibility of emboli originating from the surface or calcification of the derived layer leading to a loss of compliance [34].

Tecoflex is an example of a polyurethane developed by Thermedics in Waltham, Mass. A flocked surface is produced by attaching polyester fibrils to the polyurethane substrate. Such technology has led to the introduction of an integrated textured surface that is applied successfully in clinical LVADs made by Thermedics (Figure 8).

Textured surfaces have been introduced on metals by a sphere sintering process. These fused titanium spheres have been applied to nonmoving parts of blood pumps [35]. Such textured surfaces subsequently generate a stable pseudoneointima after long-term application. The deposited layer assures that no thrombus formation occurs (Figure 9).

Several laboratories have expanded on the texturization concept and have pursued the application of cell seeding techniques for blood pump components. Cultured human endothelial cells are used to accelerate the development of a thin organized cellular interface. Some scientists consider the formation of pseudoneointimal linings composed of native collagen and a layer of endothelial cells highly desirable since it represents an end stage in the intravascular healing process. Such techniques have been applied to vascular graft prostheses [36,37].

Calcification

In long-term studies, the literature has shown that calcification occurs on both smooth and rough surface materials [4,5,30,38]. Calcified deposits are seen preferentially in the stress concentrations areas of the moving diaphragm. The location of calcified deposits also coincides with the loci of surface imperfections or surface defects. It has been suggested that the degenerative changes in the bulk structure and surface properties of long-term mechanically active polymers may account for diminished functions or complete device failure. In studies with calves, this calcification on blood pumps and heart valves has been described as dystrophic calcification characterized by the deposit of calcium salt (calcium phosphate) in injured, degenerated or dead tissue [38]. Smooth surfaces, after contact in blood, are coated with plasma proteins. If no cellular deposition takes place, this

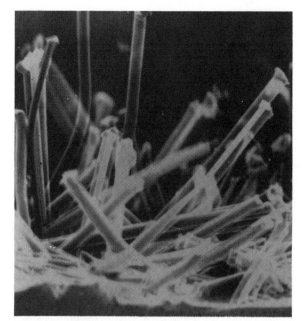

Figure 8. A cross-section of a conventional polyester flocked surface. Polyester fibrils approximately 300 μm long are bonded to the base Biomer and form a rough polymer surface (300 ×).

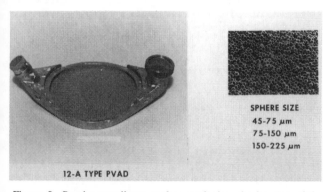

SPHERE SIZE

45-75 μm

75-150 μm

150-225 μm

12-A TYPE PVAD

Figure 9. Powder metallurgy surface applied to the housing of the parathoracic LVAD (Thermedic's, Waltham, Mass). The sintered titanium powder metal surface uses 45 to 225 μm diameter spheres.

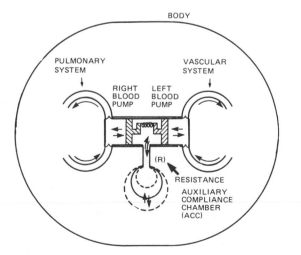

Figure 10. Auxiliary compliance chamber necessary for two alternate beating ventricles.

becomes a stable pump surface. However, if deposition occurs and if the deposited cells are not replaced by living cells, then the deposited blood cells may die, resulting in degeneration. These cells become the nuclei and center for precipitation and crystallization of calcium salt. This type of deposition can readily occur on surfaces with imperfections, contaminants such as dust, bubbles, and as a result of fatigue failure after long-term use.

Heart Valves

The Bjork–Shiley valve was introduced in 1969 and remains one of the most widely used commercially available heart valves. Basically, the valve consists of a Stellite 21 (chromium–cobalt alloy) cage with a disk which pivots around an eccentric axis in the plane of the valve orifice. Originally made of Delrin, this has been changed to pyrolytic carbon. This valve has been used in several types of blood pump prostheses. One example of a tissue valve is the dura mater valve, developed at the University of Sao Paulo Brazil, which has been used in biolized blood pumps at the Cleveland Clinic. This nonvalvular tissue is obtained from the dura mater removed from undiseased accident victims within 12 hours of death. The 3 leaflet valve is fabricated on a cloth-covered stent that assures a large contacting surface between adjacent leaflets when the valve is closed [39]. At the present time this valve is not commercially available in the U. S.

Compliance Chamber

A variable volume device is required to compensate for the volume changes which occur within pulsatile blood pumps. A totally implantable LVAD would be a "closed" system. With displacement type pumps the nonblood side of the pump undergoes a volume change equal and opposite to that of the blood side (Figure 10). Since energy to these systems is a major consideration, a variable volume device should accommodate the displaced volume with a minimum expenditure of energy. One such compliance system under evaluation includes a compliance chamber (consisting of a titanium backplate curved to fit the inside of the rib cage) and a flexing diaphragm that faces the lung. This system can be inflated with up to 150 ml of fluid which can be shuttled back and forth from the back side of the pump to the compliance chamber located elsewhere in the body. This textured series of compliance studies appears promising for totally implantable blood pump systems. Since 1983 the use of a gas-filled intrathoracic compliance chamber was conceived as a simple and practical solution to the variable volume problem. The prerequisites for this system to work properly are (1) biological compatibility that would allow stable and acceptable pressure-volume characteristics for long durations, and (2) retention of the gas mixture in an environment in which gas diffusion gradients inherently exist.

The previous, lenticular shaped, dacron velour-covered polyurethane compliance chambers showed stable, thin compliant tissue capsule formation in calves in durations of up to two years [40]. These good results were reproduced in experiments in which the polyurethane membrane was replaced by Hexsyn, which offered fabrication advantages. In addition, dynamic testing showed that energy consumption due to inflation and deflation work was quite low at volume flow rates over the range from 180 and 500 ml/sec. Therefore, the biological compatibility can be considered well-established.

Our recent permeability testing showed that sulfur hexafluoride, a nontoxic, medically-used gas, would have slow permeation rates and serve well as a buffer gas in the compliance gas mixture. In vivo experiments currently underway are being used to quantify the concentrations of the physiologic gases for equilibrium conditions in a closed system and gas diffusion rates. For these studies, sealed, nonfunctioning compliance chambers are implanted in the thorax of calves. Chambers which were initially air-filled show faster rates of volume loss than chambers initially filled with the SF_6-buffered gas mixture.

Integrated blood pump–compliance chamber in vivo experiments were initiated in which the systems were implanted as a sealed unit without external pressure or sample taps. Compliance gas volume is monitored by a Hall-effect sensor on the compliance chamber. These experiments demonstrate that buffer gas diffusion, although relatively low, is substantial enough to necessitate some gas addition for long-term implants.

CONCLUSION

In this review, we have attempted to show a growing momentum directed towards gaining an understanding of the mechanism and regulation of blood–surface reactions of materials. Physiological studies have established the sequence of protein deposition onto surfaces. Physicochemical studies have identified the surface groups whose presence or absence participate in the blood passivation process or aid in the analysis of their function. Advanced spectroscopic methods have determined the surface changes after implant, thereby facilitating studies on polymer synthesis and device fabrication. We often speak of the blood-compatible polymers in terms of a number of distinct pathways that help a surface adapt to the blood or tissue environment. However, several new choices are now available for preparing and processing new materials. This development of new polymeric synthetic and natural materials and their applications to a family of blood pump devices have permitted a new biochemical assault on the problem of blood compatibility. The impact of the future applications of these material surfaces in blood pumps will ultimately be measured by the amount of new information they bring to bear on biocompatibility issues not yet resolved by other methods available.

REFERENCES

1 ALTIERI, F. D. "Status of Implantable Energy Systems to Actuate and Control Ventricular Assist Devices," *Artif. Organs*, 7:5–20 (1983).
2 BORETOS, J. W. and M. Eden, eds. *Contemporary Biomaterials*, Park Ridge, New Jersey:Noyes Publications, p. 651–665 (1984).
3 BAIER, R., R. C. Dutton and V. L. Galt. "Surface Chemical Features of Blood Vessel Walls and of Synthetic Materials Exhibiting Thromboresistance," in *Surface Chemistry of Biological Systems*, M. Black, ed. New York:Plenum, pp. 235–260 (1970).
4 NOSE, Y., H. Harasaki and J. Murray. "Mineralization of Artificial Surfaces that Contact Blood," *Trans. Am. Soc. Artif. Intern. Organs*, 27:714–718 (1981).
5 COLEMAN, D. L., H. Hsu, D. Dong and D. Olsen. "Polymer Properties Associated with Calcification of Cardiovascular Devices," in *Calcium in Biological Systems*, R. Rubin, G. Weiss and J. Putney, Jr., eds. New York:Plenum Press, pp. 653–659 (1985).
6 McMILLAN, C. R. "Physical Testing of Elastomers for Cardiovascular Applications," *Artif Organs*, 7(1):78–91 (1983).
7 LEMM, W. "Biodegradation of Polyurethane in Polyurethanes," in *Biomedical Engineering*, H. Planek, G. Egbers and I. Syres, eds. B. V. Amsterdam:Elsevier Science Publishers, pp. 103–134 (1984).
8 LYMAN, D. J., L. C. Metcalf, D. Albo, et al. "The Effect of Chemical Structure and Surface Properties of Synthetic Polymers on the Coagulation of Blood III. In Vivo Adsorption of Proteins on Poly Surfaces," *Trans. Am. Soc. Artif. Intern. Organs*, 20:474–478 (1974).
9 SALZMAN, E. W., J. Lindan, D. Bruer and E. W. Merrill. "Surface Induced Platelet Adhesion, Aggregation and Release," in *The Behavior of Blood and Its Components at Interfaces*, L. Vroman and E. Leonard, eds. Ann N.Y. Acad. Sciences, 283:1–560 (1977).
10 BRUCK, S. D. "Considerations of Species Related Hematological Differences on the Evaluation of Biomaterials," *Biomat. Med. Dev. Artif. Organs*, 5(1):97–113 (1977).
11 DIDISHEIM, P., M. K. Dewanjee, C. S. Frisk, M. P. Kaye and D. N. Fars. "Animal Models for Predicting Clinical Performance of Biomaterials for Cardiovascular Use," in *Contemporary Biomaterials*, J. Boretos and M. Eden, eds. Park Ridge, New Jersey:Noyes Publications, pp. 132–119 (1984).
12 DODDS, W. J. "Platelet Function in Animals; Species Specificities," in *Platelets: A Multidisciplinary Approach*, G. de Faetano and S. Garattini, eds. N.Y.:Raven Press, pp. 45–49 (1978).
13 HILL, J. D., D. J. Farrar, J. J. Hershon, P. G. Compton, G. J. Avery, B. S. Levin and B. N. Brent. "Use of a Prosthetic Ventricle as a Bridge to Cardiac Transplantation for Post Infarction Cardiogenic Shock," *New Eng. J. Med.*, 314(10):626–628 (1986).
14 JOYCE, L. D., K. Johnson, C. Cabrol, et al. "Results of the First One Hundred Patients Who Received Jarvik Total Artificial Hearts as a Bridge to Cardiac Transplantation," *Circulation*, 78(4):581 (1988).
15 JOYCE, L. D., K. Johnson, C. Cabrol, et al. "Nine Year Experience with the Clinical Use of Total Artificial Hearts as Cardiac Support Devices," *Trans. Am. Soc. Artif. Intern. Organs*, 34:703–737 (1989).
16 COOLEY, D. A., D. Liotta, G. L. Hallman, et al. "First Human Implantation of Cardiac Prothesis for Staged Total Replacement of the Heart," *Trans. Am. Soc. Artif. Intern. Organs*, 15:253–266 (1969).

17 SWARTZ, M. T., G. Pennington, S. A. Ruzevich, L. R. McBride, L. W. Miller, J. E. Reedy and D. R. Termuhlen. "Incidence of Isolated Left Ventricular Failure in Bridge to Transplant Candidates," *Trans. Am. Soc. Artif. Intern. Organs*, 35:730–733 (1989).

18 STARNES, V. A., P. O. Oyer, P. M. Portner, et al. "Isolated Left Ventricular Assist as a Bridge to Cardiac Transplantation," *J. Thorac. Cardiovasc. Surg.*, 96:62–71 (1988).

19 PENNINGTON, D. G., J. P. Merjovy, M. T. Swartz, et al. "The Importance of Biventricular Failure in Patients with Postoperative Cardiogenic Shock," *Ann. Thorac. Surg.*, 39:16–26 (1985).

20 GRIFFITH, B. P. "Interim Use of the Jarvik 7 Artificial Heart: Lessons Learned at Presbyterian University Hospital of Pittsburgh," *Ann. Thorac. Surg.*, 47:158–166 (1989).

21 SHUMAKOV, V. I., G. M. Griaznov, G. N. Shemchuzhnickov, I. M. Kiselev and A. P. Osipov. "Implanted Artificial Heart with Radioisotope Power Source," *Artif Organs*, 7(1):101–106 (1983).

22 KOLFF, W., T. Akutsu, B. Dreyer and H. Norton. "Artificial Heart in the Chest and Use of Polyurethane for Making Hearts, Valves and Aortas," *Trans. Am. Soc. Artif. Intern. Organs*, 5:298–303, 959.

23 VROMAN, L. and E. F. Leonard, eds. *Behavior of Blood and Its Components at Interfaces*, New York:Ann N.Y. Acad. Sci., 283 (1977).

24 BAIER, R. "The Organization of Blood Components Near Interfaces," in *The Behavior of Blood and Its Components at Interfaces*, L. Vroman and E. Leonard, eds. New York:Ann. N.Y. Acad. of Sciences, 283:17–26 (1977).

25 KOLFF, W. J. and F. Stellwag. "Blood at Artificial Organ Surfaces: Progress to Date as Stepping Stones for the Future," in *The Behavior of Blood and Its Components at Interfaces*, L. Vroman and E. Leonard, eds. Ann. N.Y. Acad. Sci., 283:443–456 (1977).

26 IMAI, Y., K. Tajima and Y. Nose. "Biolized Materials for Cardiovascular Prostheses," *Trans. Am. Soc. Artif. Intern. Organs*, 17:6–9 (1971).

27 KAMBIC, H., S. Murabayashi and Y. Nose. "Biolized Surfaces as Chronic Blood Compatible Interfaces," in *Biocompatible Polymers, Metals and Composites*, M. Szycher, ed. Lancaster, PA:Technomic Publishing Co., Inc., pp. 179–198 (1983).

28 YOZU, R., L. A. R. Golding, G. Jacobs, S. Murabayashi, H. Harasaki, R. Kiraly and Y. Nose. "Preclinical Evaluation of a Biolized Temporary Ventricular Assist Device," *Cleve. Clin.*, 51:119–126.

29 WARD, R. S., K. A. White and C. B. Hu. "Use of Surface Modifying Additives in the Development of a New Biomedical Polyurethaneurea," in *Polyurethanes in Biomedical Engineering*, H. Planeb, G. Egbers and I. Syre, eds. Amsterdam:Elsevier Science Publishers, pp. 181–200 (1984).

30 LEVY, R. J., F. J. Schoen, S. Howard, J. T. Levy, L. Osbry and M. Hawley. "Calcification of Cardiac Valve Bioprostheses: Host and Implant Factors," in *Calcium in Biological Systems*, R. Rubin, G. Weiss and J. Putney, eds. New York:Plenum Press, pp. 661–668 (1985).

31 RATNER, B. D. and R. W. Paynter. "Polyurethane Surfaces: The Importance of Molecular Weight Distribution, Bulk Chemistry and Casting Conditions," in *Polyurethanes in Biomedical Engineering*, H. Planek, G. Egbers and I. Syre, eds. B. V. Amsterdam:Elsevier Science Publishers, pp. 41–61 (1984).

32 SA DA COSTA, V., D. Brier-Russel, E. W. Salzman and E. W. Merrill. "ESCA Studies of Polyurethanes: Blood Platelet Activation in Relation to Surface Composition," *J. Coll. Interf. Sci.*, pp. 445–452 (1981).

33 TURNER, S., M. Bosart, N. Clay and O. Frazer. "Pseudoneointimal Analysis of Cheonically Implanted Blood Pumps," in *Biocompatible Polymers, Metals and Composites*, M. Szycher, ed. Lancaster, PA:Technomic Publishing Co., Inc., pp. 213–237 (1983).

34 BERNHARD, W. F., G. G. LaFarge, R. H. Less, M. Szycher, R. I. Berger and V. Poirier. "An Appraisal of Blood Trauma and Blood Prosthetic Interface During Left Ventricular Bypass in the Calf and Humans," *Ann. Thoracic. Surg.*, 26:427–437 (1978).

35 HARASAKI, J. Snow, R. Gerrity, R. Whalen, K. Ozawa, R. Kiraly and Y. Nose. "Powdered Metal Surface for Blood Pump," *Trans. Am. Soc. Artif. Intern. Organs*, 25:225–230 (1979).

36 INES, C. L., S. Eskin and C. L. Seidel. "Adhesion of Human Umbilical Vein Endothelial Cells to Mitrathane, A Segmented Polyether Urethane, Under Conditions of Shear and Axial Stress (Strain)," *Trans 2nd and World Congress of Biomaterials*, Washington, D.C., 7:142 (April 1984).

37 HUNTER, T. J., S. P. Schmidt, W. V. Sharp and G. S. Malendzak. "Controlled Flow Studies in 4 mm Endothelialized Dacron Grafts," *Trans. Am. Soc. Artif. Intern. Organs*, 29:177–182 (1983).

38 HARASAKI, H., R. Gerrity, R. Kiraly, G. Jacobs and Y. Nose. "Calcification in Blood Pumps," *Trans. Am. Soc. Artif. Intern. Organs*, 25:305–310 (1979).

39 HARASAKI, H, J. Snow, R. Kiraly and Y. Nose. "The Dura Mater Valve. In Vitro Characteristics and Pathological Changes After Implantation in Calves," *Artif. Organs*, 3:176–183 (1979).

40 SNOW, J., H. Harasaki, J. Kasick, R. Whalen, R. Kiraly and Y. Nose. "Promising Reuslts with New Textured Surface Intrathoracic Variable Volume Device for LVAS," *Trans. Am. Soc. Artif. Intern. Organs*, 27:485–489 (1981).

CHAPTER 9

Prosthetic Heart Valves

KEVIN C. DELLSPERGER, M.D., Ph.D.[1] and
K. B. CHANDRAN, D.Sc.[1]

ABSTRACT: Since the intracardiac implantation of the first prosthetic heart valves in 1960, many investigators have studied the material composition, hydrodynamic function and clinical results with a large variety of different cardiac valve replacements. The material composition, *in vitro* hydrodynamic results and clinical results for the current widely used prostheses such as the Starr. Edwards, Bjork. Shiley, Medtronic. Hall, Omniscience, St. Jude Medical, Hancock, Carpentier. Edwards and Ionescu. Shiley prosthetic heart valves are presented. During the last three decades many major advances in design and function of prosthetic valve replacements have been made; however, the design of the "ideal" prosthetic valve has yet to be accomplished. Qualities of an "ideal" prosthetic heart valve are discussed with regard to needed scientific advances required to achieve the goal towards the same.

INTRODUCTION

The human heart consists of two fluid pumps in series, the right heart and the left heart. Each fluid pump has two chambers, the atrium, a collecting chamber, and the ventricle, a pumping chamber, in addition to two one-way valves.

The valves in the right heart are the tricuspid valve, located between the right atrium and right ventricle, and the pulmonary valve, located between the right ventricle and pulmonary artery. The mitral valve is located between the left atrium and left ventricle, while the aortic valve is located between the left ventricle and aorta. These valves normally allow fluid to pass in one direction freely while inhibiting retrograde flow. The cardiac valves play a vital role in maintaining normal cardiac output and perfusion pressures throughout the cardiovascular system.

FLOW DYNAMICS OF NATURAL AORTIC AND MITRAL VALVES

Heart valve diseases are predominantly found in the left heart, and replacement of diseased aortic and mitral valves with prostheses is a common practice today. It is therefore interesting to consider the flow past the natural valves before comparing the flow development past valve prostheses of various geometries. The natural aortic valve consists of three thin crescent-shaped leaflets (referred to as semilunar valves) of about 0.1 mm in thickness. In the full open position, the leaflets are aligned to the axis of the aorta and behind each leaflet is a sinus of valsalva. In two of the sinuses are the ostia for the left and right coronary arteries and the third is called the noncoronary sinus. In the closed position, the central margins of the three cusps come together along three radii 120° apart to seal the aortic orifice. Since the leaflets have negligible inertia, they open and close passively due to the pressure gradient across the valve. The dynamics of the natural aortic valve has been the subject of several theoretical and experimental investigations [1,2].

At the beginning of systole, the valve leaflets open with a minimal transvalvular pressure gradient (about 1 mm Hg higher in the ventricular cavity than in the aorta) and the blood is ejected into the aorta. *In vitro* model studies have shown that the velocity profile distal to the aortic valve in the aorta is relatively flat [1]. This has been subsequently confirmed by *in vivo* measurements in animals using pulsed Doppler [3] and hot-film anemometry [4]. The efficient closure of the aortic valve has been attributed to the vortex formation behind the leaflets in the sinuses [1]. These vortices, with higher pressure compared to the jet-like flow through the orifice, enable the leaflets to move towards closure during late systole when there is still flow of blood into the aorta. At the beginning of diastole, the

---

[1]Departments of Internal Medicine and Biomedical Engineering, The University of Iowa, Iowa City, Iowa 52242, U.S.A.

reverse pressure gradient immediately causes the valve leaflets to close with minimal backflow (regurgitation) of blood into the left ventricle.

The mitral valve has two leaflets, thinner than the aortic valve leaflets, which attach to from an elliptical mitral valve annulus. The anterior leaflet of the mitral valve is near the left ventricular outflow tract, and the posterior leaflet is near the left ventricular free wall. The leaflets are attached to the papillary muscles by chordea tendinea. On closure, the free edge of one cusp is pressed against the other. The attachment to the papillary muscle prevents the cusp from prolapsing into the atrium during ventricular contraction. The mechanics of the mitral valve have also been analyzed experimentally and theoretically [2,5]. As the valve opens, blood rapidly fills the left ventricle. With rapid blood flow, two vortices are formed in the ventricular cavity distal to the two leaflets [5]. During diastasis, as the mitral flow decelerates, the leaflets begin to close due to the vortices. During atrial contraction, the mitral valve again opens fully. At the beginning of ventricular contraction, the mitral flow ceases and the valve closes completely due to the adverse pressure gradient. Detailed velocity measurements within the left ventricle have not been performed to confirm the flow dynamics described above from *in vitro* experiments.

As seen from the *in vitro* flow studies and *in vivo* hemodynamic measurements, the normal heart valve opens passively with minimal transvalvular pressure gradient (TPG) and closes efficiently with minimal regurgitation. Flow development in the aorta past a normal tricuspid aortic valve consists of central flow characteristics with minimal flow disturbances [6].

HEART VALVE REPLACEMENT

Energy is efficiently used by the heart when the left ventricle and the cardiac valves are free of disease. If the aortic and mitral valves are diseased, left ventricular efficiency is lost, leading to ventricular decompensation and failure, which may ultimately lead to death. The proper timing of aortic and/or mitral valve replacement may restore overall cardiac function to near normal states.

Mitral valve replacement in patients with mitral stenosis should be performed when the mitral valve orifice area is calculated to be less than 1.0 cm²/m² body surface area using the Gorlin equation [7]. The timing of mitral valve replacement in patients with mitral regurgitation is not as clearly understood as in patients with mitral stenosis. Factors such as the rapidity of disease progression, the patient's clinical and hemodynamic status, particularly the left ventricular function, renal function and pulmonary function play a major role in determining the timing for valve replacement [7].

Aortic valve replacement in patients with aortic stenosis should be undertaken when the aortic valve area is less than 0.4 cm²/m² body surface area in symptomatic or asymptomatic patients. Aortic valve replacement in patients with aortic regurgitation should be done in symptomatic patients with chronic aortic regurgitation. However, asymptomatic patients with aortic regurgitation represent a group of patients in whom the timing of aortic valve replacement is quite controversial and beyond the scope of this chapter [7].

The typical operative procedure for aortic valve replacement requires a median sternotomy. The patient is placed on cardiopulmonary bypass, the body temperature lowered and the heart arrested with a cold potassium cardioplegia. Exposure of the aortic valve is made through an aortotomy in the ascending aorta. The diseased aortic valve is excised and a prosthetic valve is sutured into the aortic valve annulus. The aortotomy is closed, the left ventricle vented, the patient rewarmed and removed from cardiopulmonary bypass. The incision is closed and the patient taken to an intensive care unit for close observation. An incision through the left atrium is made to expose the mitral valve apparatus in mitral valve replacements. The mitral valve and the chordae tendinae are excised and the valve substitute is sutured into place. The left atrium is closed and the remainder of the surgical procedure is the same as for aortic valve replacement.

The hospital mortality, defined as death within 30 days of the operation for aortic or mitral valve replacement, is between 2 and 10% depending on the clinical condition of the patient and concomittant surgical procedures, if any, such as coronary artery bypass grafting, multiple valve replacement, and urgency of the valve replacement [8].

HEMODYNAMIC EVALUATION OF PROSTHETIC HEART VALVES

The commercially available heart valve prostheses today can be broadly classified into two categories: mechanical prostheses, and bioprostheses. The mechanical prostheses are the caged ball valves, tilting disc valves and bileaflet valves. Bioprosthetic valves consist of porcine xenografts and bovine pericardial xenografts. The details of the flow characteristics from *in vitro* evaluation and the clinical results after the implantation of the prostheses are included in the next section. In the United States, the valve prostheses are regulated by the Food and Drug Administration (FDA). Before a valve is approved for general use within the United States, *in vitro* studies, *in vivo* evaluation in animal models and evaluation after implantation in humans under controlled protocols are required. The *in vitro* evaluation of prosthetic valves includes hemodynamic measurements and accelerated fatigue testing. The hemodynamic evaluation requires measurement of transvalvular pressure gradient (TPG) and percent regurgitation (PCR) under pulsatile flow conditions in a mock circulatory loop at various heart rates and flow rates. More recently, several investigations studying the detailed measurements of velocity profile and turbulent shear stresses distal to valves have been reported in the literature [9–16].

Briefly, the pulse duplicator consists of a drive system with the capability of duplicating the pumping action of the heart with adjustments for the heart rate and systolic duration. The drive system simulates physiological pulsatile flow of a blood analog fluid in a closed-loop system. The mock circulatory loop consists of two flow chambers with mounted prosthetic mitral and aortic valves, a lumped resistance and compliance chamber simulating the systematic circulation (Figure 1). Left atrial, left ventricular and aortic pressures are monitored and maintained within physiological limits. Flows and transvalvular pressure gradients across the mitral and aortic valve prostheses are measured and analyzed. The blood analog fluid generally used for the evaluation of mechanical prostheses is a glycerol solution (30–40% by volume glycerol in distilled water) whose viscosity coefficient and density are similar to values for blood flow in large arteries. With bioprosthetic valves, physiological saline is used since many believe that glycerine is absorbed by the tissue, making the leaflets stiffer. The valve chambers used in the evaluation are rigid and made of transparent lucite. The aortic chamber has an axi-symmetric circular tube and sinus with diameters similar to the human aorta. The axi-symmetric mitral valve chamber used for prosthetic mitral valve evaluation has a diameter representing the average short axis diameter of the left ventricle.

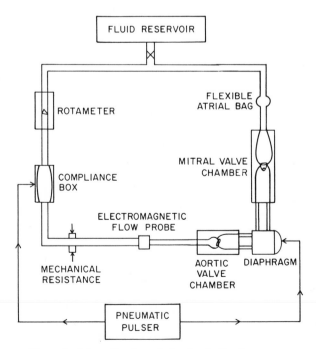

Figure 1. Schematic of a typical pulse duplicating system.

A differential pressure transducer connected to pressure taps upstream and downstream to the valve is used to measure the pressure drop across the valve. The signals from the pressure transducer and the electromagnetic flow meter are averaged over several cardiac cycles (typically 100) and the averaged signals are used to compute the PCR, cardiac output (CO), peak systolic pressure gradient (ΔP_{peak}) and the mean systolic pressure gradient (ΔP_{mean}). These values can be used to compare various prosthetic valves. Based on a modified hydraulic formula originally proposed by Gorlin and Gorlin [17], an effective aortic valve orifice area can be computed by the formula

$$VOA = MSF/44.5 \sqrt{\Delta P_{mean}} \qquad (1)$$

where MSF is the mean systolic flow rate. The constant 44.5 includes the discharge coefficient across the valve orifice as well as the conversion factor for units where pressure is expressed in mmHg and flow expressed in cm³/sec. For the mitral valve orifice area, 37.9 is used as the constant, and mean diastolic flow is used in place of MSF.

The energy loss in flow across the valve prostheses can be used to compare the performance of the valves given by the relationship

$$\Delta E = \frac{1}{\tau} \int_0^\tau \Delta P(t) Q(t) dt \qquad (2)$$

where ΔE is the energy loss, ΔP is the pressure drop across the valve, Q is the flow rate and τ is the duration of the cardiac cycle.

Velocity profiles distal to the valve are measured accurately by using Doppler anemometry (LDA). More recently, using a two-channel LDA system, turbulent shear stress magnitudes distal to the valves have also been measured [16]. To compare the *in vitro* hemodynamic results for valves of various designs, the valve sizes must be comparable. The valve sizes are usually specified by the tissue annulus diameter (TAD). The velocity profiles, TPG and PCR comparisons described below are from tests on aortic valves of 27 mm TAD.

In general, the geometry of the aortic and mitral valve prostheses are similar except for the difference in the sewing ring which conforms to the anatomy of the respective value orifice. Detailed velocity profiles distal to the mitral valve prostheses in a flow chamber simulating the human left ventricle have not been hitherto obtained. More recently, detailed velocity profiles distal to the mitral valves in an axi-symmetric chamber have been reported [16]. As can be expected, the velocity profiles are similar in shape to those measured distal to aortic valve prostheses with different velocity magnitudes due to differences in the instantaneous flow rate signals used in the experiments. Hence, in this chapter, we do not discuss the velocity profiles distal to the mitral valves separately.

In vitro accelerated life testing is the other component of prosthetic valve evaluation. Using accelerated life testing, durability data can be accumulated in a reasonable length of time [18]. Bioprosthetic valves, tested at 70 beats per minute (bpm) have shown to yield the same failure characteristics as testing at 2100 bpm [19]. Assuming an average heart rate pf 70 bpm, at 2100 bpm one calendar month of testing is equivalent to the valve opening and closing in the human body for 30 months. Such tests allow the investigator to determine the durability of the material used in the manufacture of the valves and aid in predicting the amount of wear expected within the human body.

PROSTHETIC MECHANICAL VALVES

The Starr–Edwards™ Silastic® Ball Valve Prosthesis

In 1961, Starr and Edwards reported their first successful intracardiac mitral valve replacement using an early Starr–Edwards™ Silastic® ball valve prosthesis [20]. The current Starr–Edwards™ Model 1260 aortic valve was made available in 1968 and Model 6120 mitral valve was made available in 1966 (see Figure 2).

The Starr–Edwards™ Silastic® ball valve prosthesis is made of a polished Stellite Alloy No. 21 cage. The ball is made of silicone rubber which contains 2% (by weight) barium sulfate for radiopacity. Both the mitral and aortic valve sewing rings use a silicone rubber insert under the knitted composite Teflon®/polypropylene cloth [21].

The centrally occluding caged ball valve was the first successful design of the mechanical valve prostheses. In the full open position, the ball remains at the apex of the cage with a peripheral flow of blood past the ball. Figure 3 shows a typical velocity profile in peak systole (124 ms after valve opening) at a distance 29 mm distal to the valve seat in the aortic chamber. As shown in Figure 3, jetlike flow is present near the vessel wall with a large wake region downstream to the ball. Such flows will induce relatively large wall shear stresses in the lumen of the aorta which may damage the endothelial lining. The wake region is present throughout systole in *in vitro* studies [10]. It is interesting to note that thrombi have been observed with the implanted valves in the region of the large wake. At a mean flow rate of 6 liters per minute (lpm) and heart rate of 70 bpm, a mean systolic pressure drop of 10 mmHg and a PCR of 5% were measured for this valve. At smaller mounting sizes, the pressure drop will increase making this valve more stenotic. The pressure drop and PCR for this valve are similar to those obtained for the mechanical valves of other designs at comparable flows and heart rates. Peak turbulent shear stresses of 1850 dynes/cm²

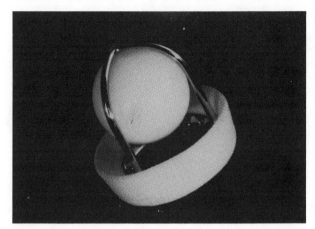

Figure 2. Photograph of a Starr–Edwards™ Prosthetic Valve (Courtesy of American Edwards).

have been measured in the immediate vicinity of these valves during peak systole [16].

The Starr–Edwards™ Silastic® ball valves have been and are currently used widely in aortic and mitral valve replacements. Dr. Albert Starr from Portland, Oregon reported on his current results with the Starr–Edwards™ Model 1260 aortic valve and Model 6120 mitral valve. He grouped his patients into valve replacement during periods of 1965 to 1972 and 1973 and 1984. The 133 patients who received the Model 1260 aortic valve had a 4.6%/patient-year (pt-yr) incidence of thromboembolism from 1965 to 1972 while the 470 patients with aortic valve replacement (AVR) between 1973 and 1984 had a 1.8%/pt-yr incidence of thromboembolism. From 1965 to 1972 the

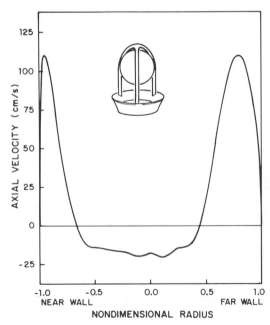

Figure 3. Velocity profile distal to a caged ball valve in peak systole.

incidence of aortic valvular thrombosis was 0.2%/pt-yr and the incidence of valve failure was 1.5%/pt-yr. Valve failure is defined as a valve-related death or complication necessitating valve replacement. From 1973 to 1984 with AVR there was no valve thrombosis and 1.1%/pt-yr incidence of valve failure. In the 84 patients with the Starr–Edwards™ Model 6120 mitral valve prosthesis the incidence of thromboembolism, thrombosis and all valve failures during the 1965 to 1972 was 6.0%/pt-yr, 0.6%/pt-yr and 1.9%/pt-yr, respectively. Mitral valve replacement (MVR) during 1973 to 1984 in 234 patients was beset with an incidence of thromboembolism, valve thrombosis and valve failure of 2.9%/pt-yr, 0.0%/pt-yr and 1.2%/pt-yr, respectively [22].

Miller and colleagues from Stanford reported an incidence of 2.7%/pt-yr for thromboembolism, 3.1%/pt-yr for anticoagulant related hemorrhage and 2.2%/pt-yr for valve related failure in 449 patients undergoing AVR with the Starr–Edwards™ Model 1260. With the Starr–Edwards™ Model 6120 mitral valve prosthesis implanted in 509 patients between 1965 and 1976, they found an incidence of thromboembolism, anticoagulant related hemorrhage and valve failure of 5.7%/pt-yr, 3.7%/pt-yr and 3.8%/pt-yr, respectively.

The Björk–Shiley® Valve Prosthesis

Since the first human use by Dr. Viking Björk in 1969, the Björk–Shiley® prosthesis has undergone several modifications [8]. The original Björk–Shiley® prosthesis was made of a Haynes 25 cobalt based alloy orifice ring with a Delrin® disc and Teflon® sewing ring [25]. In 1971, the Delrin® disc was changed to a Pyrolite® carbon disc to improve durability. Between 1971 and 1977 the inflow and outflow struts of the valve ring were welded into place. In 1977, the inflow strut was made an integral part of the valve ring and a radiopaque marker was added to the Pyrolite® disc [26,27]. In 1982, the outflow strut was made an integral part of the valve ring in the form of a monostrut [25] (see Figure 4).

Tilting disc valves, in the full open position, form a ma-

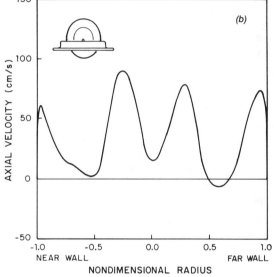

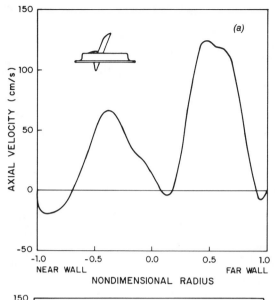

Figure 5. Velocity profile distal to a tilting disc valve in peak systole: (a) with the major orifice to the right; and (b) disc tilting to the top.

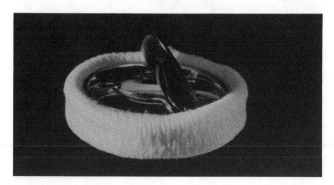

Figure 4. Photograph of a Björk–Shiley® prosthesis (Courtesy of Shiley, Incorporated).

jor and a minor flow orifice (Figure 5). Depending on the model of the tilting disc valve, the disc opens to an angle of 60–75° with the majority of flow passing through the major flow orifice. The earlier spherical disc Björk–Shiley® valve had an opening an angle of 60°. The convexo-concave Björk–Shiley® valve (concave at the inlet of the valve) opens to 70°. Velocity measurements of the two models show the convexo-concave model with relatively more flow through the minor flow orifice although no significant hemodynamic improvement is apparent. The Medtronic–Hall™ valve opens to an angle of 75° and the velocity profiles distal to this valve were also similar to those of the Björk–Shiley® valves. Velocity profiles measured distal to a tilting disc valve are shown in Figure 5(a). In Figure 5(a), the disc is oriented such that the major orifice is to the right and the velocity measurements are obtained along the center line in the minor and major flow orifices. The profile shows two peaks corresponding to the flow orifices with the higher velocity jet the major orifice flow. Near the vessel wall in the minor orifice, a flow reversal is observed and is persistent throughout systole. Deposition of thrombi and tissue ingrowth have been observed in this region after implantation in humans.

The velocity profiles with the valve rotated 90°, such that measurements were obtained parallel to the disc tilt axis along the minor flow orifice are shown in Figure 5(b). In this orientation, the disc is tilting to the top of the figure and a three peaked velocity profile is observed. The larger velocity magnitudes occur in the core region. It is interesting to note that higher turbulent shear stresses were measured in this orientation distal to the disc in the minor flow orifice when compared to the orientation shown in Figure 5(a) [10,16]. Peak turbulent shear stresses of about 3400 dynes/cm² have been reported distal to the disc valves. Since the velocity profiles distal to the tilting disc valve are markedly asymmetric, one might expect the valve orientation with respect to the aortic root to have a significant effect on the flow development in the aorta. A qualitative flow visualization study was performed with three different orientations of the valve with respect to the aortic root using a model of a human aorta mounted in the pulse duplicator [28]. This study showed that with the major orifice towards the inner wall of the primary curvature of the aorta, a region of relative stasis throughout the cardiac cycle was observed along the outer wall of primary curvature proximal to the brachio-cephalic arterial branch. Further quantitative comparisons of the effects of orientation of the tilting disc valve in the model human aorta have also been reported [29]. The mean systolic pressure drop at a flow rate of 6 lpm and heart rate of 70 bpm is about 6–8 mm Hg for a 27 mm tilting disc valve with PCR of 10–13%.

The Björk–Shiley® tilting disc prostheses have enjoyed widespread use during the last decade. Except for modifications of the convexo-concave disc and prostheses which have had opening angles of 70° instead of 60° the Björk–Shiley® prostheses have had a durable track record [8,25]. However, other complications of valve replacement exist. Aortic valve replacement with Björk–Shiley® valves was found to have a linearized rate of thromboembolism of between 0.6 and 1.0%/pt-yr [25,27,30–32] with follow-up to 9 yrs. The incidence of valve thrombosis in the experience of these authors was between 0 and 0.5%/pt-yr. Anticoagulant-related hemorrhage occurred in 1.7 to 2.4%/pt-yr of patients having aortic valve replacement with the Björk–Shiley® prosthesis [25,27,30–32]. Valve failure as defined as mechanical failure or complications requiring valve replacement occurred in 0.06 to 1.5%/pt-yr [27,30–32] of the patients having aortic valve replacement.

Mitral valve replacement with the Björk–Shiley® pros-

thesis has had similar experience as in the aortic valve replacement patients. Thromboembolic events, valve thrombosis, and anticoagulant-related hemorrhage occurred in mitral valve replacement patients with an incidence of between 1.4 and 5.8%/pt-yr, 0 and 3.0%/pt-yr and 1.1 and 2.1%/pt-yr respectively [25,27,30,31,33]. The incidence of failure for mitral valve replacement was between 0.06 and 4.0%/pt-yr [27,30,31,33].

The Medtronic–Hall™ Disc Valve Prosthesis

In 1977, the first Medtronic–Hall™ (formerly Hall–Kaster) prosthesis was implanted in humans [34]. This prosthesis was introduced as an effort to reduce the incidence of valvular thrombosis in tilting disc valves. The Medtronic–Hall™ valve has an opening angle of 75° relative to the plane of the orifice [35]. The Medtronic–Hall™ valve has a nonalloyed Titanium housing. The sewing ring is made of Teflon® knitted fabric assembled with Dacron® sutures. The disc occluder is made of Pyrolite® carbon over a substrate of graphite laced with 5% Tungsten for radiopacity [36]. The valve assembly is shown in Figure 6.

Due to the relatively recent introduction of the Medtronic–Hall™ valve into clinical use, limited data exists regarding complications from implantation. Hall, and others [37] reported in his 7-1/2 years experience a thromboembolic rate of 1.4%/pt-yr for aortic valve replacement and 1.7%/pt-yr for mitral valve replacement. The valve thrombosis rate was 0.1%/pt-yr for aortic valve replacement and 0.2%/pt-yr for mitral valve replacement. There were no reported valve failures. Matsunaga and co-workers [38] reported no episodes of valvular failure or thromboembolism in their 36 months experience with the Medtronic–Hall™ prosthesis. Beaudet and colleagues [39] reported a 1.2%/pt-yr and 2.4%/pt-yr incidence of thromboembolism for aortic and mitral valve replace-

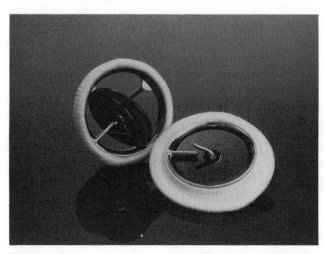

Figure 6. *Photograph of a Medtronic–Hall™ prosthesis (Courtesy of Medtronic Blood Systems, Inc.).*

ment, respectively, in 95 aortic valve replacement, 107 mitral valve replacement and 28 double valve replacement patients. No occurrences of mechanical valve failure or valvular thrombosis were reported. The authors reported 80% of their patients were free of all valve related complications at 3 years.

The Omniscience® Heart Valve Prosthesis

The Omniscience® heart valve prosthesis has been in clinical use since 1978 (see Figure 7). This valve is a modification of the Lillehei–Kaster prosthesis also manufactured by Medical, Incorporated. The Omniscience® valve housing is made of unalloyed titanium [40]. The Omniscience® occluder is made of Pyrolite® coated on graphite with a small percentage of silicon to improve wear and hardness properties. The graphite is laced with Tungsten to make it radiopaque. The occluder is curved to maximize the opening moment when open. The disc is inclined at 12° when closed and opens through an arc of 68° to 80°. The sewing ring on the Omniscience® valve is available in either Dacron® or Teflon® fabrics [40].

Mikhail [41] presented the cumulative clinical data on the Omniscience® valve used for Pre-Market Approval to the United States FDA. The data were collected over a 65 month period at seven United States and one Canadian centers. The incidence of a thrombotic complication (valve thrombosis, thromboembolism or a transient ischemic episode) was 1.8%/pt-yr for aortic valve replacement and 2.3%/pt-yr for mitral valve replacement. The incidence of anticoagulant related hemorrhage was 0.8%/pt-yr. There were no cases of mechanical valve failure. DeWall and colleagues [42] reported their five year experience with the Omniscience® prosthesis in 155 aortic valve replacement, 125 mitral valve replacement and 46 double valve replacement patients. The authors reported an incidence of transient ischemic episodes of 0.9%/pt-yr

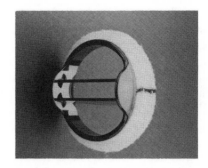

Figure 8. *Photograph of a St. Jude Medical™ prosthesis (Courtesy of St. Jude Medical, Inc.).*

(six patients). Eleven patients had serious thromboembolic events (valve thrombosis or thromboembolism with residual deficit) for a linearized rate of 1.7%/pt-yr. There were three episodes of aortic valve thrombosis (two fatal) and five episodes of nonfatal mitral valve thrombosis. There were one fatal and three nonfatal hemorrhages due to anticoagulation for a linearized rate of 0.2%/pt-yr. No case of mechanical valve failure was reported.

The St. Jude Medical™ Hinged Bileaflet Prosthesis

The St. Jude Medical™ prosthesis is a low profile, central flow, bileaflet prosthesis made entirely of Pyrolite® coated graphite laced with 5–10% tungsten for radiopacity. The two leaflets are "attached" to the valve housing by a hinge mechanism. Tolerances allow for the passage of blood through the hinge regions thus producing a mechanism for decreased thrombogenecity. When closed, the leaflets meet the valve housing at 30–35° depending on valve size. In the full open position the leaflets travel through a 50–55° arc to 85° relative to the plane of the orifice [35]. The sewing ring is made of double velour Dacron® (see Figure 8).

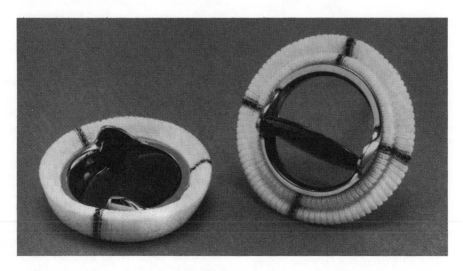

Figure 7. *Photograph of an Omni–Science® prosthesis (Courtesy of Medical Incorporated).*

Velocity profiles distal to the bileaflet valve were obtained in two orientations as shown in Figure 9. In the first orientation, the measurements were obtained perpendicular to the tilt axis as shown in Figure 9(a). In the full open position, flow through the two major flow orifices and a central minor flow orifice resulted in a three-peaked velocity profile. With the valve rotated 90°, velocity profiles were also obtained in the central flow orifice [12]. In this orientation, a relatively uniform velocity profile is observed [Figure 9(b)] with regions of flow reversal near the valve ring. This is the hinge region, where the leaflets

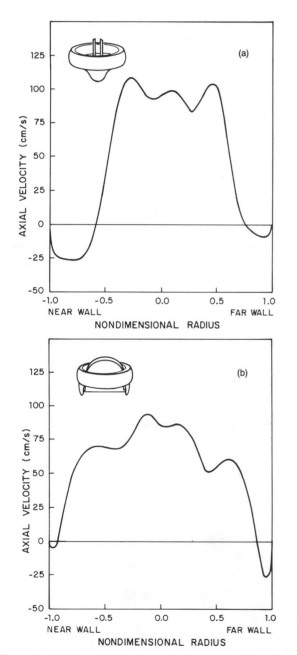

Figure 9. *Velocity profile distal to a bileaflet valve in peak systole: (a) perpendicular to the tilt axis; and (b) parallel to the tilt axis.*

attach to the valve housing and microthrombus deposition has been reported with implanted bileaflet valves. The mean systolic pressure drop and PCR measured for a bileaflet valve at a mean flow of 6 lpm and heart rate of 70 bpm were 6 mm Hg and 10% respectively. Peak turbulent shear stresses of approximately 2000 dynes/cm² have been reported for the bileaflet valve [16]. Of the mechanical valve prostheses, the bileaflet valve exhibits the smallest pressure drop for a given valve size. Studies in the model human aorta with the bileaflet valves show no significant differences in flow development with the valve oriented in two different positions [12].

The St. Jude Medical™ valve has been implanted clinically since 1977. Several of the larger clinical centers reported their results with St. Jude Medical™ valves recently. Arom et al. [43] in their six year experience with the St. Jude Medical™ valve reported an incidence of embolization of 0.7%/pt-yr for aortic valve replacement and 2.2%/pt-yr for mitral valve replacement. The incidence of anticoagulant related hemorrhage for aortic valve replacement and mitral valve replacement was 4.6 and 2.2%/pt-yr, respectively. They reported no case of valvular thrombosis or structural failure in patients undergoing isolated aortic valve or mitral valve replacement. Czer and co-workers [44] reported thromboembolic rates of 2.1%/pt-yr after aortic valve replacement and 1.7%/pt-yr after mitral valve replacement in their 6 year experience with the St. Jude Medical™ valve. They also studied thromboembolic rates in patients receiving only antiplatelet agents (aspirin and dipyridamole) compared to warfarin anticoagulation. The overall thromboembolic rate in warfarin treated patients was 2.5%/pt-yr compared to 7.7%/pt-yr in patients treated soley with antiplatelet agents. The incidence of anticoagulant related hemorrhage was 1%/pt-yr. Valvular thrombosis occurred in three patients with inadequate anticoagulation therapy for a linearized rate of 1.2%/pt-yr. No case of valve thrombosis occurred in patients with mitral valve replacement. Beaudet and colleagues [45] reported their 5-1/2 year experience with the St. Jude Medical™ prosthesis. They found an overall thromboembolic rate of 1.1%/pt-yr for patients with aortic valve, mitral valve and double valve replacement. The thromboembolic rate in patients anticoagulated with warfarin was 0.3%/pt-yr for aortic valve replacement and 0.4%/pt-yr for mitral valve replacement, while in patients treated only with antiplatelet agents the thromboembolic rate was 6.2%/pt-yr for aortic valve replacement and 16.7%/pt-yr for mitral valve replacement. Valvular thrombosis did not occur in patients anticoagulated with warfarin. In patients using antiplatelet agents the valvular thrombosis rate was 6.1%/pt-yr for aortic valve replacement and 5.5%/pt-yr for mitral valve replacement. The risk of anticoagulant related hemorrhage was 0.6%/pt-yr. There were no cases of structural failure reported.

BIOPROSTHETIC VALVES

The Hancock™ Porcine Xenograft

Since the first clinical use of a Hancock™ porcine valve in 1970, many investigators have used this prosthesis [46]. Initially, the porcine tissue, fixed by a stabilized glutaraldehyde process, was mounted in a rigid metal stent, but in 1971 the flexible polypropylene stent was introduced. The inflow aspect of the stent has a stellite ring for rigidity and radiopacity. The polypropylene stent is covered with Dacron® polyester fabric. The fixed porcine aortic valve is attached to the cloth covered stent and a sewing ring made of a silicone rubber insert covered with Dacron® polyester fabric. Recently, Wright [46] and colleagues presented the new Hancock II™ low pressure fixed porcine heart valve. The Hancock II™ valve is fixed using a stabilized glutaraldehyde process at pressures less than 2 mm Hg. The stent material is Delrin® (acetyl resin) with stellite eyelets at the apex of each post and inflow ring. Dacron® polyester fabric is used to cover the stent and make the sewing ring [47]. The inflow surface of the Hancock II® prosthesis is shown in Figure 10.

Porcine aortic valves are mounted on relatively high supporting struts and have restricted valve opening areas. An effective valve orifice area computed using Equation (1) shows the porcine valve orifice area to be about 40% less than a pericardial valve of the same size [11]. The velocity profile distal to the porcine valve shows a relatively high velocity jet (Figure 11) which is not coincident with the centerline of the flow chamber. Turbulent shear stresses of approximately 4500 dynes/cm² have been measured distal to the porcine valve in peak systole [48]. A mean systolic pressure drop of 7–10 mm Hg and a PCR of 2–4% have been measured with a 27 mm porcine valve at a mean flow of 6 lpm and heart rate of 70 bpm. The porcine valves are known to be significantly more stenotic at

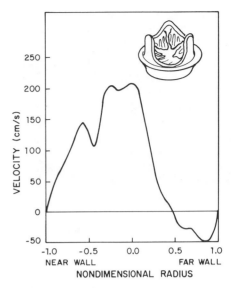

Figure 11. *Velocity profile distal to a porcine valve in peak systole.*

smaller sizes compared with the corresponding size of a mechanical prosthesis.

Many reports on the clinical effectiveness of the Hancock™ porcine valve have been published. Bolooki and colleagues [49] reported on his 4 to 9 year follow-up of 117 patients with 129 Hancock™ valves. Thromboembolism occurred at a linearized rate of 0.7%/pt-yr. Anticoagulant related hemorrhage occurred at a linearized rate of 0.3%/pt-yr. Mitral valve failure (calcification and stenosis, leaflet tear or perforation) occurred in 9.5% of the patients with mitral valve replacement for a linearized rate of 1.5%/pt-yr. No occurrence of aortic valve structural failure occurred. Gallo and associates [50] published their 5–8 year follow-up of 403 patients with Hancock™ porcine valves. The incidence of thromboembolism for aortic valve and mitral valve replacement was 1.0%/pt-yr and 1.9%/pt-yr respectively. The incidence of anticoagulant related hemorrhage occurred at a rate of 0.5%/pt-yr. Primary tissue failure occurred in patients with aortic Hancock™ valves at a linearized incidence of 1.1%/pt-yr. The incidence of mitral valve tissue failure occurred in 1.9%/pt-yr. In addition, the incidence of clinical valvular dysfunction, i.e., patients with a new stenotic or regurgitant murmur, occurred at a linearized rate of 1.4%/pt-yr. The percentage of patients free of reoperation at 8 yrs by actuarial analysis was 68% for mitral valve and 80% for aortic valve replacement by actuarial analysis.

The Carpentier–Edwards® Porcine Valve Prosthesis

The Carpentier–Edwards® porcine valve was introduced in 1975 and has a less extensive clinical evaluation compared with the Hancock™ porcine valve. The stent is

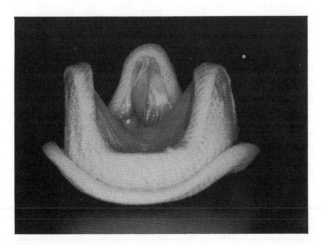

Figure 10. *Photograph of the Hancock II™ prosthesis (Courtesy of Johnson and Johnson Cardiovascular).*

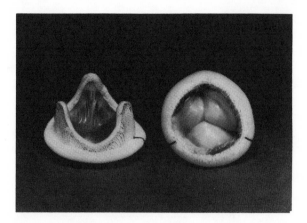

Figure 12. *Photograph of a Carpentier-Edwards® prosthesis (Courtesy of American Edwards).*

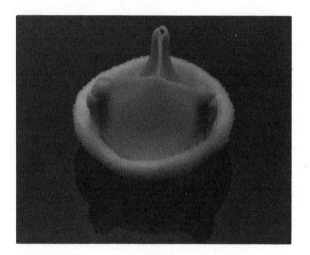

Figure 13. *Photograph of an Ionescu–Shiley® prosthesis (Courtesy of Shiley, Incorporated).*

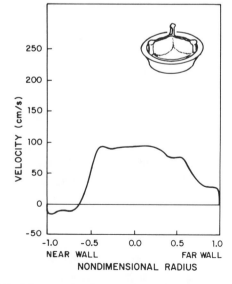

Figure 14. *Velocity profile distal to a pericardial valve in peak systole.*

made of a lightweight Elgiloy®, a corrosion resistant alloy. Elgiloy® is used in other medical applications such as pacemaker leads and vena cava filters. The stent is covered with a porous knitted Teflon® cloth. The porcine valve is fixed using a stabilized glutaraldehyde process. The sewing ring is made of a soft silicone rubber insert covered with porous, seamless Teflon® cloth [51] (see Figure 12).

Since the Carpentier–Edwards® prosthesis has been introduced in 1975, limited long-term experience with this prosthesis has been reported. Pelletier and colleagues [52] reported on their 5 year experience in 605 patients using the Carpentier–Edwards® prosthesis. The thromboembolic rate was 1.7 and 1.5%/pt-yr for aortic valve and mitral valve replacements, respectively. The risk of anticoagulant related hemorrhage was 0.5%/pt-yr. Primary tissue failure only occurred in one patient for a linearized rate of 0.1%/pt-yr. The actuarial probability of being free of all valve related complications at five years was 93%. Jamieson and others [53] published their six year experience with the Carpentier–Edwards® valve in 355 patients. They found an incidence of thromboemboli for aortic and mitral valve replacement to be 1.1 and 1.7%/pt-yr, respectively. Approximately 10% of aortic valve replacements and 45% of mitral valve replacements received anticoagulant therapy. Anticoagulant related hemorrhage occurred in one patient for a linearized rate of 0.07%/pt-yr. Primary tissue failure occurred at a linearized rate of 0.2 and 1.0%/pt-yr for aortic and mitral valve replacement, respectively. The actuarial probability of freedom from all valve related complications at six years was 84%.

The Ionescu–Shiley® Bovine Pericardial Xenograft

In 1971, Dr. Marion Ionescu and colleagues [54] began using a bovine pericardial xenograft for single valve replacements constructed in their hospital laboratory at Leeds Infirmary in Leeds, England. In 1976, all Ionescu pericardial valves were constructed using refined techniques by Shiley Incorporated. The Ionescu–Shiley® prosthesis (see Figure 13) is made from bovine pericardium. The stent is made of titanium and covered with Dacron® cloth. The sewing ring, also made of Dacron® cloth, is attached to the cloth-covered stent. The pericardium is attached to the stent, fixed using a stabilized glutaraldehyde process and sterilized using formaldehyde and glutaraldehyde. Recent modifications in the design of the Ionescu–Shiley® prosthesis consist of a lower profile prosthesis with the stent now constructed from acetyle resin (Delrin®).

Pericardial bioprostheses have a geometry similar to that of the natural aortic valve. As previously stated, the valve orifice area for the pericardial valve is significantly larger compared with the porcine valve prostheses. The velocity profile distal to the pericardial valve (Figure 14) shows a relatively uniform velocity profile with vortex formation behind the leaflets in the sinus cavity [11]. The flow development past the pericardial bioprosthesis can be expected to closely simulate the flow development past the natural aortic valve [1]. Relatively low turbulent shear stresses, about 2400 dynes/cm² in peak systole, have been reported distal to the pericardial bioprosthesis [48]. The mean systolic pressure drop and PCR of 3–6 mm Hg and 4–7% respectively have been measured with a 27 mm pericardial valve at a mean flow of 6 lpm and heart rate of 70 bpm [11].

Ionescu and colleagues [54] reported on his results with both the hospital-made and Shiley-made mitral valves. They found a linearized rate of embolism of 0.6%/pt-yr. They reported no case of valvular thrombosis. The linearized rate of tissue failure was 0.6%/pt-yr, but no Shiley made valves failed in 5.7 years of follow-up. The actuarial probability of freedom from valve failure at 11 years for mitral valve replacement was 90.4%. Gonzalez-Lavin and co-workers [55] published their five year experience in 168 patients with aortic valve replacement using the Ionescu–Shiley valve. The incidence of thromboembolism was 1.3%/pt-yr. The incidence of primary tissue failure was 0.3%/pt-yr. The actuarial probability of freedom from primary valve failure at five years was 96%.

The Ideal Prosthetic Heart Valve

It is evident from the above discussion that even though patients lead a better quality of life, there are several problems associated with the implanted prostheses. Hydrodynamic studies show the presence of regions of flow separation and relative stasis distal to the prostheses which have been clinically correlated with thrombus deposition and tissue overgrowth. The valves also induce relatively large mechanical stresses such as bulk turbulent and wall shear stresses. Relatively large wall shear stresses have been shown to damage the endothelial cells with increased risk of atherosclerotic plaque formation [56]. Bulk turbulent stresses of 1500–4000 dynes/cm² have been shown to cause hemolysis of red blood cells [57]. In the presence of foreign surfaces, turbulent shear stresses of 100 dynes/cm² have been shown to destruct the erythrocytes [58]. Platelets have also been shown to have a substantially lower tolerance to shear stresses than human erythrocytes. It is clear that the hemodynamic characteristics of the present valve designs induce significant mechanical stresses which contribute towards the thromboembolic complications as well as in tissue failure. Hence, continuing efforts to improve the valve designs to achieve desirable hemodynamic characteristics is warranted. With the recent developments in total artificial heart and left ventricular assist devices where the valve prostheses are used, the improvement of valve designs assumes added importance.

When designing prosthetic heart valves, there are several characteristics of natural heart valves one aims to mimic. These include minimal transvalvular pressure gradients, minimal regurgitant fractions, central flow characteristics and complete biocompatibility. The materials within the prosthesis should be durable, nontoxic and nonthrombogenic, i.e., ideally, the materials should *not* require the long-term use of anticoagulant therapy. The prosthetic heart valve should be surgically implanted with ease and not interfere with normal cardiac function and anatomy. The normal function of the prosthetic valve should be quiet, should not damage cellular blood elements or cause denaturing of proteins. Finally, prosthetic valves should be readily available, manufactured with ease and relatively inexpensive.

FUTURE DIRECTIONS

The choice of which valve to use in an individual patient is a difficult one confronting cardiologists and cardiovascular surgeons. They must weigh the advantage of the durability of mechanical type prostheses and the need for long-term anticoagulant therapy against the limited durability of the bioprostheses without the need for long-term anticoagulant therapy. Therefore, physicians, biomedical engineers and other inventors have yet to design the "ideal" prosthetic valve substitute.

One approach to meet the characteristics of the "ideal" prosthetic valve includes new fixing processes for bioprosthetic valves that greatly improve durability, decrease the incidence of dystrophic calcification and do not change the relatively nonthrombogenic nature of existing bioprostheses. Another approach would be the introduction of a new durable, nonthrombogenic material from which a mechanical type prosthesis could be fashioned. Some think a synthetic valve which could be constructed to copy the geometry of the natural human aortic valve would be the ideal valve substitute. The problems with currently available materials are durability and higher than acceptable transvalvular pressure gradients.

In summary, since the first use of a prosthetic heart valve in 1960, many investigators have tried to improve the many problems associated with heart valve replacement. Currently available prostheses are markedly improved over some earlier valve substitutes, but the search for the "ideal" prosthetic valve continues. To advance towards this goal, a major breakthrough in either materials science or collagen biochemistry must occur.

REFERENCES

1 BELLHOUSE, B. J. and L. Talbot. "The Fluid Mechanics of the Aortic Valve," *J. Fluid Mech.*, 35:721–735 (1979).

2 LEE, C. S. F. and L. Talbot. "A Fluid-Mechanical Study of the Closure of Heart Valves," *J. Fluid Mech.*, 91:41–63 (1979).

3 FARTHING, S. P. and P. Peronneau. "Flow in the Thoracic Aorta," *Cardiovasc. Res.*, 13:607–620 (1979).

4 SEED, W. A. and N. B. Wood. "Velocity Patterns in the Aorta," *Cardiovasc. Res.*, 5:319–330 (1971).

5 REUL, H. and N. Talukder. "Heart Valve Mechanics," in *Quantitative Cardiovascular Studies; Clinical and Research Applications of Engineering Principles*, N. H. C. Hwang, D. R. Gross and D. J. Patel, eds. Baltimore:University Park Press, (12):527–564 (1979).

6 STEIN, P. D. and H. N. Sabbah. "Turbulent Blood Flow in the Ascending Aorta of Humans with Normal and Diseased Aortic Valves," *Cir. Res.*, 39:58–65 (1976).

7 BRAUNWALD, E. "Valvular Heart Disease," in *Heart Disease: A Textbook of Cardiovascular Medicine, 2nd Edition*, E. Braunwald, ed. Philadelphia, PA:W.B. Saunders Co. (1984).

8 LEFRAK, E. and A. Starr. *Cardiac Valve Prostheses*, New York, NY:Appleton-Century-Crofts (1979).

9 YOGANATHAN, A. P., W. H. Corcoran and E. C. Harrison. "*In Vitro* Measurements in the Vicinity of Aortic Prostheses," *J. Biomechanics*, 12:135–152 (1979).

10 CHANDRAN, K. B., G. N. Cabell, B. Khalighi and C-J. Chen. "Laser Anemometry Measurements of Pulsatile Flow Aortic Valve Prostheses," *J. Biomechanics*, 16:865–873 (1983).

11 CHANDRAN, K. B., G. N. Cabell, B. Khalighi and C-J. Chen. "Pulsatile Flow Past Aortic Valve Bioprostheses in a Model Human Aorta," *J. Biomechanics*, 17:609–619 (1984).

12 CHANDRAN, K. B. "Pulsatile Flow Past St. Jude Medical Bileaflet Valve: An *In Vitro* Study, *J. Thorac. Cardiovasc. Surg.*, 89:743–749 (1985).

13 PHILLIPS, W. M., P. G. Alchas and A. J. Snyder. "Pulsatile Prosthetic Valve Flows: Laser Doppler Studies," in *Biofluid Mechanics*, D. J. Schneck, ed. Academic Press, 2:243–265 (1980).

14 BRUSS, K-H., H. Reul, J. Van Gilse and F. Knott. "Pressure Drop and Velocity Fields at Four Mechanical Heart Valve Prostheses: Björk–Shiley Standard, Björk–Shiley Concave-Convex, Hall-Kaster and St. Jude Medical Life Support Systems," 1:3–22 (1983).

15 WOO, Y-R. and A. P. Yoganathan. "*In Vitro* Pulsatile Flow Velocity and Turbulent Shear Stress Measurements in the Vicinity of Mechanical Aortic Heart Valve Prosthesis," *Life Support Systems*, 3:283–312 (1985).

16 WOO, Y-R. and A. P. Yoganathan. "*In Vitro* Pulsatile Flow Velocity and Shear Stress Measurements in the Vicinity of Mechanical Mitral Heart Valve Prostheses," *J. Biomechanics*, 19:39–51 (1986).

17 GORLIN, R. and S. G. Gorlin. "Hydraulic Formula for the Calculation of the Area of Stenotic Mitral Valve, Other Cardiac Valves and Central Circulatory Shunts," *American Heart J.*, 41:1–29 (1951).

18 FETTEL, B. E., D. R. Johnston and P. E. Morris. "Accelerated Life Testing of Prosthetic Heart Valves," *Medical Instrumentation*, 14:161–164 (1980).

19 BROOM, N. D. "The Stress/Strain and Fatigue Behavior of Gluteraldehyde Pressured Heart-Valve Tissue," *J. Biomechanics*, 10:707–724 (1977).

20 STARR, A. and M. L. Edwards. "Mitral Valve Replacement: Clinical Experience With a Ball Valve Prosthesis," *Ann. Surg.*, 154:726 (1961).

21 Starr-Edwards Clinical Report, American Edwards Laboratories (January 1984).

22 STARR, A. "The Starr Edwards Valve," *J. Am. Coll. Cardiol.*, 6:899–903 (1985).

23 MILLER, D. C., P. E. Oyer, R. S. Mitchell, E. B. Stinson, S. W. Jamieson, J. C. Baldwin and N. E. Shumway. "Performance Char-

acteristics of the Starr–Edwards Model 1260 Aortic Valve Prostheses Beyond Ten Years," *J. Thorac. Cardiovasc. Surg.*, 88:193–207 (1984).

24 MILLER, D. C., P. E. Oyer, E. B. Stinson, B. A. Reitz, S. W. Jamieson, W. A. Baumgartner, R. S. Mitchell and N. E. Shumway. "Ten to Fifteen Year Reassessment of the Performance Characteristics of the Starr–Edwards Model 6120 Mitral Valve Prothesis," *J. Thorac. Cardiovasc. Surg.*, 85:1–20 (1983).

25 BJÖRK, V. O. and D. Lindblom. "The Monostrut Björk–Shiley Heart Valve," *J. Am. Coll. Cardiol.*, 6:1142–1148 (1985).

26 BJÖRK, V. O. "The Improved Björk–Shiley Tilting Disc Valve Prosthesis," *Scand. J. Thorac. Cardiovasc. Surg.*, 12:81–84 (1978).

27 BJÖRK, V. O., A. Henze and T. Hindmarsh. "Radiopaque Marker in the Tilting Disc of the Björk–Shiley Heart Valve," *J. Thorac. Cardiovasc. Surg.*, 73:563–569 (1977).

28 CHANDRAN, K. B., B. Khalighi, C-J. Chen, H. L. Falsetti, T. L. Yearwood and L. I. Hiratzka. "Effect of Valve Orientation in Flow Development Past Aortic Valve Prostheses in a Model Human Aorta," *J. Thorac. Cardiovasc. Surg.*, 85:893–901 (1983).

29 CHANDRAN, K. B., B. Khalighi and C-J. Chen. "Experimental Study of Physiological Pulsatile Flow Past Valve Prostheses in a Model Human Aorta: II. Tilting Disc Valves and the Effect of Orientation," *J. Biomechanics*, 18:773–780 (1985).

30 DAENEN, W., A. Nevelsteen, P. van Cauwelaert, E. de Maesschalk, J. Willems and G. Stalpaert. "Nine Years' Experience with the Björk–Shiley Prosthetic Valve: Early and Late Results of 932 Valve Replacements," *Ann. Thorac. Surg.*, 35:651–663 (1983).

31 MURPHY, D. A., F. H. Levine, M. J. Buckley, L. Swinski, W. M. Daggett, C. W. Akins and W. G. Austen. "Mechanical Valves: A Comparative Analysis of the Starr–Edwards and Björk–Shiley Prostheses," *J. Thorac. Cardiovasc. Surg.*, 86:746–752 (1983).

32 PERIER, P., J. P. Bessou, J. S. Swanson, D. Bensasson, J. C. Chachques, S. Chauvaud, A. Deloche, J. N. Fabiani, P. Blondeau, C. D'Allaines and A. Carpentier. "Comparative Evaluation of Aortic Valve Replacement with Starr, Björk and Porcine Valve Prostheses," *Circulation, 72 (Suppl II)*, 2:140–145 (1985).

33 PERIER, P., A. Deloche, S. Chauvaud, J. N. Fabiani, P. Rossant, J. P. Bessou, J. Relland, H. Bourezak, F. Gomez, P. Blondeau, C. D'Allaines and A. Carpentier. "Comparative Evaluation of Mitral Valve Repair and Replacement with Starr, Björk and Porcine Valve Prostheses," *Circulation, 70 (Suppl I)*, 1:187–192 (1984).

34 NITTER-HAUGE, S., B. Semb, M. Abdelnoor and K. V. Hall. "A 5 Year Experience with the Medtronic–Hall Disc Valve Prosthesis," *Circulation, 68 (Suppl II)*, 2:169–174 (1983).

35 CARLSON, D. and L. W. Stephenson. "Mechanical Cardiac Valves: Current Status," *Cardiology Clinics*, 3:439–443 (1985).

36 JOHNSON, K. M. Personal Communication, Medtronic Blood Systems, Inc. (1986).

37 HALL, K. V., S. Nitter-Hauge and M. Abdelnoor. "Seven and One-Half Years' Experience with the Medtronic–Hall Valve," *J. Am. Coll. Cardiol.*, 6:1417–1421 (1985).

38 MATSUNAGA, H., K-I. Asano, A. Furuse, H. Maku-Uchi, T. Takayama and K. Yagyu. "Clinical Experience of Hall–Kaster Valve. Operative Results and Hemodynamic Status," *J. Cardiovasc. Surg.*, 25:138–141 (1984).

39 BEAUDET, R. L., N. L. Poirier, A. J. Guerraty and D. Doyle. "Fifty-Four Months' Experience with an Improved Tilting Disc Valve (Medtronic–Hall)," *Thoracic Cardiovasc. Surgeon*, 31:89–93 (1983).

40 PIKE, R. W. Personal Communication, Medical Incorporated (1986).

41 MIKHAIL, A. A. "Omniscience Cardiac Valve Prosthesis Compre-

hensive Clinical Review 65-Month, 8-Center Evaluation," PMAA Data Base Summary, Medical Incorporated (1984).

42 DeWall, R., L. C. Pelletier, A. Panebianco, G. Hicks, B. Schuster, R. Bonan, J-P. Martineau and L. Yip. "Five-Year Clinical Experience with the Omniscience Cardiac Valve," *Ann. Thorac. Surg.*, 38:275–280 (1984).

43 Arom, K. V., D. M. Nicoloff, T. E. Kersten, W. F. Northrup III and W. G. Lindsay. "Six Years of Experience with the St. Jude Medical Valvular Prothesis," *Circulation, 72 (Suppl II)*, 2:153–158 (1985).

44 Czer, L. S. C., J. Matloff, A. Chaux, M. DeRobertis, A. Yoganathan and R. J. Gray. "A 6 Year Experience with the St. Jude Medical Valve: Hemodynamic Performance, Surgical Results, Biocompatibility and Follow-up," *J. Am. Coll. Cardiol.*, 6:904–912 (1985).

45 Baudet, E. M., C. C. Oca, X. F. Roques, M. N. Laborde, A. S. Hafez, M. A. Collot and I. M. Ghidoni. "A 5 1/2 Year Experience with the St. Jude Medical Cardiac Valve Prosthesis," *J. Thorac. Cardiovasc. Surg.*, 90:137–144 (1985).

46 Wright, J. T. M., C. E. Eberhardt and M. L. Gibbs. "Hancock II—An Improved Bioprothesis," in *Cardiac Bioprostheses*, L. H. Cohn and V. Gallucci, eds. New York:Yorke Medical Books, pp. 425–444 (1982).

47 Gibbs, M L. Personal Communication, Johnson and Johnson Cardiovascular (1986).

48 Yoganathan, A. P., Y-R. Woo and H-W. Suns. "Turbulent Shear Stress Measurements in the Vicinity of Aortic Heart Valve Prostheses," *J. Biomechanics* (in press) (1986).

49 Bolooki, H., S. Mallon, G. A. Kaiser, R. J. Thurer and J. Kieval. "Failure of Hancock Xenograft Valve: Importance of Valve Position (4- to 9- Year Follow-up)," *Ann. Thorac. Surg.*, 36:246–252 (1983).

50 Gallo, I., B. Ruiz and C. M. G. Duran. "Five- to Eight-Year Follow-up of Patients with the Hancock Cardiac Bioprosthesis," *J. Thorac. Cardiovasc. Surg.*, 86:897–902 (1983).

51 Carpentier–Edwards Valve. American Edwards Laboratories. Technical Bulletin (1984).

52 Pelletier, C., B. R. Chaitman, R. Baillot, P. G. Val, R. Bonan and I. Dydra. "Clinical and Hemodynamic Results with the Carpentier–Edwards Porcine Bioprosthesis," *Ann. Thorac. Surg.*, 34:612–624 (1982).

53 Jamieson, W. R. E., L. C. Pelletier, M. T. Janusz, B. R. Chaitman, G. F. O. Tyers and R. T. Miyagishima. "Five-Year Evaluation of the Carpentier–Edwards Porcine Bioprosthesis," *T. Thorac. Cardiovasc. Surg.*, 88:324–333 (1984).

54 Ionescu, M. I., D. R. Smith, S. S. Hasan, M. Chidambaram and A. P. Tandon. "Clinical Durability of the Pericardial Xenograft Valve: Ten Years' Experience with Mitral Replacement," *Ann. Thorac. Surg.*, 34:265–277 (1982).

55 Gonzalez-Lavin, L., S. Chi, T. C. Blair, J. Y. Jung, A. G. Fabaz, P. M. McFadden, B. Lewis and G. Daughters. "Five-Year Experience with the Ionescu–Shiley Bovine Pericardial Valve in the Aortic Position," *Ann. Thorac. Surg.*, 36:270–280 (1983).

56 Fry, D. L. "Acute Vascular Endothelial Changes Associated with Increased Blood Velocity Gradients," *Cir. Res.*, 22:165–197 (1968).

57 Nevaril, C., J. Hellums, C. Alfrey, Jr. and E. Lynch. "Physical Effects in the Red Blood Cell Trauma," *AIChE. J.*, 15:707–711 (1969).

58 Sutera, S. P. and M. H. Mehrjardi. "Deformation and Fragmentation of Human Red Cells in Turbulent Shear Flow," *Biophysical J.*, 15:1–15 (1975).

59 Huns, J. C., R. M. Hochmuth, J. H. Joist and S. P. Sutera. "Shear Induced Aggregation and Lysis of Platelets," *Trans. ASAIO*, 22:285–291 (1976).

CHAPTER 10

Bioprosthetic Heart Valves: Tissue Mechanics and Implications for Design

J. MICHAEL LEE, Ph.D.[1] and
DEREK R. BOUGHNER, M.D., Ph.D.[2]

ABSTRACT: While a clinical success due to low thrombogenicity, bioprosthetic heart valves have an uncertain lifespan due to the coupled problems of tissue fatigue and calcification. One common factor linking these problems is the mechanical design and properties of the chemically-treated tissue leaflets. This paper discusses some problems in the understanding of the mechanical properties of the valve leaflets, the effect of chemical fixation on those properties, the use of mechanical constraints during fixation, and description of tissue viscoelastic behavior for mechanical modelling. Finally, the implications of these problems for valve design are considered.

INTRODUCTION

Over the last fifteen years, the use of bioprosthetic heart valves to replace diseased natural valves has become an important alternative to the use of completely synthetic materials. While not completely constructed from biological materials, these devices use chemically-treated tissue leaflets to occlude blood flow. The advantage of having blood predominantly in contact with these materials lies in their low thrombogenicity. Indeed, many patients receiving these valves do not require chronic systemic anticoagulation therapy. The newest generation of bioprosthetic valves features lower profiles, improvements in hemodynamic function, and an increasing sophistication of chemical treatment. Nonetheless, their functional lifetime remains an interesting question mark. The coupled problems of structural fatigue and tissue calcification remain to be understood and defeated. Until the mechanisms underlying these limitations are completely understood, the notion of a bioprosthetic valve which will last the lifetime of a young patient will remain an unattained goal; the clinician must continue to weigh freedom from anticoagulation therapy against long-term mechanical durability.

The leaflets of bioprosthetic materials, unlike their living counterparts, lack the active cellular components necessary to repair ongoing fatigue damage. Cellular invasion by the host, if any, has proven to be destructive, at least for aldehyde-fixed devices. Therefore, barring biological degradation, the designer of bioprostheses must produce valve leaflets which will endure a lifetime of cyclic loading without mechanical failure due to structural fatigue. If we consider a young patient, say thirty years old, this can mean forty-five years times thirty million loading cycles per year: an imposing total of more than 1.35 billion cycles! Structural fatigue failure without the influence of biological degradation by the host can be produced under controlled circumstances in the laboratory using accelerated pulse duplicators. The resulting damage to the leaflet collagen structure produces perforations and tears which are sometimes, but not always, similar to those seen in clinical implantation. In vivo, the relationship between mechanical fatigue and calcification is much more important. The link between fatigue and calcification is probably synergic. It has been suggested that initiation sites for calcification can be provided by the fatigue disruption of collagen bundles in high leaflet stress sites. However, once calcification has begun, the high stiffness mineral crystals must act as stress concentrators. This, in turn, would accelerate the damage to local collagen bundles, and a vicious circle results. If these mechanisms hold, then inhibition of leaflet fatigue damage should also lead to a reduction in the susceptibility of bioprostheses to calcification.

[1]Centre for Biomaterials, University of Toronto, 124 Edward St., Toronto, Ontario, Canada M5G 1G6

[2]Departments of Biophysics and Medicine, University of Western Ontario, London, Ontario, Canada N6A 5C1

In order to improve the fatigue lifetime of bioprosthetic heart valves, we can take either of two approaches: (1) we can perform stress analyses and redesign the valves to eliminate the regions of high local stress which may lead to premature fatigue damage; or (2) we can modify the mechanical properties of the leaflet material to better withstand the operating stresses. One objective of the stress analysis approach is to identify the stress patterns which are most damaging to the chemically modified tissue structure. For any stress analysis to be valid, it must incorporate detailed knowledge of the geometry of the valve during the cardiac cycle, the distribution of applied forces, and the mechanical properties of the material under in vivo deformations. On the other hand, if we wish to modify the mechanical properties of the material, we must know which stresses will exist (presumably from stress analysis); however, the results of the stress analysis, in turn, will depend on the assumed mechanical properties of the leaflet materials. Clearly, in reality both approaches must be incorporated simultaneously in the design and construction process.

In this chapter, we will consider some current problems in the study of the mechanical properties of the leaflets of bioprosthetic heart valves. We will concentrate on the effect of fixation on tissue mechanics and characterization of the mechanics of bioprosthetic rather than fresh tissue. While our remarks will principally concern the aldehyde-treated porcine aortic valve and bovine pericardial xenografts which dominate the current market, some discussion of human dura mater bioprostheses will be helpful. We will also discuss the type of mathematical description of tissue behavior that is likely to be useful to mathematical modellers performing stress analyses. Finally, we will look at some of the implications that the results of mechanical experiments on bioprosthetic tissue have for valve design.

DEVELOPMENT OF BIOPROSTHETIC HEART VALVES

Until the early 1960's, the management of patients with valvular heart disease was quite unsatisfactory. Premature death was the inevitable outcome, and medications had little ability to prolong life. Clearly, the mechanical problem of heart valve disease required a mechanical solution. This solution appeared with the introduction of prosthetic heart valves, both mechanical and bioprosthetic. Of these two varieties, the former proved quickly successful, but the latter did not.

The first biological valve implants were orthotopic homograft valves. These were cadaver valves obtained within 48 hours of death and initially implanted without special structural supports. Preservation techniques included sterilization by various means, freeze-drying or storage in antibiotic solution. Unfortunately, the long-term success of these valves was limited, with cusp rupture reported at 37% by 6 years and 50% by 8 years [1–3]. Although still utilized in a few centers and undergoing some resurgence in popularity, their initial high failure rate and limited availability resulted in a search for alternatives.

The porcine heterograft valve was first described in 1967 and had the clear advantages of abundant supply and a multiplicity of sizes [4]. The valves were harvested from 7–12 month old pigs, attached to metallic stents and rings and fixed in formaldehyde. The stent proved necessary to support the tissue in its normal cup shaped configuration and to achieve satisfactory opening and closure [5–6]. Yet again, in the long term, these valves proved unsuccessful. The original designers had hoped for tissue ingrowth to sustain the implanted material, but by 1970 their failure rate was unacceptably high, with Carpentier reporting nearly 100% failure by 4 years [7]. Examination of the recovered grafts showed the leaflet material to have a decreased tensile strength and inflammatory or immunological cellular reaction with no tissue regeneration by host fibroblasts. Clearly, any tissue valve replacement would have to depend on its own structural integrity to attain satisfactory durability.

A significant advance occurred in 1969 when Carpentier described the glutaraldehyde fixation technique for porcine bioprosthesis [8]. This five carbon dialdehyde molecule reacts with tissue proteins to form crosslinks, the crosslinking process being sensitive to a variety of conditions including temperature, pH and molecular species [9]. Largely through its reactions with collagen, it produced a substantial improvement in tissue durability and successfully reduced tissue antigenicity. By 1971 the commercial availability of porcine valve xenografts provided an acceptable functional alternative to totally synthetic valve prostheses with the distinct advantage that systemic anticoagulation therapy was not required. Several manufacturers began production and a variety of minor modifications then ensued. For example, the Carpentier–Edwards valve stents had "fully flexible" characteristics [10] which allowed the technician assembling the valve to bend the stent posts in the annulus region to match the stent to the porcine valve tissue being utilized. An alternative design concept was the Angell–Shiley [11], which allowed for anatomic variations by utilizing a large variety of stents molded from casts of "typical porcine valves." Thus, the technician mounting the porcine valve could select a suitable stent and appropriately fix the valve to it.

A further rationale for the flexible polypropylene stent was to reduce "shock loading" of the valve tissue and thence local stresses during closure, possibly improving valve longevity [12]. Changes in stent post height which produced a valve with a higher profile, resulted from the desire to incorporate more valve tissue within the stents. An anatomic problem with porcine aortic valves was addressed in 1976 with the introduction of the modified orifice valve. The normal porcine valve is asymmetric with a muscular bar formed from the outflow tract ventricular myocardium occupying a significant portion of the right coronary leaflet. This reduces the flow area of the valve. In the modified orifice valve, the right coronary cusp was excised and replaced by the noncoronary cusp from a larger porcine valve, improving valve hemodynamics [13]. However, a further increase in stent post height was necessary to accommodate the leaflet segment and the various trade-offs in valve performance continued.

Unfortunately, the mechanics of mounting porcine valve tissue inside a metal or plastic ring produced a structure with an inevitably small orifice size for small diameter aortic roots. Outflow obstruction was a problem. A second problem was insufficient porcine valve availability. Less then 10% of valves supplied to manufacturers were usable for prosthesis construction. An alternative material was suggested by Ionescu in 1971 [14]. He began to experiment with the pericardium from 6 to 18 month old calves. This 0.4 mm thick pericardium was cut and positioned over the outside, rather than the inside, of cloth covered rigid titanium stents. The early Ionescu-Shiley valves used a single piece of pericardium to form the bioprosthesis; later versions used three pieces for the three cusps and, by 1976, these valves were commercially available from several manufacturers. Various design features were promoted including the "low profile" construction and flexible plastic stents. The primary advantages over the porcine bioprosthesis, however, were low transvalvular pressure gradients and more flexible cusps [6]. These valves quickly achieved wide popularity.

The expense of commercially-available prosthetic heart valves also led Zerbini and Puig [15] to the development of human dura mater bioprostheses as an inexpensive alternative prosthesis for use in developing countries. Implanted initially in 1971 in Brazil, these valves used three individual leaflets constructed from homologous dura mater treated for up to two weeks in 98% glycerol. The leaflets were rehydrated, treated with antibiotics, and mounted on stainless steel stents. Clinical durability of these devices proved acceptable, but there has been a lack of interest in recent years.

Why do the presently available bioprosthetic valves fail? Infection, valve dehiscence and stent fracture are relatively rare problems, and the most common difficulty is tissue calcification and/or leaflet tearing or fenestration. Several authors have attempted to address these problems, and a variety of answers and suggestions have arisen. The evidence strongly suggests that immunologic processes do not contribute significantly to the calcifica-

tion and disruption of bioprosthetic valves. The concensus seems to be that mechanical stresses are in some way responsible for valve deterioration by accelerating the calcification process. When tissue disruption and failure eventually occur, the site is usually adjacent to calcium deposits; however, they may also occur alone.

Although manufacturers showed considerable interest and innovative skill in regular improvements in the mounting frame design of their valves, considerably less attention was paid to the actual leaflet materials being utilized, i.e., to their histologic features and physical properties as mechanical devices. The initial impression was that whether bovine pericardium or porcine valve tissue was used the glutaraldehyde fixation process made the materials immunologically inert, and the valves seemed to open and close well, standing up to the stress satisfactorily. However, over the past several years it has become increasingly clear that neither the porcine aortic valve nor the bovine pericardial xenografts display adequate long term durability. Serious problems with an increasing incidence of valve failure have been reported by various authors. For porcine valves, for example, Milano and coworkers [16] reported a 7% failure rate at 5 years and 29% at 9 years, while by 12 years 39% of these valves in the mitral position and 31% in the aortic position had failed. Similar failure rates have been reported by Reul and coworkers for pericardial xenografts [17]. Bortolotti [18] has commented that primary valve tissue failure is the most common indication for reoperation in patients with a porcine bioprostheses, and continued efforts should be directed toward the search for more durable biological valves.

The earliest indication of problems with long-term durability appeared when the bioprosthetic valves were implanted in children and adolescents. Such valves failed rapidly, primarily by tissue calcification, and usually required replacement within 3 years of implantation [19,20]. Results in adults were better, but in 1978 a scanning and transmission electron microscopic study of a small number of explanted valves by Ferrans and co-workers [21] showed minor changes in collagen fibrils by 2 months, and in 4 valves in place for 21 to 30 months there was evidence of severe collagen breakdown despite a macroscopically normal appearance. Under light microscopy, collagen breakdown was manifested by the disappearance of collagen fibril bundles and the appearance of a pale staining matrix free of fibrillar elements, showing no birefringence on polarizing light microscopy. In addition, there were findings of valve surface erosion and lipid accumulation. Calcific deposits were noted in one valve and, in a valve replaced after 6 years, tears of the valve cusps were present. Their impression was that the collageneous framework of glutaraldehyde-treated heterografts underwent progressive deterioration with time and might be a critical factor in determining long-term durability.

Some authors feel that valve ring and stent designs are still imperfect despite the manufacturers' best efforts and may be producing unacceptable stresses. Drury and co-workers [22] noted that some plastic support frames can develop permanent deformation or creep which may be responsible for valve failure. The original bioprosthetic valves had rigid frames but, intuitively, stent flexibility has been regarded as an asset to reduce valve stress. A variety of somewhat flexible metal or plastic frames have been utilized by the various manufacturers with the intent of duplicating the aortic root behavior. Drury examined the natural aortic root in 120 pig hearts, and he characterized the pattern of expansion of the sinuses as well as the radial and axial displacement of the commissural points during pressurization. He observed no clear pattern of motion between the three commissures or the sinuses. He then compared the load and deflection behavior of six biologic heart valve frame designs and also observed a variety of responses. Ultimately, he concluded there was simply insufficient data to make definite recommendations regarding the ideal frame geometry and stent material, but he suggested that flexible, fatigue and creep resistant titanium alloy might be the most logical material presently available.

Although most valve designs are reputed to have flexible stents, the in vivo evidence suggests that the stent posts of popular porcine and pericardial bioprostheses do not flex significantly during the cardiac cycle. Thubrikar and co-workers found no evidence of significant change in the measured commissure perimeter when the position of stent post markers was examined [23]. In contrast, the commissure perimeter of the natural aortic valve has been shown to expand with systole and decrease from systole to diastole [24,25]. Thus, although a truly flexible stent design appears desirable, present valves do not imitate the motion of the normal aortic root. Whether this failure can be implicated in the evidently limited durability of bioprosthetic valves remains uncertain.

BIOPROSTHETIC LEAFLET MATERIALS

All bioprosthetic heart valves currently available in North America have leaflets which are made from one of two types of material: (1) aldehyde-fixed porcine aortic valves or (2) aldehyde-fixed bovine pericardium. The choice of these particular tissues is based largely on their ready availability from slaughter. This is a major advantage over both the difficulties encountered in obtaining cadaveric tissue (like human dura mater) or fresh homograft tissue (like human aortic valves), and the problems of performing valve constuction from autogenous tissue (like the pericardium) during a surgical procedure. Furthermore, aldehyde fixation allows for large-scale valve manufacture with quality control testing unattainable in a hospital or operating room setting.

Bioprosthetic valves have been designed to mimic the normal trileaflet human aortic valve. Curiously, the cusps of the normal valve are seldom of equal size—half the time one cusp is of substantially different size than the other two, and one-third of the time all 3 cusps are of markedly different size [26]. Internally, the leaflets of human and porcine aortic valves are similar. They are highly differentiated connective tissue structures composed of three basic components: collagen, elastin and mucopolysaccharides. These components are arranged in various mixtures, predominantly in 3 layers within the valve leaflet: the ventricularis, spongiosa and fibrosa, all covered by a monocellular layer of endothelium. The bottom layer, the ventricularis, lies on the smooth-surfaced ventricular side of the valve and is composed mainly of radially oriented elastin with some bundles of circumferentially arranged collagen interspersed [27,28]. On the aortic side of the valve, by contrast, the load-bearing fibrosa is composed almost completely of circumferentially arranged collagen bundles that provide circumferential resistance to stress during diastole, while the leaflets more freely develop the large radial strains [29] during leaflet closure. Clark and Finke [27] found a 50% reduction in leaflet thickness as the aortic valve moved from its relaxed to stressed state, and that reduction is apparently accounted for by the reduction in amplitude of the leaflet corrugations [30]. Lying between the corrugated fibrosa and the smooth ventricularis is the spongiosa which contains a large quantity of mucopolysaccharide interspersed with loosely arranged collagen fibrils. It is presently not clear how the fibrosa is attached to the ventricularis, but the outer 2 layers can be readily split mechanically at the level of the spongiosa. The function of the spongiosa remains unclear although it likely permits substantial shear deformation of the valve during bending.

For construction of porcine aortic valve bioprostheses, aortic valves are excised from the heart with the aortic root intact. They may then be trimmed and mounted intact in a supporting stent to form the bioprosthesis. Alternatively, the muscular noncoronary leaflet and its attached third of the aortic root may be removed and be replaced with a coronary leaflet and aortic segment from another valve before mounting. The geometry and apposition of the leaflets are finally established by the application of a pressure gradient across the closed valve leaflets during the initial fixation in glutaraldehyde.

In contrast, bovine pericardium is structurally very different from normal aortic valve cusps. It is a relatively isotropic material composed of nearly identical layers of dense collagenous sheets lying parallel to the surface. The external surface is somewhat rougher than the smooth visceral surface and elastin is distributed throughout the thickness of the pericardium with increased density nearer the rough external surface. The appearance of the tissue is rather uniform and, with the exception of minimizing vascularity, valve manufacturers apparently have no particular preference for areas of the pericardial sac used for valve construction. Trowbridge and co-workers have recently warned that the central portion of the sac, in a sector emanating radially from the ligaments in that area was substantially more extensible than other regions of the calf pericardium and should be avoided in valve construction [31]. The elastin content of the pericardium in this sector is much greater than in other areas and has a much coarser appearance. Clearly, given the structural differences between pericardium and normal heart valve tissue one would reasonably expect different mechanical properties and leaflet behavior.

More choices are available to the valve designer when constructing a leaflet-type valve from a sheet of tissue such as pericardium. While the original Ionescu-Shiley valve and most other pericardial valves since have used a trileaflet construction mimicking the natural aortic valve, there is no a priori reason to adopt this construction for all applications. Indeed, both bileaflet and unileaflet valves have been developed at least experimentally with associated claims regarding naturalness of function or resistance to fatigue [32,33,34]. In cutting the leaflets, all the leaflets for one valve can be formed from a single strip of tissue without cutting, or each leaflet can be formed separately. The final shape of the valve leaflets is determined, in part, by the technique used in suturing the tissue to the supporting stent and, in part, by the application of surface stress (say, by using cotton balls) to mold the leaflets during fixation in glutaraldehyde. Pressure-fixation has not been used to our knowledge in construction of bovine pericardial bioprosthetic valves.

Dura mater is another sheetlike material available for valve construction. It also contains mostly collagen with relatively few elastin fibers, but does not show the same architecture of fiber weave that is seen in pericardium. Rather, the orientation and overlapping of the layered collagen fibers seems to change suddenly over distances of millimeters to centimeters [35,36]. For valve preparation, rectangles of tissue are obtained from the superior cranium, in the avascular regions on either side of the superior saggital sinus. The treatment of the three leaflets with glycerol rather than glutaraldehyde is unique to this valve type. No physical constraints are used during fixation of the valve; rather, the leaflets are supported by a plastic mold while they are sutured to the supporting stainless steel stent [15].

Structurally, the leaflets of all bioprostheses are made from tissues which, before excision, contained collagen fibers, elastin fibers, mucopolysaccharide, intrastitial fluid, and at least some cellular components. By the end of valve construction, however, these components have been subjected to a variety of alterations. The tissues are usually fixed in both glutaraldehyde and formaldehyde. These reagents are used in differing concentrations, for different treatment times, and are prepared in a variety of buffered solutions. It is worth noting that the choice of the fixative concentration and solution chemistry can be in-

fluenced by a variety of considerations, including inhibition of calcification, efficacy of sterilization, hydrodynamic performance, maximal saturation of crosslink sites, and in vitro fatigue lifetime. Glutaraldehyde fixation, for instance, is normally performed near pH 7.4, although its crosslinking efficiency is highest about pH 8 [37]. Where phosphate buffer was initially used with glutaraldehyde solutions, concern over calcification has led to the alternative use of organic HEPES buffer. Formaldehyde post-fixation is generally performed in a slightly acidic acetate buffer, pH 5.4. According to Woodroof [38], this choice ensures maximum sterilization of the valve, but since aldehyde crosslinking of tissue is least effective around this pH, this may also prevent formaldehyde crosslinking or its substitution for glutaraldehyde crosslinks. If fixative concentration and exposure time are chosen to ensure maximal saturation of available crosslink sites, the degree of crosslinking may be assessed by evaluation of collagen thermal shrinkage temperature or resistance to enzymatic degradation. However, as is well known in the leather industry, maximal crosslinking does not necessarily correlate with optimal mechanical properties (for instance high tensile strength) and may actually produce a more brittle material.

Since calcification has been identified as a major problem in valve bioprostheses several authors have suggested chemical treatment of the bioprosthetic material to inhibit intrinsic mineralization. Tissue treatments with surfactants or detergents, polymeric plastics, and ionic substitutes have all been described and at least some have been incorporated in the most recent generation of valves [39–41]. The evidence that collagen is a focus for calcification is strong but it remains uncertain whether it is simply a passive nucleator or whether the calcium of the matrix vesicles is an active initiating factor in the mineralization process. There has been a search for compounds unique to mineralized tissue that may be involved in the pathogenesis of the process and a class of proteins (GLA proteins) have been described. The role of these proteins remains uncertain but the concept of a biochemical instigator for the process suggests a possible biochemical solution to the problem.

While the aldehyde fixation can be expected to produce changes in mechanics as a result of crosslinks in collagen and to a lesser extent in elastin and the other protein components of the tissue, the effects of the other treatments (including the buffers) on tissue structure and the mechanical consequences of these treatments have not been examined in the literature. Some indirect evidence of extraction of mucopolysaccharides can be drawn from ultrastructural studies of the bioprosthetic material. Ishihara and co-workers [42] have noted significantly lower levels of mucopolysaccharides in processed tissue than in fresh tissue. However, aside from commenting on the loss of the endothelial layer, they did not suggest how this component was lost.

MECHANICAL FUNCTION OF BIOPROSTHETIC VALVES

In both the natural valves of the heart and bioprosthetic valves, the leaflets undergo a complex pattern of stresses and strains during the cardiac cycle. When open, the leaflets are flexed at their attachment to the stent or aortic wall and (when seen in pulsatile testers) the leaflets flap in a manner similar to a flag. (Interestingly, this leaflet flapping can also be seen echocardiographically in 5–10% of patients with normal aortic valves.) The leaflets subsequently slam shut, producing reflexure at the wall attachment, very rapid tensile loading of the leaflets and additional bending near the center of the leaflets. The tensile stresses are certainly biaxial, and the bending may incorporate both compression and shearing of the leaflet tissue.

Estimation of the stresses present in the leaflets during a given phase of the cardiac cycle presents a considerable challenge to the engineer due to (1) the difficulty in establishing the geometry of the leaflets during the entire cardiac cycle, (2) the need to adequately characterize the inhomogeneity, anisotropy, and viscoelasticity of the leaflet material, (3) the difficulty in defining boundary conditions, (4) the difference in force and pressure conditions in different valve positions (say mitral versus aortic), and (5) the very dynamic nature of the loading.

Published stress analyses of the natural aortic valve or trileaflet prosthetic valves have generally only analyzed the stresses in the leaflets during diastole. Clark and co-workers [43], for instance, established the geometry of the leaflets using silicone rubber molds of closed valves in excised intact aortic roots and close-range stereophotogrammetry. This information was combined with assumptions of uniform leaflet thickness and linear isotropic elastic behavior of the leaflet material, and was used in a stress analysis based on shell theory (thin-walled pressure vessel analysis) and finite element methods. Subsequently refined by Catalogu and co-workers [44] using smoothed geometric data, this technique showed that the maximum principal stresses in the leaflets lay in the circumferential direction. This conclusion did not rely on any assumption of greater leaflet stiffness in that direction. Additional analyses by Chong and Missirlis [45] also used silicone rubber molds, but these workers used membrane and shell analyses and a more sophisticated geometric approach with photogrammetry of small markers on actual valve leaflets subjected to simulated diastolic pressures. The leaflet tissue was still considered to be elastic, but was permitted to be inhomogeneous and nonlinearly elastic in the radial and circumferential directions. The nonlinear elasticity of the leaflets was measured in accompanying simple microtensile tests of isolated circumferential and radial strips of tissue. The results of this analysis suggested that the radial stresses in the tissue leaflets were much greater than the circumferential stresses: a curious

conclusion unique to this study. Silicone rubber molds have also been used by Ghista and Reul [46] in an effort to optimize the design of a trileaflet valve. However, since they envisioned a valve with synthetic elastomeric leaflets, they were concerned with a wider range of design variable than were considered in analyzing the stresses in natural valves. Their finite element approach therefore could reasonably use linear elastic theory and produced a map of stress levels for comparison with the fatigue limits of their polymer.

Christie and Medland [47] developed a model for the mechanical behavior of the cusps using finite element analysis. Their analysis included modelling of the leaflet material as an isotropic membrane reinforced with circumferential elastic fibres and examination of leaflet behavior under conditions simulating the presence of a constraining rigid stent. Their analysis suggested that because the net movement of the leaflet was toward the coapting surface, the area of coaptation actually increased with increasing pressure in a bioprosthetic valve. Another interesting observation has been made by Broom and Christie [48] by incorporating leaflet anisotropy into their finite element stress analytical model of the diastolic aortic valve. They showed that the calculated stresses depend greatly on the relative values of the circumferential and radial leaflet stiffnesses: the stiffer the leaflets are in the circumferential direction, the greater the relative size of the calculated principal stress in that direction. Further, the coaptation area is increased and, therefore, there is less chance of regurgitation. This work indicates firstly that sizeable errors may have been present in earlier work on natural aortic valves due to assumptions of leaflet material isotropy. Secondly, it shows that there may be real functional advantages if other bioprosthetic tissues (such as bovine pericardium) can be prepared in such a way as to produce marked leaflet anisotropy. This notion is addressed further below.

While these studies have provided useful information on the distribution of tensile stresses in the closed valve during diastole, they tell us nothing of what occurs during systole or during opening and closure. An approach to dynamic stress analysis has been employed by Thubrikar and co-workers [29,49]. They attached radiopaque tantalum markers to the leaflets of natural aortic valves of dogs and of porcine bioprostheses in calves and used geometric information obtained from fluoroscopy to calculate tensile, compressive, and bending stresses in the leaflets. They have provided the first in vivo measurements of leaflet strains and radii of curvature in both diastole and systole; however, in calculating bending properties, they made the fundamental assumption that the stress–strain curve of the leaflet material in compression is the reflection of its curve in tension. This assumption is unsupportable in a pliant composite material and is the philosophical equivalent of pushing a rope. Therefore, their calculations of compressive and bending stresses must be treated with extreme caution.

Thubrikar and co-workers have also presented evidence for a relationship between mechanical stresses and calcification of bioprosthetic valves. Calcium deposits were initially described in association with sites of collagen disorganization or disintegration [21,50] and Thubrikar's group believed that collagen breakdown was caused by "excessive wear." Using the radiopaque marker system described above, they analyzed for sites of leaflet flexion during the cardiac cycle, calculated the "elastic" properties of fresh valve material, and estimated the stresses being sustained. They suggested that bioprosthetic leaflet materials poorly withstood the bending stresses and shear deformation involved as they opened and closed during the cardiac cycle. After identifying the areas of greatest membrane and bending stress, they examined the pattern of calcification in bioprosthetic valves implanted in calves [51]. They noted that in systole acute bending occurred at the mural attachments of the cusps for both porcine and bovine pericardium valves. In addition, for the porcine leaflets, reversed bending in the central portion was noted. They observed that calcium deposits in the bioprosthetic material first occurred in the commissural region and later in the basal regions. It occurred in all pericardial valves by four weeks and all porcine valves by seven weeks. For the porcine valves there were linear streaks of mineralization from the point of leaflet attachment out into the leaflet itself but for pericardial valves the calcification was clumped rather than linear and occurred mainly at the attachment sites. Histological sections of the porcine valves showed calcification to be present within both the spongiosa and fibrosa, while for pericardium the calcium was more diffusely laid down in all layers along the bending zone, both within and especially between the collagenous sheets. The crystals of calcium for both valve types were found within or surrounding the collagen fibrils and it was evident that collagen breakdown was not necessary for a high calcium density. Despite the apparent lack of collagen disintegration as a precipitating cause it was evident that the problem was a focal abnormality primarily related to points of high bending stress and not generalized throughout the valve. They concluded that the initial stages of calcification occur in a similar pattern in all types of valves coincident with sites of high mechanical stress in the zones of leaflet flexion. They suggested that two types of local stress concentration occurred in such areas: pure bending and shear. They also suggested that if a material which has little or no resistance to compressive stress is flexed, it will buckle in the area of compression and produce internal "voids" as the material deteriorates. They felt their observations suggested this possibility.

Other finite element analyses of leaflet stresses have also been attempted and related to regions of leaflet calcification or perforation. Sabbah and co-workers [52] used this technique to estimate the effects of valve stiffening, thinning or focal calcification. They suggested that failure of valve material tends to develop in areas where mechanical forces are exerted in a highly localized manner, either due to the pattern of opening and closure of the cusps or because calcific deposits are present. To analyze these hypotheses, they made assumptions that leaflets were of equal size, symmetrical and uniformly thick, that annulus deformation under pressure was minimal, and that the valve tissue was isotropic. Bending effects were neglected and the stent was assumed to be rigid. They modelled the relaxed cusp shape as one half of an elliptic paraboloid and calculated the magnitude and distribution of stresses in normal porcine leaflets, stiffened leaflets, leaflets with focal calcification and leaflets with thinning. For the normal glutaraldehyde-treated leaflets, the maximum tension and shear stresses were highest near the leaflet commissures with overall increases when tissue stiffening was simulated. Maximal stress concentration then appeared near the center of the leaflet. Focal calcification and focal thinning produced marked stress gradients between such sites and the surrounding tissues: that is, they acted as stress concentrators. Sabbah and co-workers felt that these findings compared satisfactorily with morphologic studies of degenerated bioprosthetic valves which have shown a high incidence of tears and calcification near the commissures and in the central portion of the leaflet. As additional evidence, in a study by Stein and co-workers [53], leaflet tears or holes were associated with calcific deposits in 41% of cases. This again suggests a cause and effect relationship betweeen structural damage and calcification.

Natural heart valves are supported and constrained by the fibrous rings which separate the atria and ventricles of the heart. These rings are not inextensible: indeed, the opening of the natural aortic valve has been shown by Brewer [54] to begin with the enlargement of the aortic root under ventricular pressure so that the leaflets are at first separated without flexure. This is followed by flexure of the leaflets and complete opening of the valve. Leaflet flexure is therefore largely instigated by flow, not by transmural pressure differences. In existing bioprosthetic valves, however, the boundary conditions are quite different: the valve stent constrains the root of the valve in a basically inextensible ring. Therefore, the valve root cannot expand circumferentially and the leaflets of a porcine aortic valve bioprosthesis must flex more during opening than they would during equivalent physiological function in the pig. The result of this difference must be a greater susceptibility to flexural fatigue in a bioprosthetic valve with a rigid stent than in one with a truly flexible supporting ring. While flexible stent posts have been incorporated as a result of stress analyses, annular flexibility equivalent to that in the fibrous rings of the heart has never been incorporated in a commercially available valve. Further, we must also consider that the post-operative base of the valve is a composite of the patient's original fibrous ring, the valve stent, and the porcine fibrous ring. Therefore, some limitation of expansion may be inevitable. The only alternative may be a valve with bioprosthetic tissue leaflets (perhaps of pericardium) free-formed in situ without a supporting stent. This would, however, represent a considerable surgical problem in forming and handling the prosthesis. Finally, it is worth noting that the inflexible stent ring forms one of the boundary conditions in most stress analyses of bioprosthetic valves. Leaflet stresses predicted in these analyses may be quite different from those in valves with freely extensible rings.

The tensile stresses developed in bioprosthetic valve leaflets during the cardiac cycle are clearly biaxial, the strains in each direction being coupled by the appropriate Poisson ratios. Nonetheless, very little is known about the biaxial mechanical properties of the leaflet material. Biaxial properties are certainly required in stress analyses. However, the mechanical properties of the leaflets have typically been assumed to be those seen in uniaxial tests and to be the same in each direction. Biaxial properties of actual bioprosthetic leaflet materials have not been reported in the literature. In part, this is simply due to the experimental difficulties of biaxial testing. While in a uniaxial test the strain in a sample strip can be calculated from the simple separation of the grips (in the absence of slippage), this is not true in a biaxial test. If grips are used, the test sample must be cruciate, the long arms of the cross ensuring nearly uniform biaxial stress in the central portion of the sample. The strains must be measured in the central portion only because the extension will not be uniform from grip to grip: in this area, the strain in a given direction will be reduced by the Poisson effect if stress is applied in the second direction. Alternatively, as in the work of M-C Lee [55], multiple suture attachments can be made to each side of a square sample of tissue. The principal difficulty with this system, however, is ensuring uniform stressing of the tissue through careful adjustments of the suture ties. In either method, the monitoring of stress is accomplished by measuring directional load and dividing by the cross-sectional area of the sample in that direction. Strain measurement is more difficult: it must be performed in both directions and be non-contacting. Typically, a video extensometer (video analyzer) system is used with one or two television cameras and markers on the tissue surface. To date, two systems of this sort for biaxial testing of planar connective tissues have been described in the literature, and both have been custom-built [55,56]. Although intended for study of bioprosthetic materials, the van Noort apparatus was never used for a published biaxial study; the Fung apparatus has only been applied to fresh tissue. While biaxial testing of individual aortic valve leaflets using one of these methods would certainly be very difficult, pericardial material could be readily tested using a cruciate sample.

Given that uniaxial testing of leaflet mechanics is more easily accomplished and forms the bulk of the literature on the subject, what considerations must be given to its use in evaluating leaflet mechanical properties? Firstly, the strains predicted by uniaxial in vitro testing will certainly be overestimates of the in vivo strains. Stresses in the second principal direction, which would normally produce a reduction in strain due to Poisson coupling are absent in uniaxial tests. Secondly, while both types of tests are subject to artifacts due to the cutting of long collagen fibers during sample preparation, uniaxial testing may allow additional artifactural reorientation of fibers toward the direction of stress unopposed by stresses in the second direction. Therefore, during cyclic loading of a uniaxial test specimen, this reorientation may produce an artifactual increase in stiffness of the sample. Further, this reorientational freedom may also be expressed as increased stress relaxation, creep, and hysteresis during initial loading cycles which may decline during the course of the experiments. There is no direct way of assessing these contributions during uniaxial testing. They can be evaluated only by comparing uniaxial test results with biaxial test results on equivalent material. Such tests have not been conducted.

Given the rapidity of the opening heart valve leaflets, surprisingly little is actually known about the mechanical properties of the leaflet tissue under high strain rates. In vitro testing of leaflet materials has typically employed strain rates substantially below those estimated to occur in vivo, approximately 15,000 %/min [45]. This value is quite reasonable if 20% strain is achieved over a loading time of 0.1 sec: a mean strain rate of 12,000 %/min. In vitro strain rates have not exceeded several hundred percent per minute, generally due to equipment restrictions. Therefore, a gap in strain rate of nearly two orders of magnitude remains to be bridged. Much has been made, nonetheless, of the relative elastic–viscoelastic behavior of the leaflet materials under these lower strain rates, and this stress–strain information has been included in stress analyses, typically as "elastic" behavior. The implications of experimental strain rate for viscoelastic analysis of the leaflet material are discussed next.

The leaflets of natural heart valves have presumably been structurally optimized for their mechanical performance, especially for resistance to repeated flexure. However, with the exception of porcine aortic valve bioprostheses, the leaflets of bioprosthetic valves are made from tissues which do not undergo significant flexure during physiological function. Pericardium, for instance, undergoes very little flexure during the normal cardiac cycle; rather, it is subjected largely to planar biaxial stress. It is reasonable, therefore, to be concerned about the resistance of pericardium to flexural fatigue.

If we are to understand how normal aortic valves can withstand a lifetime of flexure in a healthy patient, we must understand both the structural features of normal valve leaflets which provide resistance to flexural fatigue, and the importance of ongoing repair of fatigue damage by connective tissue cells. The structure of normal aortic valve leaflets has been well examined and it is clear that the circumferential alignment of the major collagen bundles in the leaflet fibrosa serves at least two, possibly distinct, purposes: (1) it provides for leaflet anisotropy, the greatest strength and stiffness being aligned with the direction of greatest tensile stress, and (2) it provides for "rolling" of these major bundles by each other as the leaflet bends. Major collagen bundles do not extend in the radial direction where flexure would result in bundle buckling and disruption. This is clearly not the case for pericardium and dura mater which show crossed-fibrillar array structure: that is, major fiber bundles running in several directions, a design likely intended to produce effective planar mechanical isotropy [57]. When these materials are used as valve leaflets, at least some major collagen bundles will be aligned in the radial direction and flexure of these bundles must result. The resistance flexural fatigue of leaflets made from pericardium or dura may depend on the precise directional alignment of the collagen fibers, the size of the collagen bundles and the degree of interweaving of fibers between adjacent planes in the tissue. For instance, layers can be easily peeled away from normal aortic valve leaflets, suggesting limited attachment between layers, and freedom of adjacent layers to shear past each other during flexure. This may be critical to their resistance to flexural damage, since bending through shear would reduce compressive buckling. By contrast, the layers of pericardium are well interlaced and do not pull apart, suggesting that layer-to-layer shear is less likely during leaflet bending.

MECHANICAL EFFECTS OF FIXATION TREATMENTS ON BIOPROSTHETIC LEAFLET MATERIALS

The term "bioprosthesis" was coined by Carpentier [58] to describe tissues which had been rendered non-viable through chemical treatment, typically using a protein crosslinking agent like glutaraldehyde or formaldehyde. Carpentier and colleagues settled on the use of aldehydes early on, and the use of the dialdehydes like glutaraldehyde proved most promising in their early experimental implantations. Since then glutaraldehyde fixation has dominated the bioprosthetic industry with little investigation of alternative treatments. Indeed, glycerol has been the only alternative treatment to find large-scale use. However, as will be discussed below, this treatment is to some extent also an aldehyde treatment. In recent years research on alternative fixation agents has accelerated due to increased concern over the effects of aldehydes on mechanical properties, over cytotoxicity from release of residual or labile glutaraldehyde, and over the possible exacerbating effect of glutaraldehyde on calcification. As well, recent evidence suggests that glutaraldehyde fixation may not suppress immunological reactions as effectively as was originally believed [59]. Literature studies on the effect of fixation on the mechanical properties of bioprosthetic leaflet materials have been limited almost exclusively to aldehydes and glycerol. Much of this work has involved simple fixation without mechanical constraints on the tissue. Alternatively, aldehyde fixation has been combined with the use of physical constraints (tethering, pressure, uniaxial or biaxial strain) to develop methods for "engineering" the mechanical properties or shape of the leaflets.

Simple Fixation of Porcine Aortic Valves in Aldehydes

The effect of simple aldehyde fixation on porcine aortic valve leaflets was first examined by Tan and Holt [60]. They investigated a variety of storage techniques for allograft materials including phosphate-buffered 37% formaldehyde. Using circumferential and radial strips of porcine aortic valves, they looked at simple one-pull stress-strain responses and stress relaxation before and after treatment. They found that formaldehyde treatment increased stiffness, decreased total extension, and reduced stress relaxation in both directions. Studies by Broom [61,62] confirmed these results using a 0.625% phosphate-buffered glutaraldehyde solution and either porcine pulmonary valves [62] or bovine and porcine mitral valves [61]. He found that fixation increased the stiffness of the tissue under low strains and decreased the overall extensions of the leaflets. Using a microtensile device and Nomarski interference microscopy, he also demonstrated that, after fixation, the crimp of the collagen bundles in the tissue was "frozen in" and did not completely collapse even under high stress.

The studies outlined above painted a consistent picture of aldehydes stiffening the leaflets of bioprostheses. However, when Broom later examined the stress–strain behavior of strips of porcine aortic valve leaflets fixed in 0.625% phosphate-buffered glutaraldehyde [63], he found much greater extensibility and lower stiffnesses than had been previously reported in his experiments on other valve tissues. These were not compared with results from fresh tissue. The tensile stiffening of tissues in aldehydes has also been more substantially challenged by two separate and much more complete studies by Rousseau and co-workers [64] and ourselves [65,66]. Rousseau and co-workers examined circumferential strips of porcine aortic valves both before and after fixation in 0.625% phosphate-buffered glutaraldehyde. (Note that each strip was tested in both conditions.) The experiments involved a single extension of the tissue followed by 120 seconds of stress relaxation. This experiment was then repeated. Lee and co-workers examined radial and circumferential strips of porcine aortic valves. The strips were cut *either* from fresh valves *or* from valves fixed in 0.625% phosphate-buffered glutaraldehyde followed by 4% phosphate-buffered formaldehyde. The experiments included cyclic stress–strain testing with hysteresis measurements, stress relaxation, creep, and fracture. Both of these studies showed that simple fixation in aldehydes produced materials which were stiffer than fresh tissue under low strains (less than 10%), yet overall were much more extensible. The shape of the stress–strain curves were markedly different for the fresh and fixed tissues, a result not seen in the previous studies. Both studies also showed reductions in stress relaxation after fixation. In the additional experiments, Lee et al. also showed that fixation produced substantial differences in cyclic preconditioning responses, and reductions in creep, but no change in cyclic hysteresis. Interestingly, fixed tissue demonstrated unrecovered "plastic" deformation during cyclic loading: that is, an increase in unloaded length. This was not seen in the fresh tissue. As well, in fracture testing, fixation reduced the tissue modulus of the strips (the final stiffness under high stress), reduced the ultimate tensile strength (UTS) and increased the strain at fracture.

The discrepancies between the results of the studies outlined above (for instance, increasing or decreasing stiffness) are not easily explained. Experimental stress levels cannot be a factor since the maximum stresses in all five studies were in the range of several hundred kiloPascals. While gauge length definition or problems in measuring the cross-sectional areas of strips of irregular valve tissue may explain some of the specific differences in the observed extensibilities or stiffnesses, these factors cannot explain the marked change in the shape of the stress–strain curve after fixation observed by ourselves, by Rousseau and co-workers, and indirectly supported by Broom [63]. The consistency of the later studies, supported by work in pericardium (see below) suggests that glutaraldehyde-fixation does indeed increase tensile extensibility.

Since bending stresses have been implicated in bioprosthetic valve failure, we have examined the effect of simple fixation on the bending properties of strips of porcine aortic valve leaflets. A tissue bending machine has been constructed that allows measurement of the force required to bend a strip of aortic valve leaflet around specific radii of curvature [67]. The resultant bending moment produced in the tissue strip can then be calculated. Comparison has been made between the bending behavior of fresh tissue and tissue treated in 0.625% phosphate-buffered glutaraldehyde. The graph of bending moment versus curvature for both tissues showed low stiffness under low bending curvatures, while at higher bending curvatures the material became considerably stiffer [68]. The shape of the bending curves was similar to that of the tensile stress–strain curves. Although both normal and simply fixed tissues had bending curves which were concave upward, the treated tissue followed a substantially different curve from the fresh tissue, and demonstrated a substantially higher bending stiffness.

Given this evidence of high bending stiffness in fixed tissue, we have examined the tendency of bioprosthetic material to buckle when bent. As discussed by Thubrikar [23], any tissue being bent sustains at least some compressive stress on the inner surface of the bend and some tensile stress on the outer surface. Since glutaraldehyde fixed aortic valves are substantially stiffer than normal valves in bending, we would expect greater than normal stresses during leaflet bending and the possibility of compressive buckling, producing localized sites of high bending stress. Since buckling produces high bending stresses in individual fibers or fiber bundles, it could be the initiator for mechanical fatigue and fiber breakage. To examine the propensity of valve material to buckle when bent we examined strips of normal and simply fixed porcine aortic valve material bent to curvatures of 0.18 mm^{-1} to 6.67 mm^{-1}. Samples were embedded and sectioned in this position. Although fresh tissue showed some minor degree of tissue buckling under high bending curvatures, it was clear that the fixed tissue buckled under much lower curvatures and to a greater depth (see Figure 1). In addition to tissue buckling, we also observed collagen fibre separation in areas of high bending curvatures in the bioprosthetic material, supporting Thubrikar's contention that such buckling sites could be damaging to collagen structure, and be suitable areas for initiation of calcification.

Simple Fixation of Bovine Pericardium in Aldehydes

The effect of simple aldehyde fixation on bovine pericardium was first examined by van Noort and co-workers [69] using a custom-built, servo-driven low-speed testing machine. Examining the same strip of tissue before and after glutaraldehyde–formaldehyde treatment, their technique relied on the use of highly osmotic glycerol or sucrose solution as a non-reactive "annealing" treatment to remove the effects of the strain history applied to fresh tissue during testing. However, as will be described below, glycerol treatment has a significant effect on the mechanical properties of tissue, and the results of these tests must be viewed with caution. More recent work by Trowbridge and co-workers [70] on pericardium fixed in 0.2% phosphate-buffered glutaraldehyde has included measurement of cyclic stress–strain response and hysteresis, as well as stress relaxation. This paper was

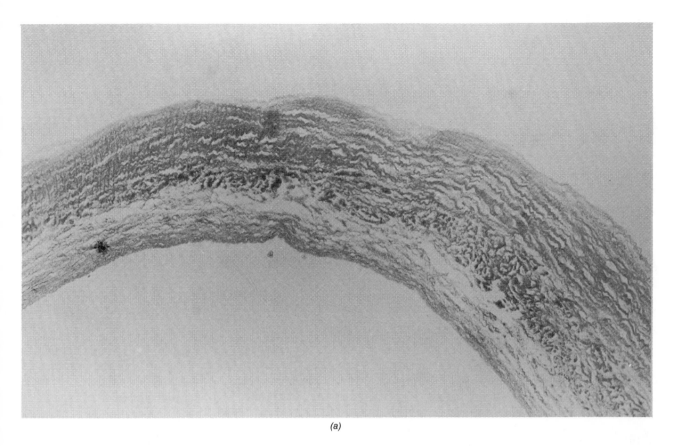

(a)

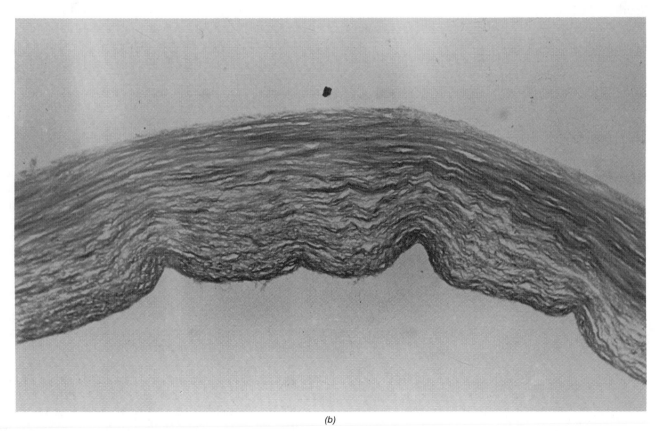

(b)

Figure 1. *Photomicrographs of tissue from fresh (a) and glutaraldehyde treated (b) porcine aortic valve leaflets. The leaflets were fixed while bent in the circumferential direction with the fibrosa near the outer surface. They were histologically processed, sectioned to the thickness of 7 um and stained with picrosirius red. The fresh tissues (a) bent to a smooth arc with no significant local deformations while the glutaraldehyde treated tissues (b) showed compressive buckling of fibres on the inner surface (photographs courtesy of Dr. Ivan Vesely).*

principally concerned with modelling of the "elastic" be-havior of fixed tissue and did not include data on fresh tissue. However, in a later work [31] the effect of similar fixation on directional strips of bovine pericardium was examined using cyclic stress–strain studies only. Their results showed an increase in the extensibility of bovine pericardium after fixation which paralleled that seen in porcine aortic valve tissue. Simply fixed bovine pericar-dium also showed increased unloaded length after cyclic loading; however, unlike porcine aortic valve tissue, "plastic" deformation was also seen in fresh tissue. The nature of this deformation has been examined by Trow-bridge and Crofts [71], who found it to be completely recoverable after 10.5 hours in fresh tissue and after 24 hours in fixed tissue. This strongly suggests that the defor-mation is viscoelastic rather than plastic.

We have recently finished a more complete study of the anisotropic viscoelastic behavior of bovine pericardium, both fresh and fixed in 0.5% phosphate-buffered glu-taraldehyde and 4% acetate-buffered formaldehyde [72]. We also found the fixed tissue to be much more extensible than the fresh tissue, with shape changes in the stress–strain curve which both confirmed the results of Trow-bridge and co-workers, and matched the results in porcine aortic valves by Rousseau [64] and ourselves [66] (see Figure 2). In agreement with Trowbridge and co-workers [31], we found that the first loading cycle produced unique changes in the stress–strain curve accompanied by a large fall in the hysteresis loss. Additionally, we confirmed the increase in unloaded length of both fresh and fixed tissue during cyclic loading. In experiments on viscoelastic be-havior, we found that simple fixation produced reductions in both stress relaxation and creep which paralleled those seen in porcine aortic valves. In fracture tests, by contrast,

fixation did not affect either the tissue modulus or UTS, but only increased the strain at fracture.

The results of these studies strongly suggest that the mechanical effect of the fixation in aldehydes is largely in-dependent of the specific architecture of the connective tissue treated. Porcine aortic valve leaflet material and bovine pericardium respond very similarly to glutaralde-hyde or glutaraldehyde–formaldehyde treatment despite quite different histologies. It is important to note that the changes in properties are basically superimposed on the original tissue properties. For instance, circumferential strips of fresh porcine aortic valve leaflets are considera-bly stiffer than radial strips; after fixation, they are still stiffer but the stress–strain curves for both types of strips have changed shape proportionally.

Simple Fixation of Dura Mater in Glycerol

Glycerol has been used as a preservative, sterilant, and fixative for treatment of human dura mater intended for use in valve construction. Its action has been suggested to be due primarily to dehydration when the typical 98% solution is used. Strong dehydration of collagenous tissues can lead to the formation of additional crosslinks when it is performed by, say, freeze-drying (lyophiliza-tion) or by the use of dry heat [37]. Indeed drying is a common, primitive way of preparing leather. Therefore, it is reasonable that strong dehydration in a solution of high osmolarity could produce a similar effect. However, it has also been shown that when glycerol is exposed to air, glyc-eraldehyde is formed and can produce crosslinks. Glyc-eraldehyde crosslinking cannot be ruled out unless the glycerol treatment was conducted under an inert at-mosphere [73]. In either case, modification of tissue mechanical behavior must be expected.

Only two studies of the effect of glycerol on the mechanical behavior of human dura mater exist. The study by van Noort and co-workers [74] used unoriented strips of human dura mater stored for 12 days in 98% glyc-erol. The fresh and treated strips were simply extended until fracture occurred. They found no statistically signifi-cant changes in the incremental modulus, failure stress or failure strain. By contrast, a much more complete study by McGarvey in our laboratory [35] examined a range of viscoelastic responses of both fresh and glycerol-treated human dura mater. Testing of oriented strips included ex-amination of stress–strain and hysteresis responses during cyclic loading, stress relaxation, creep, and fracture be-havior. They found marked changes in the stress–strain response of the tissue after treatment: the curves shifted toward lower strains and thus showed much reduced strain at fracture. The qualitative change in the stress–strain curve did not resemble that produced by glutaraldehyde treatments on other tissues. Stress relaxation and creep were both reduced in a manner similar to that produced by

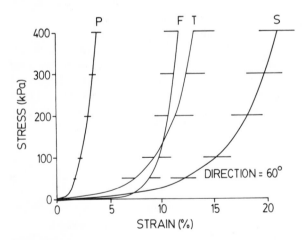

Figure 2. *Mean stress–strain curves for strips of bovine pericardium cut at 60° relative to the base-to-apex direction. n = 5 for each group. Mean ± standard error of mean. F = Fresh tissue. S = Simply fixed. T = Tethered during fixation. P = Pressure fixed. Note that for the tethered sample, the mean strains are similar to those of fresh tissue, but the curve shape is similar to that for simple fixation.*

aldehydes. Both the tissue modulus and ultimate tensile strength were also reduced by glycerol treatment.

Whether produced by drying or glyceraldehyde, glycerol fixation has a significant effect on the mechanical behavior of connective tissues. Therefore, its use as an "annealing" agent by van Noort and co-workers to remove the strain history of their test strips—a procedure based on the results of their very simple study of dura—must be discounted since the first crosslinking treatment the tested fresh tissue will receive will be that of glycerol rather than the aldehyde treatment under investigation. Interestingly, later work from Sheffield by Trowbridge and co-workers has abandoned this method. It is important to note that McGarvey and co-workers allowed the complete rehydration of the tissue samples prior to testing. This consideration is very important after dehydration treatment if one is to simulate the state of the tissue after implantation. Finally, the use of glycerol in the circulating fluid of pulsatile testers to simulate the viscosity of blood is clearly inappropriate with bioprostheses since additional crosslinking may be created during testing of the valve.

Other Crosslinking Agents

The increasing recent interest in alternative crosslinking agents has not produced any accompanying studies on the mechanical effect of these agents. Among the proposed alternative methods are new chemical agents and some physical methods which are by no means new. Chemical methods include carbodiimides (cyanimide) [37], and polyepoxy compounds such as polyethylene glycol [75]. In work with purified collagen preparations, cyanimide has been shown to produce as many as seven times more crosslinks than glutaraldehyde with the only biproduct being the release of water-soluble urea. It acts on different sites than does glutaraldehyde and has been found to produce bioprosthetic material which is much more amenable to ingrowth by host cells than is glutaraldehyde-treated tissue. This has been suggested to be due to the absence of cytotoxicity associated with labile glutaraldehyde in vivo [37]. There have been no mechanical studies on the effects of cyanimide but preliminary work in our own laboratories indicates that simple fixation by glutaraldehyde or cyanimide are mechanically indistinguishable.

Polyepoxy compounds react with amino groups on collagen producing a pliable white material. In tests on perirdium, polyepoxy-fixation produced unchanged tensile strength, increased extensions over fresh or glutaraldehyde-treated tissue, but with a shrinkage temperature considerably below that for glutaraldehyde-treated tissue [75]. Physical methods such as freeze-drying and heat-drying have been used in the leather industry but may be attractive since these methods form crosslinks at sites complementary to those formed by chemical

means. It has been suggested, for instance, that cyanimide and dry heat might be used in combination to produce a very crosslinked, noncytotoxic, collagenous material.

USE OF MECHANICAL CONSTRAINTS DURING FIXATION

The mechanical effect of chemical fixation can be significantly altered through the application of stress during the treatment. The use of pressure fixation in the preparation of porcine aortic valve xenografts is the most obvious example, but the use of leaflet molding in the construction of bovine pericardial xenograft valves is an example of the use of direct contact to produce tension and bending of the leaflets. The effect of various types of constraints on the mechanical properties of the leaflet materials has been examined for both porcine aortic valve and bovine pericardial xenografts. These are reviewed below under the headings of uniaxial stress, tethering, and pressure fixation (biaxial stress).

Effect of Uniaxial Stress During Fixation

The effect of uniaxial stress during fixation on valve leaflet material has been examined by Broom [62] and Rousseau and co-workers [64] using isolated test strips of tissue. Broom extended strips of porcine pulmonary valve tissue in a microtensile device of 460 kPa stress and fixed the tissue at that *length*. (Note: This is really the application of uniaxial *strain*, not uniaxial stress.) The stress fell to about 390 kPa over an hour while the fixation occurred. Using Nomarski interference microscopy, he found that the fixation "froze" the crimp condition and produced a 5% residual strain. (The strip was longer after fixation.) He proposed that this could be used to control the mechanical properties of the tissue. Indeed, in a simple test, the strips fixed under stress showed considerably lower strains than did those simply fixed in glutaraldehyde. He suggested that the curve was simply shifted toward lower strain by reduction of the nonlinear "incubation" region of the stress–strain curve where collagen crimp collapse and fiber migration occur.

Later, in a more extensive viscoelastic study, Rousseau and co-workers [64] fixed strips of porcine aortic valve material under no load, under 0.01 N initial load, and under 0.3 N initial load. Again, strains corresponding to these initial loads were actually applied, the loads chosen to simulate low and high pressure fixation as described below. Use of the lower load produced a material only slightly more extensible than the fresh tissue, although with an altered curve shape more similar to simply fixed tissue than to the fresh tissue. Use of the higher load, on the other hand, produced a result similar to that seen by

Broom: the stress–strain curve was shifted toward lower strains and the curve shape was very similar to that of the fresh tissue. The use of even a small load reduced stress relaxation even more than had simple fixation; large loads resulted in a further reduction.

The results of these studies suggest that even if shrinkage in aldehyde is prevented through enforcement of a small applied strain, the mechanical properties of the fresh tissue are not preserved. This is demonstrated by the change in shape of the stress–strain curve (even when the maximum strains during testing were similar) and the reductions in stress relaxation behavior. Whether the uniaxial strain had any effect on the anisotropy of the leaflet material could not be assessed since the stress was applied only along the length of a single test strip.

The effect of uniaxial strain during fixation of bovine pericardial material was initially examined by Reece and co-workers [76]. This study, however, used van Noort's glycerol annealing technique and therefore is suspect. Nonetheless, they found a shift of the stress–strain curve toward low strain with the application of increasing strains during fixation. Again, only single strips were fixed so the effect on isotropy could not be assessed.

We have recently finished a much more extensive study of the effect of genuine uniaxial stress during fixation on the viscoelastic properties of bovine pericardial xenograft material [77]. We fixed large rectangles of pericardium under uniaxial stress by suspending weights from the gripped rectangles. Strips could then be cut at angles of 0°, 30°, 60°, and 90° to the direction of stress and the effect of directional stress on anisotropy assessed. Fresh anterior bovine pericardium was found to be only mildly anisotropic, being modestly more extensible in the circumferential direction than in the other four directions. After fixation under uniaxial stress, however, the material was strongly anisotropic: the tissue was markedly stiffer in the direction of applied stress. Indeed, the effect of the directional stress completely overwhelmed the original anisotropy of the fresh tissue. Interestingly, in the direction at 90° to the applied stress where the Poisson contraction would offer no opposition to shrinkage, the stress–strain curve looked much like that of simply fixed tissue: that is, with greater extensibility and the same change in shape of the curve. In the direction of applied stress, the stress–strain curve showed the shift toward lower strains with preservation of curve shape seen in valve tissue by Broom and Rousseau. The application of directional stress did not produce anisotropy of the relaxation properties of the material, but did produce a significant increase in tensile strength in the direction of stress, and a significant increase in the strain at fracture at 90° to that direction. This work shows the importance of applying the stress condition to a sample which was large enough that the effect on anisotropy can be assessed. Little of this information could have been obtained from fixation of single strips.

Effect of Tethering During Fixation

Tethering is the enforcement of dimensions (typically the unloaded or in vivo dimensions) during some physical or chemical treatment. In the context of the aldehyde fixation, it means the enforcement of the initial dimensions of the fresh material: that is, the prevention of shrinkage in the fixative. This constraint has not been examined in porcine aortic valve tissue, and indeed it is not possible to tether an intact valve. Tethering of test strips in one direction only was examined by Reece and co-workers [76] in the study on bovine pericardium described above. Bearing the glycerol treatment in mind, their tethered tissue showed smaller strains than the simply fixed tissue, but with a similar shape to the stress–strain curve. This result was similar to that seen by Rousseau and co-workers with small imposed strains on isolated strips of porcine aortic valve tissue.

We have recently used a plexiglass clamping apparatus to tether large circular samples of bovine pericardial tissue during glutaraldehyde fixation and examined the directional effect of tethering on viscoelastic behavior [78]. Tethering produced a material which was only slightly more extensible than the fresh tissue, but with a stress–strain curve shape similar to that of simply fixed tissue (Figure 2). This again parallels the results of Rousseau et al. and Reece et al., indicating that even if most shrinkage is eliminated by tethering, the viscoelastic behavior of the tissue is still altered by the fixation process. Again, this is supported by reduction of stress relaxation behavior and an increase in UTS. Interestingly, we also found that both simple fixation and fixation with tethering removed the small anisotropy in the fresh tissue, perhaps due to directional shrinkage in the direction of greatest fibrous tissue support.

Effect of Pressure Fixation (Biaxial Stress)

Application of transmural pressure during fixation is routinely used in the construction of porcine aortic valve xenografts. Prior to the work of Broom discussed below, manufacturers had been glutaraldehyde-fixing their valves in the closed position under a pressure head in excess of 50 mm Hg, primarily to produce esthetically pleasing valves with good cusp geometry and coaptation. Pressure produces biaxial tensile stresses in the leaflet material which directly oppose the shrinkage induced by the fixation. The effect of pressure fixation in porcine aortic valves was described initially by Broom and Thomson [63] who compared the effects of one hour of fixation under (a) 100 mm Hg transvalvular pressure, (b) 4 mm Hg transvalvular pressure, and (c) slightly greater than 1 mm Hg transvalvular pressure ("0 pressure" fixation). Using Nomarski interference microscopy, they found that 100 mm Hg pressure completely collapsed the collagen crimp in the leaflets, and even 4 mm Hg significantly reduced the crimp. This result was used to hypothesize that the collagen crimp of the fresh leaflets—retained only in the "0 pressure" valves—was necessary for smooth, graded opening of the leaflets which they observed in their in vitro flow testing. The crimp was also felt to be a necessary condition to avoid kinking (buckling) of the leaflets during bending. Simple "elastic" stress–strain curves from circumferential strips of each valve type showed that increasing the transvalvular pressure during fixation produced increasing shifting of the stress–strain curve toward lower strain and a change in curve shape from that of simple fixation to that of the fresh valve tissue. Later fatigue studies were performed by Broom [79] using a specially designed high speed testing device to flex strips of tissue at 30 times the normal heart rate. These tests indicated that valves fixed under 100 mm Hg transvalvular pressure were much more susceptible to collagen bundle disruption (presumably produced by bending compression) than were valves fixed under less than 1 mm Hg transvalvular pressure. It was again suggested that maintenance of the collagen crimp during fixation was critical to resisting leaflet buckling and consequent fatigue damage.

To further expand on this thesis, Broom studied coaptation of porcine aortic valve leaflets in vitro. He found that the coaptive ratios of left and right coronary cusps in the low pressure fixed valves were much improved over those same leaflets in high pressure fixed valves. At inflation of the valve cusps with an 80 mm Hg pressure head a desirable "peeling back" at the coaptive margins of the low pressure fixed valves was noted but this was not observed for the high pressure fixed valves. When the low pressure fixed valves were constrained by a simulated mounting ring there was a reduction or elimination of the peeling back motion or occasionally even a reversal, thus increasing the coaptive margin. If the fixed valve possesses a high radial compliance the major circumferential fiber bundles can separate and the coaptive area can be increased. Concern over satisfactory coaptation of the leaflets fixed under low pressure was addressed by examining leaflet coaptive ratios. He concluded that the low pressure fixed valves were indeed better than high pressure fixed leaflets in terms of coaptive area as well. His recommendations have since been accepted by valve manufacturers and low pressure fixation of porcine aortic valve xenografts has become standard. The efficacy of this design feature in increasing the durability of bioprostheses has yet to be established.

More recently, Thubrikar and co-workers [80] compared the simple stress–strain behaviors of strips of natural canine aortic valve leaflets with those of porcine aortic valve leaflets fixed under 100 mm Hg transvalvular pressure in 2% glutaraldehyde. Setting aside the obvious problem of interspecies comparison, the fixed porcine tissue was stiffer than the fresh canine tissue and showed smaller total strains.

We have also examined the viscoelastic behavior of pressure-fixed porcine aortic valve leaflet material prepared using glutaraldehyde–formaldehyde fixation under 100 mm Hg pressure [65,66]. We found that high pressure fixation substantially shifted the stress–strain curves in both the circumferential and radial directions toward lower strain without change in shape or relative directional stiffness. It also reduced stress relaxation and creep even more than did simple fixation, and, with the exception of a reduced strain at fracture, left the fracture properties of the material unchanged. The changes in viscoelastic behavior which we observed after high pressure fixation were very similar to those seen by Rousseau and co-workers [64] when they applied strains intended to simulate high pressure fixation to isolated strips of valve material.

Taken together, the results of these experiments suggest that fixation of porcine aortic valves under increasing pressure produces an increasing collapse of collagen crimp structure which is reflected in a gradual shifting of the stress–strain curve toward lower strain. Low pressure (<1 mm Hg) produces functional strains similar to those in fresh material, but does not eliminate the change in the shape of the stress–strain curve seen after simple fixation. Higher pressures produce a significantly less extensible material but with a stress–strain curve shape more similar to the natural tissue. Increasing pressure also produces an increasing loss of viscoelastic stress relaxation and creep properties, suggesting that the collapsed fiber architecture is locked into place by the fixation and is less able to rearrange with time under stress.

Pressure fixation, while not used in construction of commercial bovine pericardial xenograft valves, can be performed on sheets of pericardial material. Indeed, a rectangle of this material could be fixed under uniform biaxial stress—a possibility not available for intact valve tissue. We have recently examined the effect of pressure fixation in 0.5% phosphate-buffered glutaraldehyde on the viscoelastic properties of bovine pericardium [78]. We clamped a circular sample of pericardium in the plexiglass clamping ring used in the tethering experiments described above, and applied a fluid column of glutaraldehyde to produce a transmural pressure of 50 mm Hg. We then cut strips at 0°, 30°, 60°, and 90° to the base-to-apex direction and tested them for cyclic stress–strain response, stress relaxation, and fracture properties. Pressure-fixation of bovine pericardium produces results which almost exactly parallel those seen with porcine aortic valve material: shifting of the stress–strain curve to lower strain with maintenance of curve shape (Figure 2), reduction of stress relaxation beyond that seen with simple fixation, and maintenance of fracture properties. In other experiments, we have reduced the pressure to 10 mm Hg and found changes intermediate between the higher pressure fixation and simple tethering.

Comparing the data for bovine pericardium and porcine aortic valve leaflets, it is clear that increasing pressure fixation of both types of leaflet materials produces equivalent viscoelastic mechanical changes. Furthermore, tethering of pericardium during fixation to prevent shrinkage produces mechanical properties equivalent to those seen with less than 1 mm Hg pressure in porcine aortic valves. These two processes in the two materials may therefore be considered to be equivalent.

VISCOELASTICITY OF BIOPROSTHETIC LEAFLET MATERIALS

Bioprosthetic heart valve leaflet materials have only been examined over a very modest range of strain rates, at most about two orders of magnitude below those experienced in vivo. Under these conditions, both porcine aortic valve leaflets and bovine pericardial xenograft leaflets display very similar viscoelastic characteristics. These can be summarized as follows:

(a) Both materials show nonlinear stress–strain curves under all available strain rates.

(b) Both materials show no dependence of stress–strain response on strain rate over the range examined.

(c) Both materials show substantial cyclic hysteresis. After fixation the hysteresis is very large on first loading, but declines with cycling to plateau between 10 and 20 percent. Hysteresis is not affected by fixation or by method of fixation.

(d) Both materials display stress relaxation and creep. Both responses are reduced by fixation and further reduced with increasing stress during fixation. Stress relaxation appears to be independent of initial strain in porcine aortic valves and to be dependent on initial strain in bovine pericardial xenografts.

(e) Both materials display increased unloaded length after cyclic loading. This deformation is greatest in simply fixed material and, in bovine pericardial material at least, appears to recover completely over hours or days.

Both of these materials are clearly viscoelastic and modelling their responses as elastic, say in a stress analysis or as a framework for analysis of in vitro mechanical test results, is at best a crude approximation. Aldehyde-fixed bioprosthetic leaflet materials are more elastic than are fresh tissues. However, while fixation under any stress level reduces stress relaxation and creep responses significantly, hysteresis losses are unchanged and greater than 10%. Trowbridge [70] has used an argument based on characteristic times to suggest that glutaraldehyde-fixed bovine pericardial tissue can be accurately treated as being elastic during in vivo function. However, as will be discussed below, a fundamental error in analyzing the relaxation behavior of the material in terms of a simple Maxwell unit invalidates his argument.

If we wish to describe the viscoelastic behavior of these materials mathematically, are appropriate models available? The only current model intended to completely describe the viscoelastic behavior of natural tissues is Fung's quasi-linear theory [81]. This model is a variation on classical linear viscoelastic theory, incorporating the principle of Boltzmann superposition, but allowing for nonlinear elastic stress–strain responses under very high strain rates: that is, under near step loading. In order to satisfy this model, the stress–strain curve must firstly shift toward lower strains with increasing strain rate under the range of experimental times where stress relaxation or hysteresis is observed. This condition is not satisfied in bioprosthetic leaflet materials since they have thus far been strain rate independent under the range of strain rates examined. Secondly, the stress relaxation curve [specifically, the reduced relaxation function, $G(t)$] must be independent of initial strain. By definition, $G(t)$ is the relaxation behavior which one observes if the material is step loaded to an initial strain, and this strain is held constant. In practice, samples are loaded over some finite time and this distorts the short relaxation time information recorded after the chosen strain is reached. Whether or not $G(t)$ is independent of strain, therefore, is difficult to assess without more rapid loading than has thus far been employed in the literature. However, under the strain rates in the literature studies, porcine aortic valve tissue appears to satisfy this requirement while bovine pericardial xenograft material does not. Thirdly, the stress–strain curve may be nonlinear even under high strain rates. The peculiarity of this condition lies in the fact that, with significant stress relaxation, even materials with linear, high strain rate elastic stress–strain responses may appear to have nonlinear stress–strain behavior under sufficiently slow loading. The requirement for consistently nonlinear stress–strain responses at least appears to be satisfied.

As outlined above, we have examined the applicability of Fung's theory in light of currently available test data [81,83]; however, final validation or invalidation of this theory must await high strain rate investigations of mechanical properties where the problems of slow loading can be controlled. Interestingly, Rousseau and co-workers [64] have used the quasi-linear model to calculate a reduced relaxation function $G(t)$ for fresh and fixed porcine aortic valve tissue. They have further analyzed the quasi-linear model for distorting effect of finite loading times on observed stress–strain and relaxation behavior [84,85]. However, they have not experimentally addressed the fundamental question of whether or not the conditions implicit in the model are satisfied: they have simply assumed its applicability.

Would simpler spring and dashpot models suffice instead? Even with nonlinear springs, the answer must be no. The reason lies in the shape of the stress relaxation curves observed experimentally. In relaxation experiments by ourselves [66,72,77] and by Trowbridge and co-workers [70], plotting of the percentage stress remaining at a given time after loading [an approximation of the reduced relaxation function $G(t)$] against the logarithm of time reveals a nearly straight line which does not flatten even past 1000 seconds (Figure 3). This curve shape is unattainable with simple models, and is evidence for a relaxation spectrum of nearly uniform density. As an illustration, Figure 3 also shows the quite different relaxation curves for the single exponential decays typical of simple Maxwell solids with either of two time constants: (a) 100 s, or (b) 10^5 years as suggested by Trowbridge for bovine pericardial material. Discrete relaxation times are characterized by strong inflection points and isolated drops in stress on the logarithmic relaxation curve: the relaxation curve is flat (that is, there is no relaxation) over times other than about one decade either side of the single characteristic relaxation time. Trowbridge's own linear relaxation curves therefore completely invalidate his Maxwell model! From this analysis, it is clear that neither one nor even a few characteristic relaxation times could adequately describe the relaxation behavior of these materials; simple spring and dashpot models are inappropriate.

The inappropriateness of the simpler available models underscores the need for a more powerful and flexible model like Fung's quasi-linear theory which can accept a wide range of relaxation spectra. This reasoning also shows that, within the range of experimental times so far—from tenths of seconds to thousands of seconds—the leaflets of bioprosthetic heart valves behave viscoelastically, without evidence of a high strain rate elastic re-

sponse (flattening of the relaxation curve for short experimental times) or a rubber equilibrium response (flattening of the relaxation curve for long experimental times).

Finally, we must also note that the strain rate independence displayed by these materials in the presence of cyclic hysteresis is evidence for nonlinear viscous behavior which is impossible to describe by linear viscoelastic methods. This type of independence is typical of materials displaying pseudoplastic (sometimes termed thixotropic) behavior; that is, decreasing viscosity with increasing shear rate. This is probably rooted in the behavior of the mucopolysaccharide matrix material and provides an interesting modelling problem. However, it is imperative that we not mistake independence of stress-strain response on strain rate for elastic behavior, but remember that a sizeable hysteresis loop is always present, clear evidence of viscoelastic, *not* elastic behavior.

IMPLICATIONS FOR DESIGN OF BIOPROSTHESES

The mechanical properties of bioprosthetic leaflet tissues as revealed by in vitro testing have several interesting implications for the construction of heart valves. The viscoelastic nature of the leaflet materials has been ignored in published stress analyses. The so-called "elastic" stress-strain behavior of the leaflet tissue has been taken to be the stress-strain curve measured in low strain rate in vitro studies. Interestingly, the stress-strain curves for preconditioned materials have thus far been strain rate independent and if this trend is valid up to in vivo strain rates the strain rate approximations employed may—by serendipity—be quite good. Further, the viscoelastic character of the fresh tissue is reduced as one examines simply fixed tissue, tissue tethered during fixation, and pressure-fixed tissue. Thus an elastic approximation is considerably better with pressure-fixed tissue than with fresh tissue. On the other hand, the observed stress-strain curves have exclusively been drawn from uniaxial studies with all their limitations. Further, the particular stress-strain response observed in vitro depends strongly on the preconditioning regimen employed and the stress relaxation or creep experiments performed. Therefore, regardless of how elastic or viscoelastic the in vitro stress-strain response may be, the in vitro stress-strain curve may only be an approximation of that in vivo.

Porcine aortic valve leaflets are strongly anisotropic and remain so after fixation with or without pressure. This anisotropy is due to histological features intimately linked both to the distribution of stress in the closed leaflets and to long-term resistance to flexural fatigue. Bovine pericardial xenograft material, by contrast, is nearly isotropic when simply fixed, fixed with tethering, or fixed under pressure. However, fixation under directional stress

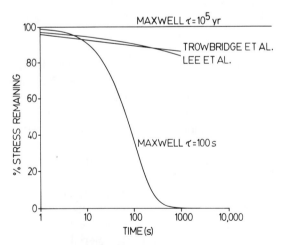

Figure 3. *Stress relaxation behavior for simply fixed calf pericardium from Lee et al. [72] and Trowbridge et al. [70]. Percent stress remaining at a given time is plotted against the $\log_{10}$ of time in seconds. Also shown are the relaxation behaviors of ideal Maxwell solids [reduced relaxation functions $G(t)$] with relaxation times (τ) of 100 seconds and of 10^5 years. The time of 10^5 years was used by Trowbridge to describe the relaxation behavior of calf pericardium. However, as can be seen from the curves, no relaxation occurs with this model over the experimental time period and therefore the model is a poor description of the actual behavior of the material.*

allows for controlled anisotropy of the fixed material. This should produce better apposition of the leaflets if the leaflets are constructed such that the direction of greatest stiffness is the circumferential direction and the direction of greatest extensibility is the radial direction. It is important to resolve whether anisotropy produced through fixation of bovine pericardial material is as significant for hemodynamic function and resistance to flexural fatigue as is the histologically-based anisotropy of porcine aortic valve leaflet. These questions must be addressed on two fronts. Firstly, the accelerated fatigue performance of valves constructed from simply fixed and from anisotropic pericardium must be compared. Secondly, we must discover the mechanism for the creation of the anisotropy. Is it due to directional increases in chemical activity of those collagen fibers under most stress, or is it due to migration of collagen toward the direction of stress and its subsequent "riveting" in place? If directional chemical activity is involved, this can be investigated by fixing the tissue under stress in one direction and comparing its anisotropy with tissue which was subsequently fixed under stress in a second direction. If fiber migration is involved, the anisotropy may be increased by uniaxially loading the tissue in saline for a period of time before fixation. This would allow additional fiber migration and should produce greater anisotropy. This latter mechanism would be most likely to produce improvement in resistance to flexural fatigue since greater alignment of fiber in the direction of principal tensile stress would better mimic the structure of natural aortic valve leaflets.

The advantages of low pressure fixation for both improved hemodynamic function and resistance to flexural fatigue in porcine aortic valve xenografts have been demonstrated by Broom and Thomson [63]. Mechanically, this treatment produces a leaflet material with operating strains very similar to those of fresh leaflets, but with a quite different shape to its stress–strain curve. The mechanical test results imply that shrinkage in aldehydes has largely been eliminated by very low pressure fixation, leaving a natural collagen crimp structure. Aldehyde fixation has still changed the stress–strain response, but the mechanism of this change and its implications are not clear. An exact parallel for low pressure fixation of porcine aortic valves is provided by two-dimensional tethering of bovine pericardium during fixation. In this preparation method, no stress has been applied: shrinkage has simply been reduced or eliminated. Exactly the same mechanical changes are produced by this technique as are produced by low pressure fixation of porcine aortic valves. It is interesting to speculate whether the maintenance of a natural degree of collagen crimp in bovine pericardial material has any implications for fatigue performance since this tissue was never intended for flexure. Gabbay [32] has claimed an improvement in flexural fatigue performance of uni-leaflet bovine pericardial xeno-

graft valves made from tissue tethered during fixation. However, details of the tethering technique have not been described.

It is clear from in vitro experiments on bioprosthetic leaflet materials that these materials display an increase in unloaded length after cyclic loading. This increase may be as little as 2% or less in fresh tissue to greater than 10% in simply fixed tissue and is apparently completely reversible after short-term loading. The implication of this data is that the leaflets of these prostheses must be larger in function than they were during construction, thus producing a larger coaptation area than was originally designed. While this may be of limited in porcine aortic valve leaflets where there are few choices which bear on leaflet coaptation, it is more interesting for bioprostheses where the leaflets are constructed from sheetlike tissues like pericardium and the designer can expect a substantial increase in leaflet size during function. The 10% figure quoted above may be an overestimate since it was obtained under uniaxial loading. On the other hand, it may be a considerable underestimate if long-term, irreversible creep of the leaflets during extended cycling is considered. The dearth of literature reports on changes in leaflet dimensions during function may simply be due to its not being expected or to the difficulty of accurately measuring the size of intact leaflets. Schoen and co-workers [86] have recently presented the first report of extensive plastic deformation of bioprosthetic valve leaflets during function. They found greatly extended leaflets in unileaflet pericardial xenograft valves after experimental implantations. This extension produced massive redundancy of leaflet material and improper valve closure. Bearing in mind that Trowbridges' group saw recovery of in vitro viscoelastic–plastic deformations produced by cyclic loading over many hours or days, this in vivo deformation was apparently both permanent and significant.

It remains a curious matter that glutaraldehyde fixation both increases the tensile extensibility of bioprosthetic valve leaflet material and increases its bending stiffness. Simple aldehyde fixation actually increases the tensile stiffness of tissue, but only in the low strain, low stiffness region of the stress–strain curve. If beam bending occurs, it is possible that this increase in tensile stiffness could contribute to increased bending stiffness. It is not known, however, how fixation affects the compressive properties of the leaflet tissue. Clearly, since the tissues are freely pliable before fixation, there cannot be any significant compressive stiffness in the fresh material. The increase in bending stiffness after fixation must therefore be an expression of the appearance of significant compressive stiffness or of increased resistance to shearing between layers in the leaflet. The occurrence of increased buckling during in vitro bending tests after fixation strongly suggests the latter mechanism.

If we are to extend the functional lifetime of bioprosthetic tissue leaflets after implantation, we must make every attempt to reduce the functional stresses—especially the bending stresses—on the tissue leaflets. When one compares the opening characteristics of stent-supported valve prostheses, fresh or fixed, with the opening characteristics of the normal aortic valve, it is clear that expansion of the valve annulus is critical in reducing the total flexure of each leaflet during opening and in determining the shape of the flow orifice. From this viewpoint, the elimination of the stent ring or the incorporation of a truly flexible stent ring into the design of the next generation of bioprosthetic heart valves must be seen as paramount. This is not a trivial matter from a technical viewpoint since placement and suturing will be much more difficult with a stentless valve or with a much reduced stent. Further, the marketing of this type of valve to the surgeon may be a commercial consideration. However, we must weigh against these arguments improved opening function and increased fatigue lifetime, and ask ourselves how important ease of placement is if we are unnecessarily facing early reoperation.

Finally, little has been made of the reductions in stress relaxation and creep produced by fixation. These viscoelastic properties are expressions of the freedom of structural components to reorient and extend slowly in response to directional stresses. If stress relaxation and creep are reduced, the ability of the fibrous components of bioprosthetic leaflets to rearrange and reduce local stress concentrations is limited; unrelieved high local stresses could then lead to premature local fatigue failure. This hypothesis is borne out by the reduction in ultimate tensile strength seen in porcine aortic valve leaflets after simple fixation. Here, the leaflets shrink in fixative and the collagen structure is at least partially locked in by the fixation. Under elongation, local stress concentrations occur but cannot be easily relieved due to limited stress relaxation properties. The result is early initial failure of fibers and loss of tensile strength. This phenomenon was first discussed by Mohanaradhakrishnan and Ramanathan [87] to explain loss of tensile strength in collagenous tissues after fixation. It is entirely possible that the utility of low pressure fixation of porcine aortic valves lies not only in maintenance of natural collagen crimp structure, but also in maintaining the collagen architecture in its natural orientation relative to the principal stresses. If an inappropriate architecture is locked into place, say by fixation under no restraints or under high pressure, this architecture may have limited freedom to rearrange and early fatigue failure may ensue.

Overall, it is clear that porcine and pericardial valves have been a substantial advance in the management of valvular heart disease. Unfortunately, clinical experience with these valves has shown their long term durability to be unsatisfactory for many patients and has decreased the surgical enthusiasm for their use. The experimental evidence to date suggests that the mechanical properties of the valve materials and the mechanical stresses imposed during the cardiac cycle are responsible for ultimate tissue failure. Future investigations of the tissue mechanics of bioprosthetic heart valve materials should provide many of the clues to the mechanisms underlying fatigue failure and accompanying calcification.

ACKNOWLEDGEMENTS

This work was supported by grants to Dr. Lee by the Natural Sciences and Engineering Research Council of Canada and to Dr. Boughner by the Heart and Stroke Foundation of Ontario.

Dr. Lee is an Ontario Ministry of Health Career Scientist. Dr. Boughner is a Research Associate of the Heart and Stroke Foundation of Ontario.

REFERENCES

1 ROSS, D. N. "Homograft Replacement of the Aortic Valve," *Lancet*, 2:487 (1962).

2 BARRATT-BOYES, B. G. "Homograft Aortic Valve Replacement in Aortic Incompetence and Stenosis," *Thorax*, 19:131 (1964).

3 BARRATT-BOYES, B. G., A. H. G. Roche and R. M. L. Whitlock. "Six Year Review of the Results of Freehand Aortic Valve Replacement Using an Antibiotic-Sterilized Homograft Valve," *Circulation*, 55:353 (1977).

4 BINET, J. P., A. Carpentier, J. Langlois, C. Duran and P. Colvez. "Implantation de Valves Heterogenes dans le Traitment des Cardiopathies Aortiques," *C. R. Acad. Sci. Paris*, 261:5733 (1965).

5 CARPENTIER, A., P. Blondeau and P. Marcel. "Remplacement de L'appareil Valvulaire Mitral par des Heterotopiques," *Presse Med.*, 75:1603 (1967).

6 WRIGHT, J. T. M. "Porcine or Pericardial Valves? Now and the Future: Design and Engineering Considerations," in *Biological and Bioprosthetic Valves*, E. Bodnar and M. Yacoub, eds. New York:Yorke Medical Books, p. 567 (1982).

7 CARPENTIER, A. "From Valvular Xenograft to Valvular Bioprosthesis (1965–1977)," *J. Assoc. Adv. Med. Instr.*, 11:98 (1977).

8 CARPENTIER, A., C. G. Lamaigre, L. Robert, S. Carpentier and C. Dubost. "Biological Factors Affecting Long-Term Results of Valvular Heterografts," *J. Thorac. Cardiovasc. Surg.*, 58:467 (1969).

9 BOWES, J. H. and C. W. Cater. "The Reaction of Glutaraldehyde with Proteins and Other Biological Materials," *J. Royal Microsc. Soc.*, 85(2):193 (1966).

10 REIS, R. L., W. D. Hancock, J. W. Yarbrough, D. L. Glancy and A. G. Morrow. "The Flexible Stent," *J. Thorac. Cardiovasc. Surg.*, 62:683 (1971).

11 ANGELL, W. W., J. D. Angell, A. Woodruff, A. Sywak, and J. C. Kosek. "The Tissue Valve as a Superior Cardiac Valve Replacement," *Surgery*, 82:875 (1977).

12 WRIGHT, J. T. M. "Hydrodynamic Evaluation of Tissue Valves," in *Tissue Heart Valves*, M. I. Ionescu, ed. London:Butterworths, p. 31 (1979).

13 WRIGHT, J. T. M. "A Pulsatile Flow Study Comparing the Hancock

Porcine Xenograft Aortic Valve Prosthesis Models 242 and 250," *Med. Instrum.*, 11:114 (1977).

14 IONESCU, M. I. and A. P. Tandon. "The Ionescu–Shiley Pericardial Xenograft Heart Valve," in *Tissue Heart Valves*, M. I. Ionescu, ed. London:Butterworths, p. 203 (1979).

15 ZERBINI, E. J. and L. B. Puig. "The Dura Mater Allograft Valve," in *Tissue Heart Valves*, M. I. Ionescu, ed. London:Butterworths, p. 253 (1979).

16 MILANO, A., U. Bortolotti and E. Talenti. "Calcific Degeneration as the Main Cause of Porcine Bioprosthetic Valve Failure," *Am. J. Cardiol.*, 53:1066 (1984).

17 REUL, G. J., Jr., D. A. Cooley, J. M. Duncan, O. H. Frazier, G. L. Hallman, J. J. Livesay, D. A. Ott and W. E. Walker. "Valve Failure with the Ionescu–Shiley Bovine Pericardial Bioprosthesis: Analysis of 2680 Patients," *J. Vasc. Surg.*, 2:192 (1985).

18 BORTOLOTTI, U., A. Milano, A. Mazzucco, C. Valfre, E. Talenti, F. Guerra, G. Thiene and V. Gallucci. "Results of Reoperation for Primary Tissue Failure of Porcine Bioprostheses," *J. Thorac. Cardiovasc. Surg.*, 90:564 (1985).

19 GEHA, A. S., H. Laks, H. C. Stansel, J. F. Cornhill, J. W. Kilman, M. J. Buckley and W. C. Roberts. "Late Failure of Porcine Valve Heterografts in Children," *J. Thorac. Cardiovasc. Surg.*, 78:351 (1979).

20 SILVER, M. M., J. Pollock, M. D. Silver, W. G. Williams and G. A. Trusler. "Calcification of Porcine Xenograft Valves in Children," *Am. J. Cardiol.*, 45:685 (1980).

21 FERRANS, V. J., T. L. Spray, M. E. Billingham and W. C. Roberts. "Structural Changes in Glutaraldehyde-Treated Porcine Heterografts used as Substitute Cardiac Valves," *Am. J. Cardiol.*, 41:1159 (1978).

22 DRURY, P. J., J. Dobrin, E. Bodnar and M. M. Black. "Distribution of Flexibility in the Porcine Aortic Root and in Cardiac Support Frames," in *Biologic and Bioprosthetic Valves*, E. Bodnar and M. Yacoub, eds. New York:Yorke Medical Books, p. 580 (1986).

23 THUBRIKAR, M. J., J. R. Skinner and S. P. Nolan. "Design and Stress Analysis of Bioprosthetic Valves In Vivo," in *Cardiac Bioprosthesis*, L. H. Cohn and V. Gallucci, eds. New York:Yorke Medical Books, p. 445 (1982).

24 THUBRIKAR, M., R. Harry and S. P. Nolan. "Normal Aortic Valve Function in Dogs," *Am. J. Cardiol.*, 40:563 (1977).

25 THUBRIKAR, H., L. P. Bosher and S. P. Nolan. "The Mechanism of Opening of the Aortic Valve," *J. Thorac. Cardiovasc. Surg.*, 77:863 (1979).

26 SILVER, M. A. and W. C. Roberts. "Detailed Anatomy of the Normally Functioning Aortic Valve in Hearts of Normal and Increased Weight," *Am. J. Cardiol.*, 55:454 (1985).

27 CLARKE, R. E. and E. H. Finke. "Scanning Electron Microscopy of Human Aortic Leaflets in Stressed and Relaxed States," *J. Thorac. Cardiovasc. Surg.*, 67:792 (1974).

28 MOHRI, H., D. D. Reichenbach and K. A. Merendino. "Biology of Homologous and Heterologous Aortic Valves," in *Biological Tissue in Heart Valve Replacement*, M. I. Ionescu, D. N. Ross and G. H. Wooler, eds. London:Butterworths, p. 137 (1972).

29 THUBRIKAR, M., W. C. Piepgrass, L. P. Bosker and S. P. Nolan. "The Elastic Modulus of Canine Aortic Valve Leaflets In Vivo and In Vitro," *Circ. Res.*, 47:792 (1980).

30 BROWN, N. and G. W. Christie. "The Structure/Function Relationship of Fresh and Glutaraldehyde-Fixed Aortic Valve Leaflets," in *Cardiac Bioprostheses*, L. H. Cohn and V. Gallucci, eds. New York:Yorke Medical Books, p. 476 (1982).

31 TROWBRIDGE, E. A., K. M. Roberts, C. E. Crofts and P. V. Lawford. "Pericardial Heterografts: Toward Quality Control of the Mechanical Properties of Glutaraldehyde Fixed Leaflets," *J. Thorac. Cardiovasc. Surg.*, 92:21 (1986).

32 GABBAY, S., U. Bortolotti, G. Cipolletti, F. Wasserman, R. W. M. Frater and S. M. Factor. "The Meadox Unicusp Pericardial Bioprosthetic Heart Valve: New Concept," *Ann. Thorac. Surg.*, 37:448 (1984).

33 BLACK, M. M., P. J. Drury, W. B. Tindale and P. V. Lawford. "The Sheffield Bicuspid Valve," in *Biologic and Bioprosthetic Valves*, E. Bodnar and M. Yacoub, eds. New York:Yorke Medical Books, p. 709 (1986).

34 WALKER, D. K., L. N. Scotton, D. E. Hewgill, R. G. Racca and K. T. Brownlee. "Development and In Vitro Assessment of a New Two Leaflet Replacement Heart Valve Designed Using Computer Generated Bubble Surfaces," *Med. Biol. Eng. Comput.*, 21:31 (1983).

35 MCGARVEY, K. A., J. M. Lee and D. R. Boughner. "Mechanical Suitability of Glycerol-Preserved Human Dura Mater for Construction of Prosthetic Cardiac Valves," *Biomaterials*, 5:109 (1984).

36 HIGHISON, G. J., D. J. Allen, L. J. A. Didio, E. J. Zerbini and L. B. Puig. "Ultrastructural Morphology of Dura Mater Aortic Allografts After 44–73 Months of Implantation in Humans," *J. Submicrosc. Cytol.*, 12:165 (1980).

37 WEADOCK, K., R. M. Olson and F. H. Silver. "Evaluation of Collagen Crosslinking Techniques," *Biomat. Med. Dev. Artif. Org.*, 11:293 (1983–1984).

38 WOODROOF, E. A. "The Chemistry and Biology of Aldehyde Treated Valve Xenografts," in *Tissue Heart Valves*, M. I. Ionescu, ed. Toronto:Butterworths, p. 347 (1979).

39 JONES, M., E. E. Eidbo, S. M. Walters, V. J. Ferrans and R. E. Clark. "Effects of 2 Types of Preimplantation Processes on Calcification of Bioprostheses," in *Biological and Bioprosthetic Valves*, E. Bodnar and M. Yacoub, eds. New York:Yorke Medical Books, p. 451 (1986).

40 LENTZ, D. J., E. M. Pollack, D. B. Olsen, E. J. Andrews, J. Murashita and W. L. Hastings. "Inhibition of Mineralization of Glutaraldehyde-Fixed Hancock Bioprosthetic Heart Valves," in *Cardiac Bioprostheses*, L. H. Cohn and V. Gallucci, eds. New York:Yorke Medical Books, p. 306 (1982).

41 CARPENTIER, A., A. Nashref, S. Carpentier, N. Goussef, J. Relland, R. J. Levy, M. C. Fishbein, B. El Asmar, M. Benomar, S. El Sayed and P. G. Donzeau-Gouge. "Prevention of Tissue Valve Calcification by Chemical Techniques," in *Cardiac Bioprostheses*, L. H. Cohn and V. Gallucci, eds. New York:Yorke Medical Books, p. 320 (1982).

42 ISHIHARA, T., V. J. Ferrans, M. Jones, S. W. Boyce and W. C. Roberts. "Structure of Bovine Parietal Pericardium and of Unimplanted Ionescu–Shiley Pericardial Valvular Bioprostheses," *J. Thorac. Cardiovasc. Surg.*, 81:747 (1981).

43 CLARK, R. E., H. M. Karara, A. Cataloglu and P. L. Gould. "Close-Range Stereophotogrammetry and Coupled Stress Analysis as Tools in the Development of Prosthetic Devices," *Trans. Am. Soc. Artif. Int. Organs*, 21:71 (1975).

44 CATALOGLU, A., R. E. Clark and P. L. Gould. "Stress Analysis of Aortic Valve Leaflets with Smoothed Geometrical Data," *J. Biomech.*, 10:153 (1977).

45 CHONG, M. and Y. F. Missirlis. "Aortic Valve Mechanics Part II: A Stress Analysis of the Porcine Aortic Valve Leaflets in Diastole," *Biomat. Med. Dev. Art. Org.*, 6:225 (1978).

46 GHISTA, D. N. and H. Reul. "Optimal Prosthetic Aortic Leaflet Valve: Design Parametric and Longevity Analyses: Development of the Avcothane-51 Leaflet Valve Based on the Optimum Design Analysis," *J. Biomech.*, 10:313 (1977).

47 CHRISTIE, G. W. and I. C. Medland. "A Non Linear Finite Element Stress Analysis of Bioprosthetic Heart Valves," in *Finite Elements in Biomechanics*, R. H. Gallagher, ed. New York:Wiley and Sons, p. 153 (1982).

48 BROOM, N. and G. W. Christie. "The Structure/Function Relationship of Fresh and Glutaraldehyde-Fixed Aortic Valve Leaflets," in *Cardiac Bioprostheses*, L. H. Cohn & V. Gallucci, eds. New York:Yorke Medical Books, p. 476 (1982).

49 THUBRIKAR, M. J., J. R. Skinner, T. R. Eppink and S. P. Nolan. "Stress Analysis of Porcine Bioprosthetic Heart Valves In Vivo," *J. Biomed. Mat. Res.*, 16:811 (1982).

50 FERRANS, V. J., S. W. Boyce, M. E. Billingham, M. Jones, T. Ishihara and W. C. Roberts. "Calcific Deposits in Porcine Bioprostheses: Structure and Pathogenesis," *Am. J. Cardiol.*, 46:721 (1980).

51 DECK, S. D., M. J. Thubrikar, S. P. Nolan and J. Aouad. "Role of Mechanical Stress in Calcification of Bioprostheses," in *Cardiac Bioprostheses*, L. H. Cohn and V.Gallucci, eds. New York:Yorke Medical Books, p. 293 (1982).

52 SABBAH, H. N., M. S. Hamid and P. D. Stein. "Estimation of Mechanical Stresses on Closed Cusps of Porcine Bioprosthetic Valves: Effects of Stiffening, Focal Calcium and Focal Thinning," *Am. J. Cardiol.*, 55:1091 (1985).

53 STEIN, P. D., S. R. Kemp, J. M. Riddle, M. W. Lee, J. W. Lewis, Jr. and D. J. Magilligan, Jr. "Relation of Calcification to Torn Leaflets of Spontaneously Degenerated Porcine Bioprosthetic Valves," *Ann. Thorac. Surg.*, 40:175 (1985).

54 BREWER, R. J., J. D. Deck, B. Capati and S. P. Nolan. "The Dynamic Aortic Root: Its Role in Aortic Valve Function," *J. Thorac. Cardiovasc. Surg.*, 72:413 (1976).

55 LEE, M.-C., M. M. LeWinter, G. Freeman, R. Shabetai and Y. C. Fung. "Biaxial Mechanical Properties of the Pericardium in Normal and Volume Overload Dogs," *Am. J. Physiol.*, 249:H222 (1985).

56 VAN NOORT, R., J. C. Stevens and M. M. Black. "A New Apparatus for the In Vitro Testing of the Mechanical Properties of Soft Tissues," *Eng. Med.*, 7:231 (1978).

57 WAINWRIGHT, S. A., W. D. Biggs, J. D. Currey and J. M. Gosline. *Mechanical Design in Organisms*, London:Edward Arnold, p. 124 (1976).

58 CARPENTIER, A. "From Valvular Xenograft to Valvular Bioprosthesis (1965-1977)," *Med. Instru.*, 11:98 (1977).

59 SALGALLER, M. L. and P. K. Bajpai. "Immunogenicity of Glutaraldehyde-Treated Bovine Pericardial Tissue Xenografts in Rabbits," *J. Biomed. Mat. Res.*, 19:1 (1985).

60 TAN, A. J. K. and D. L. Holt. "The Effects of Sterilization and Storage Treatments on the Stress–Strain Behaviour of Aortic Leaflets," *Ann. Thorac. Surg.*, 22:188 (1976).

61 BROOM, N. D. "The Stress–Strain and Fatigue Behavior of Glutaraldehyde-Preserved Heart-Valve Tissue," *J. Biomech.*, 10:707 (1977).

62 BROOM, N. D. "Simultaneous Morphological and Stress–Strain Studies of the Fibrous Components in Wet Heart Valve Leaflet Tissue," *Conn. Tiss. Res.*, 6:37 (1978).

63 BROOM, N. D. and F. J. Thompson. "Influence of Fixation Conditions on the Performance of Glutaraldehyde Treated Porcine Aortic Valves: Toward a More Scientific Basis," *Thorax*, 34:166 (1979).

64 ROUSSEAU, E. P. M., A. A. H. J. Sauren, M. C. van Hout and A. A. van Steenhoven. "Elastic and Viscoelastic Material Behavior of Fresh and Glutaraldehyde-Treated Porcine Aortic Valve Tissue," *J. Biomech.*, 16:339 (1983).

65 LEE, J. M. and D. R. Boughner. "Effect of Fixation and Pressure-Fixation on the Tissue Mechanics of Porcine Aortic Valve Cusps," Digest of papers, 8th Canadian Medical and Biological Engineering Conference, p. 78 (1980).

66 LEE, J. M., D. R. Boughner and D. W. Courtman. "The Glutaraldehyde-Stabilized Porcine Aortic Valve Xenograft: II. Effect of Fixation With or Without Pressure on the Tensile Viscoelastic Properties of the Leaflet Material," *J. Biomed. Mater. Res.*, 18:79 (1984).

67 VESELY, I. and D. R. Boughner. "A Multi Purpose Tissue Bending Machine," *J. Biomechanics*, 18:511–513 (1985).

68 VESELY, I. and D. R. Boughner. "Analysis of the Bending Behaviour of Porcine Xenograft Leaflets and of Natural Aortic Valve Material: Bending Stiffness, Neutral Axis and Shear Measurements," *J. Biomechanics*, 22:655 (1989).

69 VAN NOORT, R., S. P. Yates, T. R. P. Martin, A. T. Barker and M. M. Black. "A Study of the Effects of Glutaraldehyde and Formaldehyde on the Mechanical Behavior or Bovine Pericardium," *Biomaterials*, 3:21 (1982).

70 TROWBRIDGE, E. A., M. M. Black and C. L. Daniel. "The Mechanical Response of Glutaraldehyde-Fixed Bovine Pericardium to Uniaxial Load," *J. Mater. Sci.*, 20:114 (1985).

71 TROWBRIDGE, E. A. and C. E. Crofts. "Evidence that Deformations Which Occur During Mechanical Conditioning of Bovine Pericardium are not Permanent," *Biomaterials*, 7:49 (1986).

72 LEE, J. M., D. R. Boughner and S. A Haberer SA. "The Bovine Pericardial Xenograft: I. Effect of Fixation in Aldehydes Without Constraint on the Tensile Viscoelastic Properties of Bovine Pericardium," *J. Biomed. Mater. Res.*, 23:457 (1989).

73 BELLO, J. and H. R. Bello. "Chemical Modification and Crosslinking of Proteins by Impurities in Glycerol," *Arch. Biochem. Biophys.*, 172:608 (1976).

74 VAN NOORT, R., M. M. Black, T. R. P. Martin and S. Meanley. "A Study of the Uniaxial Mechanical Properties of Human Dura Mater Preserved in Glycerol," *Biomaterials*, 2:41 (1981).

75 MIYATA, T., Y. Noishiki, K. Kodaira and Y. Furuse. "New Cross-linking Method for Collagenous Biomaterials," *Trans. Soc. Biomat.*, 12:130 (1986).

76 REECE, I. J., R. van Noort, T. R. P. Martin and M. M. Black. "The Physical Properties of Bovine Pericardium: A Study of the Effects of Stretching During Chemical Treatment in Glutaraldehyde," *Ann. Thorac. Surg.*, 33:480 (1981).

77 LEE, J. M., R. Corrente and S. A. Haberer. "The Bovine Pericardial Xenograft: II. Effect of Tethering or Pressurization During Fixation on the Tensile Viscoelastic Properties of Bovine Pericardium," *J. Biomed. Mater. Res.*, 23:477 (1989).

78 LEE, J. M., M. Ku and S. A. Haberer. "The Bovine Pericardial Xenograft: III. Effect of Uniaxial and Sequential Biaxial Stress During Fixation on the Tensile Viscoelastic Properties of Bovine Pericardium," *J. Biomed. Mater. Res.*, 23:491 (1989).

79 BROOM, N. D. "An 'In Vitro' Study of Mechanical Fatigue in Glutaraldehyde-Treated Porcine Aortic Valve Tissue," *Biomaterials*, 1:3 (1980).

80 THUBRIKAR, M., W. C. Piepgrass, J. D. Deck and S. P. Nolan. "Stresses of Natural Versus Prosthetic Aortic Valve Leaflets In Vivo," *Ann. Thorac. Surg.*, 30:230 (1980).

81 FUNG, Y. C. "Stress–Strain–History Relations of Soft Tissues in Simple Elongation," in *Biomechanics: Its Foundations and Objectives*, Y. C. Fung, ed. Inglewood Cliffs, N.J.:Prentice Hall, p. 181 (1972).

82 LEE, J. M. and D. R. Boughner. "Uni-axial Viscoelastic Properties of Bioprosthetic Heart Valve Materials: Application of Quasi-linear Theory to Data from Instron-Type Testing," Digest of Papers, 9th

Canadian Medical and Biological Engineering Conference, p. 13 (1982).

83 LEE, J. M. and S. A. Haberer. "Unsuitability of Linear or Quasi-linear Viscoelastic Theory for Description of the Tensile Mechanical Properties of Bovine Pericardial Xenograft Material," *Proceedings, 7th Annual Conference of the Canadian Biomaterials Society*, p. 58 (1986).

84 DORTMANS, L. J. M. G., A. A. H. J. Sauren and E. P. M. Rousseau. "Parameter Estimation Using the Quasi-Linear Viscoelastic Model Proposed by Fung," *J. Biomech. Eng.*, 106:198 (1984).

85 SAUREN, A. A. H. J. and E. P. M. Rousseau. "A Concise Sensitivity Analysis of the Quasi-Linear Viscoelastic Model Proposed by Fung," *J. Biomech. Eng.*, 105:92 (1983).

86 SHEMIN, R. J., F. J. Schoen, R. Hein, J. Austin and L. H. Cohn. "Hemodynamic and Pathologic Evaluation of a Unileaflet Pericardial Bioprosthesis Valve," *J. Thorac. Cardiovasc. Surg.*, 95:912 (1988).

87 MOHANARADHAKRISHNAN, K. and N. Ramanathan. "Studies on Collagen Fibers: Part III. Strength," *Leather Sci.*, 12:12 (1965).

CHAPTER 11

Cardiac Pacing Leads

V. BARBARO, Ph.D.,[1] P. BARTOLINI,[1] S. CAIAZZA,[2]
P. CHISTOLINI,[1] and D. IALONGO[3]

ABSTRACT: The technology involving synthetic biomaterials has rapidly evolved during the last decades. It is
therefore the aim of this paper to define the state-of-the-art
in the field of cardiac pacing leads, and its prospectives.
The authors describe the device components in relation to
their function, and analyse the problems regarding design,
implantation and use with respect to mechanical, electrical
and biocompatibility requirements. An original contribution
is the investigation on electrode–tissue interface, and on the
long-term performance and durability of lead insulating
sheaths made of silicone rubber or polyurethane. As re-
gards this latter issue, and taking into account the concern
expressed in literature and the warnings of the Food and
Drug Administration about the use of polyurethane insulating sheaths, "in vitro" electrical measurements and scanning electron microscopy (S.E.M.) observations are made.

INTRODUCTION

In the framework of an electrical cardiac stimulation
system, a cardiac pacing lead has the function of electrically connecting the impulse generator to the myocardium
for cardiac pacing and for sensing of spontaneous signals
produced by the heart. In order to perform such functions,
the cardiac leads must necessarily be designed to fulfill
certain physical (mechanical and electrical) and chemical
requirements (biocompatibility). Several materials and
configurations, with different chemical, mechanical and
electrical features, are used to perform these functions.
Naturally, the final outcome has always been a compromise between the different requirements. In fact, there

is no such thing as an ideal cardiac pacing lead, but different leads have been designed to carry out different
functions. One of the factors that is normally neglected is
the fact that an individual operator may be familiar only
with a certain type of cardiac lead, so that a lead model
which has not caused any complications for one operator
may turn out to be a problem for another. However, it is
necessary to have objective reference criteria for comparing the different leads available. In the present work, we
will discuss the requirements of cardiac pacing leads, the
attempts made thus far to improve their performance,
their possible complications, and future perspectives.

A cardiac pacing lead can be positioned either endocar-
dially or epicardially. If implanted in the epicardium, surgery must be performed under total anesthesia. However,
if the lead is introduced in the endocardium, local
anesthesia will suffice. The endocardial approach is currently the most widely used technique by which cardiac
leads are introduced intravenously and, with the help of a
stylet (Figure 1), guided towards the apex of the right ventricle.

A cardiac pacing lead is schematically composed of five
sections:

- the connector, which connects the cardiac lead to
  the generator in a stable and watertight manner
- the conductor, which transmits electrical signals
  alternately (along one line) to and from the heart,
  keeping its characteristics constant in time
- the insulating sheath, which insulates the
  conductor from the outside environment, without
  interacting with the host organism
- the electrode, which establishes contact with the
  myocardium surface that will prove to be effective
  both in terms of stimulation and sensing
- the fixation system, which guarantees a stable

[1]Department of Biomedical Engineering, Istituto Superiore di Sanità,
Roma, Italy

[2]Department of Ultrastructures, Istituto Superiore di Sanità, Roma, Italy

[3]Pacemaker Center, Ospedale S. Camillo, Roma, Italy

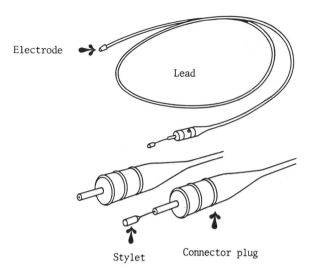

Figure 1. Cardiac pacing lead.

Electrode

Lead

Stylet

Connector plug

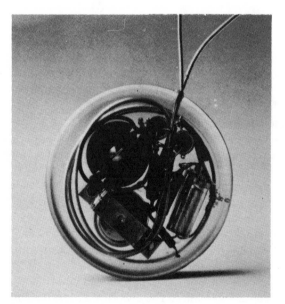

Figure 2. The first implantable pacemaker of A. Senning.

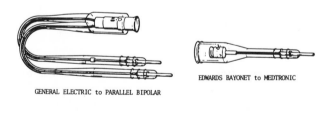

GENERAL ELECTRIC to PARALLEL BIPOLAR

EDWARDS BAYONET to MEDTRONIC

COAXIAL BIPOLAR to PARALLEL BIPOLAR

PARALLEL BIPOLAR to COAXIAL BIPOLAR

Figure 3. Lead adapters.

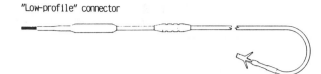

"Low-profile" connector

Figure 4. Unipolar low profile connector.

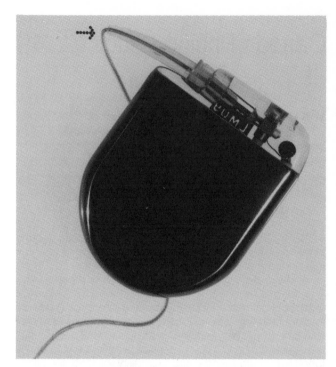

Figure 5. The arrow shows the sharp angle formed by the lead. This is a stress point for conductor coil.

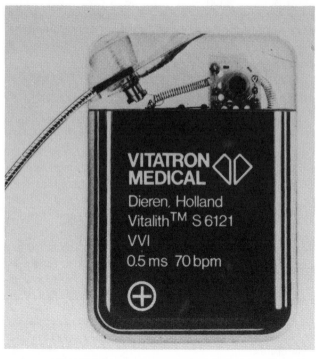

VITATRON ◇◇
MEDICAL
Dieren, Holland
Vitalith™ S 6121
VVI
0.5 ms 70 bpm
⊕

Figure 6. The Vitatron connector. The lead comes out obliquely from the pacemaker, without a sharp angle.

contact between the electrode and the myocardium.

These individual components will now be examined in greater detail in terms of their functions, state-of-the-art techniques, and possible future developments.

CONNECTOR

In the first pacemakers implanted in man, the cardiac lead was permanently affixed to the pulse generator (Figure 2). This obviously gave rise to two kinds of problems: (a) the difficulty of positioning the electrode in the right ventricle without the help of a stiff stylet; and, (b) the impossibility of changing the generator while leaving the cardiac lead *in situ*. The pacing lead and the pulse generator soon became two separate elements, but the electrode–pacemaker connection never came to be standardized. In the seventies, most cardiac pacing leads made reference to five different types of connections, each being made by a different manufacturer, with the exception of the Cordis and Medtronic types that were also used by other firms. The problem of connecting a cardiac lead and a pacemaker of different makes was solved by using adapters (Figure 3). These devices have two types of drawbacks: (a) they take up greater room in the site where the pacemaker is positioned, with the risk of inducing decubitus; and, (b) they are points of mechanical and electrical weakness along the route of the stimulus.

Over the past few years, although connectors have not actually been standardized (probably due to marketing reasons), a decrease in the different types of connectors has occurred. Moreover, several firms have introduced in their catalogues the "low-profile" connection (Figure 4), both for the unipolar and bipolar types, in addition to conventional connections. The "low-profile" connector is expected to become universal in the future, because of its mechanical and space-related features, which will be discussed later. Indeed, the point at which the cardiac lead goes out from the generator is one of the parts submitted to greatest stress. In the case of a traditional connector the cardiac lead forms a very sharp bend at its exit from the pacemaker, since the first part is kept stable by the stiff nature of the connection (Figure 5). This problem was solved by Vitatron, who developed a connection with the cardiac lead coming out from the pacemaker obliquely (Figure 6). Today, with the design of the "low-profile" connection, the stiff part of the connector has been eliminated. This makes it possible for the cardiac lead to come out from the generator without a sharp bend, thus reducing the stress on the insulating sheath and the coil.

The size of the connector was also the object of a constructive evolution (Figure 7). In unipolar systems, the connector was designed as a natural extension of the lead, without additional thickness. The "O-rings" required to guarantee watertightness were incorporated in the pacemaker connection. Similarly, in bipolar systems, the use of concentric (rather than parallel) coils, as well as the modifications performed in unipolar cardiac leads, made it possible to significantly decrease the thickness of the connector. The size of the connector is an element of great importance in terms of the total size of the pacemaker, especially for bicameral pulse generators (which are equipped with two leads for pacing and sensing of both atrium and ventricle). Once a pacemaker is approximately 5–7 mm thick, it is evident that the cardiac lead can significantly limit its reduction in terms of size. It seems unlikely that the connector will undergo further significant size reductions with the materials currently being used. Indeed, the connector size is related to the technological development of the conductor and insulating sheath.

CONDUCTOR

The cardiac pacing lead is subjected to continuous mechanical stress *in vivo*, mainly due to bending caused by heartbeat, respiration, and other bodily movements. Thus, the cardiac conductor must be highly resistant to mechanical fatigue and corrosion due to contact with any possible biological fluids. Moreover, the conductors must be characterized by a low electrical impedance. The most widely used materials are light, stainless steel alloys, of which the following are the most frequently applied:

Elgiloy	cobalt (Co)	40%
	chromium (Cr)	20%
	nickel (Ni)	15%
	molybdenum (Mo)	7%
	manganese (Mn)	2%
	carbon (C)	0.15%
	beryllium (Be)	0.04%
	iron 16 (Fe)	complement to 100%
Inox 316 L	chromium	16–18%
	nickel	10–14%
	molybdenum	2–3%
	carbon	0.03%
MP 35 N	cobalt	35%
	chromium	20%
	nickel	35%
	molybdenum	10%
	iron	0–1%
DBS	Drawn Brazed Strand	
	(strand composed of silver and MP 35 N)	

Although the heart contracts approximately 40 million times in a year, causing considerable bending of the cardiac lead, this phenomenon accounts for only 2% of coil fractures. The remaining 98% of coil fractures take place

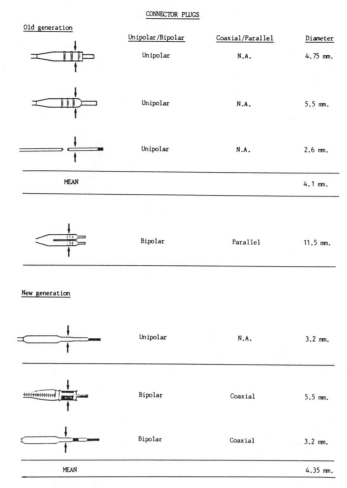

CONNECTOR PLUGS

Old generation

	Unipolar/Bipolar	Coaxial/Parallel	Diameter
	Unipolar	N.A.	4.75 mm.
	Unipolar	N.A.	5.5 mm.
	Unipolar	N.A.	2.6 mm.
MEAN			4.1 mm.
	Bipolar	Parallel	11.5 mm.

New generation

	Unipolar	N.A.	3.2 mm.
	Bipolar	Coaxial	5.5 mm.
	Bipolar	Coaxial	3.2 mm.
MEAN			4.35 mm.

Figure 7. *New and old most widely used connector plugs.*

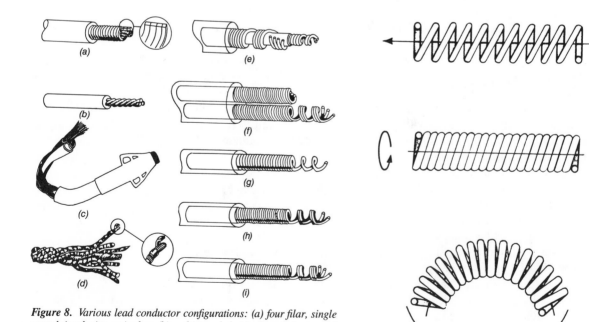

Figure 8. *Various lead conductor configurations: (a) four filar, single strand tinsel wire, unipolar; (b) multistranded unipolar conductor; (c) Elcor lead: 3000 graphite fibers; (d) six filar multistrand tinsel wire, unipolar; (e) coaxial bipolar; (f) parallel bipolar; (g) unifilar unipolar conductor; (h) bifilar unipolar conductor; and (i) trifilar unipolar conductor.*

Figure 9. *Types of lead conductor stresses.*

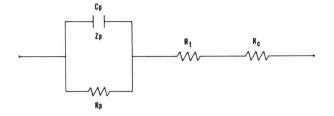

$C_p = 2\,\mu F$, $R_p = 500\,K\Omega$, $R_c = (8 \div 100)\,\Omega$, $R_t = 500\,\Omega$

Figure 10. *Simplified equivalent circuit model for pacing impedance with typical values for the components.*

in the vicinity of the pacemaker, or in the proximity of the entry into the vein [1].

The fractures of single-thread coils are statistically due to stress caused by the weight or movement of the pacemaker. One way to guarantee greater reliability is to introduce a redundant system, i.e., a system made up of parallel subsystems. In the event of one or more failures, the system continues to operate as long as one subsystem is functioning. The application of this principle to cardiac leads entails the use of multiple coils and/or multifilar multiple coil conductors. Recently, a cardiac pacing lead named "ELCOR" was released on the market. It is composed of two bundles of 3,000 graphite filaments flowing in teflon tubes, which in turn are tied around a central teflon tube also used as a guide for the stylet [2]. The graphite conductor has higher flexibility and greater traction resistance, leading to increased longevity compared to pacing leads with different conductors.

Figure 8 shows some typical configurations of pacing conductors. The analysis of all types of induced mechanical tests (i.e. fatigue tests) and the electrical resistance of coil conductors indicate the critical parameters of the coil. A coil is subjected to three types of stress (Figure 9): tension, twisting, and bending. The effect of such stresses depends upon the geometry of the coil (i.e., the diameter of the turns, diameter of the coil, number of turns, spaces between turns) [3] and upon the tensile and shear moduli of the material employed. Table 1 reports the average life expectancy data from bending tests performed on certain conductors. The table shows that life expectancy of the MP 35 N alloy in a multifilar coil configuration is approximately 1,000 times greater than that of the same alloy but having a single thread configuration. In the case of DBS multifilar coils, there is further improvement by a factor of 10.

A change in the geometry of the parameters aimed at reducing stress and increasing flexibility usually brings about an increase in electrical resistance [5]. An increase in electrical resistance, however, produces a decrease in the energy available for stimulation. Therefore, a coil designed for enhanced stress and flexibility resistance

usually has a relatively high electrical resistance. A good design requires a compromise between the two. Impedance of the electrode should also be taken into account because impedance and resistance are directly related.

CARDIAC PACING LEAD IMPEDANCE

The impedance of a cardiac pacing lead, intended as an electrode–tissue conductor, contains three contributions: the conductor resistance (Rc), the tissue resistance (Rt), and the polarization impedance (Zp). Note that the first two components are purely resistive while the third component is complex (resistive + capacitive component) and linked to the electrode-tissue interface (Figure 10).

$$\text{Zelectr} = \text{Rc} + \text{Zp} + \text{Rt}$$

This scheme is valid whether the lead has the pacing or sensing function. In particular, Rt and Rc remain the same in both cases, but the polarization impedance is much greater when the cardiac lead has a sensing function [6,7]. It is thus clear that there are two cardiac lead impedances, according to the lead function, and that sensing impedance is much greater than the impedance of the same lead that has a pacing function.

These three magnitudes may be varied to optimize the functional objectives of a cardiac pacing lead:

- maximal pacing energy of the pacemaker impulse for a given pulse width
- maximal life expectancy of the pacemaker energy source.

But since these requirements contradict each other, it is practically impossible to manufacture an ideal cardiac lead in terms of impedance. Attempts can be made, however, to obtain good compromises.

The resistance, Rc, of the conductor is that which can be measured between the two poles of the lead by means of an ohmeter. It will have to be minimized in order to obtain maximum performance (the greater the quantity of current flowing in the conductor, the greater the amount of useful energy reaching the tissue, with less energy dissipating into heat on the lead itself). One way to change the

TABLE 1. Flex Life of Some Representative Conductors

Conductor Type (Material)	In Vitro Flex Life[a] (B50 Cycles)
Single filar coil (MP35N)	2×10^5
Tinsel wire (platinum)	8×10^5
Multifilar coil (MP35N)	2.5×10^8
Multifilar coil (DBS)[b]	2×10^9

[a] Cycles to failure of 50^6 of specimens, flexed $\pm\ 90°$ at 120BPM at STP.
[b] DBS-MP35N/Silver, drawn-brazed-strand.
Modified from STOKES and Coll. [4].

resistance of the conductor is to alter the geometry of the conductor itself (for example changing the turn diameter in a coil, the diameter of the coil, the number of turns, the space in between turns, etc. . . .). However there is a limit to compromises here beyond which the improvement of performance causes detriment to the mechanical features.

Upton [3] reports an example of geometric variation performed to improve electrical resistance. By increasing the number of threads in a coil from three to four, resistance decreases by one and a half times. By performing this procedure in Medtronic the two models, 6961 and 6962, were obtained. Despite one being unipolar and the other bipolar, the two have very similar resistances for the conductor: 87 ohm for the former, and 95 ohm for the latter. Much better results may be obtained by employing particularly suitable conductor materials. Typical values for conductor resistance are currently included between 8 and 100 ohm.

The resistance R_t should be maximized for two main reasons: First, a relatively high value increases the overall impedance of the system, increasing the life expectancy of the pacemaker battery. Second, since the section of the electrode is inversely proportional to the resistance itself, a relatively high R_t value entails a small electrode radius (which is proportional to the square root of the surface area). This brings about improvements in terms of size (thus facilitating the introduction of several pacing leads into the same vein), and in terms of threshold reduction. Actually, R_t resistance, in addition to depending upon the section, also depends on the temperature and conductivity of the tissue [8,9], but *in vivo*, temperatures and conductivity may be considered as constant. A typical R_t value is about 500 ohm. Much greater R_t values, however, are not advisable since they would significantly increase the polarization impedance and consequently cause a further growth of sensing impedance as compared to pacing impedance.

The polarization impedance, Z_p, is directly proportional to the concentration of ions at the electrode–tissue interface. The separation of ions of opposite signs, which is created at the interface by the flow of current, generates a potential that is opposed to the flow of current itself. Although a greater concentration of ions at the interface (greater Z_p) does not play a particularly important role in cardiac pacing, it forces the pacemaker to provide additional voltage in order to exceed such a potential for providing good cardiac pacing. In this regard it is better to minimize the polarization impedance. This impedance is a function of several parameters, such as the electrode material, its surface area, its shape, and the correct application of pulse width. This latter element explains why the polarization impedance in sensing is greater than that in stimulation: in sensing, the R wave has a 20–140 ms duration, decisively longer than the 0.5–1.2 ms duration for stimulation. The following values for the Z_p polarization impedance components may be regarded as typical: $C_p = 2\ \mu F$, $R_p > 300\ k\Omega$.

CARDIAC PACING LEAD SIZE

The size of the pacing lead poses three kinds of problems. First, the lead must be inserted intravenously and then positioned so that it reaches the heart. There may be cases in which the size of the vein will not allow the introduction and placement of the lead, thus making it necessary to adopt other approaches which will prolong the operation. Second, there is the problem of simultaneous implantation of two leads, due to the ever-increasing need of bicameral pacemakers. It is obvious that the thinner the leads, the greater the chances of introducing them into the same vein. Finally, there is the problem of complications that would make it necessary to insert a second, a third and even fourth lead (in a bicameral system two leads are positioned at each implantation) during the life of a cardiac pacing system. In most cases cardiac leads are left on site. If the same subject is submitted to further implantations, it is preferable that the newly implanted leads are as thin as possible. Table 2 shows the size of unipolar cardiac leads used. In old generation leads the insulating sheath was made up of silicone. The use of polyurethane as an insulator (this material is stronger and stiffer than silicone) as well as other types of silicone, has made it possible to manufacture unipolar leads with an insulating sheath thinner by approximately 40%. Similar results were obtained in bipolar cardiac leads not only by modifying the insulating material, but also by abandoning the parallel configuration of the coils and resorting to the concentric configuration, thus reducing the thickness by 30% to 50%, according to the cases (Table 2).

INSULATING SHEATH

The insulating sheath is in direct contact with blood. The insulating material must therefore fulfill significant biocompatibility and biostability requirements. It must be non-toxic, non-thrombogenic, and non-carcinogenic, and these features, along with the functional characteristics, must remain unchanged in time. However, the main function of a cardiac pacing lead is to allow the correct transmission of stimulation and sensing signals from the pacemaker to the cardiac tissue, making sure that such signals are not dispersed in the surrounding tissue. The physical parameter that reflects this property is the degree of electrical insulation between the lead conductor and the surrounding tissue.

There are several causes [10] which may lead to loss of insulation:

TABLE 2. Lead Dimension

Old Generation

Model	Diameter (mm.)	C/P[a]	French	U/B[b]	Material
Sorin CVT 62	2.5		7.5	U	Silicone
CPI 4116	2.5		7.5	U	Silicone
Biotronik K	2.2		6.5	U	Silicone
MDT 6907R	2.64		8	U	Silicone
Intermedics 463-01	2.5		7.5	U	Silicone
Pacesetter 815	2.7		8	U	Silicone
Elema 288S	2.2		6.5	U	Silicone
Mean	2.5		7.5		
MDT 6962	3.12	P	9.5	B	Silicone
CPI 4230	3.2	P	9.5	B	Silicone
Intermedics 466-01	3.2	P	9.5	B	Silicone
Pacesetter 816	3.3	P	10	B	Silicone
Mean	3.2		9.5		

New Generation

Model	Diameter (mm.)	C/P	French	U/B	Material
CPI 4150	1.5		4.5	U	Silicone HP
MDT 6959	1.5		4.5	U	Urethane
Biotronik DNT	1.5		4.5	U	Silicone
Intermedics 495-01	1.3		4	U	Urethane
Cordis Encor	1.3		4	U	Urethane
Pacesetter 865	1.2		3.5	U	Urethane
Mean	1.4		4		
MDT 4012	2.29	C	7	B	Urethane
Intermedics 467-03	2	C	6	B	Urethane
Pacesetter 866	1.5	C	4.5	B	Urethane
CPI 4266	2.2	C	6.5	B	Silicone HP
Mean	2		6		

[a]C = coaxial wires; P = parallel wires.
[b]U = unipolar; B = bipolar.

- Starting from the implant time the cardiac pacing lead may be damaged by the scalpel in the zone where suturing is performed.
- The cardiac lead is submitted to continuous mechanical stress, both at the time of implantation and during the period following it.
- The contact with blood or other biological fluids may in time lead to the degradation of the insulating sheath.

In all of the above mentioned circumstances, the surface of the cardiac lead undergoes degradation, with the subsequent formation of cracks and fissues and loss of electrical insulation. This degradation may be measured directly, by using electrical-type measurements, or indirectly through scanning electron microscopy (SEM) observation. The latter technique also makes it possible to assess the size and depth of the fissures present on both the inner and outer surfaces of the cardiac lead insulating sheath.

Silicone and polyurethane are the materials currently used for manufacturing insulating sheaths. The excellent features of silicone in terms of biocompatibility, biostability and long-term performance are well known and extensively documented. The main defects resulting from the use of this material are of a mechanical nature [11]. Silicone is a relatively soft material, or more precisely, it is characterized by a low tear strength. This means that silicone is liable to be damaged by the scalpel or by sutures during the implantation procedure.

Halfway through the Seventies pacing leads with a polyurethane insulating sheath were introduced into the market. This made it possible to benefit from two advantages as compared to traditionally used silicone:

- decrease in thickness of the pacing lead
- less friction between the lead–blood, lead–vein and lead–coil interfaces

The results thus allowed the implantation quality of the lead to be improved, as well as the introduction of two

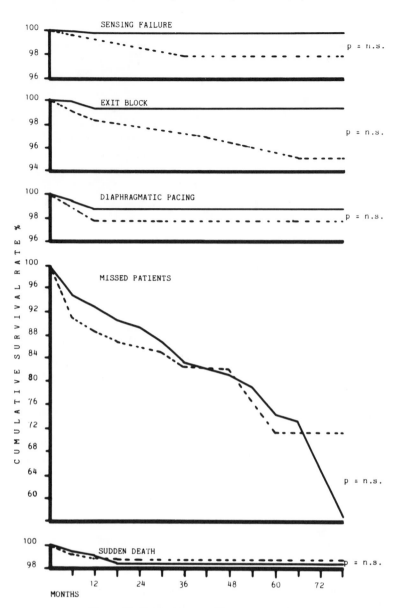

Figure 11. *Survival curves. SR (—), PU (———).*

leads in the same vein with greater ease. It was also possible to create an active fixation system by means of a retractable screw, i.e., a screw that is fastened and unfastened from the tip of the lead by imparting a rotating motion to the coil through the head of the connector. A few years after the introduction of such an insulating sheath, however, malfunctioning phenomena were reported due to damage of the polyurethane. This material thus became the object of many studies [12–19].

In order to better understand the long-term causes and the entity of such defects we have undertaken several investigations:

(a) Clinical follow-up approximately 78 months long on 647 patients, of which 384 had polyurethane (PU) leads, and the remaining 263 silicone rubber (SR) leads

(b) Electrical insulation measurements, both in new and explanted pacing leads

(c) Scanning electron microscope observations of new and explanted leads

These investigations were performed for both polyurethane and silicone in order to better compare the long-term performance of these materials. The results are discussed in the following sections.

Clinical Follow-up

The clinical studies were performed on the basis of two groups: the first comprised 384 patients with an implanted PU coated ventricular pacing lead and the second comprised 263 patients with implanted SR coated leads. The patients were reviewed daily during the first 15 days after the implant, then 1 month after dismissal and, successively, every 6 months or, if necessary, more frequently, for a maximum of 78 months. Successively, the cumulative survival rates have been examined for the following cases: exit block, sensing failure, diaphragmatic pacing, sudden deaths and missing patients. The results have also been examined using the t^2 statistical test at a 95% confidence level. The results of the clinical follow-up are outlined below and have been summarised in graphical form in Figure 11.

The sensing failure survival curves are quite similar (PU coating 99.5%; SR 97.8%). The exit block curves show that the PU coated leads present a greater number of exit blocks, showing a trend consistently lower than the SR leads (PU = 95.1%; SR = 99.1%). However, the difference is not statistically significant. The diaphragmatic pacing survival curves are quite similar (SR = 98.9%; PU = 97.9%). Sudden deaths (SR = 98.5%; PU = 98.9%) and missed patients (SR = 61%; PU = 71.1%) survival curves do not show statistical differences.

Electrical Insulation Measurements

As far as electrical measurements are concerned, a special electrolytic cell was developed which is capable of measuring electrical admittance on the insulated lead sections [15]. Admittance is the reciprocal of impedance. The greater the admittance the worse the quality of electrical insulation. Cardiac pacing leads were grouped into the following four categories:

- new silicone pacing leads
- explanted silicone pacing leads
- new polyurethane pacing leads
- explanted polyurethane pacing leads

As shown in Figure 12, both silicone and polyurethane explanted leads were reported to have a greater admittance as compared to new leads. The degradation level of explanted polyurethane leads, however, is considerable and the difference in comparison with explanted silicone leads is statistically significant (P < 0.001). In all cases, however, admittance values are relatively low and below the levels at which the average life-expectancy of leads is affected.

Scanning Electron Microscope Observations

Many SEM observations were carried out during the past years on PU and SR insulating leads in order to compare the morphological changes induced by the contact with blood. Nevertheless, many reports are conflicting due to lack of information on PU polymer, type and manufacturer of the lead. In this regard the following SEM micrographs are all related to commercially available PU and SR pacing leads of a single type and producer for each material (Medtronic for PU and LEM Biomedica for SR leads). The unimplanted leads were prepared for SEM observation as received and without cleaning treatment, while explanted leads were gently cleaned in saline in order to remove possible surface biological debris. Segments of intravenous tracts were cut by means of a new razor blade, operating in a stereomicroscope to minimize externally applied stresses on the specimens. They were glued on the stubs with a suitable inclination for better observation of both the outer surface and the cutplane. The lead segments were gold-sputtered and observed in a Philips 515 scanning electron microscope.

A highly representative picture of the morphology of an unimplanted PU insulating lead is shown in Figure 13. The outer surface of the lead appears to be clean and regular with the typical ripples due to shrinkage depending on the molding process. The cross section surface of the same lead (Figure 14) is also continuous and regular, as well as the intersection line between the outer surface and the cutplane. The intravenous PU insulated lead, having been in contact with blood for 9 months before explantation (Figure 15), does not show significant degradation of the outer surface, whose structure is well preserved. This is confirmed by the lead cross section (Figure 16), which shows just very slight signs of marginal discontinuity and minor amount of debris on the outer surface part near the cutplane intersection line.

The surface morphology is dramatically modified in a PU insulating lead explanted after 35 months (Figure 17). In this case the degradation of the outer surface is exten-

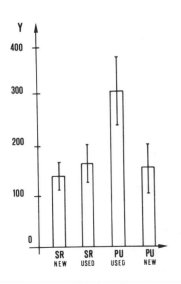

In Vitro Admittance $Y = \left[nA \cdot V^{-1} \cdot cm^{-1} \right]$

Figure 12. Admittance measurements in new and used leads.

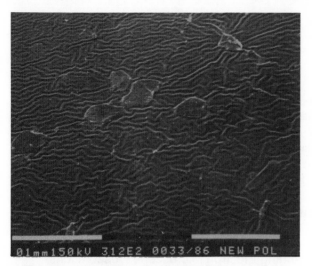

Figure 13. Outer surface of unimplanted PU insulating lead.

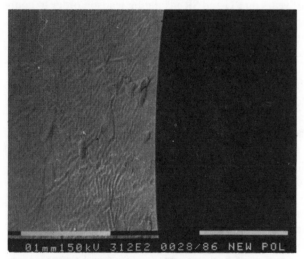

Figure 14. Cross section of the PU lead in Figure 13.

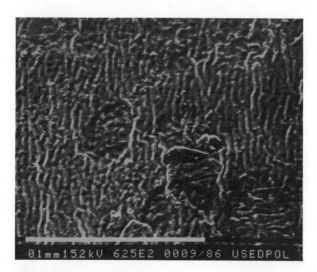

Figure 15. Outer surface of PU insulated lead explanted after 9 months.

sive, with wide cracks almost uniformly arranged, resulting in breaking away of the surface material. The cross section (Figure 18) shows that the severe surface cracks may reach a maximal depth of about 50 μm inside the lead.

The outer surface of a PU lead explanted after 56 months is shown in Figure 19. The degradation consists if the typical large cracks randomly arranged, also manifest in depressed areas of the surface. At this level, as shown in Figure 20, the depressions appear as cavities that deepen inside the material. It must be pointed out that the PU degradation does not seem to be time-dependent.

As for SR insulating leads, the following pictures are representative of the different behavior of this material: Figure 21 shows the outer surface of a new SR lead whose morphology is regular and typical of an unimplanted lead. Also, in the cross section (Figure 22) no evidence of defects is detectable, also given the stress due to sectioning of the material. The minimal presence of debris is due to specimen preparation.

The outer surface of a SR insulating lead explanted after 9 years is shown in Figure 23. In this case the surface morphology is modified by the long contact time with blood, resulting in the degradation phenomena. Erosion and mobilization of material are evident although large areas of the surface are still regular and clean. It is important to note that the degradation affects only the lead surface, without deepening inside the material (Figure 24). In order to interpret these results, and those reported in literature, three main hypotheses are formulated:

(1) Polyurethane cracking is caused by the extrusion stress of the insulating sheath and is limited in time. Moreover, in leads with a DBS conductor the infiltration of biological fluids through the insulating sheath may induce the formation of organosilver complexes, causing rapid oxidation of polyurethane [16].

(2) Cracking is also due to the extrusion process, but environmental factors come into play determining degradation; this phenomenon is time-dependent [17,18].

(3) From a clinical point of view, slight differences are observed in the complication trend between polyurethane and silicone. Such differences, however, are not yet sufficient for precise conclusions to be drawn.

The bibliographic remarks together with some polyurethane lead recalls by the FDA at the beginning were alarming for those using this kind of insulating sheath. Today, after having used polyurethane for almost ten years, attempts can be made to draw certain conclusions. We followed up cases with polyurethane and silicone leads implanted in the ventricle for up to a maximum of 7 years.

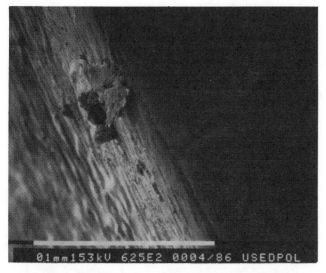

Figure 16. Cross section of the PU lead in Figure 15.

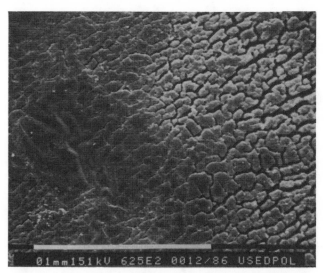

Figure 19. Outer surface of PU insulated explanted after 56 months.

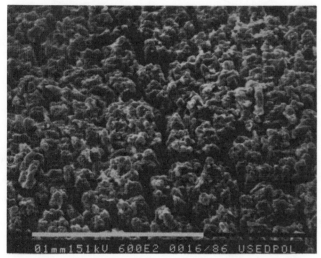

Figure 17. Outer surface of PU insulated lead explanted after 35 months.

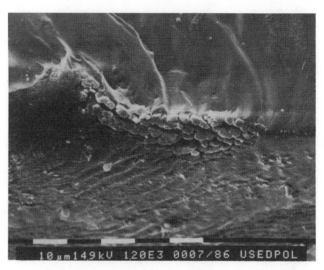

Figure 20. Cross section of the PU lead in Figure 19.

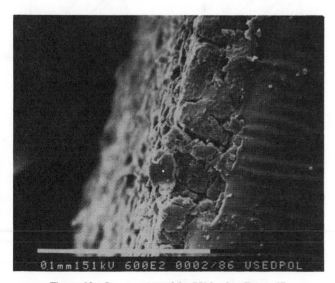

Figure 18. Cross section of the PU lead in Figure 17.

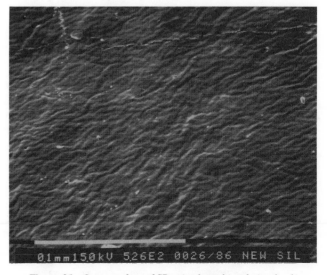

Figure 21. Outer surface of SR unimplanted insulating lead.

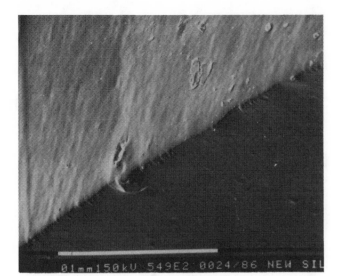

Figure 22. Cross section of the SR lead in Figure 21.

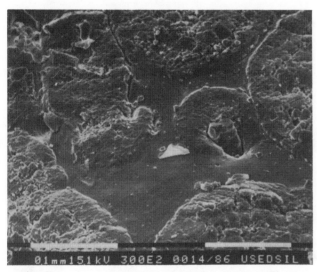

Figure 23. Outer surface of SR insulating lead explanted after 9 years.

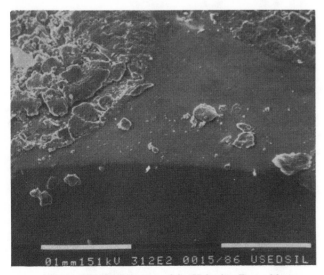

Figure 24. Cross section of the SR lead in Figure 23.

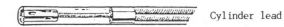 Cylinder lead

 Flanged lead

Figure 25. Cylinder and flanged leads.

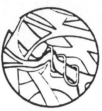 HELICAL COIL TIP

 TINED TIP

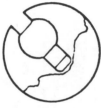 BALLOON TIP

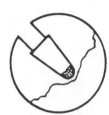 POROUS TIP

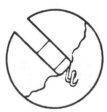 SCREW-IN TIP

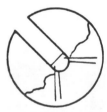 PRONGED TIP

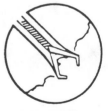 ENDOCARDIAL PINCH-ON

Figure 26. Different types of fixation systems.

TABLE 3. Urethane Types and Lead Failures

Manufacturer	Urethane	References
Medtronic	Pellethane 2363-80A	78,85
Intermedics	Pellethane 2363-80A	78,85
Telectronics	Pellethane 2363-90A	78,85
Cordis	Pellethane 2363-55D	78,85

Manufacturer	Failures		References
	n.	%	
Medtronic	72/2027	3.55	58,77–84
Intermedics	0/160	0	78
Telectronics	0/38	0	58,78
Cordis	0/64	0	78

Lead Model	Failures		References
	n.	%	
MDT 6991U MDT 6990U MDT 6972	67/658	10.18	77–83
MDT 6971 MDT 6957 MDT 4002 MDT 6857J	5/1369		58,78,80, 82–84

The analysis of survival curves, however, did not reveal significant differences in the incidence of complications between the two types of insulating sheaths.

So what accounts for the malfunction observed a few years ago and for the FDA recalls? If we analytically observe the data provided by the literature, we notice three interesting facts (Table 3):

(1) Not all producers use the same kind of polyurethane, and complications occur only in one type of polymer.

(2) Although two producers may use the same kind of polyurethane, the complications reported were found only in the leads made by one single producer, and were restricted only to certain models.

(3) FDA recalls and explanations provided by the producer underscore the fact that possible malfunctions are limited to a certain registration number of the suspected models.

It thus seems possible to conclude that polyurethane is a reliable material for the manufacture of implantable pacing leads but (especially for softer polymers) it requires greater attention during the extrusion process, as opposed to silicone. As for possible evolutions of insulating materials, it seems that currently there are no alternatives to silicone and polyurethane. A longer period of observation will be necessary, however, to elucidate which of the two will yield better long-term results and to assess if the decrease in thickness performed in the most recent models of silicone leads, to make them comparable to polyurethane leads, will cause problems in the future.

FIXATION SYSTEM

In order to assure effective cardiac pacing, a stable connection between the electrode and the cardiac wall must be established. In the past, cardiac leads were not manufactured with fixation systems. At the most, their tips were provided with a cone section (flanged cardiac leads) (Figure 25). Dislocations occurred very frequently with this type of lead (Table 4). Attempts were thus made to design fixation systems for electrodes that would be both active (screws and such), and passive (tines, porous electrodes) (Figure 26). Furthermore, given the particular position in which the electrode is located within the atrium, special

TABLE 4. Fixation Systems and Leads Dislocation

Electrode Location	Tip Characteristics	Displacements		References
		n.	%	
Atrium	Screw-in	9/314	2.9	20,21,22,&
	J-shaped + screw-in	0/48	0	&
	J-shaped	6/36	16.7	23
			20	24
	J-shaped + tines	23/440	5.2	25–32
	Helifix	13/352	3.7	31,33–36,20
	Tined	3/81	3.7	37,38,&
	Coronary sinus	19/150	12.7	33,39–41
Ventricle	Cylindric or flanged	703/5630	12.5	42–45
	Porous-surfaced	1/99	1	43,46,47
	Tined	13/1754	.7	43,48–54,&
	Helifix	16/1220	1.3	59–62
	Screw-in	25/1194	2.1	63,&
	Other active fixation	3/221	1.4	64,65

& = Our observations.

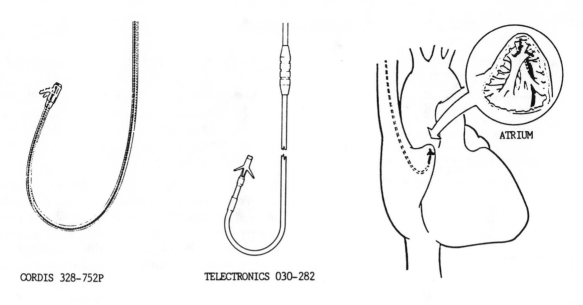

CORDIS 328–752P

TELECTRONICS 030–282

ATRIUM

Figure 27. *Atrial tined "J" shaped leads.*

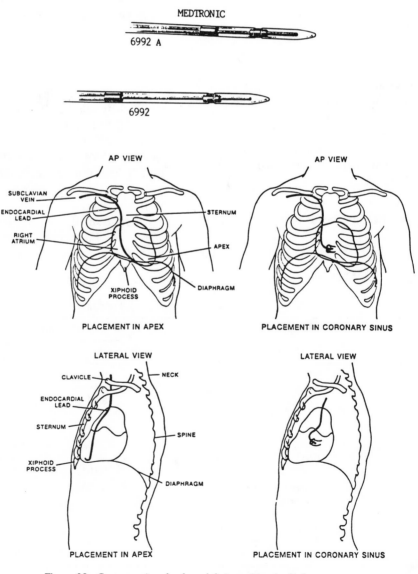

MEDTRONIC

6992 A

6992

AP VIEW

SUBCLAVIAN VEIN
ENDOCARDIAL LEAD
RIGHT ATRIUM
STERNUM
APEX
XIPHOID PROCESS
DIAPHRAGM

PLACEMENT IN APEX

AP VIEW

PLACEMENT IN CORONARY SINUS

LATERAL VIEW

CLAVICLE
NECK
ENDOCARDIAL LEAD
STERNUM
SPINE
XIPHOID PROCESS
DIAPHRAGM

PLACEMENT IN APEX

LATERAL VIEW

PLACEMENT IN CORONARY SINUS

Figure 28. *Coronary sinus leads and their position in the heart.*

leads were designed having a "J" preshaped curve to improve their stability (Figure 27). Tines allow stability by penetrating within the trabeculae of the atrium or ventricle (Figure 26,27). A similar mechanism is also used by the "Helifix" lead, which, with a rotating motion, wraps around muscles (Figure 26). Porous electrodes, on the other hand, owe their stability to the growing of a thrombus within the porous area, and to its progressive replacement by the fibrous tissue from the heart, so that the electrode is enveloped in the cardiac tissue. The screw-in, however, and other similar techniques provide stability by directly penetrating the myocardium, thus guaranteeing the electrode heart anchorage. In the atrium, further attempts were made to solve stability problems by positioning the electrode in a small vein terminating in the heart: the coronary sinus (Figure 28). Results, however, were not satisfying, as shown in Table 4, and this method is only used in exceptional cases. Thanks to active and passive fixation systems a remarkable decrease in dislocations was registered. Currently, the most widely used types are screw-in and tined leads. On the basis of our case studies, we drew survival curves for 447 ventricular screw-in leads, and for 200 ventricular tined leads (data provided at the beginning of our follow-up study).

The following complications were examined: dislocation, pacing failure and sensing failure (Figure 29). The incidence of displacements was reported to be lower than 5% and restricted to the first 12 months for both lead types. Sensing failure was similar in both cases. Only in pacing failure was a lower curve observed for screw-in leads, due to the occurrence of this complication up until the fifth year, while in tined leads it disappeared after one year. It is, however, impossible to establish with certainty that a greater incidence of pacing failure occurs in screw-in leads. As will subsequently be reported, it is other variables of the electrode that influence the stimulation threshold.

ELECTRODE

The average 5 volt output of the PM is accounted for by the need to have reserve energy in case the stimulation threshold increases. The output of the PM could be reduced by prolonging the generator life expectancy if a constantly low chronic stimulation threshold were obtained. This is clear because the electrodes have been the object of numerous investigations aimed at obtaining acute and chronic low threshold values. The increase in chronic stimulation threshold is directly proportional to the thickness of the fibrous capsule growing around the electrodes as a reaction to a foreign body, which is an inert tissue drawing the electrode away from the excitable tissue. Over the past few years investigations have been undertaken in five directions:

(1) Totally porous electrodes (Figure 30), which allow tissue to grow inside the electrode for the purpose of coupling a small stimulation surface with a large sensing surface (Figure 31), and which determine a reduction of the fibrous capsule.

(2) Electrodes with a metal microporous surface (Figure 32), for which the above-mentioned considerations hold true.

(3) Pyrocarbon electrodes with micropores (Figure 33) which, in addition to the previously described advantages, have a minimal polarization, thus making a greater amount of energy available for pacing.

(4) Black platinum with concentric circle electrodes (Figure 34). Black platinum has a microporous structure. Moreover, the presence of concentric circles provides a greater number of high current density sites as compared to a ring or cylinder-like morphology.

(5) Steroid eluting lead (Figure 35). Cortisone is a powerful anti-inflammatory drug that inhibits the growth of the fibrous capsule around the electrode.

Bobyn and coworkers [66] have observed in dogs the formation of a fibrous capsule significantly thinner in microporous surface electrodes (170 ± 59 μm) than in totally porous electrodes (297 ± 121 μm), $P < .025$. In the same cases, no differences were found in the acute stimulation threshold values, while the chronic stimulation threshold (30 weeks) was found to be lower by an average of 30% in electrodes with a microporous surface ($P < .0001$). As for the amplitude of the chronic endocardial electrogram, the microporous surfaced electrodes showed also an improvement in signal as compared to the implant (from 25.8 ± 8.5 mV to 27.0 ± 8.4 mV), with a slight increase in the sensing impedance (from 1.1 ± 0.1 kΩ to 1.2 ± 0.2 kΩ). On the contrary, an electrogram amplitude decrease was reported in totally porous electrodes (from 31.4 ± 6.1 mV to 25.1 ± 7.9 mV) with a concomitant increase in input impedance (from 0.9 ± 0.3 kΩ to 1.6 ± 0.5 kΩ). A comparative study between microporous Polycarbon and Platinum [67,68] has revealed a constantly lower threshold trend for the former. The Target TIP electrode (Figure 34), recently manufactured by MTD, has been of great interest for it presents extremely low acute and chronic threshold values (Figure 36) and may hopefully allow the PM output to be lowered in the near future. For the future, MDT has ushered in a new era in the generation of electrodes by designing a slow cortisone eluting electrode (Figure 35). The conception of an electrode has thus changed—from an inert component it has assumed a dynamic function. The experimental results [69,70] obtained in dogs have been very promising, since it was possible to maintain the stimulation threshold around 1 volt even in the chronic phase (Figure 36).

UNIPOLAR AND BIPOLAR SYSTEMS

The cardiac pacing may either be unipolar or bipolar. In both systems the cathode is represented by the lead tip, while the anode in the unipolar system is made up by the PM case, and in the bipolar system it is located along the lead, from 0.5 to 3 cm away from the cathode (Figure 37). When cardiac pacing came into being it was bipolar, but in time it has become unipolar (especially in European countries). This change has derived from the fact that it is easier to implant unipolar pacing leads, due to their being more thin and flexible.

The unipolar system, however, presents certain disadvantages as compared to the bipolar one in terms of the sensing function. In the former, in fact, the cathode and anode are separated by muscles which are sources of electrical potentials that, despite the filtration at the PM imput, may produce oversensing phenomena. However, since in the bipolar system the cathode and anode are located close to one another within the heart, more protection is assured against such phenomena (Figure 37). In the unipolar system oversensing is a rather widespread phenomenon which usually manifests itself during exercise when the muscles are in motion. At times, however, a simple arm movement may be sufficient to trigger it (Figure 38). Generally, this phenomenon produces symptoms in a small percent of the cases. In fact, the following two requirements must be fulfilled for symptomatic oversensing to occur:

(1) Oversensing must take place at a time when the spontaneous activity of the patient is not present.

(2) The cause having induced oversensing must be present long enough to produce the symptom.

However, when this problem cannot be solved by reprogramming the PM and a cause-effect relationship may be established between oversensing and symptoms, another operation must be performed in order to replace the electrode and/or the pacemaker (different passing band).

A bipolar system for picking up signals may not see the signal if its direction is perpendicular to the axis of the lead system. This does not occur if the system has a unipolar configuration (the anode being at a great distance). This was one of the most important arguments against bipolar leads over the past years. But if this is true in experimental situations, it would be very unlikely for it to occur in the heart. This is because the final depolarization vector is obtained by summing up several vectors that manifest themselves centrifugally, being projected from inside the heart towards the outside. Therefore, the following conditions should take place for the signal to be reduced to zero or to decrease significantly:

(1) All individual instantaneous activation vectors must be present along one single axis.

(2) This axis must be completely or almost completely perpendicular to that from which signals are picked up (and this is highly unlikely given the shape of the heart). In fact, Figure 39 shows that even signals of a different morphology, thus originating from different areas of the heart, are always easier to record from a bipolar lead than from a unipolar one. With regard to acute threshold values there is no difference between the unipolar and bipolar systems, except for the slew-rate of the endocavitary potential, which is reported to be considerably higher in the bipolar system (Table 5).

Another problem of unipolar systems is the anodic stimulation of pectoral muscle. This is not a common situation, but in some patients it may be a serious problem leading to reoperation. This problem does not happen with the bipolar system because the anode is inside the heart. Considering the current size of bipolar pacing leads, their better sensing function as compared to unipolar leads, the absence of muscle stimulation, and the essentially identical threshold values, it seems reasonable to expect that they will be used more extensively in the future. Their use will also be encouraged by a greater use of bicameral PM, since, theoretically, the bipolar system can more easily eliminate crosstalk problems (that is sensing in one chamber of the spike and/or evoked potential in the other chamber).

SINGLE PASS ATRIOVENTRICULAR LEAD

The factor lowering the number of bicameral PM implants is the need for the introduction of two leads (atrial and ventricular). In fact, it often is necessary to introduce the two leads by two separate veins. This lengthens implant time and makes it harder to position the electrodes in atrium and ventricle because they interfere with each other. Therefore, some authors [71,76] have investigated the feasibility of implanting a single pass atrioventricular

TABLE 5. Bipolar/Unipolar Acute Ventricular Data (in the Same Patient)

	Bipolar	Unipolar	P
Threshold (P.W. = .5 ms.) volts (26 pts.)	.64 +/− .2	.66 +/− .33	n.s.
Impedance (.5 ms./5 volts) ohms (28 pts.)	753 +/− 95	764 +/− 193	n.s.
Electrogram Amplitude millivolt (24 pts.)	6.5 +/− 3.1	6.8 +/− 3.6	n.s.
Slew-Rate m/ms (11 pts.)	1.25 +/− .69	.59 +/− .34	.005

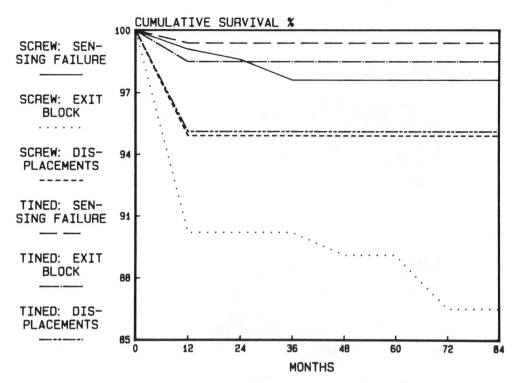

Figure 29. *Ventricular screw and tined leads (complications).*

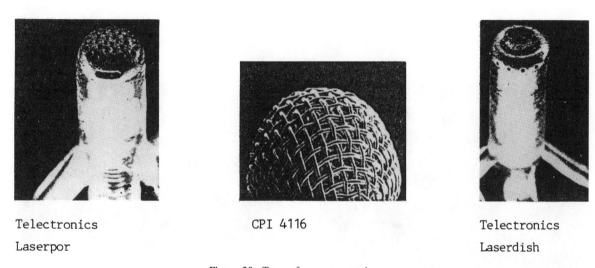

Telectronics   CPI 4116   Telectronics
Laserpor   Laserdish

Figure 30. *Types of macroporous tips.*

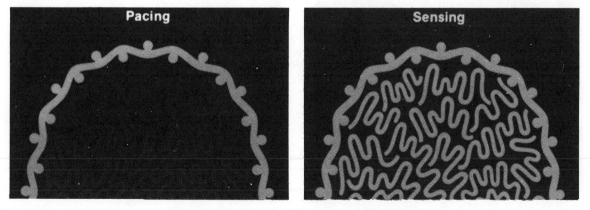

Figure 31. *Pacing and sensing surfaces of CPI 4ll6 lead.*

205

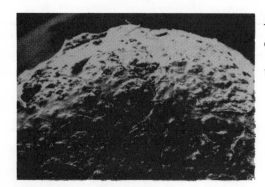

<u>Low--power view (110X).</u>

Growth of tissue into the

porous surface.

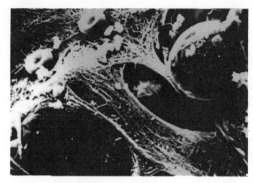

<u>High-power view (2200X).</u>

Mature fibrous connective

tissue with collagen bundles

in the interstices between

the metal spheres.

Figure 32. *Surface of Cordis Elgiloy porous. Surfaced tip.*

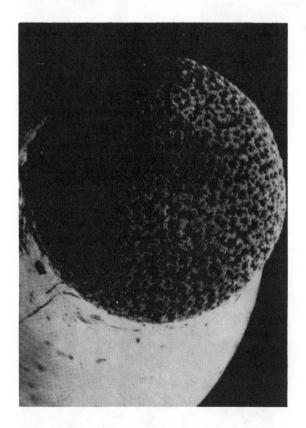

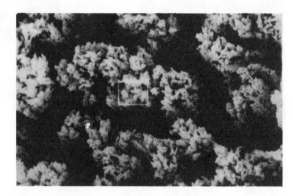

Magnification X 500

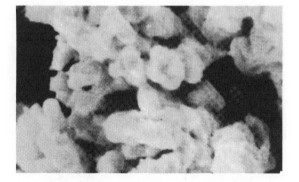

Magnification X 36

Magnification X 5000

Figure 33. *Surface of Sorin 580 pyrocarbon tip.*

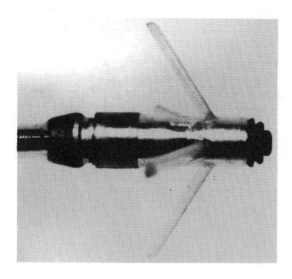
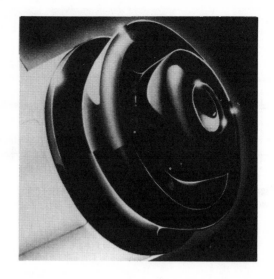

Figure 34. Surface of target tip Medtronic lead.

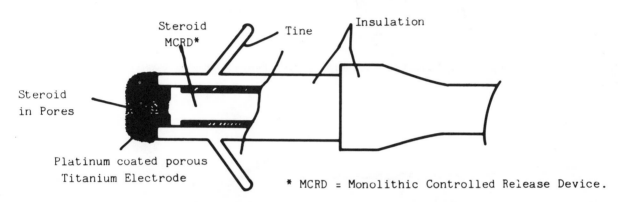

Steroid
MCRD*

Tine

Insulation

Steroid
in Pores

Platinum coated porous
Titanium Electrode

* MCRD = Monolithic Controlled Release Device.

Figure 35. The Medtronic steroid eluting lead.

THRESHOLD

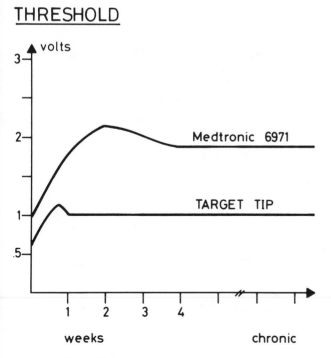

Medtronic 6971

TARGET TIP

Figure 36. Threshold values of target tip lead.

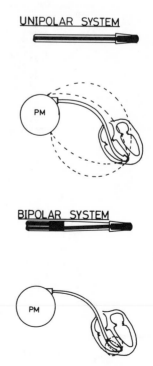

UNIPOLAR SYSTEM

BIPOLAR SYSTEM

Figure 37. Unipolar and bipolar cardiac pacing systems.

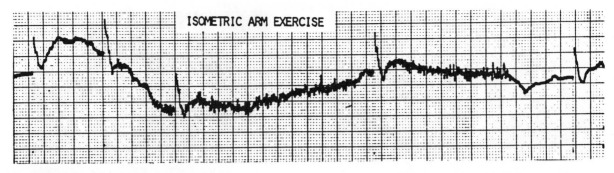

Figure 38. The artifacts in the long pause are due to isometric right arm exercise (pulse generator is right positioned), the myopotentials inhibit the PM.

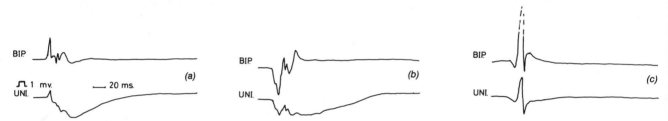

Figure 39. Three different waveforms from the same patient and from the same lead. Waveforms are simultaneously recorded by unipolar and bipolar mode.

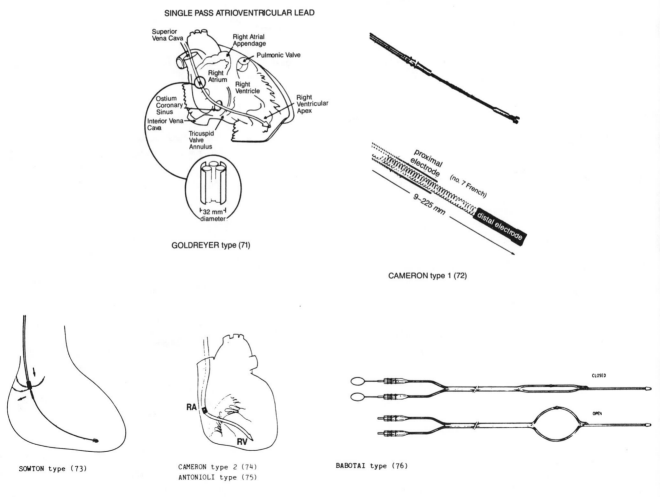

Figure 40. Different types of single pass atrioventricular leads.

lead for pacing and sensing of both atrium and ventricle (Figure 40). Atrial stability and atrio-ventricular electrodic distance are major problems. Atrial stability is necessary for atrial pacing. It was obtained by Bowton with a "crown of thorns" around the lead and by Babotai with preshaped spherical leads. The atrio-ventricular distance (the distance needed to assure the electrode stability) is variable in patients, especially in those with cardiac enlargment; therefore, Cameron [72] proposed the first type of single pass lead with a variable interelectrodic distance by shifting the ventricular lead into the atrial one. However, no definitive results have been obtained in this area.

The problem is easier to deal with when only the atrial sensing is needed. In this case the lead atrial stability can be neglected, and it is possible to obtain a good signal from a floating atrial lead as in the types used by Goldreyer [71] and Antonioli [75]. These leads have allowed the use of commercially available pacemakers for ventricular pacing triggered by atrial rate.

CONCLUSION

Despite some resistance towards wider use of bipolar pacing leads, it seems that use of such leads will nevertheless increase in the future. In fact, they make it possible to bypass anode-inhibition phenomena, anodic stimulation of the pectoral muscle, and diaphragmatic pacing—factors which represent the limits of the unipolar system.

There is still the question of single bicameral pacing leads, which, despite having been partially solved for cases requiring atrial sensing, still remains unanswered for cases in which atrial pacing is necessary. The introduction of this cardiac pacing lead would allow a greater use of bicameral pacemakers, but is seems reasonable to expect that progress in this field is linked to the improvements that will be made possible by new materials suitable for reducing the size of pacing leads. Currently, the materials that will most likely yield good results in the future are carbon in its pyrolitic form for the electrode surface, and graphite fibers for the conductor. These materials are being employed in order to reduce the amount of energy required by stimulation and to make the lead more stable in terms of conductor fracture. Silicone and polyurethane insulating sheaths have been shown to be reliable for cardiac pacing leads. To date there are no data establishing the superiority of one material over the other for long-term performance. Polyurethane allows the manufacture of thinner, stronger leads with less friction. With the improvement of the extrusion process, polyurethane would be the insulation material for the future.

ACKNOWLEDGEMENTS

The authors are very grateful to Mrs. L. Moreale and Mrs. M. Piantoni for secretarial assistance and to Dr. C. Fanizza for SEM technical assistance.

REFERENCES

1 GEBHARDT, U., W. Irnich, G. Bülles and J. Broichhausen. "Multistrand Pacemaker Leads—A Really Redundant System," in *Cardiac Pacing: Proceedings of the VIth World Symposium on Cardiac Pacing*, C. Meere, ed., Montreal:PACESYMP, chap. 29, p. 4 (1979).

2 CHISHOLM, A. W., J. R. Cameron, G. M. Froggatt and A. W. Harrison. "A New Long Life Cardiac Pacing Electrode," in *Cardiac Pacing: Electrophysiology and Pacemaker Technology*, G. A. Feruglio, ed., Padova:Piccin Medical Books, pp. 1111–1112 (1982).

3 UPTON, J. E. and J. Sydorenko. "Evaluation of Platinum Nickel and MP35N Tinsel Wire for Cardiac Pacemaker Leads," Assoc. for the Advancement of Medical Instrumentation (March 1976).

4 STOKES, K. and N. L. Stephenson. "The Implantable Cardiac Pacing Lead—Just A Simple Wire?" in *The Third Decade of Cardiac Pacing*, S. S. Barold and J. Mugica, eds., Mount Kisco, New York:Futura Publishing Company, p. 365 (1982).

5 UPTON, J. E. "New Pacing Lead Conductors," in *Cardiac Pacing: Proceedings of the VIth World Symposium on Cardiac Pacing*, C. Meere, ed., Montreal:PACESYMP, chap. 29, p. 6 (1979).

6 AMUNDSON, D. C. "Sensing Properties of Pacemaker Electrodes," *Proc. Eng. Med. Bio.*, pp. 17:83 (1975).

7 RABER, M. B., T. E. Cuddy and D. A. Israel. "Pacemaker Electrodes Act as High-Pass Filters on the Electrogram," in *Cardiac Pacing*, Amsterdam:Excerpta Medica, p. 506 (1977).

8 LIDEMANS, F. W. and J. J. Denier van der Gon. "Current Thresholds and Luminal Size in Excitation of Heart Muscle," *Cardiovasc. Res.*, 12:477 (1978).

9 IRNICH, W. and U. Gebhardt. "The Pacemaker-Electrode Combination and Its Relationship to Service Life," in *To Pace or Not to Pace, Controversial Subjects in Cardiac Pacing*, HJTh Thalen, ed., The Hague:Martinus Nijhoff, p. 209 (1978).

10 SINNAEVE, A., R. Willems and R. Stroobandt. "Requirements of the Ideal Pacemaker Lead," in *Pacemaker Leads*, A. E. Aubert, and H. Ector, eds., Amsterdam, pp. 47–55 (1985).

11 STOKES, K. "The Biostability of Polyurethane Leads," in *Modern Cardiac Pacing*, S. S. Barold, ed., Mount Kisco, N.Y.:Futura Publishing Company, pp. 173–198 (1985).

12 PARINS, D. J., M. Black, K. D. McCoy and N. J. Horvath. "In Vivo Degradation of a Polyurethane," *CPI*, 4:511 (1981).

13 PARINS, D. J., M. Black, K. D. McCoy and N. J. Horvath. "In Vivo Degradation of a Polyurethane: Further Evidence," *CPI*, 7:370 (1981).

14 WELTI, J. J. "STIMAREC Report of July 1982," *Pace*, 5:944 (1982).

15 BARBARO, V., C. Bosi, S. Caiazza, P. Chistolini, P. Dini, D. Ialongo, R. Di Mascolo, G. Messina, M. Rocchi and M. Santini. "Degradation of Polyurethane and Silicone Rubber Ventricular Leads," *Biomaterials in Artificial Organs*, J. P. Paul, J. D. S. Gaylor, J. M. Courtney and T. Gilchrist, eds., London:McMillan, 18:327–334 (1984).

16 STOKES, K. B., P. W. Urbanski, M. W. Davis and A. J. Coury. "Nine Years Human Experience with Polyurethane Leads," in *Pacemaker Leads*, A. E. Aubert and H. Ector, eds., Amsterdam pp. 279–286 (1985).

17 HELMQVIST, H. "Round Table Discussion: The Polyurethane Controversy," *Pace*, 6:460 (1983).

18 MCARTHUR, W. "Round Table Discussion: The Polyurethane Controversy," *Pace*, 6:460 (1983).

19 BARBARO, V., C. Bosi, S. Caiazza, P. Chistolini, D. Ialongo and A. Rosa. "Implant Effects on Polyurethane and Silicone Cardiac Pacing Leads in Humans: Insulation Measurements and SEM Observations," *Biomaterials*, 6:28–32 (1985).

18 McARTHUR, W. "Round Table Discussion: The Polyurethane Controversy," *Pace*, 6:460 (1983).

19 BARBARO, V., C. Bosi, S. Caiazza, P. Chistolini, D. Ialongo and A. Rosa. "Implant Effects on Polyurethane and Silicone Cardiac Pacing Leads in Humans: Insulation Measurements and SEM Observations," *Biomaterials*, 6:28–32 (1985).

20 VAN HEMEL, N. M., M. I. H. El Gamal, H. Bakema, P. Bijkerk and L. M. van Gelder. "Long-Term Results of Endocardial Atrial Electrode Employing Positive Fixation," in *Cardiac Pacing: Electrophysiology and Pacemaker Technology*, G. A. Feruglio, ed., Padova:Piccin Medical Books, pp. 627–630 (1982).

21 KASSAL, H., Th. Riss, H. G. Kern, F. Stellwag and A. Laczkovics. "Selection and Optimal Placement of Atrial Leads," in *Cardiac Pacing: Electrophysiology and Pacemaker Technology*, G. A. Feruglio, ed., Padova:Piccin Medical Books, pp. 637–638 (1982).

22 SABIN, G., G. Szurawitzki and H. H. Engel. "Reproduction of Postoperative Dislodgement Rate Using Atrial Leads," in *Cardiac Pacing: Electrophysiology and Pacemaker Technology*, G. A. Feruglio, ed., Padova:Piccin Medical Books, pp. 643–644 (1982).

23 GEDDES, J. S. "Atrial Transvenous Electrode Design," in *Cardiac Pacing: Proceedings of the VIth World Symposium on Cardiac Pacing*, C. Meere, ed., Montreal:PACESYMP, chap. 30, p. 1 (1979).

24 SMITH, N., L. Vasarhelyi, W. McNamara and G. Kakascik. "A Permanent Transvenous Atrial Electrode Catheter," *J. Thorac. Cardiovasc. Surg.*, 58:773 (1969).

25 KRUSE, I. M., L. Ryden and B. Ydse. "Electrophysiological Characteristics of a Transvenous Endocardial Atrial Lead," in *Cardiac Pacing: Proceedings of the VIth World Symposium on Cardiac Pacing*, C. Meere, ed., Montreal:PACESYMP, chap. 20, p. 4 (1979).

26 SANTINI, M., M. Rocchi, A. Alliegro, E. Adinolfi, L. Pandolfo and V. Masini. "Reliability of Screw-In Leads for Permanent Atrial Sensing and Pacing," in *Cardiac Pacing*, G. Feruglio, ed., Padova:Piccin Medical Books, pp. 631–635 (1982).

27 ZUCKER, I. R., V. Parsonnet and L. Gilbert. "A Method of Permanent Transvenous Implantation of an Atrial Electrode," *Am. Heart J.*, 85:195 (1973).

28 SMYTH, N. P. D. "Atrial Programmed Pacing," in *Cardiac Pacing: A Concise Guide to Clinical Practice*, P. Varriale and E. A. Naclerio, eds., Philadelphia:Lea & Febriger, pp. 169–184 (1979).

29 KRUSE, I., L. Ryden and B. Ydse. "Clinical and Electrophysiological Characteristics of a Transvenous Atrial Lead," *Br. Heart J.*, 42:595–602 (1979).

30 BERGDAHL, L. "Helifix, An Electrode Suitable for Transvenous Atrial and Ventricular Implantation," *J. Thorac. Cardiovasc. Surg.*, 80:794–799 (1980).

31 EL GAMAL, M. I. H., L. M. van Gelder, J. J. R. M. Bonnier and H. R. Michels. "Comparison of Transvenous Atrial Electrodes Employing Active (Helicoidal) and Passive (Tined J-Lead) Fixation in 120 Patients," in *Cardiac Pacing: Proceedings of the VIIth World Symposium on Cardiac Pacing*, K. Steinbach, ed., Darmstadt:Steinkopff Verlag, 341 (1983).

32 MESSENGER, J., M. Castellanet, N. Stephenson and S. Bernstein. "New Permanent Endocardial Atrial J-Lead: Implant Techniques and Clinical Performance," in *Cardiac Pacing: Electrophysiology and Pacemaker Technology*, G. A. Feruglio, ed., Padova:Piccin Medical Books, 1023 (1982).

33 JOSEPH, S. P. and J. White. "Permanent Atrial Pacing: Functional Characteristics of Coronary Sinus and Right Atrial Appendage Electrodes," in *Cardiac Pacing: Proceedings of the VIth World Symposium on Cardiac Pacing*, C. Meere, ed., Montreal:PACESYMP, chap. 20:6 (1979).

34 EL GAMAL, M. I. H. and L. M. van Gelder. "A New Transvenous Technique for Atrial Implantation of the Helifix Electrode," in *Cardiac Pacing: Proceedings of the VIth World Symposium on Cardiac Pacing*, C. Meere, ed., Montreal:PACESYMP, chap. 32:1 (1979).

35 KAPPENBERGER, L., I. Babotai, F. Siclari, L. Egloff and M. Turina. "Ventricular Lead in Atrial Position," in *Cardiac Pacing: Proceedings of the VIIth World Symposium on Cardiac Pacing*, K. Steinbach, ed., Darmstadt:Steinkopff Verlag, 331–334 (1983).

36 KAPPENBERGER, L., I. Babotai and M. Turina. "Modified Positioning of Helifix Transvenous Atrial Electrodes," in *Cardiac Pacing: Electrophysiology and Pacemaker Technology*, G. A. Feruglio, ed., Padova:Piccin Medical Books, 649–650 (1982).

37 KRUSE, I. B., L. Rydén and B. O. Ydse. "A New Lead for Transvenous Atrial Pacing and Sensing. Clinical and Electrophysiological Experiences," *PACE*, 3(4):395 (1980).

38 KLEINERT, M. P., H. R. Bartsch and K. G. Mühlenpfordt. "Comparative Studies of Ventricular and Atrial Stimulation Thresholds of Carbon-Tip Electrodes," in *Cardiac Pacing: Proceedings of the VIIth World Symposium on Cardiac Pacing*, K. Steinbach, ed., Darmstadt:Steinkopff Verlag, 353–360 (1983).

39 SCOTT MILLAR, R. N. and I. W. P. Obel. "Experience with Long-Term Atrial Pacing Via Coronary Sinus (CS) and Right Atrial Appendage," in *Cardiac Pacing: Electrophysiology and Pacemaker Technology*, G. A. Feruglio, ed., Padova:Piccin Medical Books, 659 (1982).

40 MOSS, A. J. and R. J. Rivers. "Atrial Pacing from the Coronary Vein: Ten-Year Experience in 50 Patients with Implanted Pervenous Pacemakers," *CIRCULATION*, 57(1):103 (1978).

41 GREENSBERG, P. and M. Castellanet. "Coronary Sinus Pacing: Clinical Follow-up," *CIRCULATION*, 57(1):98–102 (1978).

42 GOULD, L., C. V. R. Reddy, F. Maghazeh, G. Cifarelli, C. S. Shin Brevetti and S. Saadat. "Three Hundred and Fifty-Three Consecutive Patients with Permanent Transvenous Pacemakers," *PACE*, 3(4):452 (1980).

43 FURMAN, S., F. Panizzo and I. Campo. "Comparison of Active and Passive Leads for Endocardial Pacing—II," *PACE*, 4(1):78 (1981).

44 MUGICA, J., M. Rollet, B. Lazarus, L. Henry, R. Duconge, P. Laxenaire and M. T. Dubois. "Pacing Lead Performance: A Study of the Behaviour of 6,032 Leads Over a Period of Twelve Years," *Medtronom, Nr.*, 15:7 (1984).

45 DI COSTANZO, A., L. Cioffi, R. Giacobbe, F. Ferrara, A. Settembre and C. Varriale. "Comparison of Leads Complications with Polyurethane Tined, Silicone Rubber Tined, and Wedge Tip Leads: Clinical Experience with 2665 Ventricular Endocardial Leads," in *Cardiac Pacing*, F. P. Gomez, ed., Madrid:Editorial Grouz, p. 993 (1985).

46 BERMAN, N. D. and I. H. Lipton. "Early Clinical Experience with a Porous Tip Electrode," in *Cardiac Pacing: Proceedings of the VIth World Symposium on Cardiac Pacing*, C. Meere, ed., Montreal:PACESYMP, chap. 29, p. 10 (1979).

47 BERMAN, N. D., S. E. Dickson and I. H. Lipton. "Acute and Chronic Clinical Performance Comparison of a Porous and a Solid Electrode Design," *PACE*, 5(1):67 (1982).

48 PERRINS, E. J., R. Sutton, B. Kalebic, L. R. Rickards, C. Morley and B. Terpstra. "Modern Atrial and Ventricular Leads for Permanent Cardiac Pacing," *Br. Heart J.*, 46:196–201 (1981).

49 HOLMES, D. R., R. G. Nissen, J. D. Maloney, J. C. Broadbent and J. Merideth. "Transvenous Tined Electrode Systems. An Approach to Acute Dislodgement," *Mayo Clin. Proc.*, 54:219–222 (1979).

50 GOLDREYER, B. N., A. L. Olive, J. Leslie, D. S. Cannom and M. G. Wyman. "A New Orthogonal Lead for Psynchronous Pacing," *PACE*, 4:638–644 (1981).

51 MOND, H. and G. Sloman. "The Small-Tined Pacemaker Lead—Absence of Dislodgement," *PACE*, 3(2):171 (1980).

52 GOPAL RAO, M. D., F. I. C. S. "Experience with Trabeculae Lodging Endocardial Lead," in *Cardiac Pacing, Proceedings of the VIth World Symposium on Cardiac Pacing*, C. Meere, ed., Montreal:PACESYMP, chap. 31, p. 1 (1979).

53 HOLMES, D. R., J. D. Maloney, J. C. Broadbent, B. Gersh and J. Merideth. "Transvenous Tined Electrode Systems: An Approach to the Problem of Acute Dislodgement," in *Cardiac Pacing, Proceedings of the VIth World Symposium on Cardiac Pacing*, C. Meere, ed. Montreal:PACESYMP, chap. 31, p. 2 (1979).

54 GORDON, S., G. C. Timmis, R. G. Ramos, V. Gangadharan and J. Hauser. "Improved Transvenous Pacemaker Electrode Stability," in *Cardiac Pacing, Proceedings of the VIth World Symposium on Cardiac Pacing*, C. Meere, ed., Montreal:PACESYMP, chap. 31, p. 3 (1979).

55 ESTIOKO, M. R., E. Gomez, J. Camunas, R. M. Estioko, B. P. Mindich and R. A. Jurado. "Early Clinical Experience with a New Transvenous Tined Electrode Without Displacement," in *Cardiac Pacing, Proceedings of the VIth World Symposium on Cardiac Pacing*, C. Meere, ed., Montreal:PACESYMP. chap. 31. p. 4 (1979).

56 MEESE, E. H. and S. Esmaili. "Initial Clinical Experience with the Ventricular Tined Lead," in *Cardiac Pacing, Proceedings of the VIth World Symposium on Cardiac Pacing*, C. Meere, ed., Montreal:PACESYMP, chap. 31, p. 6 (1979).

57 GOULD, L., C. Patel, R. Betzu, C. Gopalaswamy and W. Becker. "Stability of Long-Term Thresholds When Utilizing Porous Tip Electrodes," *Clinical Progress in Electrophysiology and Pacing*, 3(5):365 (1985).

58 KERTES, P. J., H. G. Mond, J. K. Vohra, J. G. Sloman, C.-W. Kong and D. Hunt. "Comparison of Lead Complications with Polyurethane Tined, Silicone Rubber Tined, and Wedge Tip Ventricular Pacemaker Leads," in *Cardiac Pacing: Proceedings of the VIIth World Symposium on Cardiac Pacing*, K. Steinbach, ed., Darmstadt:Steinkopff Verlag, pp. 317–322 (1983).

59 SEQUEIRA, R. F., L. M. Clark and D. W. Barritt. "Endocardial Fixation Electrode for Permanent Cardiac Pacing," in *Cardiac Pacing, Proceedings of the VIth World Symposium on Cardiac Pacing*, C. Meere, ed., Montreal:PACESYMP, chap. 32, p. 3 (1979).

60 BOURDILLON, P. D. and A. F. Rickards. "Improved Electrode Stability with the Helifix Endocardial Fixation Electrode," in *Cardiac Pacing, Proceedings of the VIth World Symposium on Cardiac Pacing*, C. Meere, ed., Montreal:PACESYMP, chap. 32, p. 5 (1979).

61 DAHL, H. D., H. Lübbing, D. W. Behrenbeck, B. Schorne and H. Dalichau. "Clinical Experiences with Electrodes for Endocardial Implantation with Helically Coiled Tips," in *Cardiac Pacing: Electrophysiology and Pacemaker Technology*, G. A. Feruglio, ed., Padova:Piccin Medical Books, p. 1121 (1982).

62 BENNET, D., C. Bray, C. Ward, K. Shearer, V. Martin and C. Wemyss. "Comparison of Two Types of Active Fixation Electrode," in *Cardiac Pacing: Electrophysiology and Pacemaker Technology*, G. A. Feruglio, ed., Padova:Piccin Medical Books, p. 1129 (1982).

63 STENZL, W., K. H. Tscheliessnigg, D. Dacar, W. Hermann and F. Iberer. "Four Years Experience with the Bisping Transvenous Pacemaker Electrode," in *Cardiac Pacing: Proceedings of the VIIth World Symposium on Cardiac Pacing*, K. Steinbach, ed., Darmstadt:Steinkopff Verlag, pp. 327–432 (1983).

64 FURMAN, S., F. Panizzo and I. Capo. "Comparative Failure of Implantable Pronged and Standard Pacing Electrode," in *Cardiac Pacing, Proceedings of the VIth World Symposium on Cardiac Pacing*, C. Meere, ed., Montreal:PACESYMP, chap. 21, p. 5 (1979).

65 FIANDRA, O., W. Espasandin, H. A. Fiandra, D. Fiandra, F. Fernandez Barbieri and B. Erramun. "Self Fixation Electrode for Permanent Endocardial Stimulation: 10 Years Follow Up," in *Cardiac Pacing*, F. P. Gomez, ed., Madrid:Editorial Grouz, p. 1041 (1985).

66 BOBYN, J. D., G. J. Wilson, T. R. Mycyk, P. Klement, G. A. Tait, R. M. Pilliar and D. C. MacGregor. "Comparison of a Porous-Surfaced with a Totally Porous Ventricular Endocardial Pacing Electrode," *PACE*, 4(4):405 (1981).

67 BOCCADAMO, R., G. Altamura, S. Toscano, M. Pistolese, L. Cassingena and F. Lo Bianco. "Non Invasive Thresholds Follow-Up of Implanted Leads by Means of Special Radiofrequency Pacers: A Comparative Study on Activated Pyrocarbon Tip and Polished Platinum Tip Leads," Poster presented to the *VIIIth World Symposium on Cardiac Pacing, Vienna*, (May 1–5 1983).

68 LOCHAN, R., J. Hewson, V. J. Redding. "Acute, Subacute and Chronic Threshold Characteristics of Activated Carbon, Sintered and Platinum Tip Electrodes," Poster presented to *CARDIOSTIM*, (1984).

69 TIMMIS, G. C., S. Gordon, D. C. Westveer, J. R. Stewart, K. B. Stokes and J. R. Helland. "A New Steroid-Eluting Low Threshold Pacemaker Lead," in *Cardiac Pacing*, K. Steinbach, ed., Darmstadt:Steinkopff Verlag, p. 361 (1983).

70 STOKES, K. B., G. A. Bornzin and W. A. Wiebusch. "A Steroid-Eluting, Low-Threshold, Low-Polarizing Electrode," in *Cardiac Pacing: Proceedings of the VIIth World Symposium on Cardiac Pacing*, K. Steinbach, ed., Darmstadt:Steinkopff Verlag, p. 369 (1983).

71 OLIVE, A. L., B. N. Goldreyer, R. E. Brueske and D. C. Amundson. "A New Single Lead for Atrial Sensing and Ventricular Pacing," in *Cardiac Pacing: Electrophsiology and Pacemaker Technology*, G. A. Feruglio, ed., Padova:Piccin Medical Books, pp. 1101–1104 (1982).

72 CAMERON, J. R., A. W. Chisholm, A. W. Harrison and G. M. Froggatt. "A Multi-Purpose Pacing Electrode," in *Cardiac Pacing, Proceedings of the VIth World Symposium on Cardiac Pacing*, C. Meere, ed., Montreal:PACESYMP, chap. 29, p. 2 (1979).

73 SOWTON, E., J. Crick, R. J. Wainwright. "The Crown of Thorns: A Single Pass Electrode for Physiological Pacing," in *Cardiac Pacing: Electrophysiology and Pacemaker Technology*, G. A. Feruglio, ed., Padova:Piccin Medical Books, pp. 1089–1090 (1982).

74 CAMERON, J. R., A. W. Chisholm, A. W. Harrison and G. M. Groggatt. "A Single Catheter for All Modes of Pacing," in *Cardiac Pacing: Electrophysiology and Pacemaker Technology*, G. A. Feruglio, ed., Padova:Piccin Medical Books, pp. 1091–1092 (1982).

75 ANTONIOLI, G. E., G. Grassi, M. Marzaloni and S. Sermasi. "A New Implantable VDT Pacemaker Using a Single, Double-Electrode Catheter," in *Cardiac Pacing: Electrophysiology and Pacemaker Technology*, G. A. Feruglio, ed., Padova:Piccin Medical Books, pp. 1093–1100 (1982).

76 BABOTAI, I. and M. Turina. "New Atrio-Ventricular Electrode," in *Cardiac Pacing, Proceedings of the VIth World Symposium on Cardiac Pacing*, C. Meere, ed., Montreal:PACESYMP, chap. 29, p. 1 (1979).

77 van Gelder, L. M., M. I. H. El Gamal. "False Inhibition of an Atrial Demand Pacemaker Caused by an Insulation Defect in a Polyurethane Lead," *PACE*, 6(5 Part I):834–839 (1983).

78 Byrd, C. L., W. McArthur, K. Stokes, M. Sivina, W. Z. Yahr and J. Greenberg. "Implant Experience with Unipolar Polyurethane Pacing Leads," *PACE*, 6(5 Part I):868–882 (1983).

79 Fagg Sanford, C. "Self-Inhibition of an AV Sequential Demand (DVI) Pulse Generator Due to Polyurethane Lead Insulation Disruption," *PACE*, 6(5 Part I):840–844 (1983).

80 Parsonnet, V., R. Werres, T. Atherley and J. Cort. "Clinical Experience with 500 Polyurethane Insulated Pacemaker Leads," (abstract 244) *PACE* 6:A-66 (1983).

81 Welti, J. J. and J. F. Godin. "STIMAREC Report of March, April 1984," *PACE*, 7(4):773 (1984).

82 Raymond, R. D. and K. B. Nanian. "Insulation Failure with Bipolar Polyurethane Pacing Leads," *PACE*, 7(3 Part I):378 (1984).

83 Hanson, J. S. "Sixteen Failures in a Single Model of Bipolar Polyurethane-Insulated Ventricular Pacing Lead: A 44-Month Experience," *PACE*, 7(3 Part I):389 (1984).

84 Pirzada, F. A., J. Seltzer, H. Leach and P. Small. "Clinical Experience with the Medtronic 6971 Polyurethane Lead," *PACE*, 6(3 Part III):252 (1983).

CHAPTER 12

In Vitro Assessment of Prosthetic Graft Thrombogenic Potential

S. J. SHEEHAN, M.D., FRCSI,[1]
S. M. RAJAH, M.D., FRCP,[1]
and **R. C. KESTER, M.D., Ch.M., FRCS**[1]

ABSTRACT: The use of thrombogenic prosthetic materials in arterial bypass surgery has important implications for the long-term patency of these grafts. The assessment of this property outside of the clinical situation is difficult. We have used an artificial circulation to assess the thrombogenic potential of prosthetic grafts and the modification of this property by pharmacological manipulation of platelets or by altering the characteristics of the graft itself. We have found that the system produces results which are consistent and where available, are supported by clinical studies.

INTRODUCTION

Since the introduction of the tubed fabric prosthesis by Voorhees and his colleagues [1] 35 years ago, vast improvements have been made and various materials, techniques and modifications have undergone rigorous testing, many of them failing to achieve a satisfactory standard. It is noteworthy that Dacron and Teflon emerged as the most promising materials at that time [2,3] and continue as the most commonly used materials for the construction of synthetic prostheses to the present day.

Synthetic grafts have functioned well in aorto-iliac bypass surgery, but distal to the inguinal ligament nothing as yet has proved itself superior to autologous tissue [4]. All synthetic materials have some degree of thrombogenic potential, and several investigators have attempted to modify this property. The recognition of the importance of electrical charge in influencing graft patency [5] led to efforts to alter it by coating the graft with carbon [6]. Prevention of thrombus formation by the use of heparin bonding has also been studied [7]. None of these modifications appears to have influenced prosthesis behavior, and therefore none has gained clinical acceptance.

Knitted Dacron grafts possess many of the properties of the ideal prosthesis. Their porosity allows ease of handling, luminal adherence of the fibrin coagulum and the potential for tissue ingrowth, which hopefully will lead to a healed pseudointima. However, this permeability may increase blood loss in systemically heparinised patients, and therefore, these grafts must be preclotted before implantation.

The ability of Dacron to attract platelets, together with whole blood preclotting, causes deposition of activated platelets and thrombin formation which may give rise to intraluminal clotting [8]. This process may be further complicated by the detachment of the luminal layer when subjected to arterial pressure, resulting in distal embolisation. Various techniques have been developed to seal these grafts. The most commonly used techniques are single stage methods in which grafts are flushed with, or immersed in, unheparinised blood. Experience shows that these methods are unsatisfactory in terms of graft sealing and often result in the development of septae or luminal clots. The ensuing graft haemorrhage may be troublesome, increasing operating time and the need for blood transfusion. The increased thrombogenicity of grafts preclotted in this manner may be of importance in low flow, narrow caliber prostheses. The introduction of a four stage preclotting technique may overcome these problems by producing an impervious hypothrombogenic flow surface [9].

The apparent failure of modern grafts to eliminate platelet deposition has led to an interest in antiplatelet therapy. The complex process of platelet aggregation may be manipulated by a wide range of drugs. The most commonly used form of treatment is the combination of aspirin and dipyridamole. However, this regimen is asso-

[1]Cardiac Research Unit, Killingbeck Hospital and Vascular Unit, St. James's University Hospital, Leeds, U.K.

ciated with significant side effects and intolerance in up to 30% of patients [10]. Furthermore, there remains considerable debate regarding the optimum aspirin dosage required to maximize antiplatelet activity without inducing adverse effects in the patient. As an irreversible cyclooxygenase inhibitor, by its broad action, aspirin also reduces endothelial cell prostacyclin production, and this factor may be of importance in the development of intimal thickening in vein grafts [11]. These unwanted effects of aspirin have given impetus to the search for alternative antiplatelet drugs.

Assessment of platelet–prosthetic surface interactions and their modification remains difficult. Clinical studies have the disadvantage of requiring a large number of subjects and taking several years to produce meaningful results. There remains the possibility that the methods, materials and drugs used will fail to show any benefit at the end of such studies, possibly to the detriment of the participating patients. Animal studies may also be unsatisfactory due to interspecies differences in platelet, graft and endothelial cell function [12].

Therefore, we have used an artificial circulation to assess differences in many types and makes of vascular prostheses. This technique has also been utilized to study the effect of antiplatelet agents on graft–platelet interactions, both in the standard treatment regimens and in dose-ranging studies. Finally, methods of graft preclot-ting have been compared in their ability to reduce platelet deposition and activation.

MATERIALS AND METHODS

The perfusion circuit used, which is a modification of Chandler's tube [13], has been described previously [14]. Fresh heparinised human blood is pumped through twin circuits, each incorporating the test grafts (Figure 1). In the earlier experiments, one of these circuits acted as control, comprising medical grade silicone tubing throughout. Subsequently, as studies showed that there were no significant changes in haematological, biochemical or platelet parameters, the control circuit was eliminated and grafts could be compared in parallel.

Four hundred and fifty ml of blood were collected from normal, healthy volunteers into heparin bags (Fenwall Ltd.), giving a heparin concentration of 4 iu/ml of blood. Where graft properties alone were to be evaluated, donors had not taken any antiplatelet therapy in the preceding two weeks. The heparinised blood was tested for normal platelet count and aggregation and then divided into two equal volumes so that both circuits could run simultaneously. The blood, at a temperature of 37°C, was perfused through the circuits at a rate of 140 ml/minute and a pressure of 120/90 mmHg for one hour. These haemo-

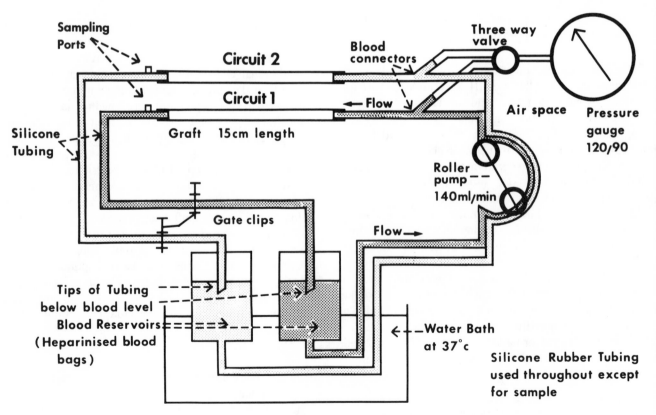

Figure 1. Schematic representation of the artificial circulation.

dynamics match the pressure and flow characteristics of the superficial femoral artery [15]. Initially, Dacron grafts were preclotted with human fibrinogen (4 g/l) using bovine thrombin solution (15 iu/ml), and then flushed with heparinised saline (100 iu/ml) for ten minutes to neutralise all excess thrombin. In all studies, platelet count and aggregation were performed at 15 minute intervals during perfusion. Blood gases, pH, plasma haemoglobin and full blood count were measured at the start and end of each study. After one hour, the grafts were flushed with 250 ml saline, fixed in 0.5% phosphate buffered glutaraldehyde (pH 7.4) for 24 hours and divided into one centimeter lengths. Comparable sections of each graft were then prepared by standard technique and examined in a Jeol T20 scanning electron microscope. To measure differences seen on scanning electron microscopy (SEM), field counts of adherent platelets were made of representative micrographs at similar magnification.

In latter studies, as differences in graft thrombogenicity became less apparent, we introduced indium-111 oxine platelet labelling. Forty millilitres of blood were taken from the same donors or Group O volunteers and the centrifuged platelets were then labelled with 100 mCi indium-111 and added to the circulating blood in the circuits. Blood radioactivity was recorded at the start and end of each experiment, and from the fall in radioactivity during perfusion we were able to determine the percentage platelet consumption. Before the graft sections underwent SEM, radioactivity counts were measured in a Phillips PW4580 automatic gammacounter. From the data obtained from both the graft and blood radioactivity, we were able to derive a graft activity index (GAI), defined as the ratio of the mean graft radioactivity to that in the blood.

The experiments can be divided into two groups. First are those comparing the thrombogenicity of commercially available grafts. In this group there are 3 studies evaluating a total of ten grafts: (a) woven Dacron (USCI Debakey), PTFE (Gore-tex) and glutaraldehyde-treated human femoral artery [14]; (b) plain knitted Dacron (Meadox Cooley), knitted double velour Dacron (Meadox Microvel), filamentous external velour Dacron (USCI Sauvage Filamentous) and a plain knitted Dacron graft with a pyrolytic carbon coating (Meadox Carboknit) [16]; and, (c) medium porosity knitted double velour Dacron (Vascutek VP1200), low porosity knitted double velour Dacron (Vascutek Triaxial) and a knitted double velour Dacron (Meadox Microvel) [17].

Second are those assessing modification of thrombogenic potential, either by antiplatelet agents or by preclotting. The latter experiment compares the effect of whole blood preclotting on Dacron graft thrombogenicity using a single stage method and the four step multistage autofibrinisation technique described by Yates and his colleagues in 1978 [9]. Grafts were preclotted by blood

donated by young, healthy volunteers and then perfused with ABO and Rhesus compatible heparinised blood [18].

Two sets of drug studies have been performed. In the first set, both in vitro and ex vivo controlled experiments were carried out [19]. The in vitro investigation entailed adding acetylsalicylic acid (ASA), diphyridamole (DPM), sulphinpyrazone (SPZ), or a combination of ASA/DPM at therapeutic concentrations to blood donated by 18 volunteers. The experiment was repeated ex vivo using blood donated by 6 volunteers after each had taken one of the following for one week: (a) no drug, (b) ASA, 300 mg three times a day, (c) DPM, 100 mg four times a day, (d) sulphinpyrazone, 200 mg four times a day, (e) ASA, 300 mg plus DPM 75 mg three times a day. Treatments were separated by a minimum interval of two weeks. The second drug study was of a randomized, double blind, crossover design in which 10 volunteers received placebo or indobufen (200 mg twice daily) for one week with a seven day washout period between treatments [20].

RESULTS

In all studies, blood gases, pH, haemoglobin and plasma haemoglobin remained unchanged during perfusion. Where control circuits were utilized, a decrease in platelet count and aggregation was noted, but the differences between the start and end of perfusion were not found to be significant.

Group I

In the graft versus graft comparisons of thrombogenicity, platelet function studies were found to be most useful where there were wide differences in graft type as shown in Study I (Table I). The results indicate that woven Dacron grafts retained more of the platelets than either Goretex or human femoral artery ($p < 0.02$).

The second experiment of this group, comparing four types of Dacron graft, shows that changes in platelet function were greatest in the filamentous external velour graft and least in the pyrolytic carbon coated prosthesis. However, these changes were not statistically significant. Assessment of scanning electron micrographs by field counts (Table 2) shows significantly greater deposition of activated platelets on the luminal surface of the filamentous prosthesis in comparison with the other grafts tested in this study ($p < 0.01$).

In comparing the three types of knitted double velour Dacron grafts, we found that there was no difference in platelet count or aggregation between any of the prostheses (Table 1). Similarly, these grafts were found to have equal thrombogenicity when assessed by isotope studies and luminal field counts.

TABLE 1. Group I: Changes in Platelet Function During Perfusion

	Platelet Count × 10⁹/1		Platelet Aggregation % Light Transmission	
	Pre	Post	Pre	Post
Study 1 [14] *Various Grafts*				
Woven dacron	195 ± 19	143 ± 11	41 ± 2	18 ± 2
PTFE	216 ± 20	178 ± 18	38 ± 4	23 ± 2
HFA	208 ± 10	163 ± 9	38 ± 2	40 ± 4
Study 2 [16] *Knitted Dacron*				
Double velour	132 ± 12	128 ± 8	78 ± 3	60 ± 9
Plain knitted	229 ± 24	142 ± 13	78 ± 3	63 ± 8
Filamentous Velour	178 ± 19	97 ± 4	73 ± 4	43 ± 10
Carbon coated	195 ± 17	148 ± 17	73 ± 4	78 ± 7
Study 3 [17] *Double Velour Dacron*				
Triaxial	183 ± 6	137 ± 9	68 ± 4	57 ± 1
VP1200	172 ± 13	133 ± 8	68 ± 1	56 ± 2
Microvel	170 ± 13	129 ± 11	72 ± 2	60 ± 2

All values are mean ± s.e.m.

Group II

In the preclotting study, there was a fall in both platelet count and aggregation during perfusion in each of the preclotting methods tested (Table 3). This occurred in both of the grafts but the changes were not found to be significant. The isotope studies (Table 4) demonstrated higher platelet consumption by those grafts preclotted by the single step method in both Bionit II and Triaxial, and for both of these grafts this difference was significant at the 5% level. The graft activity index, indicating deposition of labelled platelets on the luminal surface of these grafts, was also found to be significantly higher in those grafts prepared by the single stage technique. For Bionit

II, $p < 0.01$, and for Triaxial, $p < 0.001$. These differences found in the isotope studies were subsequently confirmed by luminal field counts of scanning electron micrographs (Table 4).

The micrograph of the single stage preclotted graft (Figure 2) illustrates the difference by showing a poor luminal surface with exposed graft fibres. Numerous clumps of deposited platelets can also be seen lying between the graft fibres. In comparison, the four step preclotted graft (Figure 3) shows a smooth fibrin base with markedly less platelet deposition.

Evaluating the anti-thrombotic activity of aspirin, dipyridamole and sulphinpyrazone in the in vitro study (Table 3, Study 2), we found that ASA and SPZ sig-

TABLE 2. Group I: Assessment of Platelet Deposition on Grafts

	Isotope Studies		
	GAI	Platelet Consumption	Scanning E.M. Cts/hp field
Study 2 [16] *Knitted Dacron*			
Double velour	not performed		126 ± 15
Plain knitted	not performed		110 ± 6
Filamentous velour	not performed		490 ± 33
Carbon coated	not performed		84 ± 10
Study 3 [17] *Double Velour Dacron*			
Triaxial	2.9 ± 1.1	23 ± 6	159 ± 11
VP1200	3.2 ± 1.3	16 ± 4	157 ± 14
Microvel	3.9 ± 1.2	19 ± 5	163 ± 7

All values are mean ± s.e.m.

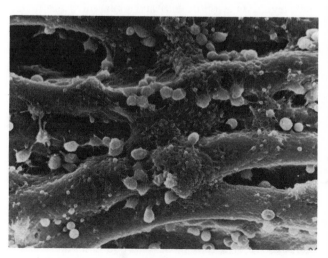

Figure 2. *Single stage preclotted graft (SEM × 750).*

TABLE 3. Group II: Changes in Platelet Function During Perfusion

	Platelet Count × 10⁹/1		Platelet Aggregation % Light Transmission	
	Pre	Post	Pre	Post
Study 1 [18]				
Preclotting Study				
Bionit II				
Single stage	210 ± 16	186 ± 14	75 ± 3	69 ± 3
Four stage	205 ± 14	173 ± 13	77 ± 4	70 ± 2
Triaxial				
Single stage	175 ± 13	175 ± 13	75 ± 3	71 ± 3
Four stage	162 ± 11	159 ± 2	79 ± 4	74 ± 4
Study 2 [19]				
Drug Study I				
(In vitro)				
Aspirin	242 ± 12	213 ± 14	44 ± 9	29 ± 8
Dipyridamole	208 ± 11	166 ± 9	55 ± 15	47 ± 14
Sulphinpyrazone	212 ± 7	174 ± 8	48 ± 12	28 ± 4
(Ex vivo)				
Control	226 ± 12	177 ± 14	84 ± 6	67 ± 13
Aspirin (ASA)	222 ± 10	204 ± 10	41 ± 6	43 ± 7
Dipyridamole (DPM)	233 ± 11	196 ± 10	67 ± 6	64 ± 9
Sulphinpyrazone	229 ± 8	185 ± 8	67 ± 5	58 ± 4
ASA/DPM	212 ± 9	189 ± 7	50 ± 10	62 ± 14
Study 3 [20]				
Drug Study II				
Placebo	236 ± 15	218 ± 17	69 ± 3	64 ± 4
Indobufen	215 ± 9	204 ± 9	56 ± 4	43 ± 6

All values are mean ± s.e.m.

nificantly reduced platelet aggregation ($p < 0.05$). Dipyridamole alone was ineffective. A single control donation was evaluated for each volunteer in the ex vivo experiment, and the test results were each compared against this common control. Again, aspirin significantly inhibited platelet aggregation ($p < 0.05$). A comparable

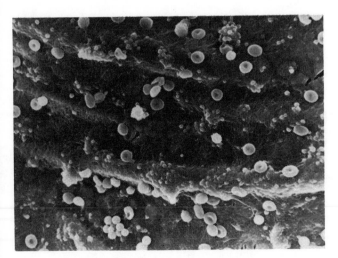

Figure 3. *Four stage preclotted graft (SEM × 750).*

result was achieved by the combination of aspirin and dipyridamole, while DPM alone and SPZ had little effect on aggregation.

Assessing platelet deposition by scanning electron microscopy, aspirin in combination with dipyridamole in the ex vivo study, and alone in both studies, was found to limit platelet deposition when compared with the control groups ($p < 0.001$). Blood from volunteers treated with dipyridamole was also found to inhibit platelet deposition ($p < 0.05$). Grafts from the SPZ experiments were found to have a similar appearance to those of the control groups.

In comparing the ability of indobufen to inhibit platelet activation, we found that there was a significant fall in platelet count in the placebo group ($p < 0.05$). This fall was not observed in the indobufen group. Indobufen was also found to significantly inhibit platelet aggregation prior to perfusion ($p < 0.02$). While platelet consumption was significantly higher in the grafts perfused with blood from the placebo group, the graft activity index in this study did not show a significant difference between the groups (Table 4). This may be a reflection of technical difficulties encountered in this experiment while introducing the labelled platelet technique to ex vivo studies.

TABLE 4. Group II: Assessment of Platelet Deposition on Grafts

	Isotope Studies		Scanning E.M. Cts/hp field
	GAI	Platelet Consumption	
Study 1 [18]			
Preclotting Study			
Bionit II			
Single stage	3.1 ± 0.7	14 ± 2	136 ± 12
Four stage	1.9 ± 0.5	7 ± 2	73 ± 7
Triaxial			
Single stage	2.6 ± 0.3	7 ± 2	126 ± 9
Four stage	1.5 ± 0.3	3 ± 1	62 ± 4
Study 2 [19]			
Drug Study I			
(In vitro)			
Control	not performed		280 ± 17
Aspirin	not performed		128 ± 10
Dipyridamole	not performed		216 ± 15
Sulphinpyrazone	not performed		191 ± 12
(In vitro)			
Control	not performed		250 ± 11
Aspirin (ASA)	not performed		73 ± 8
Dipyridamole (DPM)	not performed		145 ± 8
Sulphinpyrazone	not performed		181 ± 15
ASA/DPM	not performed		72 ± 8
Study 3 [20]			
Drug Study II			
Placebo	0.6 ± 0.1	13 ± 2	68 ± 7
Indobufen	0.5 ± 0.1	6 ± 1	42 ± 10

All values are mean ± s.e.m.

Luminal field counts in this study show a significant difference in the numbers of deposited platelets ($p < 0.01$) (Table 4).

Scanning electron microscopy of the luminal surface of the grafts in the placebo group demonstrated widespread deposition of activated platelets, with platelets displaying loss of the normal disc shape and the development of pseudopodia and cytoplasmic bridging (Figure 4). In comparison, grafts in the indobufen treated group show considerably less platelet deposition, with few platelets demonstrating significant morphological changes (Figure 5).

DISCUSSION

Prosthetic grafts have a thrombogenic potential which, by itself, influences graft patency while other factors such as surgical technique and distal run-off also play a major role. The selection of a suitable graft is vital to the success of the procedure and possibly limb survival. Platelet–graft interactions are unlikely to lead to graft occlusion in the absence of other predisposing factors in areas of high flow rates as in the aorta. However, in narrow caliber, low flow areas, platelet deposition on the graft itself may result in early graft occlusion or the formation of neointimal fibrous hyperplasia.

There is no optimal prosthetic material, and even the best material does not approach the long-term patency of autologous tissue, making adequate testing essential. Over the past eleven years, we have found that the artificial circulation, although clearly limited in its comparison to the clinical setting, provides a convenient model to study prosthetic graft interactions. The circuit itself does not exert any significant effect, either haematologically or biochemically, on the circulating blood [16,20,21]. The actual mechanics of the circuit are simple and straightforward and exclude any complicating factors such as flow restriction through the graft or occlusion of an anastomosis.

In assessing the effect of antiplatelet therapy on platelet activation and deposition by the grafts, we have found that platelet function studies and scanning electron micros-

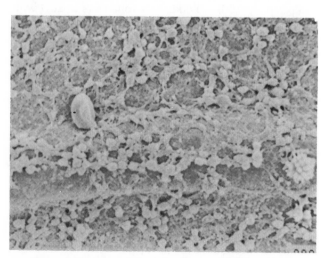

Figure 4. *Dacron graft from placebo group (SEM × 2000).*

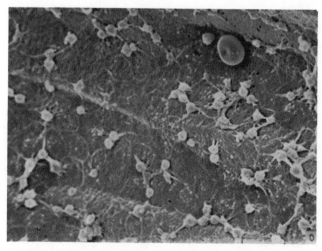

Figure 5. *Dacron graft from indobufen group (SEM × 2000).*

copy are sufficient to indicate whether a drug should be considered for clinical testing. In measuring differences between graft types, the situation becomes more complicated and requires the use of further indices of platelet activation, as in the recent studies where we have employed indium-111 labelling of platelets. The use of Indium-oxine has been shown to be a very satisfactory label, firstly on account of its high uptake and secondly as it is tightly bound in the platelet, release only occurring following cell membrane lysis [22]. Platelet labelling with indium-111 is used in clinical practice and has been shown to be accurate in identifying areas of increased platelet uptake [23].

These studies demonstrate that there is probably no difference in the thrombogenic potential of the various grafts commonly used. Hence, the selection of one over the others may be for other reasons, such as cost and ease of handling. The value of the artificial circulation has been confirmed to a large extent by the results of clinical studies. The experiments have shown that thrombogenicity may be modified, in the earlier stages at least, by differences in the preclotting technique. While the four stage preclotting technique seals knitted Dacron grafts, the use of heparinised blood in the technique significantly reduces graft thrombogenicity. The excellent short-term results achieved by Mosley and Marston in Dacron femoropopliteal bypass, without the use of antiplatelet therapy, may well be attributable to the use of this method [24].

PTFE grafts are the least thrombogenic prostheses in current general use, and their superiority to other prostheses has been demonstrated by some very good long-term patency rates [25,26]. The carbon-coated Dacron graft did not live up to its expectations, as shown in these studies, and was subsequently withdrawn due to technical difficulties in achieving an even carbon coating.

The experiments on aspirin, dipyridamole and sulphinpyrazone were performed to study the efficacy of drugs in reducing platelet activation. Several studies now attest to the usefulness of aspirin and dipyridamole in reducing the risk of graft failure, both synthetic and vein [27–32]. While sulphinpyrazone was found to alter platelet function, it was ineffective in reducing deposition of platelets on the grafts. It has been subsequently shown that sulphinpyrazone does limit platelet deposition on Dacron grafts implanted in humans [33]. As yet, there are only short-term studies available to support the use of indobufen [34,35], but we have found it effective in reducing platelet deposition. If found to be as effective as the combination of aspirin and dipyridamole in current clinical trials—it may well replace them on the grounds of tolerability.

The continuing search for the "ideal" nonthrombogenic prothesis demands accurate assessment of the material in the preclinical period. The artificial circuit can be used to predict how a graft will perform without the additional technical factors associated with implantation. It is likely that antiplatelet therapy will be required for the forseeable future, and the role of pharmacological manipulation of platelet–graft interaction will need further study. More specific intervention in the arachidonic acid metabolic pathway may well hold the key to future progress through the use of prostacyclin and its analogues or thromboxane synthetase inhibitors. The artificial circulation could, with minor modifications, be developed as a model to study the effects of these vascular prostaglandins on the platelet release reaction in graft–platelet interactions.

ACKNOWLEDGEMENTS

We are grateful to the National Heart Research Fund for its financial support in these projects. Thanks are also due to our Research Fellows over the years and to M. J. Crow, S. Puri and A. B. Latif for their expert technical assistance.

REFERENCES

1 VOORHEES, A. B., A. Jaretzki and A. H. Blakemore. "The Use of Tubes Constructed from Vinyon 'N' Cloth in Bridging Arterial Defects," *Ann. Surg.*, 135:332 (1952).

2 DETERLING, R. A. and S. B. Bhonslay. "An Evaluation of Synthetic Materials and Fabrics Suitable for Blood Vessel Replacement," *Surgery*, 38:71 (1955).

3 CREECH, O., R. A. Deterling, S. Edwards, O. C. Julian, R. R. Linton and H. Schumaker. "Vascular Prostheses. Report of the Committee for the Study of Vascular Surgery," *Surgery*, 41:62 (1957).

4 WEISEL, R. D., K. W. Johnston, R. J. Baird, A. D. Drezner, T. K. Oates and I. H. Lipton. "Comparison of Conduits for Leg Revascularization," *Surgery*, 89:8 (1981).

5 SAWYER, P. N., K. T. Wu, S. A. Wesolowski, W. H. Brattain and P. J. Boddy. "Long-Term Patency of Solid Wall Vascular Prostheses," *Arch. Surg.*, 91:735 (1965).

6 SHARP, W. V., D. L. Gardner, G. J. Andresen and J. Wright. "Electrolour: A New Vascular Interface," *Trans. Am. Soc. Artif. Intern. Organs*, 14:73 (1968).

7 HUFNAGEL, C. A. and P. W. Conrad. "A New Approach to Aortic Valve Replacement," *Ann. Surg.*, 167:791 (1968).

8 SALZMAN, E. W. "Nonthrombogenic Surfaces: Critical Review," *Blood*, 38:509 (1971).

9 YATES, S. G., A. A. B. Barros D'Sa, K. Berger, L. G. Fernandez, S. J. Wood, E. A. Rittenhouse, C. C. Davis, P. B. Mansfield and L. R. Sauvage. "The Preclotting of Porous Arterial Prostheses," *Ann. Surg.*, 188:611 (1978).

10 The Persantin-Aspirin Reinfarction Study Research Group. "Persantin and Aspirin in Coronary Heart Disease," *Circulation*, 62:449 (1980).

11 MURDAY, A. J., A. H. Gershlick, Y. D. Syndercombe-Court, P. G. Mills and C. T. Lewis. "Intimal Thickening in Autogenous Vein Grafts in Rabbits: Influence of Aspirin and Dipyridamole," *Thorax*, 39:457 (1984).

12 CLAGETT, C. P. "In Vivo Evaluation of Platelet Reactivity with Vascular Prostheses," in *Biologic and Synthetic Vascular Prostheses*, J. C. Stanley, ed. New York:Grune and Stratton, Inc., pp. 131–151 (1982).

13 CHANDLER, A. B. "In Vitro Thrombotic Coagulation of the Blood," *Lab. Invest.*, 7:110 (1958).

14 HAMLIN, G. W., S. M. Rajah, M. J. Crow and R. C. Kester. "Evaluation of the Thrombogenic Potential of Three Types of Arterial Graft Studied in an Artificial Circulation," *Br. J. Sug.*, 65:272 (1978).

15 DEDICHEN, H. and K. F. Kordt. "Blood Flow in Normal Human Ileo-femoral Arteries Studied with Electromagnetic Technique," *Acta Chir. Scand.*, 140:371 (1974).

16 DEACON, P., M. J. Crow, S. M. Rajah and R. C. Kester. "Comparison of the Thrombogenicity of Four Types of Knitted Dacron Arterial Graft in an Artificial Circulation," *Biomaterials*, 6:64 (1985).

17 COURTNEY, D. F., M. J. Crow, J. B. Fozard, S. M. Rajah and R. C. Kester. "The Thrombogenic Potential of Dacron Prostheses Investigated in an Artificial Circulation Using Indium (^{111}In)–Labelled Platelets," in *Recent Advances in Vascular Grafting: Proceedings of the International Symposium Held at the Catholic University in Nijmegen, the Netherlands, April 26–28, 1984*, S. H. Skotnicki, F. G. M. Buskens and H. H. M. Reinaerts, eds. England:System 4 Associates, pp. 91–96 (1985).

18 SHEEHAN, S. J., S. M. Rajah and R. C. Kester. "The Effect of Preclotting on the Porosity and Thrombogenicity of Knitted Dacron Grafts," *Biomaterials*, 10:75 (1989).

19 MCCOLLUM, C. N., M. J. Crow, S. M. Rajah and R. C. Kester. "Antithrombotic Therapy for Vascular Prosthesis: An Experimental Model Testing Platelet Inhibitory Drugs," *Surgery*, 87:668 (1980).

20 SHEEHAN, S. J., J. R. T. Monson, M. C. P. Salter, D. S. Rajah, S. M. Rajah and R. C. Kester. "The Effect of Indobufen on the Thrombogenic Potential of Dacron Prostheses in an Artificial Circulation," *Eur. J. Vasc. Surg.*, 2:223 (1988).

21 RAJAH, S. M., M. J. Crow, G. W. Hamlin and R. C. Kester. "Evaluation of the Thrombo-Resistant Properties of Arterial Grafts in an Artificial Circulation," *Thromb. Res.*, 12:141 (1977).

22 HAWKER, R. J., C. E. Hall, M. Goldman and C. N. McCollum. "Loss of Indium from Labelled Platelets by Ex Vivo Manipulations," *Haemostasis*, 12:116 (1982).

23 GOLDMAN, M., C. E. Hall, B. K. Gunson, R. J. Hawker and C. N. McCollum. "Indium Labelled Platelet Deposition on Prosthetic Grafts," in *Biomaterials in Artificial Organs*, J. P. Paul, J. D. S. Gaynor, J. M. Courtney and T. Gilchrist, eds., London:Macmillan, pp. 227–287 (1984).

24 MOSLEY, J. G. and A. Marston. "A 5 Year Follow-up of Dacron Femoropopliteal Bypass Grafts," *Br. J. Surg.*, 73:24 (1986).

25 YEAGER, R. A., R. W. Hobson, Z. Jamil, T. G. Lynch, B. C. Lee and K. Jain. "Differential Patency and Limb Salvage for Polytetraflouroethylene and Autogenous Saphenous Vein in Severe Lower Extremity Ischaemia," *Surgery*, 91:99 (1982).

26 GRAHAM, L. M. and J. J. Bergan. "Expanded Polytetraflouroethylene Vascular Grafts: Clinical and Experimental Observations," in *Biologic and Synthetic Vascular Prostheses*, J. C. Stanley, ed. New York:Grune and Stratton, Inc., pp. 563–586 (1982).

27 GREEN, R. M., L. R. Roedersheimer and J. A. DeWeese. "Effects of Aspirin and Dipyridamole on Expanded Polytetrafluoroethylene Graft Patency," *Surgery*, 92:1016 (1982).

28 OBLATH, R. W., F. O. Buckley, R. M. Green, S. I. Schwartz and J. A. DeWeese. "Prevention of Platelet Aggregation and Adherence to Prosthetic Vascular Grafts by Aspirin and Dipyridamole," *Surgery*, 84:37 (1978).

29 METKE, M. P., J. T. Lie, V. Fuster, M. Josa and M. P. Kaye. "Reduction of Intimal Thickening in Canine Coronary Artery Bypass Vein Grafts with Dipyridamole and Aspirin," *Am. J. Cardiol.*, 43:1144 (1979).

30 KESTER, R. C. "The Thrombogenicity of Dacron Arterial Grafts and Its Modification by Platelet Inhibitory Drugs," *Ann. R. Coll. Surg. Engl.*, 66:241 (1984).

31 CHESEBRO, J. H., V. Fuster, L. R. Elveback, I. P. Clements, H. C. Smith, D. R. Holmes, W. T. Bardsley, J. R. Pluth, R. B. Wallace, F. J. Puga, T. A. Orszulak, J. M. Piehler, G. D. Danielson, H. V. Schaff and R. L. Frye. "Effect of Dipyridamole and Aspirin on Late Vein–Graft Patency After Coronary Bypass Operations," *N. Engl. J. Med.*, 310:209 (1984).

32 RAJAH, S. M., M. C. P. Salter, D. R. Donaldson, R. Subba Rao, R. M. Boyle, J. B. Partridge and D. A. Watson. "Acetylsalicylic Acid and Dipyridamole Improve the Early Patency of Aorta-Coronary Bypass Grafts," *J. Thorac. Cardiovasc. Surg.*, 90:373 (1985).

33 STRATTON, J. R. and J. L. Ritchie. "The Effect of Sulfinpyrazone on Platelet Deposition on Dacron Vascular Grafts in Man," *Am. Heart J.*, 109:453 (1985).

34 NENCI, G. G., M. Berrettini, M. DeCunto and V. Iadevala. "Antiplatelet Activity and Safety of Indobufen (K3920): Long Term Evaluation in Patients with Vascular Disease," *ACTA Therapeutica*, 9:127 (1983).

35 SALTER, M. C. P., P. Mayor, M. J. Crow, S. M. Rajah and A. M. Davison. "Microthrombus Formation on Hemolysis Membranes; A Placebo Controlled Randomized Trial of Two Doses of Indobufen," *Clin. Nephrol.*, 24:1 (1985).

CHAPTER 13

Polyester Prostheses: The Outlook for the Future

ROBERT GUIDOIN, Ph.D.[1,2]
and **JEAN COUTURE, M.D.**[1,3]

ABSTRACT: After 30 years of experience in the fabrication of arterial prostheses, polyester manufactured by DuPont under the tradename of Dacron® is still the gold standard in terms of biostability. Despite some early weaknesses due to inappropriate concepts, the prostheses proposed today are much more stable. The outlook for the future appears to be linked to improved healing according to different methods: compound grafts, cell seeded grafts and plasma TFE grafts.

INTRODUCTION

Of all the synthetic materials proposed as arterial substitutes over the past 40 years, polyester prostheses have emerged as the material which presents the best biostability for the replacement of the large- and medium-sized vessels, since it possesses both strength and endurance [1]. Due to their extensive use as blood conduits by cardiovascular surgeons, it has been possible to evaluate their performance by analysis of the clinical results, the assessment of the patency of the graft, the limb survival, the patient rehabilitation [2,3,4], and, very importantly, by the analysis of explanted grafts [5,6] through a retrieval program such as the one existing in our laboratory since the mid-seventies [7].

Since polyester vascular prostheses have stood the test of time and thus have maintained a high level of popularity, it is accepted that their use can still increase significantly during the next decade in view of the anticipated increase in the number of patients requiring vascular surgery. Therefore, long-term patency and biostability should be the desired objectives for polyester prostheses more than any other graft, since prognoses of patients may exceed 10 or 15 years. Furthermore, implantations are done in younger and younger patients since diagnoses are more efficient as a result of the development of vascular laboratories. Therefore, the purpose of graft implantation is not only to maintain a patient autonomously, but also to keep the patient productive as a worker.

As with all prostheses, the fate of the polyester blood conduits can be affected by the progression of arteriosclerosis, the presence of associated diseases, and other risk factors which affect the thrombotic and haematological constituents of the blood (e.g., diabetes, smoking, cancer), the hemodynamic aspect of the bypass itself and the quality of the material [8]. In the most favorable conditions, a prosthesis should have the following long-term objectives:

(1) The durability of the implant should be superior to the life expectancy of the host.

(2) The insertion of the graft should not cause undesirable side effects that the host cannot overcome.

Before considering perspectives for the future of polyester protheses, we will attempt to review the available data on these devices.

HISTORICAL REVIEW

Following the favorable evaluation by Harrison in the late fifties [9,10] of a synthetic polymer known as Dacron®, vascular surgeons have also recognized its essential qualities: it is generally biocompatible, resilient, flexible, durable, and resistant to sterilization and biodegradation [11].

[1]Laboratory of Experimental Surgery, Laval University, Quebec City, Quebec, Canada

[2]Biomaterials Institute, St. François d'Assise Hospital, Quebec City, Quebec, Canada

[3]Department of Surgery, St. Sacrement Hospital, Quebec City, Quebec, Canada

This same polymer, polyethylene terephthalate, has been incorporated in the fabrication of more than 60 commercial prostheses originating in different countries. It is fair to say that most of the refinements proposed by manufacturers have not significantly improved the clinical results in patients submitted to surgical treatment. In some instances, by modifying the natural and specific characteristics of the graft, some of the prostheses have, in fact, acquired properties less than satisfactory for the patients [12]. When one considers the numerous variations, based on marketing, in the fabric construction of a number of commercial prostheses, one is not unduly surprised at the number and variety of complications such as graft dilatations, haemorrhages and the formation of false aneurysms [13].

Over the years, many contributing factors for such complications have been identified. Some factors are related to the surgical techniques, such as incorrect handling, surgical trauma, and improper anastomosis; other factors are related to the prostheses themselves—defective material, manufacturing errors, incorrect storage or sterilization and a deterioration of the polyester fibers during implantation. In addition, some authors have demonstrated that after many years, there will be some mechanical fatigue and biodegradation of the polyester material [14].

Although the experience with Dacron over the past 30 years has been very positive, it remains that in spite of changes made to the original polymer, the progress towards "the ideal vascular substitute" has been very modest, indeed. Of course, we know that the material itself is only one of the factors affecting the performance of a prosthesis; of equal importance are local and systemic factors such as the healing process, the host dependancy, and the blood compatibility. Therefore, one cannot really predict whether further refinements in the design of polyester prostheses will fulfill all the requirements of an ideal vascular graft. However, research in this field offers great possibilities because these prostheses are used so extensively, providing ample data for the evaluation of performance, both clinically and in the laboratory.

POLYESTER TEREPHTHALATE (PET)

The polyester terephthalate known under the trade name of Dacron®, manufactured by DuPont is the standard against which polyesters for vascular grafts are measured.

Chemistry

The technology for manufacturing PET resins and fibers is relatively complex. It is very unlikely that many manufacturers would be prepared to apply PET resins and fibers exclusively for medical use because this requires only small volumes of material. Consequently, the manufacturers of prostheses are more inclined to purchase materials intended for nonmedical applications and then upgrade the yarns for the fabrication of grafts.

PET has the following repeat unit, where η is in excess of 70:

$$-\left[O-CH_2-CH_2-O-C- \bigcirc -\underset{\underset{O}{\|}}{C}- \right]_{\overline{n}}$$

This polymer can be synthetized from two monomers under catalytic conditions, using either of two methods:

(a) Ethylene glycol and terephthalic acid:

$$HO-CH_2-CH_2-OH + HO-\underset{\underset{O}{\|}}{C}- \bigcirc -\underset{\underset{O}{\|}}{C}-OH \longrightarrow$$

$$HO-CH_2-CH_2-O-\underset{\underset{O}{\|}}{C}- \bigcirc -\underset{\underset{O}{\|}}{C}-OH$$

(b) Ethylene glycol and dimethyl terephthalate:

$$HO-CH_2-CH_2\,OH + CH_3-O-\underset{\underset{O}{\|}}{C}- \bigcirc -\underset{\underset{O}{\|}}{C}-O\,CH_3 \longrightarrow$$

$$CH_3OH + HO-CH_2-CH_2\,O-\underset{\underset{O}{\|}}{C}- \bigcirc -\underset{\underset{O}{\|}}{C}-OCH_3$$

In either case, a series of condensation reactions takes place under inert atmosphere or vacuum at 275°C. These reactions produce linear chains containing hydroxyl and carboxyl (or acetyl) end groups.

The polymerization is initiated by a catalyst, usually a salt of calcium or a heavy metal (antimony or manganese). These initiators are trapped in the polymer and may leach out from the filaments in-vivo and induce adverse reactions, including cytotoxicity.

The polymerization proceeds until one of the reactants is totally depleted. The average length of the polymer chains is controlled by the initial concentration of the initiator, the presence of impurities and the concentration of the minority reactant added to the process. The average molecular weights for normal PET polymers lie in the range of 15,000 to 20,000, i.e., 70 to 110 repeat units. However, there is a wide distribution of molecular weights including oligomers that are chemically more reactive.

Assessment

Identification Profile

- Infrared (IR) spectral analysis: A printout of the polyester from DuPont must be incorporated into the records to serve as reference when further batches of materials are evaluated.
- USP physicochemical tests: leachable materials and traces of heavy metals should be identified.

- Density, melt viscosity, refractive index and molecular weight distribution should be measured.
- Additives and inert-filler must be characterized.
- Mechanical, chemical and thermal investigations of the fibers are mandatory.

Cytotoxicity

Mammalian cells (human umbilical cord vein, mouse aorta, dog aorta) are cultured for a week or more in contact with the specimen. This test allows the identification of the progression of the cells, their adhesiveness and morphology. It is sensitive, rapid, economical and versatile.

Pyrogenicity

The purpose of this test is to limit to an acceptable level the risks of a febrile reaction. A volume of sterile, pyrogen-free saline is passed through the fibers. The temperature of the animals are taken hourly for 3 hours after injecting 10 ml/kg of the body weight in the vein of the ear. Temperature rises should not exceed 3.7°C.

Biostability

Candidate materials are examined for potential enzymatic degradation upon exposure to suspensions of enzymes such as trypsin, pronase, pepsin, lipase and amylase. The tests are done in a static or dynamic environment; the suspensions are subsequently examined for degradation products. The materials are studied for changes in the surface composition, tensile properties and morphology.

Primary Skin Irritation Test

It is important to predict any irritation caused by the materials application to intact and abraded rabbit skin for 72 hours.

Acute Intramuscular Implantation Test

The purpose of this test is to evaluate the reaction of living tissue to the plastic by the implantation of the test sample itself into rabbit tissue for 72 hours in the paravertebral muscles. The reactions are scored from 0 to 5, depending upon the size of the encapsulation.

Hemolysis Test

The purpose is to determine if a substance can be extracted from a material that causes hemolysis of red blood cells in rabbits.

Mutagenicity

Two tests are widely used. The accuracy of both methods for predicting carcinogenicity is considered high. The Ames bacterial mutation test is the most widely accepted. The mammalian cell transformation test utilizes baby hamster kidney cells in culture.

Cellular Immune Response

Still not widely used, it may involve post-implantation skin reaction observation and studies on lymphokines such as MIF and MAF.

Ethylene Oxide Residue Assay

It is necessary to show that the polyester does not contain deleterious amounts of ethylene oxide (EO) and its principle reaction products, ethylene chlorohydrin (ECH) and ethylene glycol (EG) after ETO sterilization.

TECHNOLOGY OF POLYESTER PROSTHESES

The Manufacturing Process

The basic stages in the production of vascular prostheses can be ascertained by a review of the pertinent literature and the analysis of samples obtained from manufacturers. Figure 1 shows the basic stages of production common to all manufacturers. The entire process is complex and requires a great deal of precision.

Following is a summary of the various steps involved in the designing of polyester vascular prostheses. For a more detailed description of all aspects of this technology, the reader is referred to our previous work on the subject [15].

Types of Yarn

Polyethyleneterephthalate (PET) is the polyester used for the production of all prostheses. It is available in a wide range of PET fibers and yarns, either as a flat or a texturized multifilament yarn. It has qualities that warrant its acceptance as an arterial substitute: it is inert, biocompatible, flexible, resilient and resistant to sterilization. Because of the complexity of the technology involved in the manufacturing of this product, and due to high costs, the yarns used are not only intended for medical applications and are liable to contain some delusterants and pigments not desirable in medical devices. Since these substances are potentially cytotoxic, they can prevent the development of endothelial cells during implantation. Therefore, designs to be implanted in humans should be upgraded from yarns containing such impurities, regardless of economic considerations.

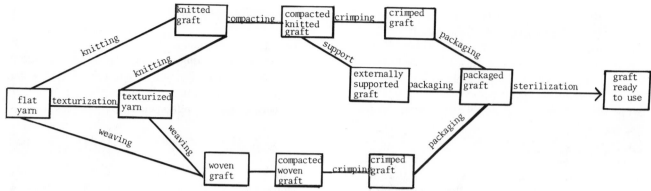

Figure 1. Technology of polyester prostheses.

From measurements made in our laboratories, it was possible to define the characteristics of the yarns used in the fabrication of prostheses by analysing the grafts received from the manufacturers [15]. This study has shown that the majority of yarns used are normal tenacity Dacron type 56 with cylindrical filaments. Occasionally, polyester filaments with trilobal sections are used: it is believed the trilobal section provides a larger surface area, increases the porosity and facilitates preclotting of the graft on a more thrombogenic surface with a better retention of the thrombotic matrix. A possible disadvantage is the fact that these filaments have exhibited some signs of fatigue and mechanical damage in implanted and retrieved prostheses [8]. Consequently, the reason for using a trilobal filament section is not convincing enough at the present time.

Fabric Construction and Properties

Although there are only two general types of fabric construction, the woven and the knitted, commercial polyester prostheses fall under four groups: woven, knitted, velour, and externally supported grafts. Most of the grafts of the third group have resulted from the development of the knitted prostheses. Consequently, it would be better to regard all velour type constructions (except Rhodergon and Microvel) as texturized knitted prostheses. In addition, the knitted fabric type has given rise to many variants over the past ten years: the basic "standard knit," the "light weight knitted," and many others.

Woven fabrics (Figure 2)—The early commercial prostheses were woven on two sets of yarns, in a plain/1.1/ weave, with a high fabric count, thus providing the surgeon with a graft which is rigid, tightly woven and of a low water permeability. Because of their stiffness and strong construction, these prostheses are prone to fraying and are more difficult to suture. However, since their water permeability is low, preclotting is not mandatory and bleeding is then reduced. They are more suitable in emergency operations involving large vessels and in elective surgery of the thoracic or abdominal aorta.

Knitted fabrics—In order to overcome the disadvantages of the woven fabrics, the knitted construction was proposed as an alternative in the late fifties with the De Bakey standard prostheses and the Milliknit prosthesis. The yarns in the knitted construction are interlooped around each other in two predominant directions: lengthwise when the fabric is "warp knit" and transverse when it is a "weft knit," as demonstrated in Figures 3 and 4. These two types bear significant differences which are important to the surgeons: the weft-knit fabrics unravels, whereas warp-knit does not. Care must be taken when cutting or suturing weft knits, especially along the lines which are not exactly parallel to the wale direction.

Specific characteristics are derived from this type of construction: they are more open than the woven types in that interstitial pores are present in the center of, or between, the loops of knitted yarn. These pores vary in size, depending on whether the yarns are non-texturized, bulk or texturized. Consequently, it is necessary to shrink the knitted tube by compaction in order to obtain an acceptable fabric count in the range of 16–39 wales/cm. This process makes it possible to alter readily the water permeability of knitted prostheses and has enabled manufacturers to design prostheses with a variable level of water permeability. However, the knitted structure is still porous at any level and generally requires preclotting prior to implantation.

The characteristics derived from an open construction and the variable level of porosity that can be obtained insure improved flexibility and compliance. Consequently, knitted prostheses are easier to handle than the woven types. They are also more prone to some elongation, a feature that can affect its dimensional stability. These structures, when exposed to lengthy and cyclic stresses, as in the arterial system, do not have the viscoelastic properties of the host artery, and can experience some dilatation, with possible consequences [16–17].

In order to improve compliance and facilitate surgical technique, the lightweight constructions were introduced by Wesolowski, Golaski and De Bakey in the sixties, giving rise to the Weavenit, Microknit and De Bakey Ultra-

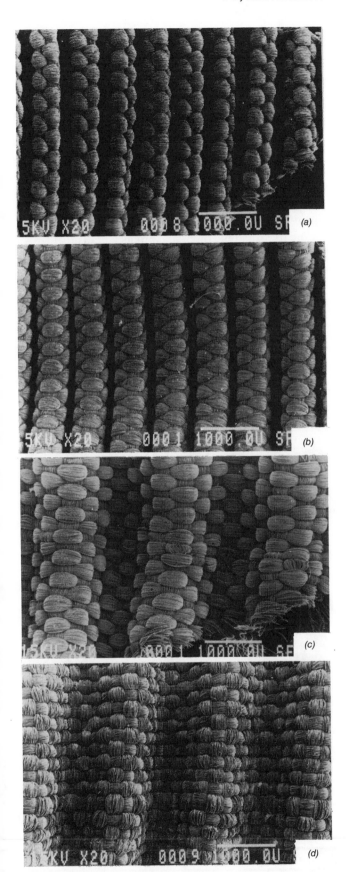

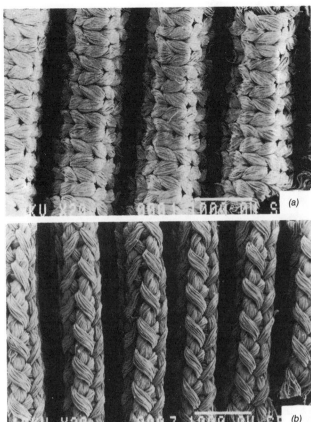

Figure 3. *SEM microphotographs of a warp-knit structure: the knitted Cooley, inside (a) and outside (b).*

Lightweight [15], respectively. These prostheses are based on the hypothesis that a thinner construction would reduce the compression–tension stress gradient across the fabric and result in more rapid preclotting, better healing and an acceptable late patency of the graft. It has been shown, however, that the thickness is not the sole factor involved. In fact, cases have been reported of lightweight knitted prostheses undergoing dilatation, false aneurysms and rupture. These findings suggest that lightweight knitted grafts cannot support cyclic stresses of the arterial circulation over extended periods. On that basis, it appears that the properties of lightweight construction do not justify their application in all locations, especially for large vessel replacements like the abdominal or thoracic aorta [18].

Velour fabrics (Figures 5 and 6)—The commercial velour grafts have a knitted construction and have been developed to improve the healing characteristics of the knitted types. To achieve this, the use of high-texturized yarns was suggested for the purpose of creating a rougher fabric surface that would improve the anchorage of the initial thrombotic matrix, the neointima to the internal wall, and also minimize blood loss during and after surgery.

This concept has led to the development of a wide range

Figure 2. *SEM microphotographs of different models of woven grafts: Woven de Bakey (a), Cooley Venisoft (b), Shanghai (c) and Indian (d).*

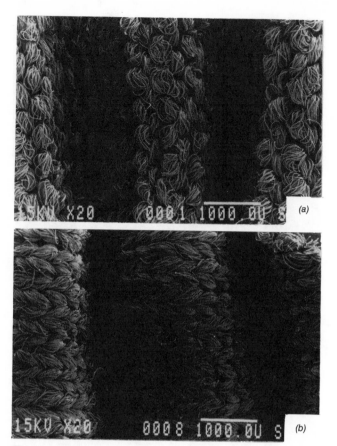

Figure 4. SEM microphotographs of a weft-knit structure: the vasculour D, inside (a) and outside (b).

rally wound monofilament of either polyester, polypropylene or teflon [20,21].

The Manufacturing Process

Compaction—This process is intended to give to the fabric an acceptable water permeability because most of the knitted structures are too porous to be used as vascular prostheses. Therefore, the fabric is shrunk either by chemical swelling agents or by a thermal process using dry or liquid steam at 120 to 155°C. Refinements of the technique have allowed the manufacturer to submit the bifurcated prostheses to differential compaction treatment for the trunk and the limbs and produce grafts that have a good anatomical trunk and limb diameter ratio, thus ensuring more uniform haemodynamic flow properties. Some undesirable effects might result from the compaction, for instance considerable swelling of the filaments, which can become distorted, either round or flattened.

The chemical compaction has resulted in some changes in the molecular orientation and crystallinity of the polymer material. According to Sawyer [22], the use of different compaction chemicals can result in changes of some characteristics, like the healing performance and the thrombogenicity of the graft surface and increase the like-

of "velour type" prostheses. The original approach has been followed with some variants as seen in the Rhodergon prosthesis which has been napped to give a raised pile and the Microvel which contains an additional set of yarns laid into a half-tricot base fabric to form a looped pile. Consequently, the accepted textile definition of the term applies only to these two types: "a thick-bodied fabric, either woven, knitted or nonwoven, that has a smooth surface by virtue of additional pile yarns or a napped fibre finish." Therefore, it would be more correct to regard all other "velour type" constructions as texturized knitted prostheses.

While this type of construction has created highly porous structures that would facilitate the growth of perigraft tissue into the graft, retain the cellular blood constituents and promote the growth of a fibre matrix, it has also raised some important concerns. For instance, it has been suggested that the growth of excessive perigraft tissue was responsible for some lumen occlusions and that the frequency of severe graft reactions is more important with velour than with other types of prostheses [19].

Externally supported grafts (Figure 7)—It is a variant of the different types of grafts whose structure is externally supported with either an adherent or nonadherent, spi-

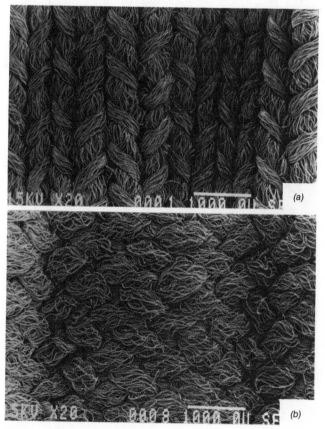

Figure 5. SEM microphotographs of a velour-type structure, the VP50K Triaxial, inside (a) and outside (b).

lihood of post-operative complications, e.g., blood oozing, haemorrhage and hematomas.

Crimping techniques—The object of crimping is to provide the surgeon with a noncollapsible prosthesis, to prevent wrinkling and kinking after implantation, to minimize local fluctuations of blood pressure, and to reduce the stress at the suture line and thrombosis at the anastomosis.

First introduced by Edwards [23], crimping is done by heat using one of two processes. After fitting the prostheses on a mandrel, it is wound spirally around the graft and heated after compression: this gives a helical crimp. Since this method is not suitable for velour and high bulk texturized fabrics, internal steam pressure in a mold is preferred for these grafts: this produces a circular crimp. It seems that these two crimped configurations are satisfactory from a clinical point of view. Measurements of the crimp level after implantation have shown a rapid loss of crimp and longitudinal compliance, particularly with circularly crimped grafts. The effects of crimping on the haemodynamics and healing properties of grafts are still open to question.

Nonetheless, crimping is essential and has contributed a lot to the improvement of the technical aspects of vascular surgery.

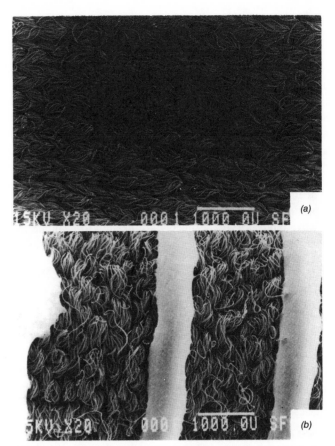

Figure 7. SEM microphotographs of an externally supported graft, the Sauvage EXS, inside (a) and outside (b).

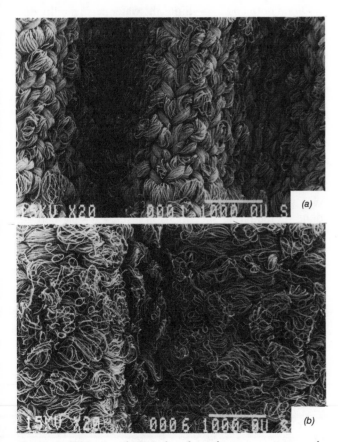

Figure 6. SEM microphotographs of a velour type structure, the Cooley double velour, inside (a) and outside (b).

Cleaning and inspection—The various stages of manufacture include many processes that can introduce some degree of contamination in the prostheses: obviously these impurities must be removed before packaging and sterilization. It is believed that specific processes for the medical device industry include hot hydrocarbon washes, mechanical or ultrasonic agitation, refluxing, caustic scouring and/or chemical bleaching.

There are very few differences between the cleaning protocols used for yarns for medical applications and those for regular apparel and furnishing. In the future, it is hoped that specialized yarns with a much lower level of impurities will be developed for medical application and the fabrication of high quality prostheses. Low power magnification is used for the inspection of the outside surface of the prostheses.

Packaging and sterilization—After a decade of industrial research and clinical evaluation, the packaging systems now in use have found wide acceptance: prostheses are packaged in semi-permeable, vacuum-formed composite sterilization systems with a rigid thermoplastic enclosure around a spun-bonded polyolefin paper (Tyvek®) cover which is heat sealed to the periphery.

Almost all prostheses are sold presterilized, and some

arise. Sterilization is done most commonly by heat, although gamma-irradiation and ethylene oxide sterilization methods are also used for certain prostheses. It was believed that polyester prostheses would not be affected by sterilization, but this is not the case. Significant changes have been observed in the chemistry and microstructural structure of PET yarns when exposed to ethylene oxide sterilization. Steam sterilization, well-recognized as an appropriate method, is believed to be responsible for some loss of mechanical compliance in some grafts. However, our laboratory studies have not shown that repeated steam sterilization makes significant changes to the water permeability and bursting strength of the grafts. Clearly, more laboratory experiments are needed to evaluate the effect of the various sterilization methods on the behavior of prostheses.

The Testing of Commercial Prostheses

The following tests are performed in order to determine the fabric and yarn characteristics before implantation. They are designed to measure the essential properties required from vascular grafts and to make sure that any new prosthesis is at least equivalent to what is already available on the market [21].

The Density Tests

Normal linear density—This test provides a measure for the coarseness or fineness of a fiber or yarn in units of decitex (decigrams per kilometer). This is done by determining the weight of a known length of yarn.

Relative density—The average relative density of the fibers can be measured using a density gradient column making it possible to measure the density of individual fibers to within 0.0001 g/cm³. For this purpose, a one-meter liquid column can be built from mixtures of carbon tetrachloride and xylene while maintaining the temperature of the column at 20.0 ± 0.1°C.

Stitch density—The tightness of a knitted structure is determined by multiplying the frequency of the columns of stitches (wales · cm⁻¹) by the frequency of the rows of stitches (courses · cm⁻¹). Measurements of stitch frequencies are obtained in both directions through an optical stereoscopic microscope at 20 to 30 magnifications with the help of a ruler. For better results, the grafts are flattened under a glass slide to remove the crimps when indicated.

The Integrity of the Fabric

Packing factor—This test is an index of the void in the textile structure and serves as a useful measurement of the potential for in vivo tissue ingrowth. It is calculated by dividing the fabric density by the relative density of the fibers: the values theoretically vary from 0 (all air and no material) to 1 (no air, as in solid plastic sheets and films). Values closer to 0 indicates greater openness, or void, in the fabric.

Filament diameter—From each type of yarn, 20 filaments are selected at random. The diameter of these filaments is determined using an optical microscope at 400 times magnification with a calibrated micrometer eye.

Fabric structure and fiber morphology—The specimens, after being exposed to osmium tetroxide vapors, are impregnated with gold palladium in order to improve their conduction. This process facilitates, through a scanning electron microscope, the observation of fabric and yarn structures and the surface morphology of the filaments.

The Permeability Tests

Water permeability—The rate of flow of water (ml/min) through one cm² of the wall of a dry prosthesis is measured using an apparatus similar to that described by Buxton and Cooley at a pressure of 120 mm Hg [25]; it provides an index of the interstitial leakage rate of the prosthesis wall prior to preclotting. Because the pressure induced by the flow of water (120 mm Hg) compacts the exposed fabric after a period of time, the test is carried out over a five minute period [26].

Blood permeability—Since the water permeability does not provide a direct indication of how quickly the wall of the prosthesis becomes impervious when exposed to blood, the blood permeability of each prosthesis is determined by the same method as mentioned above, only the water is replaced by fresh heparinized blood of a dog.

Fatigue Tests

These tests are designed to evaluate the physical properties of the prosthesis.

The crimp extension—This test measures the capacity of a graft to stretch under longitudinal tension. This is done by mounting specimens in a relaxed state between the clamps of a crimp tester, and measuring their length to the nearest 0.2 mm before and after removal of the crimp. The end point is readily attained when the fabric appears flat when viewed from above in reflected light through an optical microscope. The amount of crimp extension is defined as the difference between the extended and relaxed lengths and is expressed as a percentage of the original relaxed length.

Dilation—The Optiddiac System is used to evaluate the propensity of the grafts to dilate under static internal pressure. It involves the mounting of a tubular prosthesis over a tubular latex membrane and its fixation between two clamps: one of these clamps is fixed and supplies the air pressure, while the other, running on a low-friction track, applies a constant longitudinal tension of 113 g to the specimen. As the air pressure is increased from 0 to 340 mm Hg, the change in diameter is measured to the nearest 0.1 mm using a cathetometer. The average changes noted at a pressure of 120 mm Hg are recommended as standards [27].

Bursting strength [28]—Four alternative methods are currently proposed for the determination of different strength values. It has not been established yet whether there are significant relationships between these methods:

- Radial tensile strength: A sample in its tubular form is placed into suitable jaws (for longitudinal testing) or onto two rounded pins (for circumferential testing) and then stretched at a uniform rate (mm/mm) to reach break point. The mean tensile strength at break for the prosthesis is kN for longitudinal testing and the mean tensile strength at break/unit length is kN/mm for circumferential testing.
- Diaphragm strength: Using a flat annular clamping ring, a one cm² sample of the prosthesis to be tested is fixed over an elastic diaphragm and submitted to an increasing fluid pressure on the underside of the diaphragm until bursting of the specimen. The results are expressed in kN.
- Probe burst strength: A one cm² sample of the prosthesis to be tested is clamped over an orifice by means of a flat annular clamping ring, and a cylindrical probe with a hemispherical load being measured continuously is traversed through the specimen until it ruptures. Any test report should include the probe diameter (mm), the rate of traverse (mm/min) and the bursting load (kN).
- Balloon burst test: This test was developed at W. L. Gore and Associates. A tubular latex bladder is inserted into the graft to be tested and attached to the burst-tester water supply. The ends of the bladder and the graft are clamped off and the water pumped in to increase the internal pressure at a given rate. The results are recorded in kPa.

These various tests were used in the analysis of more than 70 commercial prostheses in our laboratory. Results are summarized in Tables 1, 2, and 3.

CLINICAL APPLICATIONS

It is generally agreed by vascular surgeons that Dacron prostheses best fulfill the requirements for an arterial substitute. Among the many types of polyester grafts available today, the knitted types have gained worldwide acceptance as vascular conduits for large- and medium-sized vessels. Over the years, some refinements in the manufacturing process have improved the flexibility and consequently the handling, suturing and compliance of these materials. The necessity for preclotting is not recognized as a major problem by most surgeons, except in emergency situations when this procedure can be time-consuming.

TABLE 1. Types of Commercial Polyester Vascular Prostheses

Type	Fabric Construction	Weave/Stitch	Commercial Name	Manufacturer	No.
Woven	Plain weave	1/1 Taffeta	Cooley Verisoft	Meadox	1
			Cooley Low Porosity	Meadox	2
			DeBakey Woven	Bard	3
			DeBakey Extra Low Porosity	Bard	4
Knitted	Weft-knit	Single jersey	DeBakey Standard	Bard	5
			Microknit	Golaski	6
			Milliknit	Golaski	7
	Warp-knit	2-bar locknit	Cooley Knitted	Meadox	8
			Cooley 2	Meadox	9
			Weavenit	Meadox	10
Velour	Weft-knit	Single jersey and texturized yarn	DeBakey Vasculour D	Bard	11
			Lopor	Golaski	12
			Sauvage Externally Supported	Bard	13
	Warp-knit	2-bar locknit and texturized yarn	Cooley Double Velour	Meadox	14
			DeBakey Vasculour II	Bard	15
			Sauvage Bionit	Bard	16
		2-bar locknit and napped pile	Rhodergon	Rhône poulenc	17
		Half-tricot and inlaid pile yarn	Microvel	Meadox	18

TABLE 2. Typical Yarn Construction of Commercial Prostheses

No.	Commercial Name	Multifilament Yarn Type	Nominal Linear Density[a] (Decitex)	Approx. Filament Count	Filament Cross-Section	Mean Filament Diameter (µm)	Delustrant Level
1	Cooley Verisoft	Warp: flat	180	108	Round	12.4	Semi-dull
		Weft: texturized	110	54	Trilobal	—	Semi-dull
2	Cooley Low Porosity	Warp: flat	96	54	Round	12.8	Semi-dull
		Weft: flat	170	108	Round	12.0	Semi-dull
3	DeBakey Woven	texturized	180	108	Round	12.5	Semi-dull
4	DeBakey Extra Low Porosity	texturized	170	108	Round	12.1	Semi-dull
5	DeBakey Standard	texturized	190	108	Round	12.6	Semi-dull
6	Microknit	2-ply flat	2 × 28	2 × 21	Round	11.1	Semi-dull
7	Milliknit	2-ply flat	2 × 56	2 × 27	Round	13.9	Semi-dull
8	Cooley Knitted	flat	170	60	Round	16.2	Semi-dull
9	Cooley 2	texturized	180	68	Round	15.5	Semi-dull
10	Weavenit	flat	100	50	Round	13.6	Semi-dull
11	DeBakey Vasculour D	texturized	170	85	Round	13.8	Semi-dull
12	Lopor	2-ply texturized	2 × 30	2 × 15	Round	13.5	Semi-dull
13	Sauvage Externally Supported	2-ply texturized	2 × 80	2 × 40	Round	13.6	Semi-dull
14	Cooley Double Velour	Pile: texturized	100	44	Trilobal	—	Semi-dull
		Base: flat	52	27	Round	13.6	Semi-dull
15	DeBakey Vasculour II	texturized	2 × 80	2 × 42	Round	13.2	Semi-dull
16	Sauvage Bionit	texturized	190	96	Round	13.4	Semi-dull
17	Rhodergon	flat	115	32	Round	18.2	Dull
18	Microvel	texturized	48	24	Trilobal	—	Semi-dull
		flat	46	27	Round	12.5	Semi-dull

[a]Calculated from filament count, filament diameter and relative density.

TABLE 3. Typical Fabric Construction and Properties of Commercial Prostheses

No.	Commercial Name		Fabric Count (cm⁻¹) Ends/Wales	Picks/Courses	Stitch Density (cm⁻²)	Thickness (mm)	Fabric Weight (g/m²)	Packing Factor	Crimp Elongation (%)	Bursting Strength (kPa)	Water Permeability (m¹/min/cm²)
1	Cooley Verisoft	Plain weave	58	35	—	0.27	160	0.43	80	2630	250
2	Cooley Low Porosity		53	40	—	0.26	144	0.40	210	3240	60
3	DeBakey Woven		56	34	—	0.33	165	0.36	30	4900	350
4	DeBakey Extra Low Porosity		55	40	—	0.36	195	0.39	110	4830	50
5	DeBakey Standard	Weft-knit	22	31	680	0.46	200	0.32	160	3030	2530
6	Microknit		39	43	1680	0.27	103	0.28	490	1490	3340
7	Milliknit		26	35	910	0.33	140	0.31	475	1890	5300
8	Cooley Knitted	Warp-knit	20	28	560	0.55	220	0.29	150	2710	2300
9	Cooley 2		16	24	380	0.45	185	0.30	225	2110	2500
10	Weaveknit		26	33	860	0.36	165	0.33	275	1500	2920
11	DeBakey Vasculour D	Weft-knit	20	26	520	0.55	195	0.26	225	1720	2250
12	Lopor		24	27	650	0.36	130	0.26	335	1640	3000
13	Sauvage Externally Supported		22	27	594	0.68	258	0.27	180	1750	3100
14	Cooley Double Velour	Warp-knit	20	28	560	0.69	280	0.29	95	1160	1660
15	DeBakey Vasculour II		15	24	360	0.55	226	0.30	295	2420	2800
16	Sauvage Bionit		14	24	336	0.55	230	0.30	255	2370	2400
17	Rhodergon		19	29	550	0.39	155	0.29	0	1980	5790
18	Microvel		22	32	700	0.89	200	0.16	160	1110	2400

To promote better healing of the prostheses, Wesolowski submitted that porosity would stimulate tissue in-growth that would support the pseudo-intima and maintain its stability [29]. This would be achieved mainly by the in-growth through the graft's interstices across the suture line and into the prosthesis. Experience has shown that the desirable level of porosity is difficult to achieve because on one hand, a high porosity graft can produce excessive perigraft tissue in-growth and cause some intra-luminal occlusion and haemorrhaging, and on the other hand, a low porosity graft can interfere with or delay healing [30]. While a certain level of porosity is considered desirable, there is still no agreement as to the proper level. Furthermore, the long-term effects of quantitative changes in the material are still unknown. In general, surgeons feel that high porosity grafts can present problems and lead to complications. However, it is not established whether the risk is higher with porous grafts of the type developed by Wesolowski or with the porous grafts designed like a trellis and advocated by Sauvage and associates [30,32].

The same comments apply to the velour type prostheses, which, because of their construction, are weaker, less stable and can dilate quite rapidly. These grafts are not well-suited for large vessel replacements or for high located anastomoses. Also, since they are highly porous structures, the same concerns expressed for the more traditional knitted prostheses also apply to these. Therefore, caution should be exercised in their use in vascular surgery.

The percentage of complications associated with the use of polyesters is perceived to be low considering the fact that Dacron is used in the majority of patients operated upon for abdominal aneurysms or aorto-iliac and femoral obstructions. The patency rates are indeed satisfactory, 80% or more at five years for aorto-iliac reconstructions and 65 to 70% for more peripheral operations. The incidence of Dacron graft-related complications is difficult to ascertain, as most reports deal with various types of grafts and with specific complications like anastomotic aneurysms, enteric fistulae, graft occlusion, infection and rupture [33].

While it is fair to say that the incidence of anastomotic aneurysms is about 5.5%, the infection rate varies between 1.9% and 5% [34,35]. Fiber deterioration in Dacron grafts can occur in 4.9 to 5.8% of patients [13]; these percentages are probably conservative for the following reasons. First, the complications reported probably represent only a small percentage of the total number. Since patients operated upon for arterial obstruction are often affected by associated diseases involving vital organs, the advent of complications in these patients is often attributed to a failure of vital organs. If no autopsy is done following a sudden death, it is likely that the possibility of an acute cardiac condition, rather than the rupture of a previously inserted aortic graft, will be considered the cause of death. Also, very few institutions proceed to a systematic analysis of the explanted prostheses at autopsy or following a surgical intervention. Consequently, because of a lack of valuable information, it is difficult to identify less dramatic graft-related complications such as partial occlusion and dilatation.

One should also realize that the complications reported cover a follow-up period extending to an average of 5 years and do not reflect the true incidence of complications that can occur many more years after implantation. Lynn reported dilatation requiring operation in two cases, six and nine years after insertion of a Knitted Ultraweight graft [36]. Edwards reported the rupture of a Lightweight Dacron aortic graft with fatal haemorrhage at ten years [37]. There have been reports of aneurysmal dilatation and bleeding through the graft interstices with knitted or woven Dacron up to 7 years after implantation [13].

These findings underline the fact that fiber deterioration develops progressively over the years and that structural deficiencies, with ensuing complications, may increase markedly as long-term follow-up becomes available. Therefore, the percentage of graft-related complications might be much higher than the level normally accepted for vascular prostheses in general. Consequently, long-term clinical follow-up studies are essential in order to record all documented cases of graft failure. For that purpose, some authors have recommended the formation of a central registry that would also define the guidelines for the study of these grafts [38].

Such a project would require the active participation of vascular surgeons. They would be asked to keep detailed records of the grafts (manufacturers, size, lot number, date), the conditions of sterilization and storage, the handling of the graft before and during surgery, and its behavior during the post-operative period. Also, virgin samples of each implanted graft should be stored for the purpose of comparison if, in the course of subsequent years, this graft is removed at surgery or autopsy. Of course, in such a case, analysis of the explanted graft should be done thoroughly by the usual testing methods described previously [7].

A careful follow-up of patients and a study of the implanted prostheses will contribute not only to a better knowledge of the behavior of Dacron® prostheses, but also to the protection of patients submitted to surgery. Deterling has stated "that when using manufactured devices for human spare parts, one must commit himself to a follow-up of such a patient for his remaining life" [39]. This statement is as pertinent today as it was 11 years ago: the objectives of long-term follow-up and evaluation are well accepted but will require a heavy commitment from all persons involved—the manufacturers, technicians, researchers and, of course, the vascular surgeons.

From these observations, one can conclude there is a great deal of interest generated for the continuous assessment of the behavior of polyester prostheses. This should be a source of encouragement to those more directly involved: the surgeons, the technicians and, very importantly, the patients themselves. Since it is expected that the use of these implants will increase markedly over the next decade, it is important that all efforts are made to maintain, by good research and proper clinical evaluation, the level of confidence given to polyester prostheses for the past 25 years.

BIOSTABILITY OF VASCULAR POLYESTER GRAFTS

A key property of vascular prostheses is durability, particularly in large-diameter grafts that sustain the highest pressures and seldom fail through occlusion. The most common mode of failure is by fatigue brought about by material flaws, damage to the material, the environment and the structure where the material is used. In addition, the polymer is susceptible to chemical attack and hydrolysis [40–42].

Surgical Trauma

Filaments can be flattened by improperly selected clamps, and can be broken or cut by cutting tip needles. The proper placement of sutures is dictated by the textile structure. Because woven grafts are more prone to fraying, a bigger bite must be taken in, and excessive friction must be avoided because it can damage the material.

Fatigue

Structural Fatigue

Structural fatigue occurs in textile structures that are loosely knitted or woven. The base structure is stabilized by the friction between yarns and by yarn tension. If this tension is too low and the friction is overcome, the structure may shift or stretch. However, this can be partially prevented by in-growth in the implanted textile. If this in-growth is insufficient, the structure can shift; consequently, dilatation and shortening of the graft can occur.

Classical fatigue

Classical fatigue occurs when the stresses in individual filaments exceed the endurance limit for PET. This is seen mainly in damaged filaments or thin walled prostheses; typical failures include splintered or fuzzy filament ends, blunt ends and tapered ends. These various configurations are caused by the different types of initial damage and/or different subsequent filament loading patterns.

Chemical Degradation

Besides the loss in strength caused by surgical trauma or fatigue, there is a chemical degradation of the polymer due to salts, tissue electrolytes, enzymes, or absorption of biological species. SEM studies show a loss in the molecular weight of the polymer and an increase in the carboxyl group concentration. It is estimated that 25% of the initial molecular weight is lost after 120 ± 15 months of implantation in humans.

PERSPECTIVES FOR THE FUTURE

The late improvements of arterial grafts concern mainly the choice of the material and the construction of the grafts. Compound prostheses [43], cell seeding [44], and plasma treatment [45] are probably the areas where further developments can be expected.

Compound Prostheses

Preclotting to reduce blood loss during vascular surgery is mandatory for knitted and velour grafts and is recommended for woven models. Preclotting is time-consuming, and can produce an irregular flow surface and the subsequent liberation of peripheral emboli, especially if the patient is not adequately heparinized or has impaired blood properties. The prosthetic wall can be made impervious by pretreatment.

Gel Coating

Graft impregnation was introduced by Bascom, who used baked gelatin. In the sixties, Humphries, Jordan and Wesolowski developed a gelatin-coated model concept. However, their studies never led to a commercial product, mainly because of the unpredictable healing characteristics. Collagen cross-linked with glutaraldehyde becomes hard and should be rehydrated prior to implantation. Bovine collagen cross-linked with formalin and softened with glycerol produces a graft which is soft and pliable [46]. This coating can be impregnated with antibiotics that are progressively released during the biolized material degradation [47]. This type of material needs further refinements since the healing process is unpredictable because of the variable degradation rate of the collagen. Furthermore, it has to be demonstrated that these grafts do not cause immunological reactions. However, commercial products available appear highly promising.

Albumin Coating

In the early 70's, Gyurko and Domurado proposed the impregnation of polyester prostheses with glutaraldehyde cross-linked albumin. The grafts resulting from this preparation become stiff when preserved dried [48] but become softer when glycerol is added [49]. Improved biocompatibility and healing could be obtained with carbodiimide cross-linking. Prostheses of the second generation can be made available by the impregnation of growth-promoting factors such as fibronectins within the albumin matrix and by the incorporation of antibiotics.

Polytetrapeptide of Elastin Compounding

The precursor protein of fibrous elastin contains repeating peptide sequences. The high polymers can be polymerized over a polyester support. It has been found to be elastomeric and capable of an elastic modulus similar to that of the natural elastic fiber. Experiments in dogs indicate that this approach requires further refinements [50].

Bioerodible Compound

The materials of biological origin, such as chitosan, might be of unpredictable degradation, healing, and immunological reaction [51]. Synthetic polypeptides based on glutamic acid could be better, but need to be investigated. They are already used by the pharmaceuticals companies for the controlled release of macromolecules and may be suitable for use on grafts [52]. These properties can be applied to the fabrication of grafts.

Presealing of Vascular Prostheses

Introduced in the mid-seventies, this technique consists of gluing fibrin into the wall of the prosthesis. The control of bleeding is then easier for the surgeon, even in heparinized patients. However, this method is sensitive to shock and acidosis, which can cause the lysis of the sealing process.

Cell Seeding

The luminal surface of polyester grafts never heals completely and thus remains thrombogenic. Cell seeding is likely to promote complete endothelial lining and the thrombogenicity is reduced accordingly.

Mechanical Derivation of Endothelial Cells

This approach was first described by Herring in 1978 [53]. Endothelial cells were harvested by passing a steel wool pledget through canine vein segments. The cells were then seeded into polyester prostheses by incorporating them in the thrombotic matrix during preclotting. At 4 weeks post-implantation, 76% of the flow surface was found to be thrombus-free, as compared to only 22% in preclotted grafts. Furthermore, pathological investigations confirmed the genuine endothelial features of the surface cells.

Enzymatic Derivation of Endothelial Cells [54]

This concept was introduced by Stanley. Harvesting of the cells involved sequential incubation of venous endothelium in collagenase and trypsin solutions. Both freshly harvested and cultured autologous endothelial cells were seeded. Four weeks after implantation, 80% of the flow surface of polyester-seeded grafts was lined with endothelium.

Incorporation of Peritoneal Mesothelial Cells [55]

Mesothelial cells can be harvested more readily and in larger numbers than endothelial cells; it has been demonstrated that they can also adequately support the blood flow. Those cells are closely related embryologically to endothelial cells, both being derived from the mesenchyme. Polyester prostheses seeded with autologous peritoneal mesothelial cells prior to implantation in the abdominal aorta of dogs led to a 90% coverage of the flow surface. This is probably a more practical alternative to the seeding of prostheses by endothelial cells.

Plasma Treatment (Figure 8)

The grafts are treated by a base discharge that deposits a thin coating on the graft surface, significantly changing its surface chemistry but without measurable changes in porosity, compliance or surface topography. This method can be applied with silicone [56], polypropylene [57] and tetrafluoroethylene [58]. Preliminary results were encouraging, but will have to be further confirmed in humans.

CONCLUSION

The progress in the development of polyester prostheses, after 30 years of use in vascular surgery, has not been as significant as expected. The necessity for indepth research did not seem justified until a number of graft failures was reported in the literature. Assessment of the performances were limited to in vivo evaluation in animals, with occasional mechanical testing. Healing char-

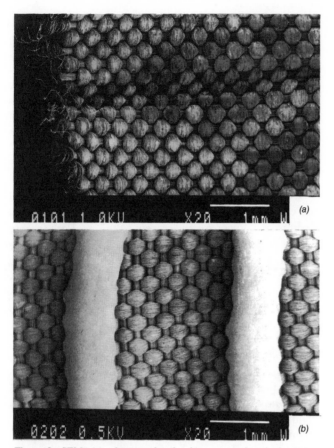

Figure 8. SEM microphotographs of a plasma coated graft, the Atrium Plasma TFE, inside (a) and outside (b).

acteristics have been disappointing and are probably related to the patients' physiological conditions. New attempts to better evaluate all aspects of the prostheses will certainly be made in the future.

ACKNOWLEDGEMENTS

This work has been supported, in part, by the Medical Research Council of Canada, Health and Welfare Canada, and Supplies and Services Canada. The authors are indebted to D. Lafrenière-Gagnon, Nicole Massicotte, Gilles Mongrain and Jacques Rodrigue for technical assistance. The guidance of Camille Gosselin, Martin King and Allan Downs is gratefully acknowledged.

REFERENCES

1 SNYDER, R. W., B. Tenney and R. Guidoin. "Strength and Endurance of Vascular Grafts," in *Vascular Graft Update—Safety and Performance*, H. E. Kambic, A. Kantrowitz and P. Sung, eds. ASTM publication STP898, pp. 108–121 (1986).

2 DEBAKEY, M. E. "The Development of Vascular Surgery," *Am. J. Surg.*, 137:697 (1979).

3 THOMPSON, J. E. and W. V. Garrett. "Peripheral Arterial Surgery," *New England, J. Med.*, 302:491 (1980).

4 SPITTELL, JR., J. A. and L. H. Hollier. "Aortic and Peripheral Arterial Disease: When is Surgery Warranted?" *Geriatrics*, 37:85 (1982).

5 POURDEYHIMI, B. and D. Wagner. "On the Correlation Between the Failure of Vascular Grafts and Their Structural and Material Properties. A Critical Analysis," *J. Biomed. Mat. Res.*, 20:375 (1986).

6 WALTON, K. W., G. Slaney and F. Ashton. "Atherosclerosis in Vascular Grafts for Peripheral Vascular Disease Part 2: Synthetic Arterial Prostheses," *Atherosclerosis*, 61:155 (1986).

7 GUIDOIN, R., M. King, P. Blais, M. Marois, C. Gosselin, P. Roy, R. Courbier, M. David and H. P. Noël. "A Biological and Structural Evaluation of Retrieved Dacron Arterial Prostheses," in *Implant Retrieval: Material and Biological Analysis*, A. Weinstein, D. Gibbons, S. Brown and W. Ruff, eds. NBS Special Publication, 601:29–129 (1981).

8 GUIDOIN, R., P. Levaillant, M. Marois, C. Gosselin, L. Martin, C. Rouleau, P. Blais, P. Garneau, H. P. Noël, D. Gagnon and S. Bourassa. "Les prothèses en polyethylene terephtalate (Dacron®) comme substituts artériels: évaluation des greffes commerciales comme substituts de l'aorte abdominale de chien," *J. Mal. Vasc.*, 5:3 (1980).

9 HARRISON, J. H. "Synthetic Materials as Vascular Prostheses. I. A Comparative Study in Small Vessels of Nylon, Dacron, Orlon, Ivalon, Sponge and Teflon," *Am. J. Surg.*, 95:3 (1958).

10 HARRISON, J. H. "Synthetic Materials as Vascular Prostheses. II. A Comparative Study of Nylon, Dacron, Orlon, Ivalon, Sponge and Teflon in Large Blood Vessels with Tensile Strength Studies," *Am. J. Surg.*, 95:16 (1958).

11 GUIDOIN, R., M. King, C. Gosselin, P. Blais, K. Gunaskera, M. Marois and A. Cardou. "Les prothèses artérielles en polyester," *Rev. Eur. Tech. Biomed.*, 4:21 (1982).

12 WESOLOWSKI, S. A. "A Plea for Early Recognition of Late Vascular Prostheses Failure," *Surgery*, 11:575 (1978).

13 BERGER, K. and L. R. Sauvage. "Late Fiber Deterioration in Dacron Arterial Grafts," *Ann. Surg.*, 193:477 (1981).

14 KING, M. W., R. Guidoin, P. Blais, A. Garton and W. Gunasekera. "Degradation of Polyester Arterial Prostheses: A Physical or Chemical Mechanism?" in *Corrosion and Degradation of Implant Materials: Second Symposium*, A. C. Fraker and C. D. Griffin, eds. ASTM Publication STP 859:294–307 (1985).

15 KING, M., P. Blais, R. Guidoin, E. Prowse, M. Marois, C. Gosselin and H. P. Noël. "Polyethelene Terephtalate (Dacron®) Vascular Prostheses: Material and Fabric Construction Aspects," in *Biocompatibility of Clinical Implant Materials*, D. F. Williams, ed. CRC Press, 2:177–207 (1981).

16 KINLEY, C. E. and A. E. Marble. "Compliance: A Continuing Problem with Vascular Grafts," *J. Cardiovasc. Surg.*, 21:163 (1980).

17 NUNN, D. B., M. H. Freeman and P. C. Hudgins. "Post-Operative Alterations in Size of Dacron Aortic Grafts. An Ultrasonic Evaluation," *Ann. Surg.*, 189:741 (1979).

18 OTTINGER, L. W., R. C. Darling, L. Withlin and R. R. Linton. "Failure of Ultralight Weight Knitted Dacron Grafts in Arterial Reconstruction," *Arch. Surg.*, 111:146 (1976).

19 KAUPP, H. A., T. J. Matulewicz, G. L. Lattimer, J. E. Kremen and V. J. Celani. "Graft Infection or Graft Reaction?" *Arch. Surg.*, 114:1419 (1979).

20 KENNEY, D. A., L. R. Sauvage, S. J. Wood, K. Berger, C. C. Davis, J. C. Smith, E. A. Rittenhouse, D. G. Hall and P. B. Mansfield. "Comparison of Non Crimped Externally Supported (EXS) and Crimped Non Supported Dacron Prostheses for Axillo

Femoral and Above-Knee Femoro-Popliteal Bypass," *Surgery*, 92:931 (1982).

21 KING, M. W., R. Guidoin, K. Gunasekera, L. Martin, M. Marois, P. Blais, J. M. Maarek and C. Gosselin. "An Evaluation of Czechoslovakian Polyester Arterial Prostheses," *ASAIO J.*, 7:114 (1984).

22 SAWYER, P. N., B. Stanczewski, R. Turner and H. Hoffman. "Evaluation of Chemical Compacting Techniques on the Performance, Thrombosis Rate, Histology and Healing of Experimental Similarly Fabricated Dacron Prostheses," *Trans. Am. Soc. Artif. Intern. Organs*, 24:215 (1978).

23 EDWARDS, W. S. "Progress in Synthetic Graft Development: An Improved Crimped Graft of Teflon," *Surgery*, 45:298 (1959).

24 GUIDOIN, R., C. Gosselin, L. Martin, M. Marois, F. Laroche, M. King, K. Gunasekera, D. Domurado, M. F. Sigot-Luizard and P. Blais. "Polyester Prostheses as Substitutes in the Thoracic Aorta of Dogs. I. Evaluation of Commercial Prostheses," *J. Biomed. Mat. Res.*, 17:1049 (1983).

25 BUXTON, B. F., C. C. Wukasch, C. Martin, W. J. Liebig, G. L. Hallman and D. A. Cooley. "Practical Consideration in Fabric Vascular Grafts: Introduction of a New Bifurcated Graft," *Am. J. Surg.*, 125:288 (1973).

26 GUIDOIN, R., M. King, D. Marceau, A. Cardou, D. De la Faye, J. M. Legendre and P. Blais. "Textile Arterial Prostheses: Is Water Permeability Equivalent to Porosity?" *J. Biomed. Mat. Res.*, 21:65 (1987).

27 MARCEAU, D., A. Cardou, R. Guidoin, C. Gosselin and M. King. "Etude de la déformation circonférentielle des prothèses artérielles en polytetrafluoroethylène," *Rev. Europ. Biotech. Med.*, 4:114 (1982).

28 NILSEN, E. J. "A Comparison of Two Bursting Strength Testers for Knitted Fabrics: A Mini-Diaphragm Versus a Mini-Probe Tester MSc Dissertation," University of Manitoba, Canada (1981).

29 WESOLOWSKI, S. A., C. C. Fries, K. E. Karlson, M. DeBakey and P. N. Sawyer. "Porosity: Primary Determinant of the Ultimate Fate of Synthetic Vascular Grafts," *Surgery*, 50:91 (1961).

30 MATHISEN, S. R., H. D. Wu, L. R. Sauvage, S. B. Robel, A. R. Wechezak and M. Walker. "The Influence of Denier and Porosity on Performance of a Warp-Knit Dacron Arterial Prosthesis," *Ann. Surg.*, 203:382 (1986).

31 WESOLOWSKI, S. A. "Performance of Materials as Prosthetic Blood Vessels," *Bull. N.Y. Acad. Med.*, 48:331 (1972).

32 SAUVAGE, L. R., K. E. Berger and P. B. Mansfield. "Future Directions in Development of Artificial Prostheses for Small and Medium Caliber Arteries," *Surg. Clin. North Am.*, 54:213 (1974).

33 SZILAGYI, D. E., R. F. Smith, J. P. Elliott, J. M. Hageman and C. A. Dall'Olmo. "Anastomotic False Aneurysms After Vascular Reconstruction: Problems of Incidence, Etiology and Treatment," *Surgery*, 78:800 (1975).

34 SZILAGYI, D. E., R. F. Smith, J. P. Elliott and M. P. Vrandecic. "Infection in Arterial Reconstruction with Synthetic Grafts," *Ann. Surg.*, 176:321 (1972).

35 HOFFERT, P. W., S. Gensler and M. Haimovici. "Infection Complicating Arterial Grafts," *Arch. Surg.*, 90:427 (1965).

36 LYNN, R. B. "Knitted Dacron Ultralightweight Grafts: A Warning," *Can. J. Surg.*, 22:593 (1979).

37 EDWARDS, W. S. "Arterial Grafts of Teflon," in *Vascular Grafts*, P. N. Sawyer and M. J. Kaplitt, eds. New York: Appleton-Century Crofts, pp. 173–176 (1977).

38 MORTENSEN, J. D. "Vascular Replacements: A Study of Safety and Performance," Final Report TR 1533-003, Silver Springs, MD, Food and Drug Administration (1980).

39 DETERLING, R. A., JR. "Failure of Dacron Arterial Prostheses," *Arch. Surg.*, 108:13 (1974).

40 KING, M. W., R. Guidoin, P. Blais, A. Garton and K. R. Gunasekera. "Degradation of Polyester Arterial Prostheses: A Physical or Chemical Mechanism?" in *Corrosion and Degradation of Implant Materials: Second Symposium*, A. C. Fraker and C. D. Griffin, eds. ASTM STP 859:294–307 (1985).

41 RUDAKOVA, T. E., G. E. Zaikov, O. S. Voronkova, T. T. Daurova and S. M. Degtyareva. "The Kinetic Specificity of Polyethylene Terephthalate Degradation in the Living Body," *J. Polym. Sci. Polym. Symp.*, 66:277 (1979).

42 MAAREK, J. M., R. Guidoin, M. Aubin and R. E. Prud'homme. "Molecular Weight Characterization of Virgin and Explained Polyester Arterial Prostheses," *J. Biomed. Mat. Res.*, 18:881 (1984).

43 JONAS, R. A., F. J. Schoen, R. J. Levy and A. R. Castaneda. "Biological Sealants and Knitted Dacron: Porosity and Histological Comparisons of Vascular Graft Materials With and Without Collagen and Fibrin Glue Pretreatments," *Ann. Thorac. Surg.*, 41:657 (1986).

44 STANLEY, J. C. "Endothelial Cell-Seeding of Prosthetic Vascular Grafts," in *Recent Advances in Vascular Grafting*, S. M. Skotnicki, F. G. M. Buskens and H. H. M. Reinaerts, eds. System 4, Associates (London), pp. 255–262 (1985).

45 HOFFMAN, A. S., B. D. Ratner, A. M. Garfinkle, L. O. Reynolds, T. A Horbett and S. R. Hanson. "The Importance of Vascular Graft Surface Composition as Demonstrated by a New Gas Discharge Treatment for Small Diameter Grafts," in *Vascular Graft Update: Safety and Performance*, H. E. Kambic, A. Kantrowitz and P. Sung, eds. Philadelphia:ASTM, pp. 137–155 (1986).

46 QUINONES-BALDRICH, W. J., W. S. Moore, S. Ziomek and M. Chvapil. "Development of a Leak-Proof Knitted Dacron Vascular Prosthesis," *J. Vasc. Surg.*, 3:895 (1986).

47 MOORE, W. S. and M. Chvapil. "Development of an Infection Resistant Vascular Graft," in *Recent Advances in Vascular Grafting*, S. H. Skotnicki, F. G. M. Buskens and H. H. M. Reinaerts, eds. System 4, Associates (London), pp. 216–219 (1985).

48 ROY, J., M. King, R. Snyder, R. Guidoin, L. Martin, K. Botzko, M. Marois, J. Awad and C. Gosselin. "Polyester (Dacron®) Arterial Prostheses Treated with Cross-Linked and Freeze-Dried Albumin," *ASAIO J.*, 8:166 (1985).

49 BENSLIMANE, S., R. Guidoin, D. Marceau, M. King, Y. Mehri, T. J. Rao, L Martin, D. Lafreniere-Gagnon and C. Gosselin. "Albumin-Coated Polyester Arterial Prostheses: Is Xenogenic Albumin Safe?" *Biomat. Art. Cells Art. Org.*, 15:453 (1987).

50 URRY, D. N., R. D. Harris and M. M. Long. "Compounding of Elastin Polypentapeptide to Collagen Analogue: A Potential Elastomeric Prosthetic Material," *Biomat. Med. Dev. Artif. Org.*, 9:181 (1981).

51 MALETTE, W. G., M. J. Quigley, R. D. Gaines, N. D. Johnson and W. G. Rainer. "Chitosan: A New Hemostatic," *Ann. Thorac. Surg.*, 36:55 (1983).

52 HELMUS, M. N., D. F. Gibbons and R. D. Jones. "Surface Analysis of a Series of Copolymers of L-Glutamic Acid and L-Leucine," *J. Coll. Inter. Sc.*, 89:567 (1982).

53 HERRING, M., A. Gardner and J. Glover. "A Single-Staged Technique for Seeding Vascular Grafts with Autogenous Endothelium," *Surgery*, 84:498 (1978).

54 BURKEL, W. E., J. W. Ford, D. W. Vinter, R. H. Kahn, L. M. Graham and J. C. Stanley. "Sequential Studies of Healing in Endothelial Seeded Vascular Prostheses. Histologic and Ultrastructure Characteristics of Vascular Incorporation," *J. Surg. Res.*, 30:305 (1981).

55 CLARKE, J. M. F., R. M. Pittilo, C. J. Nicholson, N. Woolf and

A. Marston. "Seeding Dacron Arterial Prostheses with Peritoneal Mesothelial Cells: A Preliminary Morphological Study," *Brit. J. Surg.*, 71:492 (1984).

56 CHAWLA, A. S. and R. Siphehia. "Characterization of Plasma Polymerized Silicone Coatings Useful as Biomaterials," *J. Biomed. Mat. Res.*, 18:537 (1984).

57 SIPHEHIA, R. and A. S. Chawla. "Characterization of Plasma Polymerized Polypropylene Coatings," *Biomaterials*, 7:155 (1986).

58 YASUDA, H. and N. Morosoff. "Plasma Polymerization of Tetrafluoroethylene II. Capacitive Radiofrequency Discharge," *J. Appl. Polym. Sc.*, 23:1003 (1979).

CHAPTER 14

Hemocompatible Fluorocarbon Emulsions

JEAN G. RIESS, Ph.D. [1]

INTRODUCTION

Fluorocarbon-based oxygen carriers injectable intravascularly are multi-component preparations. The fluorocarbons, being insoluble in water, must be used in emulsified form, which implies the presence of one or more surfactants to stabilize these emulsions. Mineral salts, a buffer system and an oncotic agent are added to adjust the osmotic and oncotic pressures and pH. A cryoprotector is needed when the emulsion has to be frozen for storage. Other substances, including nutrients, vitamins, steroids, antibiotics, thrombolytic agents and other drugs, may be added. It is therefore essential, when assessing the hemo- and, more generally, the bio-compatibility of such emulsions, to examine the innocuity of each one of their ingredients, as well as of the completed final preparation. Several of the latter's physical characteristics, including the size of the dispersed fluorocarbon particles and the osmotic pressure of the continuous aqueous phase, may indeed have determining effects on the biocompatibility of the whole, even if all the individual ingredients taken separately are innocuous.

Fluorocarbon emulsions are expected to find numerous biomedical applications, not only as temporary substitutes for blood to complement blood transfusion, as in case of non-availability or delayed delivery of compatible blood, or to permit the on-site rescue of accident victims, especially in the case of mass casualties, but also in a range of situations where oxygen is required while the transfusion of blood is ineffective or contra-indicated. They are expected, for example, to provide a means of rescuing ischemic myocardial and cerebral tissues, as in the case of coronary occlusion or stroke. Still other indications and uses include anemia, shock, CO-poisoning, perioperative hemodilution, extracorporeal oxygenation, cardioplegia, oxygenation of the cardiac muscle during coronary angioplasty, isolated organs, tissues and limbs preservation, cancer therapy where the presence of oxygen was shown to enhance the cytotoxic action of radio- and chemo-therapy; their perfusion through the ventriculo-subarachnoid spaces shows promise for brain resuscitation after ischemic insult, etc. Fluorocarbons and fluorocarbon emulsions also have considerable potential as contrast agents in diagnosis using NMR or ultrasound imaging and, when brominated and radiopaque, X-ray radiography.

Being based on synthetic compounds, these oxygenating media will be available at will, and their administration will be devoid of any risk of transmission of diseases. No typing and cross-matching will be required, and there will therefore be no delay in their utilization. Not being perishable, they will not require such sophisticated handling and storage precautions as does blood, and their long-term conservation can be envisaged.

Major historical landmarks [1] in the development of fluorocarbon emulsions for intravascular oxygen transport include the initial utilization of a fluorocarbon by Gollan and Clark in 1966 to deliver oxygen to an isolated rat heart [2], its first use in emulsified form by Sloviter in 1967 [3], the definitive survival of Geyer's "bloodless rats" in 1973 [4], the finding that F-decalin is excreted fairly rapidly [5], the development of the first generation of clinically tested emulsions, "Fluosol-DA," in Japan in 1978 [6], followed by "Ftorosan" in the USSR [7] and "Emulsion n° II" in China [8], the approval of Fluosol-DA by the FDA, and the recent development of highly concentrated emulsions of a rapidly excreted fluorocarbon, F-octylbromide (see Addendum).

Present research is aimed at developing improved

[1]Unite de Chimie Moléculaire, Associeé an CNRS, Université de Nice, Parc Valrose, 06034 Nice Cedex, France

"second-generation" blood substitutes, based on more reliable, better defined, more efficient O₂-carriers and surfactants, and having increased O₂-transport capacities, increased intravascular persistence, longer shelf-life, and minimal side effects. It also endeavors to explore their interactions with the organism and assess their therapeutic efficacy in each one of their numerous indications.

Only the most recent papers, i.e., with few exceptions those from 1982 on, will be discussed in this review. For earlier work and further literature, the reader is referred to the Proceedings of Symposia which reflect the state-of-the-art [9–12] and to two recently published collections of reviews and research accounts [13,14]. Other reviews from the author are available, which focus more particularly on the synthesis of the relevant fluorocarbons [15,16], their gas dissolving and transporting properties [17], and the criteria for their selection for biomedical uses [18]. Simultaneous presentations of the fluorocarbon and modified hemoglobin approaches to intravascular oxygen transport may be found in References [12,19,20] (See also the December 1989 Addendum).

PRINCIPLES OF O₂-TRANSPORT AND DELIVERY BY FLUOROCARBON EMULSIONS

Fluorocarbons formally derive from hydrocarbons by substitution of all their hydrogen atoms by fluorine atoms. Thus formulas 1 and 2 represent decalin and perfluoro-

1

or

2

decalin, respectively. The prefix F-, before the name of the parent hydrocarbon, as in F-decalin, and the F inside the rings of the structural formula, indicate that the compound is perfluorinated. The terms "fluorocarbons," "perfluoro-" and "perfluorinated" are, however, customarily extended to other highly fluorinated compounds, even when they also contain some occasional oxygen, nitrogen, hydrogen, chlorine or bromine atoms.

The electron-rich fluorine atoms tend to repel each other, resulting in very weak interactions between the fluorocarbon molecules in the liquid—as reflected by high

TABLE 1. Solubility of O₂ and CO₂ in Some Fluorocarbons and Fluorocarbon Emulsions (vol.%, 37°C, 1 atm.)

		O₂	CO₂
Water, Plasma		2.3	65
Blood		20	70
FC-43	$N(n—C_4F_9)_3$	40.3	142
FTPA	$N(n—C_3F_7)_3$	41.3	166
FDC		42.3	130
F-44E	$C_4F_9CH=CHC_4F_9$	50.1	247
PFOB	$C_8F_{17}Br$	50	247
Fluosol-43 (25%)	Emulsion	8.7	72
Fluosol-DA (20%)	Emulsion	7.1	70
PFOB or F-44E (50%)	Emulsion	15.3	

For additional data see Reference [17] and Table 2.

compressibilities and low surface tensions—and this facilitates the insertion of the oxygen, nitrogen, carbon dioxide and other gaseous molecules between the molecules of fluorocarbons. These materials, indeed, display the highest-known physical oxygen-dissolving capacities [17]: 40 to 50 vol % at 37°C for those acceptable for intravascular administration, compared to ca 2.3 vol % for water or blood plasma (Table 1).

The principle and mechanism of dissolution, transport and delivery of O₂ and CO₂ by fluorocarbon emulsions are fundamentally different from those which operate for blood. In contrast to hemoglobin or hemoglobin-based preparations, in which the oxygen molecule is chemically bound to the iron atom of the receptor site, there is no specific bonding interaction, but only physical dissolution of the gas in the liquid fluorocarbons [17]. Instead of the steep sigmoid O₂-intake vs O₂-partial pressure curve characteristic of hemoglobin (Figure 1), which practically

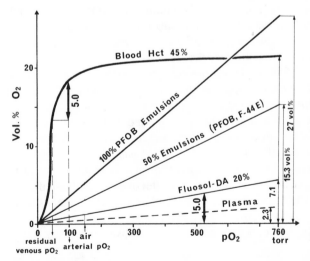

Figure 1. Oxygen uptake vs. oxygen partial pressure for blood and 20% and 50% fluorocarbon emulsions.

reaches a plateau when the partial pressure of O_2 in air is reached, there is a continuous linear increase in the amount of oxygen dissolved in fluorocarbons, which follows Henry's law.

From a practical standpoint, the O_2-dissolving capacity of a typical 20% weight/volume ($\sim$11% by volume) fluorocarbon emulsion is only of ca 1.5 vol % in room air, but it increases about four times faster than for water when the oxygen partial pressure rises above 150 mm Hg. While blood is able to release ca 5 vol % of oxygen (ca one fourth of its O_2-content) in normal physiological conditions in air, such a demand can only be met with a 20% w/v fluorocarbon emulsion if the oxygen fraction in the atmosphere inspired by the patients (FiO_2) is close to unity. This is one of the major limitations of the present fluorocarbon emulsions. This situation may be improved, as will be seen later, by using more concentrated emulsions, as the amount of oxygen dissolved will be roughly proportional to the fluorocarbon content (minus the corresponding diminution of the fraction transported by the reduced continuous plasma phase).

But the O_2-fixation or dissolution capacity of a carrier is not the sole parameter that determines the consumption of oxygen by the tissues. For the fluorocarbons, the absence of chemical fixation (there is no off-loading pO_2 requirement, in contrast with hemoglobin), the higher rate of the oxygenation/deoxygenation process, and the enormous surface for exchanges (several orders of magnitude larger than with red blood cells) relative to the small size of the particles, all contribute to facilitating the extraction of O_2, which can reach very high levels, 90% and more.

Furthermore, high PaO_2 values (300–500 mm Hg) can easily be attained under high FiO_2, which leads to high pO_2 gradients between capillaries and tissues, and hence to high initial diffusion rates in the tissues, thus providing a means of "forcing" oxygen into tissues. The smaller size of the particles results in improved microcirculatory flux, which is also propitious to the recuperation of ischemic tissues. More generally, fluorocarbon emulsions appear to be particularly indicated when high oxygen tensions rather than oxygen content are required.

Other valuable features of the fluorocarbon emulsions when compared to blood are their resistance to the mechanical effects of pumps and filters (as in extracorporeal circulation, isolated organ perfusion, etc.) and their insensitivity to chemical agents such as carbon monoxide or cyanides. It is also noteworthy that their oxygen-delivering capacity is not reduced—by contrast with that of blood—by a change of pH (as in shock) or by refrigeration. In fact, the solubility of oxygen in fluorocarbons increases when temperature decreases, and its availability remains essentially the same, while it becomes more difficult for hemoglobin to unload its oxygen when temperature decreases, as the sigmoid curve of Figure 1 is shifted to the left. A priori, this makes the fluorocarbon

emulsions better suited than blood when oxygen delivery is required in low-temperature open-heart surgery, cardioplegia, or organ preservation.

That these principles apply is supported by numerous experimental observations. As examples, one should recall Sloviter's early demonstration that a fluorocarbon emulsion can adequately supply O_2 and remove CO_2 from isolated rat brain preparations [3], and Geyer's spectacular survival of rats after close-to-total exchange-perfusion (hematocrit $\leq$3 vol %) by such an emulsion, even in atmospheres containing strong proportions of carbon monoxide [21], i.e., in conditions in which hemoglobin's oxygen transport function is totally suppressed (the control animals die in a matter of minutes).

Aerobic cell cultures were shown to grow in the virtual absence of atmosphere over an oxygenated layer of fluorocarbons [22]. Higher oxygen consumption and metabolic activity were measured when rat livers were perfused with a fluorocarbon emulsion rather than with an erythrocyte suspension, in spite of the significantly lower O_2-content and delivery, because of the elevated (95%) extraction level [23]. Effective tissue oxygenation of liver, pancreas, kidney and skeletal muscle, with a very pronounced increase of local pO_2, was observed in dogs after isovolemic hemodilution to Hct 9% with a hydroxyethylstarch solution, then with a 35% fluorocarbon emulsion under pure oxygen [24]. An improvement of myocardial tissue oxygenation and microflow were found after hemodilution by a 20% emulsion of fluorocarbons [25]. Such an emulsion was significantly more effective than blood, dextran or hemoglobin solutions in the oxygenation of the myocardium of hemodiluted dogs [26]. Survival of dogs having undergone experimental hemorrhagic shock was higher when they were infused with a 20% fluorocarbon emulsion than with blood or a hydroxyethyl starch solution [27]. Further data on O_2-delivery, and examples of improved organ and limb preservation and of protection or recuperation of ischemic cardiac or cerebral tissues will be found in the section on Biomedical Applications, Experimental and Clinical Studies.

Where clinical trials with Fluosol-DA 20% are concerned, although the authors usually report that the administration of the emulsion was beneficial to their patients (see section on Biomedical Applications: Experimental and Clinical Studies), one must be cautious in interpreting the data, in view of the widely different indications and status of the patients, frequent absence of appropriate protocols and controls, low fluorocarbon content of the emulsion and low dose administered. Some well-planned trials offering comprehensive data were nevertheless reported, which show that the emulsion fulfilled the expectations where O_2-transport and delivery was concerned, but for a limited time only, owing to limited intravascular persistence.

Thus, when five severely anemic patients were administered, preoperatively, a 20 ml/kg body weight dose of Fluosol-DA 20%, which resulted in a fluorocrit (vol % of fluorocarbon in the vascular fluid) of only 2.9%, it was shown that when the patients inspired 100% pure oxygen the fluorocarbons contributed $24 \pm 7\%$ of the oxygen consumed (a 22% increase) although they transported only 0.8 vol % of oxygen and contributed only $7 \pm 3\%$ of the total arterial O_2-content [28]. PaO_2 and PvO_2 were high (361 ± 65 and 70 ± 27 mm Hg) and the oxygen was extracted at 75–80% from the fluorocarbon, while hemoglobin remained close to saturated ($90 \pm 6\%$). But the intravascular half-life of the fluorocarbon was less than 24 hrs. Comparable results were obtained in Japan [29].

It must, however, also be realized that at high FiO_2s, the share of oxygen transported by the plasma also becomes significant, and can easily reach half of the total [28–30]. It is even possible to keep rats or baboons alive with plasma alone for several hours in the virtual absence of red blood cells when ventilated with 100% pure oxygen, but not to assure their definitive survival. Similarly, the administration of a volume expander to a group of severely anemic patients was shown to be sufficient to restore stable physiologic conditions under pure oxygen, but not at a safe FiO_2 of 0.6; administration of an additional O_2-carrier then became necessary, for which the 20% w/v fluorocarbon emulsion proved efficient—temporarily [30].

CO_2 is even more soluble than O_2 in fluorocarbons (Table 1), and no adverse reaction due to acidosis resulting from CO_2 accumulation has been reported after administration of fluorocarbon emulsions.

SELECTION OF FLUOROCARBONS FOR INTRAVASCULAR USE

To be acceptable for intravascular use, fluorocarbons must obviously obey severe requirements. These include reliability, absence of toxicity, high oxygen-dissolving capacity, large-scale industrial feasibility, acceptable excretion rate, and ease of emulsification [18]. Numerous fluorocarbons have been screened for the purpose of preparing blood substitutes [15,18,31–41]. Those few selected for further evaluation are collected in Table 2.

Purity and Reliability of the Fluorocarbons

Particular concern must be given to the reliability, and hence to the purity, definition and reproducibility of the fluorocarbons. This must be reaffirmed in view of the size of the dose—in the liter range, each liter containing several hundred grams of the fluorocarbon—that is to be administered to the patient. A glance at Table 2 will show that this criterion is far from always having been met, even

by the more recently developed "second generation" O_2-carriers. Most of them are still ill-defined complex mixtures that contain considerable amounts of unidentified components. Although these may be harmless, it is difficult to accept that they should not be properly and individually identified and their innocuity assured. Further concern is raised by the variability in composition that may occur from one batch to another.

At this point it must be recalled that there exist two basically distinct approaches to the synthesis of fluorocarbons [15,18]. One is to start from preformed hydrocarbon compounds and exchange the hydrogens for fluorine atoms; the other is to build up the fluorocarbon molecules from smaller, already perfluorinated building blocks.

The hydrogen-vs-fluorine exchange approach can be achieved through several well-developed industrial processes, such as electrofluorination or fluorination by cobalt trifluoride [42]. Unfortunately, this exchange approach is difficult to control for diverse, uncircumventable thermodynamic and mechanistic reasons [43], and therefore usually yields complex mixtures resulting from incomplete fluorination, isomerization, fragmentation, hydrogen fluoride elimination, etc. [44]. All the cyclic compounds as well as the acyclic amines shown in Table 2 were prepared by such methods, and among them only F-decalin appears to be obtained in an acceptable grade of purity as a mixture of the cis and trans isomers. The others come as multicomponent mixtures (Figure 2), whose exact composition is usually not precisely documented. The isolation of pure compounds from these mixtures is difficult, and in any event appears to be economically unrealistic on an industrial scale.

The stepwise assemblage of already perfluorinated building blocks such as tetrafluoroethylene (the precursor of Teflon) or hexafluoropropylene oxide through selective chemical routes is more suited to obtaining the well-defined, pure, reproducible materials required for intravascular administration.

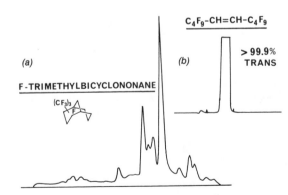

Figure 2. *Gas chromatograms of samples of (a) "F-trimethylbicyclononane" produced by the CoF_3 fluorination method and (b) bis(F-butyl)ethene prepared from tetrafluoroethylene telomerisation products.*

TABLE 2. Perfluorochemicals Most Extensively Investigated for Blood Substitution

Perfluorochemical	Code or trade names |Molec. Weight|	Preparation definition purity	vp(mmHg)37°	solub. O_2 CO_2 (vol.%, 37°C)	Stability of emulsions	Retention[a] 1/2 time (days)	Observations
(furan structure) C_4F_9	FX-80 FC-75 |418|	electrochem. mixture	58		fair	long	too high vapor pressure (lung emphysema)
$N(C_4F_9)_3$	FC-43 |671|	electrochem. mixture 80–85%	1.1	40 142	excellent	>500	for isolated organ perfusion (in Oxypherol and Emulsion n°I)
$C_8F_{17}Br$	PFOB |499|	telomerisation >99%	18	50	very good	2–6	radiopaque
(decalin structure)	FDC PP5 |462|	CoF_3 ~97%	12.5	42 142	low	7	insufficient stability of emulsions (in Fluosol-DA, Ftorosan, Emulsion n°II)
$N(C_3F_7)_3$	FTPA |521|	electrochem. mixture >95%	18.5	45 166	very good	65	long retention time (present in Fluosol-DA and Emulsion n°II)
$C_4F_9CH{=}CHC_4F_9$	F-44E |462|	telomerisation >99.9%	12.6	50 247	fair	7	
CF_3 CF_3 $CFCH{=}CHC_6F_{13}$	F-i36E |512|	telomerisation >99.9%	7.6	50 224	good	20–25	
$C_6F_{13}CH{=}CHC_6F_{13}$	F-66E |664|	telomerisation >99.9%	2.3	42.8 181	excellent	>400	for isolated organ perfusion, CEC, cell cultures, etc.
(bicyclic structure)	FBC |462|	CoF_3 67–87%	13.5	43.5	fair–poor[b]	5	limited industrial feasibility
$3CF_3$ (structure)	FTN |562|	CoF_3 50–55%	2.9	40	fair–good[b]	11–14 30[b]	too complex mixture
$(C_6F_{13})_2O$	FHE |654|	electrochem. 90–98%	2.0	43.7	excellent	>500	overlong retention
(structure with N)	FMA |483|	electrochem. 80–94%	17	40	poor–fair[b]	10–11 30[b]	remains slightly toxic even after 5 days reflux with KOH 8N/HN(^{i}Bu)$_2$
(quinoline structure)	FMOQ |495|	electrochem. 95%(cis + trans)	10.7	43	good	7	
(quinoline structure)	FHQ |495|	electrochem. 65% (major constituent 30%)	8.1	40	good	9	require multi-step complex detoxification
(quinoline structure)	FMIQ |495|	electrochem. 95%(cis + trans)			good	11	Green Cross Corp. selection for 2nd generation
(structure)	FCHP |495|	electrochem. 87%	8.6	46	fair	16	
(structure)	FMCP |595|	electrochem. 75%			excellent	60	long retention time (present in Ftorosan)

[a]For comparable doses of ~4g/kg weight in rats.
[b]Evaluations vary with method and research team.

The latter approach can be used for the preparation of F-octyl bromide [34], and is further exemplified by the synthesis of a series of bis(F-alkyl)ethenes, $C_nF_{2n+1}CH = CHC_n'F_{2n'+1}$ [33,39,40], developed as shown in Figure 3. These constitute a family of homologous linear and branched compounds, code-named F-nn'E, where the variation of the numbers, n and n', of carbon atoms in the fluorinated chains grafted onto the ethene center E, allows stepwise modification of their properties. Of the 20 compounds that were prepared, two (F-44E and F-i36E) were selected for intravascular use on account of their acceptable organ half-retention times (7 and 20–25 days, respectively), and one (F-66E) for non-intravascular use (extracorporeal circulation, organ and tissue preservation, cell cultures, etc.) because of the excellent stability of its emulsions. Besides the high degree of purity of F-44E and F-i36E, one must stress their large-scale industrial feasibility. Their above average oxygen solubility is also noteworthy: for comparable molecular weight that of F-44E is ~20% superior to that of F-decalin; this may in part be related to the structural accident linked to the presence of the double bond and to its location inside the molecule [46]. The absence of chemical reactivity and of metabolism, which could have arisen from the presence of an insaturation, was also carefully determined; it was shown that the highly shielded ethylenic bond buried inside the structure resists, for example, the action of diethylamine (3 days at 120°C), bromine (3 days at 120°C), m-chloroperbenzoic acid, or the "biomimetic" iodosylbenzene/tetraphenylporphiriniron(III) oxidative system [39,40,45].

The question of the biological inertness of the fluorocarbons will be discussed in the section on Hemocompatibility, Biocompatiblity and Side Effects of the Fluorocarbons, Surfactants and Emulsions. Their identification and quantitative analysis in blood and organs can be conveniently and precisely achieved by ^{19}F NMR [47,48], as well as, after extraction, by GC.

Excretion Rate vs Molecular Weight

A condition sine qua non for their intravascular use is that fluorocarbons ultimately leave the body. The current

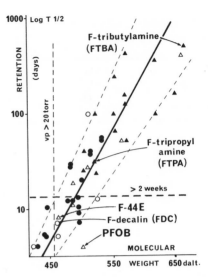

Figure 4. Retention of the fluorocarbons in the organs (on a log scale) vs. molecular weight; triangles = acyclic, circles = cyclic, open and full signs = without and with heteroatoms. For details see ref. [18].

view is that half-residence times in the organs, which is dose-dependent, should not exceed 2–3 weeks for a normal therapeutic dose. No evidence of metabolism has ever been reported for the fluorocarbons listed in Table 2. Part of their excretion, which takes place by exhalation, occurs while the fluorocarbons are present in the blood stream and circulating through the lung; the rest is taken up by the circulating macrophages, which carry them and store them in various organs, principally the liver and spleen, whence they are excreted at slower, widely differing rates, depending on the individual fluorocarbons. Some are retained in these organs for years; this was unfortunately the case for F-tributylamine, the fluorocarbon that allowed Geyer to achieve the first successful total exchange-perfusion of rats [4]. It was therefore a decisive breakthrough when Clark [5,49] and Naito [50] independently showed in 1973 that F-decalin was excreted from the body after a half-residence time of about one week only, but it turned out to be impossible to prepare stable F-decalin emulsions with the available surfactants. Somehow the belief then developed that cyclic structures (such as F-decalin) lead to improved excretion rates, and that heteroatoms (as in F-tributylamine), on the contrary, retard excretion, while the effect on the emulsion's stability is the reverse [51].

It was these notions that led to the design of the "second-generation" carriers which incorporate both cycles and nitrogen atoms in the same molecular structure. Upon closer analysis of the available excretion data, this conception is seen to be unfounded [17,18]. Figure 4 shows that the excretion rates are primarily a steep, exponential function of the fluorocarbon's molecular weight. The data available do *not* permit the assignment of any significant

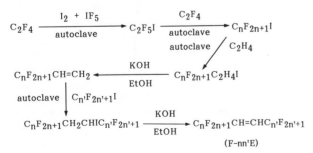

Figure 3. Example of selective synthesis of fluorocarbon-based oxygen carriers avoiding the traumatic and hard-to-control fluorine vs. hydrogen exchange reaction: the bis(F-alkyl)ethene family.

influence of the presence of cycles or of heteroatoms on the excretion rates. For a given molecular weight the excretion rates of cyclic and acyclic compounds, with or without heteroatoms, are randomly scattered within the area delineated by the dotted lines in Figure 4. The presence of cycles or heteroatoms appears to have no effect *per se*, but only in so far as it affects the molecular weight: the excretion rate being sharply dependent on the molecular weight, the effect of each cyclisation, by eliminating two fluorine atoms, i.e., 38 mass units, or the addition of a nitrogen atom, and consequently of an extra fluorine atom, i.e., 33 mass units, on this rate is considerable. Similarly, the critical solution temperatures in hexane for mono, di and tricyclic species, which appear to reflect differences in excretion rates [52], were shown to simply parallel their molecular weights; the same correlation is indeed found for cyclic and for acyclic species [53].

The individual data points given in Figure 4 should be considered with caution, as the retention time depends on the share of the fluorocarbon that is captured by the macrophages and transported to the organs, which in turn strongly depends on the dose given and on the size of the particles in the emulsions [54]. In addition, no two research groups used the same evaluation method; some data measured on mixtures probably have little meaning, and standard errors are seldom given. Nevertheless, these data considered *collectively* establish that the molecular range pertinent to intravascular use is narrow, and can be set at 500 ± 40 mass units for the fluorocarbons usually tested so far. An interesting exception is found with F-octylbromide, for which the excretion rate is considerably faster (2.1 days for a 2.5 g/kg dose; 8.4 days for a 10 g/kg dose in rats) than would be expected from its molecular weight [55]. This is undoubtedly due to the presence of the more lipophilic and exposed bromine atom in end position on the chain.

More recently, Yokoyama et al. analyzed the retention data collected on 52 compounds [56] and basically confirmed our views [17,18], since they found that neither the connectivity (cyclizations and ramifications) nor the presence of heteroatoms such as oxygen or nitrogen had significant effects on the fluorocarbons' half-retention times ($T\frac{1}{2}$) in vivo. They also confirm the excellent correlation between $T\frac{1}{2}$ and critical solution temperatures (correlation factor $r = 0.92$), or the number of fluorine atoms ($r = 0.91$), which both essentially reflect the fluorocar-

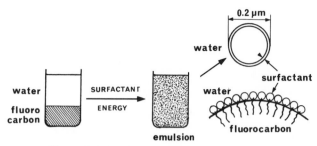

Figure 6. *Schematic constitution of an emulsion.*

bons' molecular weight (between molecular weight and number of fluorine atoms: $r = 0.98$). The introduction of the fluorocarbon's vapor pressure as a correction factor does not improve the correlation, and appears pointless in view of the uncertainty which accompanies the $T\frac{1}{2}$ measurements ($\sim 15\%$), to which one must add that, difficult to appreciate, which results from the low purity and definition of most electrochemically produced samples.

THE FORMULATION OF FLUOROCARBON EMULSIONS

Principles and Preparation Methods

Fluorocarbons are insoluble in water and do not dissolve mineral salts, proteins, metabolites, or lipids in any significant amounts [57] (Figure 5); they must therefore be dispersed as very small droplets, ca 0.1 μm in diameter (about 1/70 the size of red blood cells), in a plasma, before being infused into the vascular system. The preparation of such dispersions—or emulsions—requires the addition of surface-active agents and an input of energy, usually by ultrasonication or high-pressure homogenization.

One role of the surfactants is to reduce the interfacial tension that opposes the considerable increase in surface area associated with the dispersion of one of the phases as small droplets in the other (Figure 6). The surfactants are amphiphilic molecules, i.e., have both a hydrophilic end that interacts often through hydrogen bonding, with the water molecules and a hydrophobic tail that is more like the fluorocarbon phase. These features cause them to adsorb at the interface between the two immiscible liquids, where they tend to form a monomolecular layer.

The number of surfactants reported to have been evaluated for the preparation of fluorocarbon-based O_2-carriers is astonishingly limited compared to that of the fluorocarbons. Those used in the emulsions tested so far are essentially Pluronic F-68, a neutral synthetic polydisperse polyoxyethylenepolyoxypropylene block polymer [58], and natural egg yolk phospholipids, separately or mixed (Table 3). When injected intravenously, lecithins are rapidly metabolized, while Pluronics are excreted unmodified in the urine.

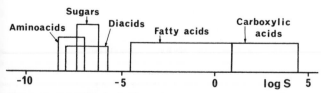

Figure 5. *Solubility (mol. % on a log scale) of some biologically relevant compounds in bis(F-hexyl)ethene at 37°C. Adapted from ref. [57].*

TABLE 3. *Surfactants Used in Blood Substitutes*

Pluronic F-68	$HO(CH_2CH_2O)_n(CHCH_2O)_p(CH_2CH_2O)_{n'}H$ CH_3 synthetic, polydisperse block-polymer, average molec. weight 8300, neutral.
Egg yolk phospholipids	R_1COOCH_2 R_2COOCH $O-$ $H_2C-O-P(O)-OCH_2CH_2N^+(CH_3)_3$ natural, polydisperse, R_1 and R_2 = various fatty acids chains, saturated and unsaturated, amphoteric, also other polar heads
Potassium oleate	$cis-CH_3(CH_2)_7CH=CH(CH_2)_7COOK$ soap derived from natural product, anionic.

The stability of the emulsions obtained with these surfactants for the excretable, i.e., relatively low molecular weight, fluorocarbons, is limited [18]. At room temperature the particles tend to coarsen with time, and the emulsions eventually break down into two separate phases. One must, however, clearly distinguish between particle aggregation and coalescence. Aggregation is favored by the high density of the fluorocarbons, but preserves the individual particles and is reversible. It is observed even with very stable emulsions, which may thus show apparent phase separation, but their initial characteristics can be restored by gentle stirring, which will resuspend the particles. On the contrary, coalescence results in the formation of larger droplets, and eventually in true phase separation; it is irreversible unless a fresh amount of energy is put in to divide the particles again. Coalescence is favored by collisions, but depends also on the particle size and size dispersion, structure of the interfacial film, viscosity of the continuous phase, etc.

Another major cause of deterioration of fine emulsions results from the increase in vapor pressure and solubility of a liquid as the size of the droplets decreases (Kelvin effect), which provides a mechanism for the fluorocarbon molecules to leave the smaller droplets and join the larger ones, progressively increasing the average particle size in the emulsion (Ostwald ripening). This molecular diffusion effect increases with increasing temperature, decreasing particle size, increasing dispersion of the size-distribution and, strongly, with increasing vapor pressure of the fluorocarbon, hence with decreasing molecular weights. Molecular diffusion is probably the major reason for the considerable difference in stability found, for example, between the F-tributylamine and F-decalin emulsions [18] or, within the same homologous series, between the bis(F-butyl) and the bis(F-hexyl) ethenes (F-44E and F-66E) [40].

Molecular diffusion can be slowed down by the addition of relatively small amounts of fluorocarbons having a higher molecular weight [59,60], but at the expense of a lengthy organ retention of this added heavy fluorocarbon.

So far no evidence supports the view that the presence of heteroatoms in the fluorocarbons contributes to stabilizing the emulsions. On the other hand, for similar molecular weights linear compounds may give more stable emulsions than cyclic ones. Thus the particle size was found to increase more slowly in emulsions of F-44E than in similarly formulated and prepared emulsions of F-decalin [40].

Emulsification has usually been achieved by sonication or by high pressure homogenization; more recently, a hydroshear process has been evaluated [61], and a new technique, based on an impinging jet principle termed 'microfluidization,' has been offered [62]. Figure 7 compares the results obtained for the same emulsion formulation with three of these procedures. The high pressure homogenization process gave the finest emulsions, and narrowest particle size distribution; however, it requires large amounts of fluorocarbon, which are not always

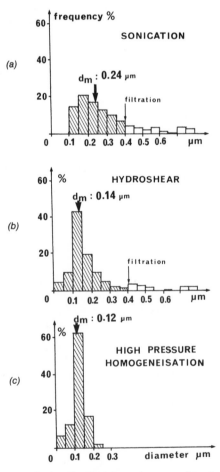

Figure 7. *Particle size distributions and average diameter, μm, of 30 w/v % emulsions of F-44E with 4% Pluronic F-68 prepared at 20°C by (a) sonication (15 min), (b) hydroshear (40 bar, 30 min), and (c) high-pressure homogenization (350 bar, 30 min).*

available when the screening of new compounds is concerned. The hydroshear process yielded somewhat larger average particle sizes, and left more large-size particles that had to be filtered out; the minimum emulsion volume to be prepared is similar. Sonication has the advantage of being applicable even when only very small samples of the fluorocarbon or surfactant are available. But it tends to give rather wide particle size distributions, and suffers from poor reproducibility since the results depend on such parameters as size and shape of the ultrasonic probe, size, shape and filling of the container, position of the sonic probe in the liquid, etc.; furthermore, it tends to provoke some degradation of the fluorocarbons, as evidenced by the formation of fluorine ions (which can be suppressed by working in the absence of oxygen), and to release titanium particles from the probe into the media.

For long the emulsions investigated have been only poorly characterized: particle size distributions have seldom been reported. This is unfortunate, expecially since many emulsions were prepared by sonication, a method which suffers from very poor reproducibility. As a consequence the appreciation of emulsion stability has often been highly subjective, and dependent on the research group. The optical density and degree of opacity of an emulsion, since they depend on how close the refractive indexes of the fluorocarbon, surfactants and water are, do not provide any reliable notion of the particle sizes; some translucent emulsions turn out to have larger particle sizes than some milky-white ones. Only the actual comparative measurement of the evolution of particle size distributions with time provides a sound basis for evaluation of the emulsion's stability. The situation should now improve rapidly, owing to the commercial availability of automated devices based on centrifugal sedimentation and light adsorption, or by laser light photon correlation spectroscopy [16].

First-Generation Fluorocarbon Emulsions

The first generation of fluorocarbon emulsions for intravascular use to have reached the clinical trial stage is essentially represented by "Fluosol-DA 20%," which was developed in 1978 by the Green Cross Corporation (Osaka, Japan) [6]. Then came "Ftorosan" in the Soviet Union (Acad. Sciences USSR, Pushchino) [7] and "Emulsion $n°$ II" in China (Acad. Sinica, Inst. Org. Chem., Shanghai) [8]. All three emulsions (Table 3) use F-decalin as the principal oxygen-carrier (70%), to which a F-trialkylamine of higher molecular weight is added (30%) in order to improve the stability of the emulsion. The primary or sole surfactant is a polyoxyethylenepolyoxypropylene block-polymer [58] of the Pluronic F-68 type. The stem emulsions are obtained by high-pressure homogenization, and the final preparations are of comparable formulation. A new emulsion, of different formulation,

based on F-octylbromide and egg yolk phospholipids, which has both oxygen-carrying and radiopaque properties, is now being investigated [63].

Of the three F-decalin-based emulsions, Fluosol is the best documented in the literature, and will be discussed below; the data available on Ftorosan and Emulsion $n°$ II basically confirm the findings made on Fluosol. In view of the close similarity of the three emulsions, it is probable that their performances and their limitations are comparable.

The formulation of Fluosol-DA [64] was dictated by the need to find a compromise between insufficient emulsion stability and excessive retention in the organs: F-decalin had been shown to be excreted reasonably rapidly ($T\frac{1}{2} \sim$ 7 days), but it turned out to be impossible to obtain stable emulsions with the available surfactants; on the other hand, F-tripropylamine allowed considerably stabler emulsions to be prepared, but was retained for an overlong period of time in the organs ($T\frac{1}{2} \sim$ 65 days). The dilemma was "solved" by adding F-tripropylamine to F-decalin in a 3:7 ratio. A more stable emulsion— although it still needs to be stored in the frozen state— resulted from this compromise, but at the expense of a prolonged retention of part of the fluorocarbon in the organs. Emulsion $n°$ II is also based on a 70:30 F-decalin/F-tripropylamine mixture, while in Ftorosan the latter compound is replaced by F-methylcyclohexylpiperidine, an electrochemically produced nitrogen-containing bicyclic compound (Table 2), for which a retention half-time of 60 days has been reported; this is surprisingly low in view of its molecular weight, which would suggest a figure closer to 200 days.

The advent of Fluosol-DA was an important milestone in the history of fluorocarbon-based biomedical O_2-carriers, but this first emulsion also has many drawbacks. Besides the prolonged organ-retention of one of the O_2-carriers, and its being based on two O_2-carriers of widely different characteristics, there are also several other problems, including: the presence of several % impurities in the F-tripropylamine employed; the use of two poly-dispersed, ill-defined surfactants, including, principally, the Pluronic F-68, which has been found responsible for an acute, though transient, anaphylactic reaction with some patients (see the later discussion on Hemocompatibility, Biocompatibility and Side Effects of the Fluorocarbons, Surfactants and Emulsions); its limited storage stability unless frozen; its relatively low oxygen-dissolving capacity, related to its low fluorocarbon content; its low intravascular persistence; and a certain lack of reproducibility from one batch to the other. Besides, no sufficient data could be offered to prove durable efficacy when it was submitted to FDA for approval in the treatment of anemia, an indication which indeed requires prolonged intravascular persistence of the fluorocarbon. The FDA's conclusion that the preparation was not ready for approval [65] is therefore logical.

The commercial availability of Fluosol-DA 20% has initially given considerable impetus to the development of the field. It had the merit of showing at a still early stage that huge amounts of a fluorocarbon emulsion can be administered intravenously and are tolerated by the organism, and that the fluorocarbons contribute significantly to the delivery of oxygen to the tissues. In a second stage, its insufficiencies and the dependence of the biomedical research community on this single preparation may have hindered the collection of significant data; moreover, people have tended to associate fluorocarbon emulsions in general with Fluosol-DA, and to systematically credit the former with the drawbacks of the latter.

Emulsions for non-intravascular use (extracorporeal circulation, organ perfusion, biomedical research) based on F-tributylamine, have also been developed under the names "Oxypherol" or "Fluosol-43" [6] by the Green Cross Corporation in Japan, and "Emulsion n° I" in China.

Towards Improved Second-Generation Emulsions

Improvement over the first-generation emulsions should primarily concern the reliability of the constituents, fluorocarbons and surfactants, the oxygen transport capacity, the intravascular persistence, the storage stability, and the minimization of side-effects.

As previously mentioned, fluorocarbons should be chosen in the 460–540 molecular weight range to assure reasonably fast excretion. F-tripropylamine, which is strongly retained in the spleen [66], where it has been detected two years after infusion of Fluosol-DA [67], should be abandoned for intravascular use.

Obtaining pure, well-defined fluorocarbons is no longer a problem, provided the telomerization route is chosen. This route is usually also associated with lower costs when both preparation and purification are taken into account.

Pluronic F-68 may have to be discarded, in view of its side effects (see the discussion on Hemocompatibility, Biocompatibility and Side Effects of the Fluorocarbons, Surfactants and Emulsions) and polydisperse nature. The development of new, biocompatible surfactants, more particularly designed for the emulsification of fluorocarbons, has become a major necessity.

Improvement of the O_2-carrying capacity of the emulsions is necessary, if only to allow safer FiO_2's to be used. This can be achieved primarily by increasing their fluorocarbon content, and then, to a limited (10–20%) extent, by choosing the compounds that have the highest O_2-solubility coefficients; here, for a given molecular weight, the linear compounds seem to have a definite edge over the cyclic ones (Figure 8) [68].

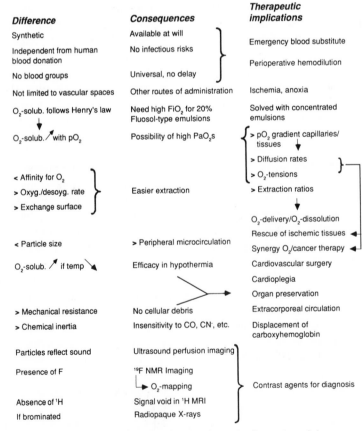

Figure 8. Potential of fluorocarbon emulsions in diagnosis and therapy.

Where the concentration is concerned, it must be realized that the Fluosol-DA 20% w/v-type emulsions contain only ca 11% of fluorocarbons by volume, and that the administration of a typical 20 ml/kilo body weight dose will then result in an intravascular fluorocarbon content (fluorocrit) of less than 3 vol %.

Considerably more concentrated emulsions are feasible. The once-offered Fluosol-DA 35% w/v preparation unfortunately received only limited attention. Yet baboons that underwent isovolemic total exchange perfusion with this preparation to hematocrit <2% survived at a safe FiO_2 of 0.6 [69]. The arterial O_2-content was then essentially the same as with Fluosol-DA 20% at $FiO_2 = 1$. Normal hemodynamics and O_2 transport were maintained, in spite of a marked fall in arterial O_2-content and total O_2-delivery. It was concluded that Fluosol-DA 35% is an effective O_2-carrier at a safe FiO_2 of 0.6. Why the 20% and not the 35% emulsion was favored for development is therefore not clear; a possible reason is that the viscosity of the emulsions increases rapidly with concentration when Pluronic is the surfactant.

Even more concentrated emulsions (50% w/v, or 27% by volume) of PFOB or F-66E with egg yolk phospholipids as the surfactant have been shown to be perfectly well tolerated by exchange-transfused (Hct ~3%) conscious rats [70]. These rats were seen to be remarkably alert under $FiO_2 = 0.6$, and their hematocrit was restored within 8–10 days. 100% w/v emulsions (52% by volume) of PFOB, more specifically designed for diagnosis purposes, have been administered to various species [71].

Intravascular persistence is another decisive issue, since it determines the efficacy of the O_2-carrying preparations. Indeed, while improvement in patients has been reported in cases of anemia after administration of Fluosol-DA, these beneficial effects were only short-lasting [28,30]. Intravascular persistence appears to depend on the size of the particles, dose given to the patients, administration mode—by fractions or all at once—nature and possible re-injection of the surfactant, and, in animals, the species. Thus for example half-residence-time in circulation in rabbits was found to increase from 30 to 85 h when the average particle size for a given formulation and dose decreased from 0.25 to 0.09 μm [6]. Half-residence times of Fluosol-DA 20% in surgical patients for 10, 20 and 30 ml/kg body weight doses were estimated at 7.5, 14.5 and 22 h, respectively [37]. A significant 3-times-longer intravascular residence of F-decalin in rats by subsequent injections of additional doses of the surfactant, in this case lecithins, has been reported [72]. Unfortunately these F-decalin/lecithin emulsions do not appear to be stable enough to stand sterilization and storage. Clearly the question of the intravascular persistence of the preparations is linked to the mastering of the emulsions, and hence to the availability of adequate surfactants.

Obtaining more stable emulsions that can be shipped and stored for several months or years without particular precautions is another important challenge. Once the fluorocarbon is chosen the stability of the emulsion will depend primarily on the surfactant(s). Pluronic F-68 and egg yolk phospholipids have obviously not been specifically designed for the emulsification of fluorocarbons, and the characteristics and stability that they confer to the emulsions of the relevant fluorocarbons appear to have reached a limit, whatever the emulsification procedure. Fluorocarbon "oils" are very different in nature from the usual hydrocarbon oil phases; they are not only considerably more hydrophobic than hydrocarbons, but they are even *oleo*phobic, and hence require surfactants with more fluorophilic ends, i.e., F-alkyl chains, in order to reduce the fluorocarbon/water interfacial tension enough to give stable emulsions. Interesting synergistic stabilization effects can also be expected from the combination of two surfactants, one of which is perfluoroalkylated [16].

A striking exception is again provided by the PFOB/lecithin emulsions, which appear to be significantly more stable than those obtained with lecithins and fluorocarbons without functional groups or heteroatoms, or where such groups or atoms are hidden inside the molecule [70]; the bromine atom at the end of the chain is likely to increase the lipophilicity of PFOB, hence its affinity for the lecithins.

A few attempts at using perfluoroalkylated surfactants have already been reported [73,74], but failed because the surfactants or preparations were toxic. However, fairly stable but still poorly defined emulsions of various fluorocarbons were obtained using a perfluoroalkylated amine oxide (XMO-10, Table 3) as the surfactant, which were only moderately toxic upon injection [75]; but this toxicity still appears to be too high to authorize intravascular use, and the fate of this surfactant and its possible retention in organs such as the spleen is not yet documented. Pluronic-type surfactants, modified by the introduction of perfluoroalkyl chains at both ends, have recently been shown to reduce surface tension significantly; but toxicity data have not yet been made available [76].

Another approach, in order to achieve long-term storage stability, may be provided by *micro*emulsions. In contradistinction to normal emulsions—or macroemulsions—microemulsions form spontaneously when the appropriate proportions of fluorocarbon, aqueous phase and surfactant(s) are present [77]. Therefore, a microemulsion is usually considered as a thermodynamically stable state of the oil/water/surfactant(s) mixture, with the interfacial tension reaching zero. The formation of microemulsions is dependent on specific interactions among the constituent molecules, and it occurs within a well defined, temperature-dependent domain of composition. An input of mechanical work will not produce a microemulsion if these interactions are not realized, while on the other hand, once these conditions are present, their formation usually occurs spontaneously. Moreover, the individual droplets of the dispersed phase are very small, with an average radius significantly lower than the wave-length of light, which makes them transparent, or at least translucent to the eye. Transparency by itself is however no proof of the occurrence of a microemulsion, as it can result from comparable refractive indexes of the two phases and surfactant film. Being essentially independent of preparation procedures, the characteristics of microemulsions are, for a given composition, highly reproducible. Microemulsions, if biocompatibility can be achieved, would be an attractive solution to the problem of long-term shelf stability of the fluorocarbon preparations.

The development of injectable microemulsions is, however, bristling with obstacles: their formulation requires considerable amounts of perfluoroalkylated surfactants, while none sufficiently biocompatible are available yet; their physical characteristics and stability domain are strongly dependent on their composition, which is destined to evolve as they are injected into the blood stream; finally, nothing is known yet of the particular physiological action that may be related to the smallness of the droplets' sizes.

The use of microemulsions of fluorocarbons as blood substitutes for the preservation of organs was first suggested by Rosano and Geracia in 1973 [78]. Perfluoroalkylated amine oxides and alcohols were mentioned among the suitable surfactants and co-surfactants, but no toxicity data were made available. Another patent reports the obtaining of clear, spontaneously formed dispersions of fluorocarbons by using a mixture of two polydisperse perfluoroalkylated polyoxyethylene surfactants [79]. These preparations unfortunately turned out to be toxic, and thus unfit for biomedical use. Delpuech et al. have shown that microemulsions can be obtained with a single monodisperse neutral perfluoroalkylpolyoxyethylene surfactant; but biocompatibility was not achieved here either [74,80]. Further work is needed to evaluate this approach; the principal difficulties here, besides the biocompatibility problem, are linked to the large amount of surface-active material required, to the narrowness of the stability domains described so far, and to the fact that their position in the phase diagram is sensitive to temperature, to dilution and to the other components present.

HEMOCOMPATIBILITY, BIOCOMPATIBILITY AND SIDE EFFECTS OF THE FLUOROCARBONS, SURFACTANTS AND EMULSIONS

The absence of acute as well as long-term toxicity is an obvious prerequisite to the routine clinical use of fluorocarbon emulsions. As noted in the Introduction, the question of the biocompatibility of fluorocarbon emulsions concerns each of their ingredients *plus* the final preparation. Unfortunately, the reported observations of side-effects are not always exploitable. For example, it is not always clear whether the indispensable control of the purity and absence of toxicity of the various ingredients, including the commercially available ones, or of the state of conservation of the emulsions has been properly done. Moreover, when side-effects of the emulsions have been noticed, it has seldom been established which ingredient or parameter was responsible. Finally, it should be clear that biocompatibility is by no means synonymous with biological inertness; the problem is to assess whether or not the beneficial O_2-delivering effect largely outweighs the undesirable other effects and possible risks for the patient, and to reduce these to a minimum.

Fluorocarbons, Surfactants, Oncotic Agents

During the earlier period of this research, there was a definite tendency to blame the fluorocarbons for any untoward reaction observed upon administration of their emulsions. As the work progressed, it was usually found that these reactions had to be imputed to the presence of impurities or to another ingredient, primarily the surfactant, or to some inappropriate physical characteristic of the emulsion, such as too-coarse particle size or inadequate osmotic pressure. Presently, it appears that the fluorocarbons themselves are biologically the most inert (besides their O_2/CO_2 delivering capacity!) of the constituents of the preparation. No one has demonstrated any toxic effect directly due to the fluorocarbons when pure and chosen in the appropriate molecular weight range. Typically, the lung emphysema observed in the early experiments with FC-80 was related to its too-low molecular weight and too-high vapor pressure (MW 418; 58 mm Hg); it was no longer found when the molecular weight was in the 460 to 540 range, defined in a previous section. A puzzling observation is that F-tributylamine appears to affect the in vitro deformability of human red cells, but only in the presence of plasma, while F-tripropylamine and F-decalin do not [81].

Unrefined fluorocarbons, crude from synthesis, often display some toxicity, especially when prepared by fluorocarbon-vs-hydrogen exchange procedures. Cell cultures, rather than analytical or spectroscopic data, provide an easy-to-perform, sensitive initial test for assessing this toxicity and for monitoring the progress of purification and detoxification procedures [82]. The measurement, with respect to controls, of the growth-rate and viability of Namalva lymphoblastoid cell cultures in the presence of the fluorocarbon, and of their growth after resowing, has for example been used for this purpose [83]. The toxic effects are usually seen to decrease when treatments such as washing with diluted aqueous potassium hydroxide, shaking with charcoal or filtration over alumina are applied. This clearly shows that the initial toxicity is not due to the fluorocarbons themselves, but to some impurities, excess reactants or side products present in the crude reaction product. Detoxification of some of the nitrogen-containing cyclic compounds, whose toxicity has been attributed to the presence of fluoroamine-containing side-products, appears to be particularly arduous, requiring lengthy heating with KOH/HNEt$_2$ to achieve it [44,84]. The observation that toxic impurities may be temporarily masked by dilution in a fluorocarbon further shows that cautious purification and control of the O$_2$-carrier must be performed before use [32].

Detoxification can also be achieved on the completed emulsion. For example, Oxypherol, the F-tributylamine emulsion marketed by the Green Cross Corp., was shown to inhibit insulin [85] and testosterone [86] secretion. It was demonstrated in the latter case that the endocrine function was no longer affected when the emulsion was first submitted to an ion-exchange and dialysis cleaning procedure [87], again establishing that it was not the fluorocarbon, but some toxic impurities present in the emulsion, which included fluoride ions, which were responsible for the deleterious effects observed.

The occasional presence of nitrogen, oxygen, bromine or hydrogen atoms, tertiary carbon atoms or hydrogenated double bonds does not appear to confer any toxicity on otherwise perfluorinated compounds. No evidence exists either for their favoring enzymatic attack or metabolism.

A report on the state of health of plant workers routinely exposed to fluorochemicals indicates that, although considerably higher than normal organic fluorine levels were found in their blood, there were no ill effects attributable to this exposure [88].

Paradoxically, much less concern has been devoted to the toxicity and possible side-effects of the surfactants, although surface-active agents by their very nature cannot be expected to be biologically innocent [89,90], especially with regard to membranes. In spite of a high LD$_{50}$ of about 8 g/kg body weight i.v. in rats [37], Pluronic F-68 has been found responsible for the unpredictable anaphylactic reaction observed in some patients in response to the injection of Fluosol-DA (vide infra). Pluronic F-68 was also shown to cause an impairment of phospholipase A$_2$ activity and to have an in vitro inhibitory effect on the chemotactic, phagocytic and metabolic functions of human neutrophils [91–94], accompanied by an impairment of host resistance to bacterial infection [95]. Other studies suggest that the Pluronic-containing emulsions Fluosol-DA and Fluosol-43 activate monocyte procoagulant generation, although no significant cytotoxicity was observed, and may impair normal monocyte oxidative metabolism [96]. Inhibition by Fluosol-DA of the growth of cultured human embryonic lung cells [97] and of macrophages obtained from peritoneal exudates of mice

[98] could also be due to this surfactant. Contradictory reports have appeared on the influence of fluorocarbon emulsions on platelet aggregation and coagulation [67, 99–101]; when effects were observed, they also appeared to be due to the surfactant and not to the fluorocarbon. No effect on platelets were noted, for example, when lecithins were used as surfactants instead of Pluronic F-68 or albumin [72].

It is clear that surfactants also require careful purification and control before use, but this is seldom documented in the publications. Commercial grade Pluronic F-68, for example, must be treated with activated charcoal or ion-exchanging resins until it no longer affects cell cultures. In any event additional effort is needed to fully assess its side effects, whether they are due to the compound itself or to an impurity, their gravity, and whether the risk they represent is acceptable or not. Some of these "side-effects" of Pluronic F-68 may have therapeutic utility. Thus it has been used to reduce fat embolism [102], and as a protective agent against hemolysis during extracorporeal circulation [103].

Compared to Pluronic F-68, egg yolk phospholipids are much less controverted—although they also come as mixtures—because of their natural origin and current wide use in intravascularly injectable fat preparations for parenteral nutrition. If the problem of the fluorocarbon/lecithin emulsion stability were resolved (which appears to be the case with the recently developed PFOB emulsions [70]), such emulsions should cause less concern than the fat emulsions, in view of the considerably greater biological inertness of fluorocarbons compared to lipids. Proper precautions should however be taken to assure constant quality and purity of the lecithins. A methanol soluble extract of Fluosol-DA, which was subsequently shown to contain lysophospholipids was shown, for example, to stimulate histamine release from rat peritoneal mast cells in vitro [104]. Such an effect, if it happened in vivo, could account for the hypotension sometimes observed in rats, when close-to-total exchange perfusion was performed with Fluosol-DA.

No perfluoroalkylated surfactant sufficiently atoxic for intravascular administration has been reported yet, but it must be said that those tested so far are very few, little was usually known about their purity, and no explanation has been offered for their toxicity. The fact that the toxicity of Clark's XMO-10-based preparations [75] is only mild is an encouraging indication that perfluoroalkylated surfactants are not necessarily toxic, and chemists are now actively working on the synthesis of new ones.

The currently-used, approved oncotic agents (such as dextrans, gelatins and hydroxyethylstarch) themselves are not devoid of risks and intolerance accidents of the anaphylactic type. Interferences with hemostasis and renal complications, rare but sometimes severe, are observed with preparations that have been commonly employed for many years [105–108]. The same fluorocarbon stem-emulsion to which different oncotic agents, including gelatins, hydroxyethylstarch and albumin, were added to adjust oncotic pressure resulted in different survival ratios of totally exchange-perfused rats, the best results being obtained with albumin [109].

Emulsions

Where the completed emulsions are concerned, it is the merit of Fluosol-DA and similar preparations to have shown that patients could tolerate considerable amounts of fluorocarbon emulsions given intravascularly. Some adverse reactions were however reported, mostly by the American authors after infusion of Fluosol-DA, including transient chest pain and respiratory distress, decrease in leukocyte counts, hypotension and abnormal hepatic and pulmonary function [28,29,110–113]. Thus, a few patients responded to the injection of a small test-dose of Fluosol-DA by a short-term hypersensitivity reaction with tachycardia, an increase in pulmonary artery pressure, a rise in histamine and serotonine levels, and a drop in neutrophils and platelets. These effects lasted only a few minutes. Vercelotti et al. described this reaction as due to an activation of the complement cascade, and traced its origin to the emulsifying agent Pluronic F-68 [111–113]. This reaction could be almost completely suppressed by corticosteroid pre-treatment. Such effects were not observed when egg yolk phospholipids were used as the surfactant [72,114]. A sudden unexplained drop in mean arterial blood pressure has also been observed in some cases; it resolved spontaneously and was no longer observed when infusion of Fluosol was resumed [115]. More recently, pulmonary complications with fever, increased alveolar-arterial oxygen gradient, and chest X-ray abnormalities were observed in a group of three patients 3–4 days after administration of Fluosol-DA, but the etiology for these reactions is not yet known [116]. An abnormal response of pulmonary arterial endothelium to Fluosol-DA was attributed in part to improper pH adjustment [117], whereas a study of pulmonary fluid balance and hemodynamics after infusion of the F-butylamine/Pluronic F-68 emulsion Oxypherol in isolated dog lung lobes showed no significant change in pulmonary microvascular permeability [118].

All three first-generation F-decalin-based emulsions (see the discussion on Towards Improved Second-Generation Emulsions) were subjected to extensive pharmacological studies, including some on acute and chronic toxicity, retention and elimination of the fluorocarbons, influence on hemodynamics, hematopoietic activity, immune system, effect on the reticuloendothelial system, liver and kidney function, carcinogenicity and teratogenicity [6,7,119].

The LD_{50} of Fluosol-DA in rats was estimated at 130 ml

(i.e., 26 g of fluorocarbons)/kilo body weight [37], i.e., a volume twice as large as that of the circulating blood volume—a figure so high that it probably becomes meaningless since it is no longer possible to distinguish between an acute toxicity effect and a volume effect. A three-month chronic toxicity test was shown to cause hepatic dysfunction and histopathological alterations of the liver and spleen, although return to normal indicated that no irreversible change occurred. Ten ml/kg doses of Fluosol-DA administered intravenously in rats repeatedly on the 1st, 3rd, 8th, 10th and 15th days (i.e., a total of 50 ml/kg) were claimed to cause no markedly adverse effects [66]. All changes observed were said to be reversible, leaving no structural damage to tissues. It should however be noted that F-tripropylamine was still abundantly present in the spleen 183 days later, indicating that the half-residence time of this particular fluorocarbon in this specific organ is well over 100 days for such a dose. No signs of mutagenicity, teratogenicity, carcinogenicity or inflammatory reactions were found [37,119]. No toxicity was reported following administration of 5 weekly doses of 8 ml/kg each during a Phase I clinical trial of Fluosol and O_2-breathing with radiation therapy [120].

Total isovolemic blood exchange in the conscious animal [121,122] provides one of the most drastic tests for evaluating the biocompatibility of fluorocarbon emulsions. Some alterations are certainly expected in tissue and organ functioning when blood is close-to-totally replaced by a fluorocarbon emulsion! That animals tolerate such near-total (to Hct of $\leq 3\%$) replacement of their blood by such emulsions is by itself astounding. The responses that occur during the exchange perfusion with Fluosol-DA have been examined in detail by Lowe et al. in the chronically catheterized conscious rat [123]. The apparently unconcerned manner with which the rats move about their cage and take food and water, while the composition of their intravascular fluid undergoes dramatic changes, and the stability of cardiovascular and respiratory indices, were taken to indicate that the functioning of the central nervous system was unimpaired. Both red and white cell numbers decreased exponentially, but at different rates, the difference presumably reflecting the larger size of the white cell compartment and the effect of reservoirs of high lymphocyte concentrations such as lymph nodes. Later on, the animals exchange-perfused with Fluosol-DA showed progressive deterioration of hemodynamic control, and all died within 48h, after a mean post-perfusion survival time of 13 ± 2h [124]; changes in plasma enzyme concentrations were noted [125]. When the animals survive—i.e., when the emulsion is satisfactory [4,70]—the normal plasma protein and white blood cell levels recover within three days after exchange perfusion to 1–3 vol.%, and the regeneration of the hematocrit takes about 8–10 days [21,70]. No impairment of neural activities (EEG, reflexogenic control of respiratory and circulatory systems, and auditory, visual and somatosensory cortical evoked potentials) was noted after close-to-total exchange perfusion of cats with Fluosol-DA-35% or Fluosol-43 [126]. No abnormal tendency to bleed has been reported when bloodless animals underwent surgery. Organs perfused with fluorocarbon emulsions maintain normal functions (see section on Organs, Limb and Tissue Preservation).

The possible deleterious effects of the fluorocarbon emulsions on the reticuloendothelial system (RES) have been a matter of concern; these effects appear to be primarily linked to the particulate nature of emulsions. Part of the fluorocarbon particles, when injected intravenously, is gradually cleared from the circulation and stored by the RES in the liver and spleen and other tissues (none was detected in the brain). The uptake and morphological changes provoked in the liver, spleen, lung and kidney by emulsions of fluorocarbons, including the practically non-excretable F-tributylamine, have been described by numerous authors [37,67,127–133]. The liver and spleen can undergo enormous enlargement that could reach 7-fold (liver) and 20-fold (spleen) —non-lethal— increases in weight when 30 daily doses of 30 ml/kg body weight (a total of 900 ml/kg!) of a 20% F-dimethyl-adamantane/F-trimethylnonane emulsion were administered to rats [133], the most marked morphological changes in these organs being the appearance of foamy cells containing large vacuoles of fluorocarbons, with persistences depending on the fluorocarbon's molecular weight.

Partial, though transient, strongly dose-dependent depression of RES function was consistently observed [134–139] following infusion of Fluosol-DA, resulting in weakened defense against bacterial challenge. Increased mortality has been observed, for example, when Fluosol-DA-treated mice were injected with toxins from *E.Coli* [139]. The same result followed septic challenge given 48 hrs after acute hemorrhagic shock in rats when resuscitation was performed with Fluosol-DA 20% [140]. Fluosol-DA administration prolonged the intravascular survival of human erythrocytes transfused to chimpanzees [137]. Clearance of blood plasma from injected carbon particles and from indocyanine green has been used as a relative measure of phagocytosis and of liver excretory function, respectively, and pentobarbital sleeping time as a global measure for the detoxifying function of the liver [139]; these functions were all depressed, but returned to control values within 2 to 4 days. One should in this context mention that there is increasing evidence that blood transfusion may also produce immunosuppression and markedly impair the recipient's host defenses, provoking increased sensitivity to infection as well as increased recurrence and decreased survival after tumor surgery [141].

On the other hand, RES hyperfunction was sometimes noted in a later stage [142]. Treatment of rats by intraperi-

toneal injection with pure or emulsified F-hexyl or F-octylbromide prior to microbial challenge was reported to result in a significant increase in survival with respect to controls [143]. Lymphoid tissue response and antibody production against intraperitoneally-injected sheep red blood cells were observed after injection of Fluosol-DA into the peritoneal cavity of rats [144]. The lack of observation of infection in experimental and clinical studies with fluorocarbon emulsions is certainly remarkable.

No fluorocarbon was found in the fetus when pregnant ewes were close-to-totally exchange-perfused with Fluosol-DA, indicating that the emulsion does not cross the placenta [145].

Again, most of these investigations concern fluorocarbon emulsions formulated with Pluronic F-68, and some contained long-retained compounds that cannot be considered for intravascular administration. Cautious work is still needed to assess possible side-effects and to determine their etiology before widespread clinical use is legalized, and this for each new formulation that will be developed.

BIOMEDICAL APPLICATIONS: EXPERIMENTAL AND CLINICAL STUDIES

Fluorocarbon emulsions are expected to find both transfusional (as blood substitutes) and non-transfusional applications, the latter being based on profound differences from blood (see discussion on Principles of O_2-Transport and Delivery by Fluorocarbon Emulsions and Figure 8): easier extraction of O_2, even at low temperature, smaller particle sizes, lower viscosity, possibility of attaining high O_2-tensions, insensitivity to chemical agents, drugs, pH, temperature and mechanical devices, capacity to act as contrast agents in echography, NMR-imaging and, when brominated, X-ray radiography, etc. Some of the experiments and clinical trials that were done to explore these possibilities—principally with Fluosol-DA 20%—are discussed here.

All-Purpose Blood Substitutes— Trauma, Hemorrhagic Shock and Anemia

Several reports suggest that fluorocarbon emulsions may be useful for emergency treatment of hemorrhagic shock, a situation which is associated with severe microcirculatory disturbance. Madjidi et al. have shown the superiority of a Fluosol-DA 20% plus Dextran 40 association over the two constituents taken separately, and over autologous blood in the treatment of experimental hemorrhagic shock in the rabbit [146]. Biro reported that Fluosol-DA could effectively be used in resuscitation of dogs from moderately severe hemorrhage, and providing an adequate O_2-supply to the heart, which bears the central burden of hypovolemic shock [27,147]. The most favorable outcome was observed with Fluosol-DA 20% with 8 dogs out of 10 surviving 48 h later, compared to 5 out of 10 with Fluosol-DA 35% and 2 out of 10 with blood or hydroxyethylstarch solution as resuscitation media. On the other hand, no significant difference was found by Proctor et al. between a blood–saline mixture, an albumin solution and a fluorocarbon emulsion (Fluosol-43) in the resuscitation of rats subjected to hypoxic hypotension [148].

The first investigation on the tolerance of Fluosol-DA 20% in humans was achieved in 1978 by Makowsky et al. on seven brain-dead casualty victims [149]; no abnormal observations were made. Then ten healthy adult volunteers from the staff of the Green Cross Corporation were infused intravenously with 20 to 500 ml of this emulsion [150]; blood pressure, ECG, liver and kidney functions, hematological and coagulation parameters were controlled, and no adverse effects were noted. By the end of 1985, more than 500 patients in Japan, and ca. 90 in the U.S. and Canada, had received Fluosol-DA. Clinical studies of Ftorosan and Emulsion n° II were achieved in the Soviet Union [41] and China [8], where the number of patients had reached 720 and 200, respectively, by mid-1985.

The first published summary of clinical studies, concerning 186 cases of therapeutic use of Fluosol-DA 20% in 26 hospitals in Japan, appeared in 1981 [100,101]. The indications included non-availability or delayed delivery of compatible blood, refusal of blood transfusion for religious reasons, risk of hepatitis in surgery, cerebral hypoxia, CO-intoxication, etc. Doses were usually in the 6 to 25 ml/kg body weight range, and the infusion rates around 10 ml/min. The patient's arterial blood oxygen content and arterial oxygen tension rose markedly when $FiO_2 > 0.5$. It was concluded that the emulsion had both a beneficial plasma-expander effect and made a significant contribution to oxygen delivery. No anaphylactic or other ill effects attributable to the emulsion were reported then. No hemorrhagic tendencies were noted during or after surgery; the liver functions were apparently not affected; the biological parameters measured in blood, serum and urine remained within normal range.

About ten other reports on clinical use of Fluosol-DA 20% in Japan, each on a group of 6 to 24 mainly surgical patients, were presented in 1981 and 1982, but often with little detail [11,12]. Although generally no adverse effects (not even an early and transient anaphylactic reaction) were reported, and authors estimate that the administration of Fluosol-DA was safe and beneficial to their patients, these reports do not allow definitive conclusions to be drawn, because of the widely different physical conditions of the patients, paucity of data or statistical treatment, or absence of appropriate standard protocols and randomized evaluation.

The state of clinical studies of Fluosol-DA 20% in Japan over the period from 1979 to 1982 (401 patients) has been reviewed more recently by Mitsuno and Ohyanagi [151]. As an example, 1 litre of Fluosol-DA 20% (2 litres in one case), was given to seven Jehovah's Witnesses suffering from severe anemia in anticipation of blood loss during operation; FiO_2 was maintained between 0.5 and 0.6. An acute but transient reaction, with a drop in neutrophiles and platelets, was observed in four patients after the injection of a 1 ml test dose. It was estimated that the amount of arterial O_2 *transported* by the fluorocarbon was only 7% of that transported by hemoglobin, but that the contribution of the fluorocarbon to the O_2 *consumed* by the tissues was 25–30% of that provided by hemoglobin. No abnormal hematological changes, effects on hepatic functions or other untoward reactions were noticed for doses up to 30 ml/kg body weight, leading the authors to conclude that Fluosol-DA was safe and effective as a blood gas carrier.

U.S. clinical evaluation of Fluosol-DA 20% in the treatment of anemia has been reviewed by Tremper et al. [28,152]. An important contribution was also presented by Gould et al. [30,153,154]. The studies were restricted to patients suffering acute anemia who refused blood transfusion on religious grounds. The first protocol, referrred to as a "humanitarian protocol," was initiated in 1979; it concerned six patients who were considered to have a lethal degree of anemia, and did not impose collection of specific data. It was followed by a "medical-use protocol" in which hemodynamic and oxygen-transport data were collected, while patients breathed either room air or 100% oxygen. Five severely anemic patients with hemoglobin levels from 1.9 to 7.5 g/dl who needed surgery received 20 ml/kg body weight doses of Fluosol-DA 20%, i.e., a total of one to two liters [28]. The fluorocarbon emulsion transported the expected amount of oxygen, as evidenced by an improvement of the cardiac index and increased oxygen consumption index, arterial and mixed venous blood oxygenation and transcutaneous oxygen tensions with respect to pre-treatment values. The authors concluded that in spite of the small amount of emulsion administered, resulting in a fluorocrit of only 2.8%, it contributed significantly to oxygen delivery when FiO_2 was high, and that this contribution could be vital for severely anemic patients; the intravascular persistence half-time was, however, reported to be less than 24 hours.

It should be noted that the amount of oxygen transported by the plasma becomes significant at high FiO_2 levels, and—in Fluosol-DA 20%-type emulsions—is larger than that carried by the fluorocarbon, which, in these emulsions, accounts for only 11% of the volume infused. It was estimated in Fluosol-treated anemic patients that the plasma contributed to 38% of the oxygen consumed, compared to 22% for the fluorocarbon [110,154].

Recently eight severely anemic surgical patients who

had a definite need for increased arterial O_2-content (mean Hb level 3.0 ± 0.4 g/dl and/or oxygen extraction level >50%), which did not disappear at FiO_2 = 0.6, were infused with Fluosol-DA 20% until the need for additional oxygen disappeared [154]. No adverse reactions were observed. The emulsion carried the expected amount of oxygen and unloaded it effectively. The maximal arterial O_2-content added by Fluosol-DA was only 0.7 ± 0.1 vol %, compared to 2.8 ± 0.6 and 1.3 ± 0.1 vol % for the red cells and plasma, respectively, while their contributions to total O_2-consumption were 28%, 22% and 50%, respectively. But Fluosol-DA was ineffective in improving the outcome in these patients, owing to the limited increase in arterial O_2-content linked to its low fluorocarbon content, to the limited doses administered, and, above all, to its insufficient intravascular persistence. This last shortcoming obviously renders such emulsions inadequate for the treatment of anemiae other than for setting a short-term unavailability of red cells. It is noteworthy that when the hemoglobin level was above 3, neither Fluosol-DA nor blood was required.

Several isolated case reports have also appeared [155–157]. Thus the vital importance of an additional 1 or 2 vol % oxygen carriage has again been underlined, when two patients with severe postpartum hemorrhage, whose hemoglobin levels had dropped to 2.6 and 3%, were infused with Fluosol-DA 20% [155]. In these cases the treatment was judged successful, as vital signs stabilized and hemoglobin levels increased, and no side reactions were noted. An improvement of cardiac index and significant increase in oxygen consumption after infusion of Fluosol-DA, reported as representative of a study on 11 anemic patients, allowed reconstructive surgery to be undertaken on a patient with a 6 g/dl hemoglobin level [156].

There is obviously a need for additional well-designed and -controlled trials, if possible with significantly more concentrated emulsions, to assess in which cases and at which doses fluorocarbon emulsions are effective as substitutes for blood, i.e., present a definite advantage over classical crystalloid or colloid solutions. No clinical trials appear to have been performed with Fluosol-DA 35%.

Cardiovascular Diseases

In view of the frequency and seriousness of heart attacks—the major cause of death in the western countries—any therapy that might reduce the extent of myocardial ischemia and infarction, and improve the prognosis, would be priceless. Fluorocarbon emulsions have potential in this respect, because of the small size of the fluorocarbon particles, which allows them to reach areas of ischemic tissues that are no longer accessible to the red cells (which furthermore are stiffened by the increase in pH associated with ischemia), and their ability to deliver

oxygen under high tensions. These characteristics are propitious to reducing the size of the infarct by increasing oxygen delivery in the ischemic zone. The infusion of the emulsion may further contribute to facilitating the diffusion of oxygen in these regions, to dissolving CO_2—thus decreasing the pH—and washing out other noxious metabolites, as well as to reducing cardiac rhythm and effort, hence oxygen demand.

Fluorocarbon emulsions may also find uses during open heart surgery as media for priming extracorporeal circulation systems, as improved oxygen-carrying cardioplegic and reperfusion solutions and during balloon coronary angioplasty to bring oxygen beyond the obstructed zone.

Several studies were aimed at assessing the efficacy of fluorocarbon emulsions in reducing the extent of tissue damage following myocardial ischemia. Kloner, Glogar et al. evaluated the effect of a 15 vol % emulsion of a 60:40 mixture of F-decalin and F-tributylamine with 10% Pluronic F-68 on actual myocardial infarct provoked by permanent coronary artery occlusion in dogs [158,159]. The dogs were exchange-perfused with either 40 ml/kg of the emulsion, or Ringer's solution, and were in both cases ventilated with 100% oxygen, or received no treatment and were ventilated with room air. The extent of myocardial infarction after 6 hours of occlusion was estimated to be considerably smaller in the fluorocarbon-treated group (70 ± 5% of the area at risk compared to 104 ± 2 and 97 ± 2% for the other groups). When brief coronary occlusions not associated with necrosis were inflicted, the administration of the emulsion reduced ischemia, as assessed by a smaller rise in intramyocardial pCO_2 level, whether the dogs breathed pure oxygen or room air [160,161]. On the other hand, the intramyocardial pO_2, as measured by a mass spectrometric probe implanted in the ischemic zone, improved only when the emulsion was administered in combination with 100% oxygen ventilation. Significant reduction of heart rate was observed. Administration of the emulsion and ventilation with room air also reduced infarct size, although not as significantly as with 100% oxygen. Similar but longer-term experiments further suggest that fluorocarbon emulsions could be useful in the treatment of acute myocardial infarction [162]. The infarct size was also significantly reduced when dogs were partially exchange-transfused with Fluosol-DA 20% rather than with saline and ventilated with 100% oxygen one hour after coronary occlusion [163]. On the other hand, Menasché et al. found no significant reduction in infarct size, compared to untreated controls, when non-exchange-transfused dogs were subjected either to a 3-hour occlusion of the left anterior descending coronary artery followed by a 2-hour reperfusion with a 20 w/v % F-tributylamine/Pluronic F-68 emulsion, or to a 5-hour permanent occlusion during which the emulsion was administered. The results suggested, however, that the fluorocarbons may offer some protection against reperfusion injury. The disparity between these results and those of the other research groups may arise from large differences in the experimental protocols [164].

Data on the oxygen tension in the myocardium were collected by Faithfull et al. in experiments on pigs that underwent occlusion of a branch of the left anterior descending coronary artery, then one hour later received 20 ml/kg of Fluosol-DA 20%, or 20 ml/kg of an isotonic dextran solution in isovolemic replacement, or no treatment, and were breathing 100% oxygen [165]. A marked steady rise of the intramyocardial pO_2 in the hypoxic area was observed when fluorocarbon treatment was instituted, while it drastically decreased in the dextran-treated animals. Biro also found increased O_2-transport and a marked improvement of blood flow to the ischemic zone when dogs with coronary artery occlusion were treated with Fluosol-DA rather than with a dextran solution, but the ischemic zone was only marginally smaller than in the untreated control group [166]. Perfusion with an F-tributylamine emulsion was found to be significantly superior to perfusion with blood in preserving both systolic and diastolic myocardial function of isolated rabbit hearts after occlusion of a major coronary artery [167]. Prevention of ischemia for up to 45 min has been achieved by Spears et al. during percutaneous transluminal coronary balloon occlusion in dogs having received Fluosol-DA [168].

Although hypothermia during extracorporeal circulation and surgery [169] decreases the heart's energy requirements, a supplement of oxygen appears to be desirable for protecting the ischemic myocardium, and this cannot be achieved by using blood as a cardioplegic liquid, because oxygen release from hemoglobin decreases with temperature [170]. Kanter and coll. established the superiority of potassium-enriched Fluosol-43 over blood or crystalloid cardioplegia in isolated rabbit heart undergoing global ischemia [171]. The intramyocardial pO_2 increased markedly more, and the oxygen consumption of the myocardium was 10 times greater in the fluorocarbon-emulsion-treated group of hearts than in the crystalloid group and 5 times greater than in the blood cardioplegia group, and resulted in improved functional recovery. Another study concerning the effect of temperature on Fluosol-43 cardioplegia in dog hearts submitted to a 90 min global ischemia [172–173] showed significantly higher recovery of left ventricular function following post-ischemic reperfusion at 4° or 10° than at 20°C, and suggested that the beneficial effects of hypothermia and fluorocarbon cardioplegia are cumulative. Almost complete preservation of myocardial ATP levels in the Fluosol-43-treated hearts was evidenced by ^{31}P NMR [174]. Only O_2-saturated and not N_2-saturated fluorocarbon cardioplegia was efficient [175]. Rousou et al. also concluded to significantly better results with Fluosol-DA than the crystalloid or blood cardioplegia during ischemic arrest in

pigs, while they found no advantage during reperfusion [176,177]. Experimental evaluations on dogs of fluorocarbon emulsions for heart perfusion through the coronary vessels (Perfuzol) and for cardioplegia (Ftorum) have also been achieved by Soviet researchers [178]; the effects on myocardial protection were judged beneficial, and clinical application was said to have begun.

Reperfusion solutions are employed to limit the myocardial lesions that may occur during heart reperfusion following surgical-type global ischemia. Menasché and coll. used globally ischemic isolated rat hearts to test magnesium-rich, calcium-poor crystalloid reperfusion solutions to which a low 2 to 10 w/v% of F-tri-n-butylamine had been added [179]. The recovery of the cardiac output and stroke volume after 2 hours of ischemia under cardioplegia increased with the fluorocarbon concentration. The cardiac output was notably superior with the 10% fluorocarbon emulsion to that observed on hearts that were treated with a cardioplegic solution during the ischemia but did not receive the reperfusion solution. In another experimental model the left anterior descending coronary artery of dogs was occluded for 4 hours before the ischemic area was reperfused with the fluorocarbon preparation [180]. These dogs had significantly smaller infarcts than the control group that had been perfused by autologous blood. The authors suggest that an appropriate perfusate could contribute to reducing the ultimate infarct size and constitute useful therapeutic adjuncts to early intra-coronary selective thrombolysis. Reperfusion of isolated rabbit hearts subjected to a 30 min ischemia gave better results with a F-tributylamine emulsion than with blood [181]. Forman et al. observed, using a canine occlusion/reperfusion preparation, that Fluosol-DA, administered intracoronarily, reduced by about 50% the size of the infarct provoked by a 1.5-hour occlusion, and significantly improved the contractile function of the heart, by comparison with the same treatment with saline [182]. It has been suggested that fluorocarbon emulsions reduce reperfusion injury by preventing formation of free radicals and/or leucocyte plugging of the microcirculation [183].

Kessler et al. established the improvement of myocardial tissue oxygenation and microflow after extreme hemodilution with Fluosol-DA in dogs [25]. Ochi et al. found no adverse effects on micro-circulatory hemodynamics when Fluosol-DA 35% was used as a priming solution in cardiovascular bypass [184]. Rousou et al. compared Fluosol-DA and blood in a similar experiment in pigs [185]; adequate O_2 and CO_2 exchanges were maintained, but pulmonary complications were experienced in both cases during the recovery period.

Cerebral Ischemia

The fluidity of the emulsions, the small size of the fluorocarbon droplets and the ready availability of the oxygen they carry suggested that they might also prove efficacious in the treatment of cerebral ischemia [186]. Using a canine model of ischemic brain regulated with a perfusion method in which it is possible to control at will the amount of blood-flow to a cerebral hemisphere, Suzuki et al. investigated the effects of a 20% mannitol solution and of Fluosol-DA 20% on cerebral ischemia [187,188]. They found that their combined administration is effective in protecting the brain from cerebral ischemia, while the treatment with either mannitol or the emulsion alone showed only limited recovery of electrical activity compared to the control group, for which no recovery was seen. The same infarct model was used to evaluate the effects of mannitol, fluorocarbons and oxygen inhalation in various combinations on the brain swelling produced after 6 h of vascular occlusion followed by recirculation of blood [189]. No signs of swelling were found when all three components were administered, whereas the animals that had received only mannitol or Fluosol suffered from severe edema. The blood–brain barrier appears to be preserved, as shown by the absence of extravasation of Evans blue in the animals given mannitol, fluorocarbon and oxygen simultaneously. A 30 to 60% decrease in the size of the infarcts was observed by Han et al. when experimentally produced focal cerebral ischemia in cats was treated by intravenously administered Fluosol-DA rather than with normal saline [190].

Peerless et al. compared the protective effects of treatment with mannitol, Fluosol-DA 35% or isotonic saline on acute ischemia following complete and permanent occlusion of the middle cerebral artery in cats breathing 95% pure oxygen [191]. Macroscopic and histological examination of the brain suggested that Fluosol-DA had a definite protective effect, which was in keeping with the observed neurological outcome. The mean PaO_2 levels were significantly higher, and the degree of ischemic neuronal damage after 6 h of complete occlusion was statistically less severe and less extensive in the Fluosol-treated animals than in the controls or mannitol-treated ones. The Fluosol-treated animals also had significantly less brain swelling than the mannitol-treated ones. However, when the occlusion was only temporary (4 h) and followed by reperfusion, all the animals showed swelling and neurologic deterioration, with no obvious difference between the control and Fluosol-DA or mannitol-treated animals [192]. Finally, Fluosol-DA could not prevent the usual damage caused by reperfusion on a damaged vascular bed. The protective effect of Fluosol-DA against ischemic injury was less marked when larger doses (2 or 3 times 15 ml/kg body weight periodically) of the emulsion were administered over longer periods (24 h) of acute ischemia [193]. Fluosol treatment apparently helped to slow the development of pathological changes, but was far from providing complete protection from ischemic injury. Fluorocarbon emulsions have also been proposed as a

means of reducing brain damage which may be created by arterial air embolism after open heart surgery [194,195]. A protective effect was indeed observed when rats or rabbits were infused with a fluorocarbon emulsion prior to receiving a bolus air injection into the carotid artery. Rats having received 30 ml/kg body weight of a 20 w/v% F-tributylamine/Pluronic F-68 emulsion, breathing 100% oxygen, tolerated a 3-times larger amount of air bubbles than did the untreated or saline- and Pluronic-treated controls.

The first clinical uses of Fluosol-DA in situations of acute cerebral ischemia were reported in 1981 by Handa, Oda et al. [196]; improvement was shown in 65% of the patients following subarachnoid hemorrhage and subsequent vasospasm. A more extensive report in 1982 mentions the administration of Fluosol-DA 20% to 107 patients suffering from cerebral ischemia of various origins [197,198]. For example, fifteen patients out of 24 suffering from symptomatic cerebral vasospasm due to ruptured aneurism, to whom Fluosol-DA 20% had been administered in doses of 10 ml/kg, showed improvement of disturbed consciousness and/or motor weakness. Cerebral blood flow increased significantly. The relief was however only temporary, and lasted about 24 h, which is consistent with the intravascular persistence of the fluorocarbon. Transient (24 h) improvement was observed in two other cases of patients treated with Fluosol-DA 20% for acute cerebral ischemia, but no definite conclusion could be drawn on the efficacy of the treatment [199].

Suzuki et al. administered a 20% mannitol solution, then Fluosol-DA 20%, to 15 patients with brain infarct, while reconstructive surgery was undertaken [200,201]. No case of aggravation nor of death among the patients occurred. Two months later, 11 of the patients had returned to normal productive activity.

Although some of the observations reported so far in human clinical trials are encouraging, others remain inconclusive; it will not be possible to assert the merits of this treatment until comparison has been made between larger and randomized groups of treated and untreated patients, using better defined, rationally devised protocols. Here again emulsions having higher O_2-carrying capacity and longer intravascular persistence will be welcome.

Another promising new method for brain resuscitation after acute ischemic insult has recently been developed, in which an oxygenated fluorocarbon emulsion is perfused through the ventriculo-subarachnoid spaces. Osterholm et al. reported a marked restoration of the electrocerebral activity and oxidative brain metabolism of cats subjected to global hemispheric ischemia for 15 minutes when perfused with an oxygenated fluorocarbon [13 w/v F-butyltetrahydrofurane (FC-80)] and nutrient-containing emulsion rather than with a non-fluorocarbon-containing preparation [202]. Analysis of the perfusate showed that O_2 was delivered and CO_2, lactate and pyruvate removed.

In another protocol a significant 70% reduction of the size of the experimental cerebral infarct was obtained when cats were subjected to a focal cerebral ischemic insult for a duration of two hours, then perfused after another hour with a 20% w/v F-butyltetrahydrofurane emulsion through this ventriculo-cisternal route [203]. This astonishingly long therapeutic window of at least three hours following the initial ischemic insult, if confirmed, will lead to questioning the commonly accepted concept that it is not possible to obtain substantial recovery of neuronal function after brain ischemia of more than 5 to 7 minutes' duration. The idea was put forward that ischemic changes in the vasculature may be the primary cause of cerebral vascular diseases and that neuronal changes are only secondary to these vascular effects. This alternative perfusion route would thus be an efficient way of preventing irreversible damage to the vasculature, and hence to the neural tissues. Whatever the mechanism(s) involved, the drastic difference in results observed between the fluorocarbon- and non-fluorocarbon-charged perfusates attest to the efficacy of the former to transport and deliver a significant amount of oxygen.

The intrathecal administration of an oxygenated fluorocarbon emulsion was also proposed as a treatment of spinal cord injury. Experiments on dogs and cats resulted in lesser edema and necrosis and in improved recovery of motor function [204,205].

Organs, Limb and Tissue Preservation

Isolated organ (including heart, kidney, liver, pancreas and stomach) [37,206] or sectioned limb preservation before reimplantation, tissue cultures, semen and embryo conservation can be improved with the help of oxygen-carrying media. Fluosol-43 was for example found to be superior to physiological salt solutions in maintaining the hemodynamic and mechanical function of isolated working rat heart [207]. Isolated guinea pig hearts showed lower coronary flow and better mechanical performances when perfused with a 20% F-tributylamine emulsion than with a Krebs-Henseleit solution [208].

Isolated rat livers perfused with an F-tributylamine emulsion, generated factors II, V, VII, IX–XII antithrombin III and plasminogene as well as when they are perfused with blood components [209]. Honda reported that kidney and liver in mongrel dogs were better preserved by intracadaver perfusion with Fluosol-DA than with a Ringer lactate solution, while blood perfusion was inadequate [210]. Significantly higher tissular pO_2's were attained when canine kidneys were perfused at 22°C with an F-tributylamine emulsion saturated with 95% O_2 and 5% CO_2 rather than with blood, allowing the metabolic processes to continue for 10 h without damage to the tissues [211]. Orthotopic transplantation of rat livers after 25

h-long perfusion with the same emulsion was successful [212]. The responsiveness of cervical spinal cord of rats was maintained for prolonged periods when perfused through the supplying arteries with an oxygenated F-tributylamine/Pluronic F-68 emulsion [213]; the alternative intrathecal route also appears to be effective [204,205]. Hypoxic pulmonary vasoconstriction response (a regulatory mechanism of arterial oxygenation) was maintained in isolated rat lungs perfused with an F-tributylamine emulsion, as effectively as with blood [214], and the perfusion of isolated dog lung lobes with Oxypherol did not provoke any marked increase in microvascular permeability (i.e., lung edema) [118]. The isolated upper gastrointestinal tract, including liver, stomach, pancreas and duodenum of dogs, remained functionally viable, with normal bile and pancreatic secretions, for 6 h during perfusion by a fluorocarbon emulsion [215]. Electrical and mechanical activity of isolated canine stomach could also be preserved [216].

Tauber et al. reimplanted the hind limbs of rabbits that had been amputated and stored for 4 h at 4°C, and found that the extremities developed a lower peripheral resistance and a higher blood flow when they were perfused for 30 min with Fluosol-43 prior to recirculation with blood than in non-Fluosol-perfused controls [217]. The recipient animals also exhibited higher arterial blood pressures and lower electrolytic and pH disturbances when the reimplanted member had received the emulsion. Similar conclusions were reached by Schindler et al. as to the beneficial effect of perfusion with Fluosol-43 of lower limbs that had been maintained anoxic for 75 min by occlusion of the abdominal aorta and inferior vena cava in rats [218], indicating that such emulsions may have a future in tiding over the time between injury and reimplantation of accidentally amputated limbs.

In man, two kidney transplantations after intracadaveric preservation of the organs with Fluosol-DA 20% have been reported [210]. Eight successful cases of kidney transplantation in humans have also been disclosed in China after preservation, in one case for 35 hours, by perfusion with Emulsion n° I (F-tributylamine) [219]. The replantation of amputated limbs after they had been perfused with Fluosol-DA at 5°C for 16 to 46 h was attempted on five patients, and was successful in two, for whom the amputation had been clean; tissue oxygenation and microcirculation were adequate during the perfusion [220].

The fact that fluorocarbon emulsions retain and even increase their capacity of carrying and delivering oxygen at low temperatures is here an important asset. Even a modest increase of the duration of viability of the isolated organs, hence of the time available for removing and shipping them (this time is presently only of 4–6 hours for the human heart, for example) would considerably increase the number of transplantations made possible.

Diagnostic

The use of fluorocarbon emulsions as contrast agents was initiated by Long, Mattrey et al. [34,221]. Both F-hexylbromide (PFHB) and F-octylbromide (PFOB) are appropriate for use in the lungs and gastrointestinal tract, while the more volatile PFHB is contraindicated for intravascular use and in fluid-filled spaces of the central nervous system.

PFOB emulsions have been investigated extensively, especially for blood pool and liver and spleen imaging by standard radiography and computed tomography [222,223]. PFOB emulsions have decisive advantages over the presently used water-soluble iodine-based contrast agents: lower toxicity, absence of diffusion into the interstitial spaces and consequent loss of radiographic contrast, resulting in reduced risk for the patient. Their much longer intravascular persistence allows imaging of the whole body, adbomen and chest, at the same sitting, which cannot be achieved with the iodine-based agents, if only because the dose required could cause renal toxicity. Significantly, the dilution of the latter contrast agents with Fluosol-DA has been suggested as a means of protecting the coronary endothelium against their damaging effects [224].

When administered intravascularly, PFOB emulsions first allow the imaging of the vascular structures [225]. The dose of PFOB required for proper blood pool imaging is in the range of 1 to 3 g/kg body weight, i.e., of 1–3 ml/kg of a 100 w/v% emulsion. It produces specific uniform enhancement of normal liver tissues, leaving tumors and other lesions the only unopacified structures within the organ [222,227]. The spleen, which accumulates 3 to 5 times as much PFOB as the liver in rats or rabbits, is even easier to image.

Fluorocarbons being also taken up by the circulating macrophages, they may serve to detect any region where phagocytes are found, such as around tumors, or infarcted and injured tissues and abcesses [228,229]. PFOB has for example been shown to accumulate at the periphery of VX2 tumors implanted in rabbit livers, thus producing a dense rim around them, clear on the photographic plates. Similar results have been obtained with brain tumors in rats [230]. Over 20 different types of experimental tumors have been imaged so far in 5 different species [71]. The clear imaging of intrahepatic and intraperitoneal abscesses was also obtained [223], related to the intense accumulation of PFOB-filled macrophages in the abscess walls.

Over a hundred non-intravascular human studies have been performed with PFOB, including 88 pulmonary and 29 gastrointestinal imaging studies with conventional X-rays [71].

Fluorocarbons also have potential as ultrasound contrast agents, mainly because the fluorocarbon droplets reflect the ultrasounds, in part perhaps also because they decrease acoustic velocity relative to water as a consequence of their high compressibilities. Echogenic enhancement of the liver and of VX2 tumors implanted in rabbit livers, for example, was observed following the administration of a PFOB emulsion or of Fluosol-DA 20% [226,231]. Preliminary human clinical trials using Fluosol-DA 20% gave encouraging results [232]. Echogenic rims were observed in patients with metastatic pancreatic, breast and gastric carcinoma, and multiple lesions in the liver were detected which could not be seen prior to Fluosol administration. Further studies with more concentrated emulsions are needed to evaluate the extent of this application and to determine the appropriate diagnostic dose.

The ^{19}F nucleus, which occurs in 100% natural abundance, and ranks second only to proton in sensitivity, also appears to be a promising probe for in vivo nuclear magnetic resonance imaging. Preliminary results indeed allowed the in vivo imaging of liver, tumor and abscess in rats after administration of a 16% v/v emulsion of F-tributylamine [233], and the evaluation of ischemic and infarcted myocardium [234]. Other results suggest that advantage could be taken of the perturbation of the T_1 relaxation time of the ^{19}F nuclei provoked by the paramagnetic oxygen molecule for imaging and monitoring oxygen in the body [48,235,236].

Yet another application of fluorocarbons in diagnosis is illustrated by the use of a translucent fluorocarbon emulsion in conjunction with a high resolution fiberoptic scope, to achieve the direct visualization and evaluation of coronary anatomy [237].

Cancer Therapy

Cancer therapy is a further area in which the oxygen delivering fluorocarbon emulsions show promise, either through their ability to activate the RES or because of their capacity of carrying O_2 to the tumors, which has been shown to enhance the tumoricidal effects of radiations or of cytotoxic drugs.

Clark et al. observed that the injection of fluorocarbon emulsions into mice conferred long lasting in vitro tumoricidal potential upon peritoneal exudate cells, probably as a result of partial blockage of the RES which provokes an increased production of macrophages [142]. Kuwamura et al. gave evidence for a synergistic effect of oxygen-carrying Fluosol-43 administration and 1,3-bis(2-chloroethyl)-1-nitrosourea (BCNU) therapy [238]. Survival of rats implanted with 9L tumor cells in the brain increased to 32 ± 5 days when the rats were treated with BCNU and Fluosol-43 and breathed 95% O_2, compared to 21 to 23 ± 3 days when they received BCNU alone or with either oxygen or Fluosol (but in room air), and to 15 ± 3 days in the untreated control group. Ohyanagi et al. reported that the administration of Fluosol-DA and oxygen enhanced the efficacy of several cytotoxic drugs in rats that had been implanted with three types of carcinoma [239]. Delay in tumor growth, with a 10-fold increase in tumor-cell killing, was found by Teicher et al. when melphalan treatment of a fibrocarcinoma was preceded by the administration of Fluosol-DA combined with 95% O_2/5% CO_2 breathing. No increase in toxicity to bone marrow, the dose-limiting side-effect of melphalan, was observed [240]. Similar increase in therapeutic efficacy was described for another chemotherapeutic agent, etoposide [241]. These effects of the fluorocarbon emulsion and oxygen combination may result from a better access of the drug to the tumor and from the increase in intratumoral pO_2 and subsequent sensitization of hypoxic cells, which are often resistant to chemotherapy. The largest effects so far, with Fluosol-DA and carbogen breathing, appear to have been observed with the alkylating chemotherapeutic agents busulfan and procarbazine with a 10-fold delay in tumor growth [242].

Several authors reported that the administration, prior to radiation therapy, of low doses of Fluosol-DA, and of 95% oxygen, to mice implanted with solid tumors of several lines led to significant delays in tumor growth [243–247]. Since no effect was observed in the absence of oxygen treatment, the radiosensitization that occurred was primarily assigned to the emulsion's ability to oxygenate the hypoxic cells of solid tumors more efficiently than blood. The treatment did not increase the radiosensitivity of the hematopoietic stem cells of the marrow or spleen, indicating that therapeutic gain could be obtained when hematologic toxicity is the dose limiting factor [247]. There may however be a danger of overloading the liver and spleen when the emulsion is administered repeatedly over a long period of time [133]. Combined administration of a fluorocarbon emulsion and of hyperbaric oxygen prior to irradiation has been advocated [120]. Phase I clinical trials of a Fluosol-DA/oxygen/radiation therapy in the treatment of advanced head and neck cancer is now underway.

Miscellaneous Applications

The possibility of using fluorocarbon vesicles as a drug transport system aimed at specific targets, including liver tumors and abscesses, has been suggested repeatedly. This use may however be limited by the low solubility of most compounds in fluorocarbons, and by their high extraction ratio by water or ligands [57]. Exceptions to this are of course gases and highly-halogenated compounds such as the halothane anesthesics [248]. On the other hand, interferences may occur; thus for example the infu-

sion in rats of either Fluosol-DA 20% or stroma-free hemoglobin was shown to alter the pharmacodynamics of penicillin and diazepan [249], indicating that the simultaneous use of O_2-carriers and drugs requires caution, but may also lead to beneficial effects.

Many other uses have been suggested for fluorocarbon emulsions in medicine [6,13,250]. Fluosol-DA was reported not to leak out when administered i.v. to five major burn patients, and to stabilize their cardiovascular state [251]. It may have contributed to saving two CO-poisoned patients [252]; little detail is given, however, on these cases. The use of fluorocarbon emulsions may also be envisaged for total body washout [253] in cases of drug overdose or toxin poisoning, or to remove myocardial depressor factors following inversible shock [254], and in the treatment of anaerobic infections such as tetanus or clostridial myonecrosis [255], which respond to an increase in oxygen tension.

Fluorocarbon emulsions were shown to reverse the sickling process of sickled erythrocytes. This may help diminish the risk that patients with sickle cell disease may develop alloimmunization as a result of repeated transfusions [254]. A synergic effect of Fluosol-DA and stroma-free hemoglobin sickling has been reported [256].

The administration of fluorocarbon emulsions through the intestinal tract was shown to reduce the rate of necrosis of intestinal villi in case of gastrointestinal ischemia [257,258]. Intraperitoneal perfusion of an oxygenated fluorocarbon emulsion has been suggested by Faithfull et al. as a means of supplementing oxygenation of the whole body [259]. Applied to rabbits, it resulted in significant improvement of the arterial pO_2. An advantage of this original procedure should be that the fluorocarbon can be removed once it is no longer needed. The administration of Fluosol-DA and oxygen was also proposed as a possible treatment of acute pancreatitis [260].

Further potential applications concern liquid membrane oxygenators, to avoid the trauma caused to blood by direct blood–gas contact. Liquid breathing could provide a means of preventing decompression hazards [261]; improved survival of rats from decompression was also observed when Fluosol-DA was administered intravascularly after compression to 8 atmospheres [262]. Light fluorocarbons were proposed in the treatment of retinal detachment [263], and F-tributylamine as a replacement medium for the vitreous humor of the eye [264].

Fluorocarbon-based gas-carriers and bloodless animals provide unique new means of investigation in biomedical research [265], for example to suppress the interference caused by hemoglobin during in situ optical measurements [266], or to assess the contribution of blood components in a given physiological or pathophysiological event [267].

The use of a fluorocarbon was even suggested as a means of keeping fleas alive while bathing in a vaccine solution destined to be inoculated into wild rabbits affected by myxomatosis! [268].

PROSPECTS

Although the transfusion of blood or red cell suspensions has become a routine procedure, it is still accompanied by problems of availability and immunological and infectious risks—among which hepatitis and AIDS are of particular concern—that provide an increasingly strong incentive for developing hemocompatible, non-antigenic, disease-free, readily transportable and storable oxygen-carrying preparations that do not require human donors.

Fluorocarbon-based O_2/CO_2 carriers have potential both for such transfusional and for many other, non-transfusional applications, especially in those situations where high oxygen tension, ready availability of oxygen, small particle size, low-temperature effectiveness, mechanical resistance, or contrast properties, are required.

The Fluosol-DA 20%-*type* emulsions, which have by now been administered to more than 1500 patients in Japan, the United States, the Soviet Union and China, provided a first prototype of such preparations. They allowed the demonstration that large amounts of intravascularly administered fluorocarbon emulsions are in general well tolerated and deliver the expected amount of oxygen to tissues and organs.

This first generation of emulsions, however, needs serious improvements where purity, reliability and excretion of the constituent fluorocarbons and surfactants, side-effects, oxygen transport capacity, intravascular persistence and long-term stability are concerned. The efficacy of these particular preparations in certain indications, such as anemia, is questionable in view of their low fluorocarbon content and low intravascular persistence. The very recognition of these insufficiencies has provided a basis for directing the present research efforts. The increased basic knowledge that has developed in the past few years indicates that the potential of fluorocarbons as oxygen carriers stands intact, and the bases for future progress are now clearly set.

Several significant improvements have already been achieved or appear to be within reach. The insufficient purity and definition of the fluorocarbons can be remedied by selective synthesis utilizing the telomerisation route. Today it is the authors' opinion that only a few compounds can be considered for intravascular use where reliability, excretion rate and cost-effective industrial feasibility are concerned. Among these are F-decalin, F-octylbromide, bis(F-butyl)ethene and F-isopropylhexylethene. F-decalin is the best documented, but no biocompatible, stable, sterilizable emulsion appears to have been obtained so far with this compound and the presently available surfactants; far better results have been gained with the other three candidate fluorocarbons, and F-octyl bromide stands out where fast excretion is considered.

The use of pure, well-defined, monodisperse fluorocarbons and surfactants will reduce the risk of immunological and other reactions. F-tripropylamine and F-methylcyclohexylpiperidine will have to be discarded, owing to their overlong retention in the organs, and probably Pluronic F-68 because of its side-effects. The effects of the emulsions on the RES, and how they can be minimized by an appropriate choice of surfactant(s) and formulation need further investigation; these effects seem to be primarily related to the particulate nature of the system, and appear to be similar to those initially found with injectable lipid emulsions such as those currently used in parenteral nutrition.

Efficacy depends on O_2-carrying capacity as well as on intravascular persistence. The feasibility of considerably more concentrated emulsions has recently been established, providing 2–4 times larger O_2-transport capacity. Smaller particles were shown to stay longer in the vascular system. Prolonged intravascular persistence has also been obtained by the administration of additional amounts of the surfactant.

Greater emulsion stability is needed. This stringently depends on the availability of new, biocompatible surfactants and co-surfactants, better adapted to the emulsification of fluorocarbons; further improvements in emulsification technology may also play a role here.

A further trend is to focus and optimize the emulsions for a given indication or application rather than to aim at an all-purpose preparation. Among those applications which appear closest to development are diagnosis, percutaneous transluminal coronary angioplasty, sensitization of tumors to X-rays, ischemia and organ preservation.

Whether it is to avoid the side-effects of Pluronic F-68, to achieve more stable and more concentrated emulsions, to prolong their intravascular persistence, to master their characteristics better in order to optimize them for a given indication, or to explore the possibility of obtaining injectable microemulsions, it has become clear that the synthesis and evaluation of new surfactants and/or co-surfactants is the necessary key to improved future generations of preparations. These surface agents will have to be monodisperse and pure in order to guarantee their reliability, facilitate their evaluation and ease their acceptance.

The question of the biocompatibility of the fluorocarbon preparations addresses all their components (and not solely the fluorocarbons, which appear to be by far the most inert of them), and also the final injectable emulsion. It must be clear that "biocompatible" does not mean biologically inert. No intravenous injection will ever be totally innocuous, and no one will want to administer any volume expander or transfuse blood to a healthy person who does not need any. On the other hand, when the life of a patient is at risk, any treatment that may improve the prognosis significantly is welcome, even it if bears some risk of side-effects. Such risk is present, even in the routinely administered dextran, hydroxyethyl starch or gelatin solutions, or with blood transfusion. The intravenous injection of massive quantities of a fluorocarbon emulsion cannot be expected to be without *any* biological effect, as it introduces foreign matter into the organism, and is expected to . . . deliver oxygen. It is the benefit-vs-risk balance that has then to be considered, and all possible precautions obviously have to be taken to reduce the risk to a minimum when developing new, second-generation fluorocarbon emulsions. This will also require further efforts where the standardization and control of the preparations and defining of the experimental and clinical protocols for their evaluation are concerned.

There is little doubt that man-made injectable oxygen carriers will sometime be developed; it is the authors' opinion that this time is now close.

ADDENDUM (December 1989)

Progress in the field of injectable fluorocarbon based oxygen carriers has proceeded at a steady pace since this review was initially written. This progress was dominated by two major events, the approval of Fluosol-DA by the American Food and Drug Administration (FDA) for use during high risk percutaneous transluminal coronary angioplasty (PTCA, Figure 9) and the development of more concentrated and more efficient fluorocarbon emulsions [269–273].

The significance of the first event is that the regulatory agencies have now recognized fluorocarbons as safe for intravenous administration in man; fluorocarbons are thus entering medical practice. This also means that efficacy has been proven by Fluosol-DA in spite of its low ca. 11% by volume fluorocarbon content, and that the benefit for patients outweighs this preparation's other limitations, inconveniences and side-effects, including the presence of a long organ-dwelling fluorocarbon and the presence of the complement-activating surfactant Pluronic F-68. Finally, the approval of Fluosol-DA eliminates the concerns which

clouded the picture of the fluorocarbon approach to oxygen carriage since Fluosol-DA's initial rejection after it had been submitted for a quite inappropriate indication.

The significance of the second event, the development of highly concentrated, room temperature stable, injectable fluorocarbon emulsions is that of a major technological breakthrough. It means that the principal shortcomings and drawbacks of Fluosol-DA (which limit its general use) have been surmounted. The new second generation emulsions contain up to five times more fluorocarbon (100% by weight or 52% by volume) than Fluosol-DA, are stable at room temperature, ready for use and contain a surfactant (egg yolk phospholipids) which is well accepted and routinely employed in injectable preparations [271–274].

The fluorocarbon used in the new high-concentration emulsions, perfluorooctyl-bromide (PFOB), itself presents two unique advantages over all the previously evaluated ones: (1) it has an exceptionally low organ half-life, for example with the same 4 g/kg body weight dose in rats the half-life of PFOB is only 4 days instead of 7 days for F-decalin and 65 days for F-tripropylamine, the two fluorocarbons present in Fluosol-DA, and (2) it is radiopaque which allows its use as a contrast agent in diagnosis and for accurate biodistribution studies. Both of these properties are related to the presence of the bromine atom at the end of the fluorocarbon chain.

In fact, PFOB was originally selected for its radiopacity for use as a contrast agent for X-ray radiography. The more concentrated emulsions were also developed to meet the requirements of this application. As it turned out, PFOB also is an ideal candidate as an oxygen carrier for blood subsitutes and other oxygen delivery applications. It can be synthesized by the very clean telomerisation route which allows the manufacture of large tonnages of highly pure material. It has among the highest known O_2 and CO_2-dissolving capacities of any perfluorocarbon, is chemically and biologically inert, and forms stable emulsions with egg yolk phospholipids.

The successful development of the new concentrated and highly efficacious emulsions allows renewed consideration for many applications which were beyond the capabilities of the dilute first generation Fluosol-type emulsions. It should be reemphasized that a satisfactory oxygen carrier has extensive potential, not only as a substitute for red blood cells in their usual transfusion indications, but also as a means of treating myocardial and cerebral ischemia, for use in preoperative hemodilution, for use in heart surgery (for external circulation, cardioplegia, prevention of reperfusion injury), as an adjuvant to radio- and chemotherapy when tumors contain resistant hypoxic cells, and as a medium for isolated organ perfusion, i.e., whenever oxygen is needed to preserve or salvage living tissues. With the advent of such highly efficacious, concentrated emulsions the full potential of "injectable oxygen" can be explored [275–277].

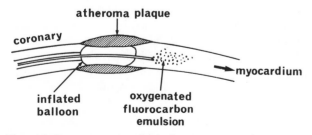

Figure 9. Percutaneous transluminal coronary angioplasty (PTCA). The oxygenated fluorocarbon emulsion is injected downstream of the inflated balloon thus preventing the myocardium from becoming ischemic.

The radiopaque properties of PFOB have also brought into the limelight the potential of fluorocarbons in diagnosis, since PFOB emulsions have the unique characteristic of being the first contrast agent capable of being detected by the three primary imaging modalities. These include X-ray/CT and ultra-sounds for which a 100% w/v PFOB emulsion will be used principally for blood pool, liver and spleen imaging. Magnetic resonance imaging is also effective either directly by detecting the ^{19}F nuclei resonance, or employing the usual ^{1}H MRI for observing signal void, or indirectly by analyzing the perturbation caused to the signal by the paramagnetic O_2 molecule, which allows oxygen imaging. Finally, imaging with ultrasound using duplex sound wave and/or color Doppler is also possible since the fluorocarbon droplets reflect the sound waves; this condition makes it possible among others to have a remarkably clear real time view of organ perfusion. One primary advantage of PFOB emulsions is that the contrast medium does not leak out of the vascular spaces and that it allows for imaging over much longer periods of time than the conventional water-soluble iodinated contrast agents [278–282].

The development of concentrated PFOB emulsions represents the single most important breakthrough achieved in the field of fluorocarbon emulsions for biomedical use in the last decade. It occurs at a time when the present practice of blood transfusion is facing increasingly serious difficulties due to public awareness of the risk of transmission of infectious diseases and other problems associated with this practice. This situation has been obviously brought to light by the propagation of AIDS.

Further progress in the field and the evolvement of future generations of products undoubtedly lies in the synthesis and evaluation of new surfactants tailor-made for developing specifically targeted fluorocarbon emulsions. The objective is to create surfactants especially designed for the emulsification of fluorocarbons. These surfactants should lead to increased emulsion stability and to the possibility of varying to a large extent the emulsions' characteristics relevant to in vivo use, including particle size, intravascular persistence, in vivo particle recognition, potential biodistribution, etc., so as to optimize these characteristics for each one of the potential therapeutic uses [283].

A modular molecular design was devised for this purpose which permits the progressive stepwise variation of these parameters. Several families of such new surfactants have already been synthesized, whose polar heads are derived from, or analogous to atoxic natural products, including sugars, polyols, amino acids and phospholipids. These compounds are now in the process of being evaluated. They display strong surfactant properties, and significant emulsion stabilization effects have already been obtained. When the biological aspect is examined, the most remarkable observation so far is that in spite of their much higher surface activity when compared to their hydrocarbon analogs, their hemolytic activity is considerably lower [284–287].

Additional literature and articles about the current advances in the field may be found in abstracts and proceedings from various recent international conferences and symposia, particularly those held in Montreal, Canada (May 87) [288], Bari, Italy (June 87) [289], Lancaster, England (March 88) [290], Brussels, Belgium (Sept. 89) [291], Sapporo, Japan (Oct. 89) [292], San Francisco, U.S.A. (Nov. 89) [293] and Honolulu, U.S.A. (Dec. 89) [294], (the increasing frequency of which demonstrates the increasing activity of the blood substitute field), as well as in some recently published reviews and papers of particular significance [295–306].

ACKNOWLEDGEMENTS

I wish to thank my co-workers whose names are listed in the references, E. Lepage, C. Onteniente and M. Rose for preparing manuscript and figures, and the Centre National de la Recherche Scientifique for support.

REFERENCES

1 RIESS, J. G. and M. Le Blanc. "Perfluorocompounds in Blood Substitutes," *Angew. Chem. Int. Ed. Engl.*, 17:621 (1978).

2 GOLLAN, F. and L. C. Clark. "Organ Perfusion with Fluorocarbon Fluid," *Physiologist*, 9:191 (1966).

3 SLOVITER, H. and T. Kamimoto. "Erythrocyte Substitute for Perfusion of Brain," *Nature*, 216:458 (1967).

4 GEYER, R. P. "Fluorocarbon Polyol Artificial Blood Substitutes," *New Eng. J. Med.*, 289:1077 (1973).

5 CLARK, L. C. "Perfluorodecalin as a Red Cell Substitute," in *Blood Substitutes and Plasma Expanders*, New York:Alan R. Liss, Inc., p. 69 (1978).

6 NAITO, R. and K. Yokoyama. "Perfluorochemical Blood Substitutes," *Technical Information Series*, n° 5 (1978) et n° 7 (1981), Osaka, Japan:The Green Cross Corp.

7 BELOYARTSEV, F. F., E. I. Mayevsky and B. I. Islamov. *Ftorosan-Oxygen Carrying Perfluorochemical Plasma Substitute*, Acad. Sci. U.S.S.R., Pushchino (1983). K. N. Makarov, *11th Intl. Symp. Fluorine Chem.*, Berlin, DDR (1985).

8 XIONG, R., R. Zhang, H. Chen, W. Huang, C. Luo and W. Cao. "A Clinical Application of Fluorocarbon Artificial Blood in 10 Cases," *Chin. J. Surg.*, 19:213 (1981).

9 *Proc. Int. Symp. Research on Perfluorochemicals in Medicine and Biology*, V. Novakova and L. O. Plantin, eds., Huddinge, Sweden:Karolinska Research Center (1978).

10 *Proc. 4th Int. Symp. Perfluorochemical Blood Substitutes*, Kyoto, Japan (October 1978), Excerpta Medica, Amsterdam (1979).

11 *"Oxygen Carrying Colloidal Blood Substitutes," Proc. 5th Int. Symp. Perfluorochemical Blood Substitutes, FRG, April 1981*, R. Frey, H. Beisbarth and K. Stosseck, eds., Munich:W. Zuckschwerdt Verlag (1982).

12 *"Advances in Blood Substitute Research," Proc. Int. Symp. Blood Substitutes, San Francisco, October 1982*, R. Bolin, R. P. Geyer and G. Nemo, eds., in *Prog. Clin. Biol. Res.*, 122 (1983).

13 In *Artif. Organs*, (n° 1), H. Ohyanagi and R. P. Geyer, eds., 8 (February 1984).

14 *Intl. Anesth. Clin.*, (n° 1), K. K. Tremper, ed., 23 (1985).

15 LE BLANC, M and J. G. Riess. "Artificial Blood Substitutes Based on Perfluorochemicals," in *Preparation, Properties and Industrial Applications of Organofluorine Compounds*, R. E. Banks, ed., Chichester:Ellis Horwood, Chap. 3. (1982).

16 RIESS, J. G. and M. Le Blanc. "Preparation of Fluorocarbon Emulsions for Biomedical Applications. Principles, Materials and Methods," in *Blood Substitutes: Preparation, Physiology and Medical Applications*, K. C. Lowe, ed., Chichester:Ellis Horwood, Chap. 5 (1988).

17 RIESS, J. G. and M. Le Blanc. "Solubility and Transport Phenomena in Perfluorochemicals Relevant to Blood Substitution and Other Biomedical Applications," *Pure and Appl. Chem.*, 54:2382 (1982).

18 RIESS, J. G. "Reassessment of Criteria for the Selection of Perfluorochemicals for Second Generation Blood Substitutes," *Artificial Organs*, 8:44 (1984); Riess, J. G. "Present Trends in Fluorocarbon-based Blood Substitutes," *Life Support Systems*, 2(4):273 (1984).

19 DELLACHERIE, E., P. Labrude, J. G. Riess and C. Vigneron. "Synthetic Carriers of Oxygen," in *Critical Reviews in Therapeutic Drug Carrier Systems*, CRC Press, 3:41 (1987).

20 TREMPER, K. K. and S. T. Anderson. "Perfluorochemical Emulsion Oxygen Transport Fluids: A Clinical Review," *Ann. Rev. Med.*, 36:309 (1985).

21 GEYER, R. P. "Studies and Uses of Perfluorochemical Emulsions as Blood Substitutes," in *Ref. 9*, p. 229 (1978).

22 GREC, J.-J., B. Devallez, H. Marcovich and J. G. Riess. "Use of Fluorocarbons to Control Cell Cultures," *Abstracts Colloque Nat. de Génie Biol. et Méd.*, Toulouse, 1982, H. Marcovich, Fr. Patent N°25, 13:264 (1983).

23 LUTZ, J., B. Decke, M. Bauml and H. G. Schulze. "High Oxygen Extraction Combined with Extensive Oxygen Consumption in the Rat Liver Perfused with Fluosol-DA, A New Perfluorocompound Emulsion," *Pflügers Arch.*, 376:1 (1978).

24 KESSLER, M., J. Höper and U. Pohl. "Tissue Oxygen Supply of Liver, Pancreas, Kidney and Skeletal Muscle," in *Ref. 11*, p. 99 (1982).

25 KESSLER, M., H. Vogel, H. Günther, D. K. Harrison and J. Höper. "Local Oxygen Supply of the Myocardium After Extreme Hemodilution with Fluosol-DA," *Prog. Clin. Biol. Res.*, 122:237 (1983).

26 BIRO, G. P. "Comparisons of Acute Cardiovascular Effects and Oxygen Supply Following Haemodilution with Dextran, Stroma-Free Haemoglobin and Fluorocarbon Suspension," *Cardiovasc. Res.*, 16:194 (1982).

27 BIRO, G. P. "Fluorocarbons in the Resuscitation of Hemorrhage," *Intl. Anesth. Clin.*, 23:143 (1985).

28 TREMPER, K. K., A. E. Friedman, E. M. Levine, R. Lapin and D. Camarillo. "The Preoperative Treatment of Severely Anemic Patients with a Perfluorochemical Oxygen-Transport Fluid, Fluosol-DA," *New Engl. J. Med.*, 307:277 (1982). Tremper, K. K. and B. F. Cullen. "U.S. Clinical Studies of the Treatment of Anemia with Fluosol-DA 20%," *Artif. Organs*, 8:19 (1984).

29 OHYANAGI, H., S. Nakaya, S. Okumura and Y. Saitoh. "Surgical Use of Fluosol-DA in Jehovah's Witness Patients," *Artif. Organs*, 8:10 (1984).

30 GOULD, S. A., A. L. Rosen, L. R. Sehgal, H. L. Sehgal and G. S. Moss. "Clinical Experience with Fluosol-DA," *Prog. Clin. Biol. Res.*, 122:331 (1983).

31 MOORE, R. E. and L. C. Clark. "Synthesis and Physical Properties of Perfluorocompounds Useful as Synthetic Blood Candidates," in *Ref. 11*, p. 50 (1982).

32 GEYER, R. P. "Recent Development in Research with Perfluorochemical Artificial Blood Substitutes," in *Ref. 11*, p. 19 (1982).

33 LE BLANC, M and J. G. Riess. "A Strategy for the Synthesis of Pure, Inert Perfluoroalkylated Derivatives Designed for Blood Substitution," in *Ref. 11*, p. 43 (1982).

34 LONG, D. M., C. B. Higgins, R. F. Mattrey, R. M. Mitten and F. K. Multer. "Is There a Time and Place for Radiopaque Fluorocarbons?" in *Preparation, Properties and Industrial Applications of Organofluorine Compounds*, R. E. Banks, ed. Chichester:Ellis Horwood, Chap. 4 (1982).

35 HELDEBRANT, C. M., H. Okamoto, M. Watanabe, A. M. McLaughlin and K. Yokoyama. "Evaluation of Four New Perfluorochemicals in Oxygen Transporting Emulsions," *Abstract. Symp. on Organofluorine Compounds in Medicine and Biology*, Amer. Chem. Soc. Natl. Meeting, Las Vegas (March 1982).

36 YOKOYAMA, K., R. Naito, Y. Tsuda, C. Fukaya, M. Watanabe, S. Hanada and T. Suyama. "Selection of 53 PFC Substances for Better Stability of Emulsion and Improved Artificial Blood Substitutes," *Progr. Clin. Biol. Res.*, 122:189 (1983).

37 YOKOYAMA, K., K. Yamanouchi and T. Suyama. "Recent Advances in a Perfluorochemical Blood Substitute and Its Biomedical Application," *Life Chem. Reports*, 2:35 (1983).

38 YOKOYAMA, K., T. Suyama, H. Okamoto, M. Watanabe, H. Ohyanagi and Y. Saitoh. "A Perfluorochemical Emulsion as an Oxygen Carrier," *Artif. Organs*, 8:34 (1984).

39 JEANNEAUX, F., M. Le Blanc, J. G. Riess and K. Yokoyama. "Fluorocarbons as Gas Carriers for Biomedical Applications 1,2-bis(F-butyl)ethene as a Candidate O_2/CO_2 Carrier for Second-Generation Blood Substitutes," *Nouv. J. Chim.*, 8:251 (1984).

40 ARLEN, C., Y. Gauffreteau, F. Jeanneaux, M. Le Blanc and J. G. Riess. "Le F-isopropyl-1, F-hexyl-2 éthène comme Transporteur des Gaz Respiratoires à Rsage Intravasculaire," *Bull. Soc. Chim. Fr.*, 562 (1985).

41 MAKAROV, K. N. "Perfluorocarbons. Their Structure and Physical Properties," *11th Intl. Symp. Fluorine Chem.*, Berlin, DDR (August 1985).

42 *Preparation, Properties and Industrial Applications of Organofluorine Compounds*, R. E. Banks, ed., Chichester:Ellis Horwood (1982).

43 ABE, T. and S. Nagase. "Electrochemical Fluorination (Simons Process) as a Route to Perfluorinated Organic Compounds of Industrial Interest," in *Ref. 41*, Chap. 1 (1982). Rendell, R. W. and B. Wright. "Fluorination of Trimethylamine Over Cobalt(III) Fluoride," *Tetrahedron*, 35:2405 (1979). Burden, J. and I. W. Parsons. "The Consequences of Cation Radical Fluorination Theory II," *Tetrahedron*, 36:1423 (1980).

44 See for ex. *Ref. 31*, Naito, Y., Y. Inoue, T. Ono, Y. Arakawa, C. Fukaya and K. Yokoyama. "Synthesis of Perfluorochemicals for Use as Blood Substitutes, Part I. Electrochemical Fluorination of N-Methyldecahydroquinoline and N-Methyldecahydroisoquinoline," *J. Fluor. Chem.*, 26:485 (1984), and Ono, T., Y. Inoue, C. Fukaya, Y. Arakawa, Y. Naito and K. Yokoyama. "Synthesis of Perfluorochemicals for Use as Blood Substitutes, Part II: Electrochemical Fluorination of Partly Fluorinated Compounds," *J. Fluorine Chem.*, 27:333 (1985).

45 RIESS, J. G. and R. Follana. "Les fluorocarbures comme substituts de l'hémoglobine pour le transport des gaz respiratoires," *Rev. Fr. Transf. et Immuno-hématol.*, 27:191 (1984).

46 HAMZA, M. A., G. Serratrice, M. J. Stébé and J. J. Delpuech. "Solute–Solvent Interactions in Perfluorocarbon Solutions of Oxygen," an NMR study, *J. Am. Chem. Soc.*, 103:3733 (1981).

47 MALET-MARTINO, M. C., D. Betbeder, A. Lattes, A. Lopez, R. Martino, G. Francois and S. Cros. "Fluosol-43 Intravascular Persistence in Mice Measured by ^{19}F nmr," *J. Pharm. Pharmacol.*, 36:556 (1984).

48 CLARK, L. C., J. L. Ackerman, S. R. Thomas, R. W. Millard, R. E. Hoffman, R. G. Pratt, H. Ragle-Cole, R. A. Kinsey and R. Janakiraman. "Perfluorinated Organic Liquids and Emulsions as Biocompatible NMR Imaging Agents for ^{19}F and Dissolved Oxygen," *Adv. Exp. Med. Biol.*, 180:835 (1984).

49 CLARK, L. C., F. Becattini, S. Kaplan, V. Obrock, D. Cohen and C. Becker. "Perfluorocarbons Having a Short Dwell Time in the Liver," *Science*, 181:680 (1973).

50 OKAMOTO, H., K. Yamanouchi, T. Imagawa, R. Murashima, K. Yokoyama, M. Watanabe and R. Naito. "Persistence of Fluorocarbons in Circulating Blood and Organs," *Proc. IInd Intercompany Conf.*, Osaka (1973).

51 See for ex. *Ref. 35*, and Clark, L. C. "Theoretical and Practical Considerations of Fluorocarbon Emulsions in the Treatment of Shock," in *Pathophysiology of Shock, Anoxia, and Ischemia*, R. A. Cowley and B. F. Trump, eds., Baltimore:Williams & Wilkins, Chap. 37 (1982).

52 MOORE, R. E. and L. C. Clark. "Chemistry of Fluorocarbons in Biomedical Use," *Intl. Anesth. Clin.*, 23:11 (1985).

53 GREC, J.-J., J. G. Riess and B. Devallez. "Etude de solvants perfluoroalkylés à usage biomédical: températures critiques supérieures de solubilité de bis (F-alkyl)éthenes dans l'hexane. Paramètres de solubilité, grandeurs d'excès de mélanges d'acides carboxyliques et de composés perfluoroalkylés," *Nouv. J. Chim.*, 9:637 (1985).

54 YOKOYAMA, K., T. Suyama and R. Naito. "Development of Perfluorochemical (PFC) Emulsion as an Artificial Blood Substitute," in *Biomedical Aspects of Fluorine Chemistry*, R. Filler and Y. Kobayashi, eds., Amsterdam:Elsevier, p. 191 (1982).

55 LONG, D. M., E. C. Lasser, C. M. Sharts, F. K. Multer and M. Nielson. "Experiments with Radiopaque Perfluorocarbon Emulsions for Selective Opacification of Organs and Total Body Angiography," *Invest. Radiol.*, 15:242 (1980).

56 YAMANOUCHI, K., M. Tanaka, Y. Tsuda, K. Yokoyama, S. Awazu and Y. Kobayashi. "Quantitative Structure—In Vivo Half-life Relationships of Perfluorochemicals for Use as Oxygen Transporters," *Chem. Pharm. Bull.*, 33:1221 (1985).

57 GREC, J.-J., J. G. Riess and B. Devallez. "Solubilité d'acides carboxyliques, acides gras, acides aminés et autres substances d'intérêt biologique dans les fluorocarbures. Phénomènes d'entrainement et de partage," *Nouv. J. Chim.*, 9:109 (1985).

58 SCHMOLKA, I. R. "A Review of Block Polymer Surfactants," *J. Am. Oil Chem. Soc.*, 54:110 (1977).

59 DAVIS, S. S., H. P. Round and T. S. Purewal. "Ostwald Ripening and the Stability of Emulsion Systems: An Explanation for the Effect of an Added Third Component," *J. Colloid and Interf. Sci.*, 80:508 (1981).

60 KABAL'NOV, A. S., Yu. D. Aprosin, O. B. Pavlova-Verevkina, A. V. Pertsov and E. D. Shcukin. "Influence of the Nature and Composition of the Disperse Phase of Emulsions of Perfluoro-Organic Compounds on the Kinetics of Reducing Their Dispersity," *Kolloidnyi Z. Akad. Nauk. SSSR*, 48:27 (1986).

61 ARLEN, C., M. Le Blanc and J. G. Riess. unpubl. results.

62 MAYHEW, E., G. T. Nikolopoulos, J. J. King and A. A. Siciliano. "A Practical Method for the Large Scale Manufacture of Liposomes," *Pharmaceutical Manufacturing*, p. 18 (1985).

63 Investigational New Drug Applications, n° 9521, Sponsor D. M. Long.

64 MITSUNO, T., H. Ohyanagi and K. Yokoyama. "Development of a Perfluorochemical Emulsion as a Blood Gas Carrier," *Artif. Organs*, 8:25 (1984).

65 *FDC Reports*, p. 12 (October 31, 1983).

66 WEST, L., N. McIntosh, S. Gendler, C. Seymour and C. Wisdom. "Effects of Intravenously Infused Fluosol-DA 20% in Rats," *Int. J. Rad. Oncol. Biol. Phys.*, 12:1319 (1986).

67 KITAZAMA, M. and Y. Ohnishi. "Long-Term Experiment of Perfluorochemicals Using Rabbits," *Virchows Arch. Pathol Anat.*, 398:1 (1982).

68 DEVALLEZ, B., Y. Gauffreteau, M. Le Blanc and J. G. Riess. in preparation.

69 GOULD, S. A., L. R. Sehgal, A. L. Rosen, L. A. Langdale, H. L. Sehgal, L. Krause and G. S. Moss. "Assessment of a 35% Fluorocarbon Emulsion," *J. Trauma*, 23:720 (1983).

70 LONG, D., C. Long, C. Arlen, M. Le Blanc, J. G. Riess, R. Follana and A. Valla. "Total Exchange Perfusion of Rats with Highly Concentrated Fluorocarbon Emulsions," *Colloq. on Red Blood Cells and Other Oxygen-Carriers*, Lyon (April 1986), *Intl. Symp. Centenary of Discovery of Fluorine*, Paris (August 1986).

71 LONG, D. C., A. R. Burgan, A. R. Long, R. A. Mattrey, D. M. Long, J. G. Riess and R. Follana. "Preparation and Evaluation of Concentrated F-octylbromide Emulsions for Contrast Agents and Synthetic Oxygen Carriers," *Intl. Symp. Centenary of Discovery of Fluorine*, Paris (August 1986).

72 SLOVITER, H. A. and B. Mukherji. "Prolonged Retention in the Circulation of Emulsified Lipid-Coated Perfluorochemicals," *Progr. Clin. Biol. Res.*, 122:181 (1983).

73 FARADJI, A., M. Giunta, Y. Dayan, L. Foulletier and F. Oberling. "Les fluorocarbures comme substitut sanguin," *Rev. Franc. de Transf. et d'Immunohématol.*, 22:119 (1979).

74 DELPUECH, J-J., G. Mathis, J. C. Ravey, C. Selve, G. Serratrice and M. J. Stebe. "La perfluorodécaline comme transporteur de gaz respiratoires: préparation et propriétés physico-chimiques de ses microémulsions aqueuses," *Bull. Soc. Chim. Fr.*, 578 (1985).

75 CLARK, L. C., E. W. Clark, R. E. Moore and D. G. I. Kinnett. "Room Temperature-Stable Biocompatible Fluorocarbon Emulsions," *Progr. Clin. Biol. Res.*, 122:169 (1983).

76 GROSS, U. and H. Meinert. "New Surfactants for Preparing Perfluorocarbon Emulsions," *11th Symp. Fluor. Chem.*, Berlin, DDR (August 1985).

77 OVERBEEK, J. T. G., P. L. de Bruyn and F. Verhoeckx. "Microemulsions," in *Surfactants*, Th. F. Tadros, ed., London:Academic, p. 111 (1984).

78 ROSANO, H. L. and W. E. Gerbacia. "Fluorocarbon Microemulsions," U.S. Patent 3,778,381 (1973).

79 CHABERT, P., L. Foulletier and A. Lantz. "Procédé de préparation de liquides á applications biologiques et transporteurs d'oxygène," *Ger. Offen.*, 2:452,513 (1975).

80 MATHIS, G., P. Leempoel, J-C. Ravey, C. Selve and J.-J. Delpuech. "A Novel Class of Nonionic Microemulsions: Fluorocarbons in Aqueous Solutions of Fluorinated Poly(oxyethylene) Surfactants," *J. Am. Chem. Soc.*, 106:6162 (1984).

81 HOLLOWAY, G. M., E. A. O'Rear and B. M. Fung. "Plasma-Mediated Alterations of Erythrocyte Deformability by Perfluorochemical Blood Substitutes," *Blood*, 67:173 (1986).

82 GEYER, R. P. "Perfluorochemical Blood Replacement Preparations," in *Ref. 10*, p. 3 (1979).

83 LE BLANC, M., J. G. Riess, D. Poggi and R. Follana. "Use of Lymphoblastoid Namalva Cell Cultures in a Toxicity Test. Application to the Monitoring of Detoxification Procedures for Fluorocarbons to be Used as Intravascular Oxygen-Carriers," *Pharm. Res.*, 195 (1985).

84 YOKOYAMA, K., C. Fukaya, Y. Tsuda, T. Suyama, R. Naito, K. Yamanouchi and K. Scherer. "Screening of New Perfluorochemicals (PFC's) as Candidates for Use in Fluorochemical Emulsion Blood Substitutes—Structures and Biological Properties," *Abstr. Symp. on Organofluorine Compounds in Medicine and Biology*, Amer. Chem. Soc. Natl. Meeting, Las Vegas (March 1982).

85 IKEDA, T., N. Hamasake, Y. Ando and H. Mashiba. "Perfusion of Isolated Rat Pancreas with Fluosol-43," in *Ref. 10*, p. 173 (1979)

86 CHUBB, C. and P. Draper. "Steroid Secretion by Rat Testes Perfused with Perfluorochemicals as Oxygen Carriers," *Am. J. Physiol.*, 248:E432 (1985).

87 CHUBB, C. "Reversal of the Endocrine Toxicity of Commercially Produced Perfluorochemical Emulsion," *Biol. of Reproduction*, 33:854 (1985).

88 UBEL, F. A., S. D. Sorenson and D. E. Roach. "Health Status of Plant Workers Exposed to Fluorochemicals—A Preliminary Report," *Am. Ind. Hyg. Assoc. J.*, 41:584 (1980).

89 ATTWOOD, D. and A. T. Florence. "Aspects of Surfactant Toxicity," in *Surfactant Systems*, London:Chapman and Hall, Chap. 10 (1985).

90 Galenica 5. I Agents de surface et Emulsions, F. Puisieux et M. Seiller, eds., Paris:Lavoisier (1983).

91 SHAKIR, K. M. M. and T. J. Williams. "Inhibition of Phospholipase A₂ Activity by Fluosol®, An Artificial Blood Substitute," *Prostaglandins*, 23:919 (1982).

92 LANE, T. A. and G. Lampkin. "Paralysis of Phagocyte Migration Due to an Artificial Blood Substitute," *Blood*, 64:400 (1984).

93 VIRMANI, R., D. Warren, R. Rees, L. Fink and D. English. "Effects of Perfluorochemical on Phagocytic Function of Leukocytes," *Transfusion*, 23:512 (1983).

94 VIRMANI, R., L. M. Fink, K. Gunter and D. English. "Effect of Perfluorochemical Blood Substitutes on Human Neutrophil Function," *Transfusion*, 24:343 (1984).

95 LANE, T. A. and G. E. Lamkin. "Increased Infection Mortality and Decreased Neutrophil Migration Due to a Component of an Artificial Blood Substitute," *Blood*, 68:351 (1986).

96 JANCO, R. L., R. Virmani, P. J. Morris and K. Gunter. "Perfluorochemical Blood Substitutes Differentially Alter Human Monocyte Procoagulant Generation and Oxidative Metabolism," *Transfusion*, 25:578 (1985).

97 WAKE, E. J., G. P. Studzinski and A. Bhandal. "Changes in Human Cultured Cells Exposed to a Perfluorocarbon Emulsion," *Transfusion*, 25(1):73 (1985).

98 BUCALA, R., M. Kawakami and A. Cerami. "Cytotoxicity of a Perfluorocarbon Blood Substitute to Macrophages In Vitro," *Science*, 220:965 (1983).

99 COLMAN, R. W., L. K. Chang, B. Mukherji and H. A. Sloviter. "Effects of a Perfluoro Erythrocyte Substitute on Platelets In Vitro In Vivo," *J. Lab. Clin. Med.*, 95(4):553 (1980).

100 YOSHIMURA, N., T. Gushiken, N. Horinokuchi, K. Kawasaki and I. Maruyama. "Effect of Fluosol-DA on the Blood Coagulation/Fibrinolytic System and the Renin-angiotensin System in Man," *Progr. Clin. Biol. Res.*, 122:343 (1983).

101 MITSUNO, T., H. Ohyanagi and R. Naito. "Clinical Studies of Perfluorochemical Whole Blood Substitute (Fluosol-DA): Summary of 186 Cases," *Ann. Surg.*, 195:60 (1982); Mitsuno, T., H. Ohyanagi and R. Naito. "Clinical Studies of a Perfluorochemical Whole Blood Substitute (Fluosol-DA)," in *Ref. 11*, p. 30 (1982).

102 ADAMS, J. E., G. Owens, J. R. Headrick, A. Munoz and H. W. Scott. "Experimental Evaluation of Pluronic F68 (A Non-Ionic Detergent) as a Method of Diminishing Systemic Fat Emboli Resulting from Prolonged Cardiopulmonary Bypass," *Surg. Forum*, 10:585 (1959).

103 MIYAUCHI, Y., J. Inoue and B. C. Paton. *Circulation*, 33:171 (1966).

104 LOWE, K. C. "Whole Blood Substitutes," *Clin. Res. Rev.*, 4:126 (1984).

105 Intl. Forum "To Which Extent Is the Clinical Use of Dextran, Gelatin and Hydroxyethyl Starch Influenced by the Incidence and Severity of Anaphylactoid Reactions?" *Vox Sang.*, 36:39 (1979).

106 TREMPER, K. K. and K. Waxman. "Artificial Plasma Expanders," in *Year Book Medical Publishers*, p. 293 (1985).

107 MOSS, G. S. and C. S. Rice. "Shock and Resuscitation," in *Edema*, N. C. Staub and A. E. Taylor, eds., New York:Raven Press, p. 563 (1984).

108 RICHTER, W. and H. Hedin. in *Allergic Reactions to Drugs*, A. L. Weck and H. Bungard, eds., Berlin:Springer Verlag (1983).

109 ARLEN, C., R. Follana, M. Le Blanc, J. G. Riess and A. Valla. unpublished results.

110 WAXMAN, K., K. Tremper, B. Cullen and G. Mason. "Perfluorocarbon Infusion in Bleeding Patients Refusing Blood Transfusions," *Arch. Surg.*, 119:721 (1984).

111 VERCELLOTTI, G. M., D. E. Hammerschmidt, P. R. Craddock and H. S. Jacob. "Activation of Plasma Complement by Perfluorocarbon Artificial Blood: Probable Mechanism of Adverse Pulmonary Reactions in Treated Patients and Rationale for Corticosteroid Prophylaxis," *Blood*, 59:1299 (1982).

112 TREMPER, K., G. Vercellotti and D. E. Hammerschmidt. "Hemodynamic Profile of Adverse Clinical Reactions to Fluosol-DA 20%," *Crit. Care Med.*, 12:428 (1984).

113 VERCELOTTI, G. M. and D. E. Hammerschmidt. "Immunological Biocompatibility in Blood Substitutes," *Intl. Anesth. Clin.*, 23:47 (1985).

114 MATTREY, R. F., D. M. Long, W. W. Peck, R. A. Slutsky and C. B. Higgins. "Perfluorooctylbromide as a Blood Pool Contrast Agent for Liver, Spleen, and Vascular Imaging in Computed Tomography," *J. Comp. Assist. Tomogr.*, 8:739 (1984).

115 NISHIMURA, N. and T. Sugi. "Changes of Hemodynamics and O₂ Transport Associated with the Perfluorochemical Blood Substitute, Fluosol-DA," *Crit. Care Med.*, 12:36 (1984).

116 POLICE, A., K. Waxman and G. Tominaga. "Pulmonary Complications After Fluosol Administration to Patients with Life-Threatening Blood Loss," *Crit. Care Med.*, 13:96 (1985).

117 McCOY, L. E., C. A. Becker, T. H. Goodin and M. I. Barnhart. "Endothelial Response to Perfluorochemical Perfusion," *Scan. Electron Micros.*, 1:311 (1984).

118 HALL, J. E., I. C. Ehrhart and W. F. Hofman. "Pulmonary Fluid Balance and Hemodynamics After Perfluorocarbon Infusion in the Dog Lung," *Crit. Care Med.*, 13:1015 (1985).

119 ZHONG, B., Q. Tang, Y. Zhou, P. Xin and X. Ding. "Mutagenicity of Fluorocarbon Blood Substitute," *Acta Pharmacol. Sin.*, 4:35 (1983). Ding, X., B. Chen, J. Shen and W. Gu. "Pharmacokinetics of Fluorocarbon Blood Substitute," *Acta Pharmacol. Sin.*, 4:262 (1983). Ding, X., S. Zhang, C. Liu, G. Wang, L. Zhou, G. Zhuang and B. Wang. "Effects of Fluorocarbon Blood Substitute on Marrow Erythropoietic Function and Phagocytic Activity," *Acta Pharmacol. Sin.*, 5:42 (1984). Wang, B. and X. Ding. "Chronic Toxic-pathologic Investigation of Fluorocarbon Blood Substitute," *Chin. J. Pathol.*, 1:64 (1985). Ding, X., B. Wang, Q. Tang, G. Wang, Y. Qin and Y. Liu. "Long Term Effects of Intravenous Infusion of Fluorocarbon Blood Substitute in Dogs," *Acta Pharmacol. Sin.*, 6:270 (1985); and ref. therein.

120 FISCHER, J. J., S. Rockwell and D. F. Martin. "Perfluorochemicals and Hyperbaric Oxygen in Radiation Therapy," *Int. J. Rad. Oncol. Biol. Phys.*, 12:95 (1986).

121 LOWE, K. C., D. C. McNaughton and R. N. Hardy. "Observations on the Physiological Responses to Blood Substitution in the Conscious Chronically Catheterized Rat," in *Ref. 11*, p. 91 (1982).

122 GOODIN, T. H., W. P. Clarke, K. Taylor, R. Eccles, R. P. Geyer and L. E. McCoy. "A Method for Evaluation of Blood Substitutes in the Conscious Animal," *Am. J. Physiol.*, H519 (1983).

123 HARDY, R. N., K. C. Lowe and D. C. McNaughton. "Acute Responses During Blood Substitution in the Conscious Rat," *J. Physiol.*, 338:451 (1983).

124 LOWE, K. C., D. C. McNaughton and R. N. Hardy. "Changes in Intravascular Fluid Composition Following Blood Replacement with Perfluorocarbon Emulsion in the Rat," *Klin. Wochenschr.*, 63:1028 (1985).

125 LOWE, K. C. and D. C. McNaughton. "Changes in Plasma Enzyme Concentrations in Response to Blood Substitution with Perfluorocarbon Emulsion in the Conscious Rat," *Experientia*, 42:1228 (1986).

126 MINOWA, K. and Y. Hayashida. "Neural Activities During Replacement of Blood with Fluorocarbon Emulsion," *Neurosurgery*, 13:402 (1983).

127 ROSENBLUM, W. I., M. G. Hadfield and J. Martinez. "Alterations of Liver and Spleen Following Intravenous Infusion of Fluorocarbon Emulsions," *Arch. Pathol. Lab. Med.*, 100:213 (1976).

128 MILLER, M. L., R. E. Moore and L. C. Clark. "Morphology and Porphometry of the Liver After Infusion of Perfluorochemical Emulsion: An Assessment of 19 Selected Compounds," in *Ref. 10*, p. 81 (1979).

129 LUTZ, J. "Studies on RES Function in Rats and Mice after Different Doses of Fluosol," *Progr. Clin. Biol. Res.*, 122:197 (1983).

130 PFANNKUCH, F. and N. Schnoy. "Long-Term Observation of PFC Storage in Organs of Rats After Various Dosages," *Progr. Clin. Biol. Res.*, 122:209 (1983).

131 NANNEY, L., L. M. Fink and R. Virmani. "Perfluorochemicals—Morphologic Changes in Infused Liver, Spleen, Lung, and Kidney of Rabbits," *Arch. Pathol. Lab. Med.*, 108:631 (1984).

132 CAIAZZA, S., C. Fanizza and M. Ferrari. "Fluosol-43 Particle Localization Pattern in Target Organs of Rats," *Virchows Arch. Pathol. Anal.*, 404:127 (1984).

133 YUHAS, J. M., R. L. Goodman and R. E. Moore. "Potential Application of Perfluorochemicals in Cancer Therapy," *Intl. Anesthes. Clin.*, 23:199 (1985).

134 LUTZ, J. "Effect of Perfluorochemicals on Host Defense, Especially on the Reticuloendothelial System," *Intl. Anesth. Clin.*, 23:63 (1985).

135 FUJITA, T., C. Suzuki and R. Ogawa. "Effect of Fluosol-DA on the Reticuloendothelial System Function in Surgical Patients," *Progr. Clin. Biol. Res.*, 122:265 (1983).

136 MITSUNO, T., Y. Tabuchi, H. Ohyanagi and T. Sugiyama. "Intake and Retention of Perfluorochemical Substance of Fluosol-DA in RES in Human," in *Ref. 11*, p. 220 (1982).

137 CASTRO, O., C. A. Reindorf, W. W. Socha and A. H. Rowe. "Perfluorocarbon Enhancement of Heterologous Red Cell Survival: A Reticuloendothelial Block Effect?" *Int. Arch. Allergy Appl. Immunol.*, 70:88 (1983).

138 CASTRO, O., A. Nesbitt and D. Lyles. "Effect of a Perfluorocarbon Emulsion (Fluosol-DA) on Reticuloendothelial System Clearance Function," *Am. J. Hematol.*, 16:15 (1984).

139 LUTZ, J. and M. Wagner. "Recovery From Pentobarbital-Induced Sleep After Administration of Perfluorinated Blood Substitutes," *Artif. Organs*, 8:41 (1984).

140 HOYT, D. B., A. G. Greensburg, S. Forbes, S. Lin and J. C. Mendelsohn. "Resuscitation with Fluosol-DA 20%—Tolerance to Sepsis," *J. Trauma*, 26:713 (1986).

141 GEORGE, C. D. and P. J. Morello. "Immunologic Effects of Blood Transfusion Upon Renal Transplantation, Tumor Operations and Bacterial Infections," *Am. J. Surg.*, 152:329 (1986).

142 MILLER, M. L., J. D. Stinnett and L. C. Clark. "Ultrastructure of Tumoricidal Peritoneal Exudate Cells Stimulated *In Vivo* by Perfluorochemical Emulsions," *J. Reticuloendothel. Soc.*, 27:105 (1980).

143 HOYT, D. B., A. G. Greensburg, F. Molter, J. J. Coyle, R. P. Saik and D. M. Long. "Perfluorocarbons and Intra-Abdominal Sepsis," *Curr. Surg.* 38:283 (1981).

144 SPRATT, J. S. "Blood Transfusions and Surgery for Cancer," *Am. J. Surg.*, 152:337 (1986).

145 CEFALO, R. C., J. W. Seeds, H. J. Proctor and V. V. Baker. "Maternal and Fetal Effects of Exchange Transfusion with a Red Blood Cell Substitute," *Am. J. Obstet. Gynecol.*, 148:859 (1984).

146 MADJIDI, A., H. Beisbarth and R. Frey. "Comparative Studies with Fluosol, Dextran, Their Mixture, or Autologous Blood in Experimental Hypovolemic Shock," *Progr. Clin. Biol. Res.*, 122:391 (1983).

147 BIRO, G. P. "Current Status of Erythrocyte Substitutes," *Can. Med. Assoc. J.*, 129:237 (1983).

148 PROCTOR, H. J., G. W. Palladino, C. Cairus and F. F. Jobsis. "An Evaluation of Perfluorochemical Resuscitation After Hypoxic Hypotension," *J. Trauma*, 23:79 (1983).

149 MAKOWSKI, H., P. Tentschev, P. Frey, St. Necek, H. Bergmann and B. Blauhut. "Tolerance of an Oxygen-Carrying Colloidal Plasma Substitute in Human Beings," in *Ref. 10*, p. 47 (1979).

150 OHYANAGI, H., K. Toshima, M. Sekita, M. Okamoto, T. Itoh, T. Mitsuno, R. Naito, T. Suyama and K. Yokoyama. "Clinical Studies of Perfluorochemical Whole Blood Substitutes: Safety of Fluosol-DA (20%) in Normal Human Volunteers," *Clin. Ther.*, 2:306 (1979).

151 MITSUNO, T. and H. Ohyanagi. "Present Status of Clinical Studies of Fluosol-DA (20%) in Japan, Clinical Experience with Fluosol-DA (20%) in the United States," *Intl. Anesth. Clin.*, 23:169 (1985).

152 TREMPER, K. K., E. M. Levine and K. Waxman. "Clinical Experience with Fluosol-DA (20%) in the United States," *Intl. Anesth. Clin.*, 23:185 (1985).

153 GOULD, S. A., A. L. Rosen, L. R. Sehgal, H. L. Sehgal, C. L. Rice and G. S. Moss. "Red Cell Substitutes: Hemoglobin Solution or Fluorocarbon?" *J. Trauma*, 22:618 (1982).

154 GOULD, S. A., A. L. Rosen, L. R. Sehgal, H. L. Sehgal, L. A. Langdale, L. M. Krause, C. L. Rice, W. H. Chamberlin and G. S. Moss. "Fluosol-DA as a Red-Cell Substitute in Acute Anemia," *New Engl. J. Med.*, 314:1653 (1986), and the correspondence this paper has aroused in the same Journal, 315:1677 (1987).

155 KARN, K. E., P. L. Ogburn, T. Julian, F. B. Cerra, D. E. Hammerschmidt and G. Vercellotti. "Use of a Whole Blood Substitute, Fluosol-DA 20%, After Massive Postpartum Hemorrhage," *Obstetrics & Gynecology*, 65:127 (1985).

156 BROWN, A. S., J. H. Reichman and R. K. Spence. "Fluosol-DA, A Perfluorochemical Oxygen-Transport Fluid for the Management of a Trochanteric Pressure Sore in a Jehovah's Witness," *Ann. Plast. Surg.*, 8412:449 (1984).

157 STEFANISZYN, H. J., J. E. Wynands and T. A. Salerno. "Initial Canadian Experience with Artificial Blood (Fluosol-DA-20%) in Severely Anemic Patients," *J. Cardiovasc. Surg.*, 26:337 (1985).

158 GLOGAR, D. H., R. A. Klonar, J. Muller, L. W. V. De Boer and E. Braunwold. "Fluorocarbons Reduce Myocardial Ischemic Damage After Coronary Occlusion," *Science*, 211:1439 (1981).

159 KLONER, R. A. and D. H. Glogar. "Overview of the Use of Perfluorochemicals for Myocardial Ischemic Rescue," *Intl. Anesth. Clin.*, 23:115 (1985).

160 KLONER, R. A., D. Glogar, R. E. Rude, S. F. Khuri, J. A. Muller, L. C. Clark and E. Braunwald. "The Effect of Perfluorocarbons on Experimental Myocardial Ischemia and Infarction," *Progr. Clin. Biol. Res.*, 122:381 (1983).

161 RUDE, R. E., D. Glogar, S. F. Khuri, R. A. Kloner, S. Karaffa, J. E. Muller, L. C. Clark and E. Braunwald. "Effects of Intravenous Fluorocarbons on Acute Myocardial Ischemic Injury Assessed by Measurement of Intramyocardial Gas Tensions," *Am. Heart J.*, 103:986 (1982).

162 KOLODGIE, F. D., A. K. Dawson, M. B. Forman and R. Virmani. "Effect of Perfluorochemical (Fluosol-DA) on Infarct Morphology in Dogs," *Virchow's Arch. (Cell Pathol.)*, 50:119 (1985).

163 NUNN, G. R., G. Dance, J. Peters and L. H. Cohn. "Effect of Fluorocarbon Echange Transfusion on Myocardial Size in Dogs," *Am. J. Cardiol.*, 52:203 (1983).

164 MENASHÉ, P., M. Escorsin, P. Birkui, A. Lavergne, M. Fauchet, P. Commin, P. Lorente, R. P. Geyer and A. Piwnica. "Limitations of Fluorocarbons in Reducing Myocardial Infarct Size," *Am. J. Cardiology*, 55:830 (1985).

165 FAITHFULL, N. S., M. Fennema, C. E. Essed, W. Erdmann, H. Jeekel and R. Lapin. "Collateral Oxygenation of the Ischemic Myocardium: The Effect of Viscosity and Oxygen Carrying Fluorocarbons," *Progr. Clin. Biol. Res.*, 122:229 (1983).

166 BIRO, G. P. "Fluorocarbon and Dextran Hemodilution in Myocardial Ischemia," *Can. J. Surg.*, 26:163 (1983).

167 MUSHLIN, P. S., R. J. Boucek, M. D. Parrish, T. P. Graham and R. D. Olson. "Beneficial Effects of Perfluorochemical Artificial Blood on Cardiac Function Following Coronary Occlusion," *Life Sciences*, 36:2093 (1985).

168 SPEARS, J. R., J. Serur, D. S. Baim, W. Grossman and S. Paulin. *Circulation*, 68(3):80 (1983).

169 KANTER, K. R. and T. J. Gardner. "The Use of Perfluorochemicals During Open Heart Surgery," *Intl. Anesth. Clin.*, 23:105 (1985).

170 MAGOVERN, G. J., J. T. Flaherty, V. L. Gott, B. H. Bulkey and T. J. Gardner. "Failure of Blood Cardioplegia to Protect Myocardium at Lower Temperatures," *Circulation*, 66(suppl. 1):60 (1982).

171 KANTER, K. R., J. H. Jaffin, R. J. Erlichman, J. T. Flaherty, V. L. Gott and T. J. Gardner. "Superiority of Perfluorocarbon Cardioplegia Over Blood or Crystalloid Cardioplegia," *Circulation*, 64:74 (1981).

172 MAGOVERN, G. J., J. T. Flaherty, V. L. Gott, B. H. Bulkey and T. J. Gardner. "Optimal Myocardial Protection with Fluosol Cardioplegia," *Ann. Thorac. Surg.*, 34:249 (1982).

173 GARDNER, T. J., J. T. Flaherty, K. R. Kanter and G. J. Magovern. "Improved Myocardial Protection with Perfluorocarbon Cardioplegia," *Progr. Clin. Biol. Res.*, 122:405 (1983).

174 FLAHERTY, J. T., W. E. Jacobus, M. L. Weisfeldt, D. L. Hollis, T. J. Gardner and V. L. Gott. "Use of ^{31}Phosphorus Nuclear Magnetic Resonance to Assess Myocardial Protection During Global Ischemia," *Am. J. Cardiol.*, 43:362 (1979).

175 FLAHERTY, J. T., J. H. Jaffin, G. J. Magovern, K. R. Kanter, T. J. Gardner, M. V. Miceli and W. E. Jacobus. "Maintenance of Aerobic Metabolism During Global Ischemia with Perfluorocarbon Cardioplegia Improves Myocardial Preservation," *Circulation*, 69:585 (1984).

176 ROUSOU, J. H., W. A. Dobbs and R. M. Engelman. "Fluosol Cardioplegia—A Method of Optimizing Aerobic Metabolism During Arrest," *Circulation*, 66(suppl. 1):55 (1982).

177 ROUSOU, J. A., R. M. Engelman, L. Anisimowicz, S. Lemeshow, W. A. Dobbs, R. H. Breyer and D. K. Das. "Metabolic Enhancement of Myocardial Preservation During Cardioplegic Arrest," *J. Thorac. Cardiovasc. Surg.*, 91:270 (1986).

178 BELOYARTSEV, F. F., B. I. Islamov and E. I. Mayevsky. *Information on Perfusion and Nonperfusion Methods of Myocardium Protection with Perfluorocarbon Emulsion*, Acad. Sci., U.S.S.R., Puschchino (1983).

179 MENASCHÉ, Ph., M. Fauchet, A. Lavergne, P. Commin, C. Masquet, P. Birkui, P. Lorente, R. P. Geyer and A. Piwnica. "Applications of a Perfluorocarbon to Heart Ischemia," *Progr. Clin. Biol. Res.*, 122:363 (1983).

180 MENASCHÉ, P., M. Fauchet, A. Lavergne, P. Commin, C. Masquet, P. Lorente, P. Birkui, P. Geyer and A. Piwnica. "Reduction of Myocardial Infarct Size by a Fluorocarbon-Oxygenated Reperfusate," *Am. J. Cardiology*, 53:608 (1984).

181 PARRISH, M. D., R. D. Olson, P. S. Mushlin, M. Artman and R. J. Boucek. "Treatment of Postischemic Reperfusion Cardiac Injury with a Perfluorochemical Solution," *J. Cardiovasc. Pharmacol.*, 6:159 (1984).

182 FORMAN, M. B., S. Bingham, H. A. Kopelman, C. Wehr, M. P. Sandler, F. Kolodgie, W. K. Vaughn, G. C. Friesinger and R. Virmani. "Reduction of Infarct Size with Intracoronary Perfluorochemical in a Canine Preparation of Reperfusion," *Circulation*, 71:1060 (1985).

183 CASALE, A. S., P. J. Horneffer, G. L. Gott and T. J. Gardner. "Oxygenated Perfluorocarbon Cardioplegia Prevents Oxygen Free Radical Reperfusion," *Surg. Forum*, 35:283 (1984).

184 OCHI, S., Y. Sasaki, H. Sakabe, Y. Wada, S. Nakaji and I. Hashimoto. "Effects of Fluorocarbon Infusion on Microcirculation During Cardiopulmonary Bypass," *Clin. Therap.*, 4:465 (1982).

185 ROUSOU, J. A., R. M. Engelman, L. Anisimowicz and W. A. Dobbs. "A Comparison of Blood and Fluosol-DA for Cardiopulmonary Bypass," *J. Cardiovasc. Surg.*, 26:447 (1985).

186 KUSSKE, J. A., M. B. Pritz and K. K. Tremper. "Perfluorochemical Emulsions for the Treatment of Cerebral Ischemia," *Intl. Anesth. Clin.*, 23:131 (1985).

187 MIZOI, K., T. Yoshimoto and J. Suzuki. "Experimental Study of New Cerebral Protective Substances. Functional Recovery of Severe Incomplete Ischemic Brain Lesions, Pretreated with Mannitol and Fluorocarbon Emulsion," *Acta Neurochir.* (Wien), 56:157 (1981).

188 KAGAWA, S., K. Koshna, T. Yoshimoto and J. Suzuki. "The Protective Effect of Mannitol and Perfluorochemicals on Hemorrhagic Infarction: An Experimental Study," *Surg. Neurol.*, 17:66 (1982).

189 SUZUKI, J., S. Tanaka and T. Yoshimoto. "Suppression of Brain Swelling with Mannitol and Perfluorochemicals—Experimental Study," *Acta Neurochir.* (Wien), 58:149 (1981).

190 HAN, D. H., N. T. Zervus, R. P. Geyer, et al. "Can Perfluorochemicals Reduce Cerebral Ischemia?" in *Cerebrovascular Diseases*, M. Reivich and H. I. Hurtig, eds., New York:Raven Press, p. 409 (1983).

191 PEERLESS, S. J., R. Ishikawa, I. G. Hunter and M. J. Peerless. "Protective Effect of Fluosol-DA in Acute Cerebral Ischemia," *Stroke*, 12:558 (1981).

192 PEERLESS, S. J. "The Use of Perfluorochemicals in the Treatment of Acute Cerebral Ischemia," *Progr. Clin. Biol. Res.*, 122:353 (1983).

193 PEERLESS, S. J., R. Nakamura, A. Rodriguez-Salazar and I. G. Hunter. "Modification of Cerebral Ischemia with Fluosol," *Stroke*, 16:38 (1985).

194 MENASCHÉ, P., E. Pinard, A-M. Desroches, J. Seylaz, P. Laget, R. P. Geyer and A. Piwnica. "Fluorocarbons: A Potential Treatment of Cerebral Air Embolism in Open-Heart Surgery," *Ann. Thorac. Surg.*, 40:494 (1985). Pinard, E., A. M. Desroches, M. Le Blanc, R. Charbonne, J. G. Riess and J. Seylaz. "Influence des fluorocarbures sur l'oxygénation et la circulation sanguine du cerveau," *Proc. Colloq. Le Globule Rouge et Autres Transporteurs d'Oxygene*, Lyon, France:Fondation Merieux, p. 161 (1987).

195 SPIESS, B. D., B. Braverman, A. W. Woronowicz and A. D. Ivankovich. "Protection from Cerebral Air Emboli with Perfluorocarbons in Rabbits," *Stroke*, 17:1146 (1986).

196 HANDA, H., Y. Oda and S. Nagasawa. "Effect of Fluosol-DA on Cerebral Circulation in Human," in *Ref. 11*, p. 204 (1982).

197 ODA, Y., T. Murata, Y. Uchida, K. Mori, S. Nagasawa, Y. Naruo, R. Asato and H. Hande. "Clinical Evaluation of Artificial Blood Substitute (Fluosol-DA 20%) in Patients of Cerebral Ischemia," *Neurol. Surg.*, 10:637 (1982).

198 HANDA, H., S. Nagasawa, Y. Yonekawa, Y. Naruo and Y. Oda. "New Treatment of Cerebral Vasospasm with Fluosol-DA 20%: Protective Effect on Cerebral Ischemia and Change of Cerebral Blood Flow (CBF)," *Progr. Clin. Biol. Res.*, 122:299 (1983).

199 SWANN, K. W., A. H. Ropper and N. T. Zervas. "Initial Results of a Clinical Trial of Fluosol-DA 20% in Acute Cerebral Ischemia, *Progr. Clin. Biol. Res.*, 122:399 (1983).

200 SUZUKI, J., T. Yoshimoto, N. Kodama, Y. Sakurai and A. Ogawa. "A New Therapeutic Method for Acute Brain Infarction: Revascularization Following the Administration of Mannitol and Perfluorochemicals. A Preliminary Report," *Surg. Neurol.*, 17:325 (1982).

201 SUZUKI, J., T. Yoshimoto and A. Ogawa. "A New Therapy for Acute Brain Infarction: Revascularization Following the Administration of Mannitol and Perfluorochemicals," *Progr. Clin. Biol. Res.*, 122:321 (1983).

202 OSTERHOLM, J. L., J. B. Alderman, A. J. Triolo, B. R. D'Amore, H. D. Williams and G. Frazer. "Severe Cerebral Ischemia Treatment by Ventriculosubarachnoid Perfusion with an Oxygenated Fluorocarbon Emulsion," *Neurosurgery*, 13:381 (1983).

203 BOSE, B., J. L. Osterholm and A. Triolo. "Focal Cerebral Ischemia: Reduction in Size of Infarcts by Ventriculo-Subarachnoid Perfusion with Fluorocarbon Emulsion," *Brain Research*, 328:223 (1985).

204 HANSEBOUT, R. R., R. H. C. Vanderjagt, S. S. Sohal and J. R. Little. "Oxygenated Fluorocarbon Perfusion as Treatment of Acute Spinal Cord Compression Injury in Dogs," *J. Neurosurg.*, 55:725 (1981).

205 OSTERHOLM, J. H., J. B. Alderman, A. J. Triolo, B. R. D'Amore and H. D. Williams. "Oxygenated Fluorocarbon Nutrient Solution in the Treatment of Experimental Spinal Cord Injury," *Neurosurgery*, 15:373 (1984).

206 SLOVITER, H. A. "Perfluorochemical Emulsions and Perfusion of Isolated Organs," *Intl. Anesth. Clinics*, 23:37 (1985).

207 SEGEL, L. D. and S. V. Rendig. "Isolated Working Rat Heart Perfusion with Perfluorochemical Emulsion Fluosol-43," *Am. J. Physiol.*, 242:H485 (1982).

208 DEUTSCHMANN, W., E. Lindner and N. Deutschlander. "Perfluorochemical Perfusion of the Isolated Guinea Pig Heart," *Pharmacology*, 28:336 (1984).

209 OWEN, C. A. and E. J. W. Bowie. "Generation of Plasmatic Coagulation Factors by the Isolated Rat Liver Perfused with Completely Synthetic Blood Substitute," *Thrombosis Research*, 22:259 (1981).

210 HONDA, K. "Fundamental and Clinical Studies on Intracadaveric Organ Perfusion with Fluosol-DA," *Progr. Clin. Biol. Res.*, 122:327 (1983).

211 RULAND, O., J. Hauss, H.-U. Spiegel and K. Schoenleben. "Comparative pO$_2$ Histograms and Other Parameters in Canine Kidneys During Perfusion with Oxypherol," *Progr. Clin. Biol. Res.*, 122:221 (1983).

212 KAMADA, N., R. Y. Calne, D. G. D. Wight and J. G. Lines. "Orthotopic Rat Liver Transplantation After Long-Term Preservation by Continuous Perfusion with Fluorocarbon Emulsion," *Transplantation*, 30:43 (1980).

213 DEUTSCHMANN, W., H. H. Wellhöner and G. Erdmann. "Perfusion of the Cervical Spinal Cord In Situ of Adult Rats Using a Perfluorocarbon Emulsion," *Brain Research*, 280:239 (1983).

214 LINDGREN, L., C. Marshall, and B. E. Marshall. "Hypoxic Pulmonary Vasoconstriction in Isolated Rat Lungs Perfused with Perfluorocarbon Emulsion," *Acta Physiol Scand.*, 123:335 (1985).

215 KOWALEWSKI, K., A. Kolodej and W. Otto. "Simultaneous Study of Canine Hepatic, Gastric and Pancreatic Function in an Isolated Preparation Perfused Ex-Vivo with Fluorocarbon Emulsion," *Surg. Gynecol. Obstet.*, 148:687 (1979).

216 KOWALEWSKI, K. and A. Kolodej. "Electrical and Mechanical Activity of Isolated Canine Stomach Perfused with Fluorocarbon Emulsion," *Surg. Gynecol. Obstet.*, 145:347 (1977).

217 TAUBER, A., P. Wentd, T. Mittlmeier, C. Stamapoulos, H. Beisbarth, P. Maurer and G. Blumel. "Initial Perfusion of Extremities with Fluosol-43 Prior to Replantation—Metabolic and Hemodynamic Investigations in Rabbits, in *Ref. 11*, p. 245 (1982).

218 SCHLINDLER, H.-G., D. Pennig, W. Schlake, K. Schönleben and E. Brug. "The Use of Fluosol-43 for Intermediary Perfusion in Amputated Limbs; Preliminary Results," in *Ref. 11*, p. 255 (1982).

219 ZHANG, R., R. C. Xiong, B. J. Su, et al. "Pharmacological Study and Clinical Application of Fluorocarbon Artificial Blood," *Chin. J. Surg.*, 23:395 (1985).

220 SMITH, A. R., B. van Alphen, S. Faithfull and M. Fennema. "Limb Preservation in Replantation Surgery," *Plastic Reconstruct. Surg.*, 75:227 (1985).

221 LONG, D. M., M. Liu, P. S. Szanto, D. P. Alrenga, M. M. Patel, M. V. Rios and L. M. Nyhus. "Efficacy and Toxicity Studies with Radiopaque Perfluorocarbon," *Radiology*, 105:323 (1972).

222 MATTREY, R. F., D. M. Long, F. Multer, R. Mitten and C. B. Higgins. "Perfluorooctylbromide: A Reticuloendothelial Specific and a Tumor Imaging Agent for Computed Tomography," *Radiology*, 145:755 (1982).

223 MATTREY, R. F., M. Andre, J. Campbell, R. Mitten, F. Multer, D. Hackney, D. M. Long and C. B. Higgins. "Specific Enhancement of Intra-Abdominal Abscesses with Perfluorooctylbromide for Computed Tomography," *Inv. Radiology*, 19:438 (1984).

224 HARJULA, A. L. J., S. Mattila, H. Myllärniemi, I. Mattila, P. Mattila and E. Merikallio. "Effects of Synthetic Blood Combined with Contrast Medium on Coronary Endothelium: An Experimental Study," *Angiology*, 37:41 (1986).

225 MATTREY, R. F., W. W. Peck, R. A. Slutsky and C. B. Higgins, Perfluorooctylbromide as a Blood Pool Contrast Agent for Liver, Spleen, and Vascular Imaging in Computed Tomography," *J. Comput. Assist. Tomogr.*, 8:739 (1984).

226 MATTREY, R. F., F. W. Scheible, B. B. Gosink, G. R. Leopold, D. M. Long and C. B. Higgins. "Perfluorooctylbromide: A Liver and Spleen Specific and a Tumor Imaging Ultrasound Contrast Material," *Radiology*, 145:759 (1982).

227 PATRONAS, N., D. L. Miller and M. Girton. "Experimental Comparison of EOE-13 and Perfluorooctylbromide for the CT Detection of Hepatic Metastases," *Inv. Radiology*, 19:570 (1984).

228 YOUNG, S. W., D. R. Enzmann, D. M. Long and H. H. Muller. "Perfluorooctylbromide Contrast Enhancement of Malignant Neoplasms: Preliminary Observations," *Amer. J. Radiol.*, 137:141 (1981).

229 MATTREY, R. F. and M. P. Andre. "Ultrasonic Enhancement of Myocardial Infarction with Perfluorocarbon Compounds," *Amer. J. Cardiology*, 54:206 (1984).

230 PATRONAS, N. J., J. Hekmatpanah and K. Doi. "Brain Tumor Imaging Using Radiopaque Perfluorocarbon: A Preliminary Report," *J. Neurosurg.*, 58:650 (1983).

231 MATTREY, R. F., G. R. Leopold, E. van Sonnenberg, B. B. Gosink, F. W. Scheible and D. M. Long. "Perfluorochemicals as Liver- and Spleen-Seeking Ultrasound Contrast Agents," *J. Ultrasound Med.*, 2:173 (1983).

232 MATTREY, R. F., G. Strich, R. E. Shelton, B. B. Gosink, G. L. Leopold, T. Lee, M. Green and C. Wisdom. "Perfluorochemicals as Ultrasound Contrast Agents for Tumor Imaging and Hepatosplenography: Preliminary Clinical Results," *Radiology*, 167:339 (1987).

233 LONGMAID III, H. E., D. F. Adams, R. D. Neirinckx, C. G. Harrison, P. Brunner, S. E. Seltzer, M. A. Davis, L. Neuringer and R. P. Geyer. "In Vivo ¹⁹F NMR Imaging of Liver, Tumor, and Abscess in Rats," *Investigative Radiol.*, 20:141 (1985).

234 GOLDMAN, M. R., E. T. Fossel, J. S. Ingwall and G. M. Pohost. "Use of the ¹⁹F NMR Evaluation of Ischemic and Infarcted Myocardium," *J. Comput. Assist. Tomogr.*, 5:304 (1981).

235 THOMAS, S. R., L. C. Clark, J. L. Ackerman, R. G. Pratt, R. E. Hoffman, L. J. Busse, R. A. Kinsey and R. C. Samaratunga. "MR Imaging of the Lung Using Liquid Perfluorocarbons," *J. Comp. Ass. Tomogr.*, 10:1 (1986).

236 REID, R. S., C. J. Koch, M. E. Castro, J. A. Lunt, E. O. Treiber, D. J. Boisvert and P. S. Allen. "The Influence of Oxygenation on the ¹⁹F Spin-Lattice Relaxation Rates of Fluosol-DA," *Phys. Med. Biol.*, 30:677 (1985).

237 SPEARS, J. R., H. J. Marais, J. Serur, et al. "In Vivo Coronary Angioscopy," *J. Am. Coll. Cardiol.*, 1:1311 (1983).

238 KUWAMURA, K. and T. Kokunai. "Effect of Perfluorochemicals on BCNU Chemotherapy: Preliminary Study in a Rat Brain Tumor Model," *Surg. Neurol.*, 18:258 (1982); Kuwamura, K., T. Kokunai, N. Tamaki and S. Matsumoto. "Synergistic Effect of Perfluorochemicals on BCNU Chemotherapy. Experimental Study in a 9L Brain Tumor Model," *J. Neurosurg.*, 57:467 (1982).

239 OHYANAGI, H., M. Nishijima, M. Usami, S. Nishimatsu, E. Matsui and Y. Saitoh. "Experimental Studies on the Possible Combined Chemotherapy to Neoplasms with Fluosol-DA Infusion," *Progr. Clin. Biol. Res.*, 122:315 (1983).

240 TEICHER, B. A., S. A. Holden and C. M. Rose. "Differential Enhancement of Melphalan Cytotoxicity in Tumor and Normal Tissue by Fluosol-DA and Oxygen Breathing," *Int. J. Cancer*, 36:585 (1985).

241 TEICHER, B. A., S. A. Holden and C. M. Rose. "Effect of Oxygen on the Cytotoxicity and Antitumor Activity of Etoposide," *J. Natl. Cancer Inst.*, 75:1129 (1985).

242 TEICHER, B. A. and S. A. Holden. "Survey of the Effect of Adding Fluosol-DA 20%/O₂ to Treatment with Various Chemotherapeutic Agents," *Cancer Treat. Rep.*, 71:173 (1987).

243 TEICHER, B. A. and C. M. Rose. "Perfluorochemical Emulsions Can Increase Tumor Radiosensitivity," *Science*, 223:934 (1984).

244 TEICHER, B. A. and C. M. Rose. "Oxygen-Carrying Perfluorochemical Emulsion as an Adjuvant to Radiation Therapy in Mice," *Cancer Research*, 44:4285 (1984); Teicher, B. A. and C. M. Rose. "Effects of Dose and Scheduling on Growth Delay of the Lewis Lung Carcinoma Produced by the Perfluorochemical Emulsion, Fluosol-DA," *Int. J. Radiat. Oncol. Biol. Phys.*, 12:1311 (1986).

245 ROCKWELL, S. "Use of a Perfluorochemical Emulsion to Improve Oxygenation in a Solid Tumor," *Int. J. Radiation Oncology Biol. Phys.*, 11:97 (1985).

246 ROCKWELL, S., T. P. Mate, C. G. Irvin and M. Nierenburg. "Reactions of Tumors and Normal Tissues in Mice to Irradiation in the Presence and Absence of a Perfluorochemical Emulsion," *Int. J. Radiation Oncology Biol. Phys.*, 12:1315 (1986).

247 SONG, C. W., W. L. Zhang, D. M. Pence, I. Lee and S. H. Levitt. "Increased Radiosensitivity of Tumors by Perfluorochemicals and Carbogen," *Int. J. Radiation Oncology Biol. Phys.*, 11:1833 (1986).

248 TREMPER, K. K., J. Zaccari, B. F. Cullen and S. M. Hufstedler. "Liquid Gas Partition Coefficients of Halothane and Isoflurane in Perfluorodecalin, Fluosol-DA and Blood/Fluosol-DA Mixtures," *Anesth. Analg.*, 63:690 (1984).

249 HODGES, G. R., J. S. Reed, C. E. Hignite and W. R. Snodgrass. "Blood Substitutes: Effects on Drug Pharmacokinetics," *Progr. Clin. Biol. Res.*, 122:430 (1983).

250 LEVINE, E. M. and K. K. Tremper. "Perfluorochemical Emulsions: Potential Clinical Uses and New Developments," *Intl. Anesth. Clin.*, 23:211 (1985).

251 NISHIMURA, N. and T. Sugi. "Fluosol-DA in Hypovolemic States of Acute Myocardial Infarction and Extensive Burn Injuries," in *Ref. 11*, p. 196 (1982).

252 MATSUKI, A., T. Jin, S. Fukushi, H. Ishihara, Y. Satoh, M. Toyota and T. Oyama. "Therapeutic Experience with Fluosol-DA 20% (FDA) in Carbon Monoxide Poisoning," *Progr. Clin. Biol. Res.*, 122:445 (1983).

253 AGISHI, T., K. Yamagata, M. A. Kobayashi, S. Teraoka, H. Honda and K. Ota. "Normothermic Whole Body Rinse-Out Utilizing Perfluorochemical-Containing Artificial Blood," *Trans. Am. Soc. Artif. Int. Organs*, 30:295 (1984).

254 REINDORF, C. A. "Blood Substitutes," *Progr. Clin. Biol. Res.*, 98:129 (1982).

255 CLINE, K. A. and T. L. Turnbull. "Clostridial Myonecrosis," *Ann. Emerg. Med.*, 14:459/129 (1985).

256 REINDORF, C. A., J. Barber, F. Dickson, T. William and W. A. Anderson. "Synergistic Effects of Perfluorochemicals and Stroma Free Hemoglobin," *Progr. Clin. Biol. Res.*, 122:435 (1983).

257 BABA, S. and K. Mizutani. "The Intraluminal Administration of Perfluorochemicals to the Ischaemic Gastrointestinal Tract," *Aust. NZ. J. Surg.*, 51:468 (1981).

258 RICCI, J. L., H. A. Sloviter and M. M. Ziegler. "Intestinal Ischemia: Reduction of Mortality Utilizing Perfluorochemical," *Am. J. Surg.*, 149:84 (1985).

259 FAITHFULL, N. S., J. Klein, H. T. Van der Zee and P. J. Salt. "Whole Body Oxygenation Using Intraperitoneal Perfusion of Fluorocarbons," *Br. J. Anaesth.*, 56:867 (1984).

260 YAMAMOTO, M., S. Okumura, H. Ohyanagi and Y. Saitoh. "Treatment of Acute Pancreatitis in Relation to the Changes of Pancreatic Enzymes," in *Pancreatitis: Its Pathophysiology and Clinical Aspects*, T. Sato and H. Yamauchi, eds., Tokyo:Univ. Tokyo Press, p. 253 (1985).

261 HARRIS, D. J., R. R. Coggin, J. Roby, G. Feezor, G. Turner and P. B. Bennett. "Liquid Ventilation in Dogs: An Apparatus for Normobaric and Hyperbaric Studies," *J. Appl. Physiol.*, 54:1141 (1983).

262 LUTZ, J. and G. Herrman. "Perfluorochemicals as a Treatment of Decompression Sickness in Rats," *Pflügers Arch.*, 401:174 (1984).

263 LINCOFF, H., J. Coleman, I. Kreissig, G. Richard, S. Chang and L. M. Wilcox. "The Perfluorocarbon Gases in the Treatment of Retinal Detachment," *Ophthalmology*, 90:546 (1983).

264 CHANG, S., N. J. Zimmerman, T. Iwamoto, R. Ortiz and D. Faris. "Experimental Vitreous Replacement with Perfluorotributylamine," *Amer. J. Ophthalm.*, 103:29 (1987).

265 GEYER, R. P. "Substitutes for Blood and Its Components," in *Blood Substitutes and Plasma Expanders*, New York:Alan R. Liss, Inc., p. 1 (1978).

266 MAYEVSKY, A., I. Mizawa and H. A. Sloviter. "Surface Fluorometry and Electrical Activity of the Isolated Rat Brain Perfused with Artificial Blood," *Neurolog. Res.*, 3:307 (1981).

267 COOK, J. A., W. C. Wise, G. E. Tempel and P. V. Halushka. "Exchange Transfusions in Rats with a Perfluorated Blood Substitute: Effect on Thromboxane B$_2$ Levels During Endotoxemia," *Circulatory Shock*, 15:193 (1985).

268 SAURAT, P. "Procédé de vaccination de lapins sauvages (oryctolagus cuniculi) contre la myxomatose à l'aide d'insectes vecteurs porteurs d'un virus vaccin non pathogène," Fr. Pat. Appl. n° 86 00851, 22.01.86.

269 RIESS, J. G. "Post-Fluosol Progress in Fluorocarbon Emulsions for In Vivo Delivery," *Proceed. Intl. Symp. Artif. Blood Substitutes (Bari, Italy, 1987) La Trasf. del Sangue*, 32:316 (1987)

270 YAMANOUCHI, Y. T. and K. Yokoyama. "Perfluorochemical Emulsions: The Industrial View," *Symp. on Biologically Active Organofluorine Compounds*, (abst. #698) (1989).

271 RIESS, J. G. "Fluorocarbons and Surfactants for In Vivo Oxygen Delivery, Recent Advances," *Symp. on Biologically Active Organofluorine Compounds*, (abst. #699) (1989).

272 LONG, D. C., D. M. Long, J. G. Riess, R. Follana, A. Burgan and R. F. Mattrey. "Preparation and Applications of Highly Concentrated Perfluorooctylbromide Fluorocarbon Emulsions," *Biomat. Artif. Cells, Artif. Org.*, 16:441 (1988).

273 LONG, D. M., C. D. Long, R. F. Mattrey, R. A. Long, A. R. Burgan, W. C. Herrick, D. F. Shellhamer. "An Overview of Perfluorooctylbromide. Application as a Synthetic Oxygen Carrier and Imaging Agent for X-ray, Ultrasound and Nuclear Magnetic Resonance," *Biomat. Artif. Cells, Artif. Org.*, 16:411 (1988).

274 MATTREY, R. F., P. L. Hilpert, D. C. Long, D. M. Long, R. M. Mitten, T. Peterson. "Hemodynamic Effects of Intravenously Administered Lecithin-Based Perfluorocarbon Emulsions in Dogs," *Crit. Care Med.*, 17:652 (1989).

275 RIESS, J. G. "Current Orientations with Regard to In Vivo Oxygen Carriers. The Fluorocarbon Emulsions," *J. Chim. Phys.*, 84:12 (1987).

276 RIESS, J. G. "Blood Substitutes: Where Do We Stand at Present With the Fluorocarbon Approach?" *Curr. Surg.*, 45:265 (1988).

277 FAITHFULL, N. S. "Potential Applications of Perfluorochemical Emulsions in Medicine and Research," in *Blood Substitutes. Preparation, Physiology and Medical Applications*, Lowe, K. C., ed., Chichester, U.K.:Ellis Horwood, p. 130 (1988).

278 MATTREY, R. F. "Potential Role of Perfluorooctylbromide in the Detection and Characterization of Liver Lesions with CT," *Radiology*, 170:18 (1988).

279 BRUNETON, J. N., M. N. Falewee, E. Francois, P. Cambon, C. Philip, J. G. Riess, C. Balu-Maestro and A. Rogopoulos. "Preliminary Clinical Results Using Perfluorooctylbromide (PFOB) for CT Imaging of the Liver, Spleen and Vessels," *Radiology*, 170:179 (1989).

280 MATTREY, R. F. "Perfluorooctylbromide: A New Contrast Agent for CT, Sonography and MR Imaging," *Am. J. Radiol.*, 152:274 (1989).

281 MATTREY, R. F., P. C. Hajek, V. M. Gylys-Morin, L. L. Baker, J. Martin, D. C. Long, D. M. Long. "Perfluorochemicals as Gastrointestinal Contrast Agents for MR Imaging: Preliminary Studies in Rats and Humans," *Am J. Radiol.*, 148:1259 (1987).

282 RATNER, D. V., H. H. Muller, B. Bradley-Simpson, D. E. Johnson, R. E. Hurd, C. Sotak and S. W. Young. "Detection of Tumors with ^{19}F Magnetic Resonance Imaging," *Invest. Radiol.*, 23:361 (1988).

283 RIESS, J. G. "Fluorocarbon Emulsions for In Vivo Oxygen Delivery. The Decisive Role Expected of the Surfactant in Future Progress," *Proceed. 2nd World Surfactant Congress*, 4:256 (1988).

284 RIESS, J. G., C. Arlen, J. Greiner, M. Le Blanc, A. Manfredi, S. Pace, C. Varescon and L. Zarif. "Design, Synthesis and Evaluation of Fluorocarbons and Surfactants for In Vivo Applications. New Perfluoroalkylated Polyhydroxylated Surfactants," *Biomat. Artif. Cells, Artif. Org.*, 16:421 (1988).

285 RIESS, J. G., J. Greiner, M. Le Blanc, Y. S. Lin, A. Manfredi, S. Pace, C. Varescon and L. Zarif. "New Polyhydroxylated Perfluoroalkylated Surfactants Derived from Sugars and Related Compounds—Applications to the Formulation of O$_2$-Carriers for In Vivo Use," *Actual. Chim. Therap.*, 15:247 (1988).

286 BLAIGNON, C., M. Le Blanc and J. G. Riess. "Synthesis and Evaluation of New F-alkylated Surface Active Agents Derived from Amino-Acids. Application to the Formulation of O$_2$-Carriers for In Vivo Use," *Proceed. 2nd World Surfactant Congress*, 2:127 (1988).

287 RIESS, J. G., S. Pace and L. Zarif. "Protective Effect Against Hemolysis of Perfluoroalkylated Chains in Surfactants," *Artif. Organs* (1990).

288 *Proceed Intl. Symp. Artificial Blood Substitutes, Montreal, Canada, May 1987*, T. M. S. Chang and R. P. Geyer, eds., *Biomat., Artif. Cells, Artif. Org.*, 16 (1988).

289 *Proceed Intl. Symp. Artificial Blood Substitute*, G. De Stasio, F. De Venuto, M. Lancieri, eds., Bari, Italy (June 1987). Servizio di Immunoematologia e Trasfusione, Presidio Ospedaliero "Di Venere," Bari/Carbonara, Italy, 1987; also in *La Trasfusione del Sangue*, II Pensiero Scientifico, 32 and 33 (1987).

290 Abstracts, Symp. on Oxygen-Carrying Preparations, *Ann. Meeting Soc. Exp. Biol.*, Lancaster, U.K. (March 1988).

291 Abstracts, Workshop on Blood Substitutes, *Ann. Meeting Europ. Soc. Artif. Org.*, Brussels, Belgium (Sept. 1989).

292 Abstracts, Intl. Symp. on Red Blood Cell Substitutes (Sapporo, Oct. 1989) in *Artif. Organs*, 13:402 (1989).

293 Abstracts, *Am. Inst. Chem. Engineers, Symp. on Blood Cell Substitute and Artificial Cells*, San Francisco (Nov. 1989).

294 Abstracts, *Pacifichem 1989, Symp. on Biologically Active Organofluorine Compounds*, Honolulu (Dec. 1989).

295 MITSUNO, T., H. Ohyanagi, K. Yokoyama and T. Suyama. "Recent Studies on Perfluorochemical (PFC) Emulsions as an Oxygen Carrier in Japan," *Biomat., Artif. Cells, Artif. Organs*, 16:365 (1988).

296 RIESS, J. G. "Oxygen-Carrying Blood Substitutes with Fluorocarbons and Blood Transfusion," United Nations Organization Industrial Development, *Symposium Report US/RAS*, 85:230/27 (1987).

297 CLEMAN, M., C. Jaffee and D. Wohlgelernter. "Prevention of Ischemia During Percutaneous Transluminal Coronary Angioplasty by Transcatheter Infusion of Oxygenated Fluosol DA 20%," *Therapy and Prevention, Coronary Angioplasty*, 74:3,555 (1986).

298 SLOVITER, H. A. "The Safety and Efficacy of Perfluorochemical Emulsions as Blood Substitutes," *Biomat., Artif. Cells, Artif. Organs*, 16:459 (1988).

299 HAMMERSCHMIDT, D. E. and G. M. Vercellotti, "Limitation of Complement Activation by Perfluorocarbon Emulsions. Superiority of Lecithin-Emulsified Preparations," *Biomat., Artif. Cells, Artif. Org.*, 16:431 (1988).

300 TSUDA, Y., K. Nakura, K. Yamanouchi, K. Yokoyama, M. Watanabe, H. Ohyanagi and Y. Saitoh. "Study of the Excretion Mechanism of a Perfluorochemical Emulsion," *Artif. Organs*, 13:197 (1989).

301 BIRO, G. P. "Blood Substitutes and the Heart: A Critical View," *La Traf. del Sangue*, 33:35 (1988).

302 BIRO, G. P. "Blood Substitutes and the Cardiovascular System," *Biomat., Artif. Cells, Artif. Org.*, 16:595 (1988).

303 ROCKWELL, S. "Perfluorochemical Emulsions as Adjuncts to Radiotherapy," *Biomat., Artif. Cells, Artif. Org.*, 16:519 (1988).

304 TEICHER, B. A., T. S. Herman, S. A. Holden and S. M. Jones. "Addition of Misonidazole, Etanidazole, or Hyperthermia to Treatment with Fluosol-DA/Carbogen/Radiation," *J. Natl. Cancer Inst.*, 81:929 (1989).

305 LUSTIG, R., N. McIntosh-Lowe, C. Rose, J. Haas, S. Krasnow, M. Spaulding and L. Prosnitz. "Phase I/II Study of Fluosol-DA and 100% Oxygen as an Adjuvant to Radiation in the Treatment of Advanced Squamous Cell Tumors of the Head and Neck," *Int. J. Radiat. Oncol. Biol. Phys.*, 16:1587 (1989).

306 RIESS, J. G. "Therapeutic Oxygen Carriage: Coordinated or Dissolved," *New J. Chem.* (in press).

CHAPTER 15

The Hemodynamic Manifestations of Blood Dialyzer Interactions

J. FRANK WALKER, M.D.[1]

INTRODUCTION

Blood–foreign surface interactions that occur when using extracorporeal devices such as the artificial kidney, haemo or plasma filters, or membrane oxygenators may lead to clinically significant problems. Dialyzer hypersensitivity (also called new dialyzer syndrome, first-use syndrome, and Cuprophan hypersensitivity) is one infrequent example, with serious consequences of complications that may occur during interaction between blood and a foreign surface [1–12]. It is clinically recognized within the first ten minutes of commencing haemodialysis and is accompanied by a range of symptoms of varying severity. The typical manifestations consist of the development of acute chest and back pain, dyspnoea, and diaphoresis with hypotension. Rarely, an acute severe anaphylactic reaction occurs with cardiopulmonary arrest. These reactions account for five deaths a year in the U.S.A. [13]. The incidence rate is 4.3 reactions per 100,000 artificial kidneys of hollow fiber construction and has remained constant between 1982 and 1984 [13]. However, minor adverse symptoms are experienced by up to 5% of the dialysis population [6,14].

The majority of reports in the United States and France describe patients dialyzed for the first time by a new (not reused) artificial kidney containing cupra ammonium cellulose (Cuprophan), in hollow fiber configuration [13,15]. In Britain, these reports are predominantly related to the use of Cuprophan in plate form. Adverse reactions develop most frequently during the first year of dialysis. The incidence declines with length of time on dialysis. However, reactions still may occur after 10 years. Infrequent reactions have been encountered when using new artificial kidneys containing cellulose acetate, polysulphone, polyacrylonitrile and even with reused dialyzers. Evidence is accumulating that certain groups may be at particular risk of developing this reaction during dialysis. Patients less than 29 years old have twice as many reactions as patients in the 30 to 49 year old range. An additional risk factor appears to be race, as Negroes or other minority groups experience three times as many reactions as Caucasians [13]. A history of Atopy may be evident in up to one-third of cases [15]. In spite of these identified risk groups, it is impossible to predict the majority of patients who will develop this manifestation of blood–dialyzer contact, or whether it will recur on subsequent dialysis.

THEORIES

The pathogenesis of dialyzer hypersensitivity has not been fully determined. Activation of the complement cascade [16] and/or sensitivity to ethylene oxide [17–21] have both been suggested as probable factors in the genesis of this reaction. However, the evidence supporting the role of these two theories remains incomplete. It remains speculative, but appears probable, that either or both of these two identified factors play a role in a significant number of cases. Whether other factors are also involved remains an open question.

Complement Activation

Activation of the complement cascade through the alternate pathway occurs regularly during the initial stages of haemodialysis [22,23]. As a result, formation of the anaphylotoxins C3a and C5a occurs, which apparently results in pulmonary sequestration of the activated neutrophils with development of the characteristic peripheral

[1]Department of Medicine, Royal College of Surgeons in Ireland and Jervis Street and St. Laurence's Hospitals, Dublin, Ireland

EVENTS FOLLOWING INTRODUCTION OF CUPROPHAN H.F. DIALYSER
INTO EXTRACORPOREAL CIRCUIT

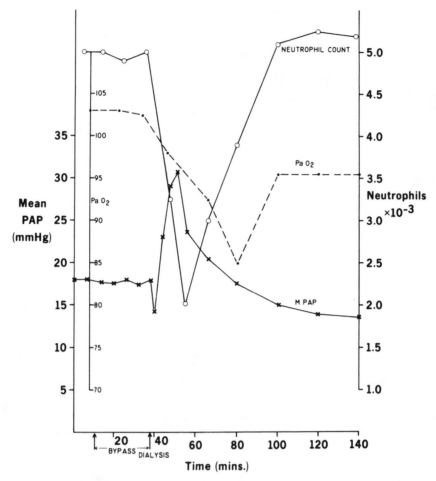

Figure 1. Changes in mean pulmonary artery pressure (mean PAP), arterial oxygen concentration (PaO2) and neutrophil count before, during and after introduction of a cupra ammonium cellulose hollow fiber dialyzer into the extracorporeal circuit. Reproduced by permission of the editor of the ASAIO Journal (from Ref. 29).

leukopenia. This pulmonary leukosequestration is accompanied by an increase in the arterial alveolar gradient with the development of hypoxemia [22,23]. Haemodialysis with artificial kidneys containing cupra ammonium cellulose is associated with greater degrees of complement activation, neutropenia, hypoxemia and more intradialytic symptoms than occurs with the use of dialyzers containing cellulose acetate, polyacrylonitrile or polymethylmethacrylate [24–28]. The quantity of complement activated in vivo during dialysis or in vitro following exposure to Zymosan has been correlated with the development of adverse intradialytic symptoms [16,28].

Clinical signs of acute pulmonary hypertension have been described in one patient during successive dialysis which was accompanied by evidence of complement activation [10]. During experimental dialysis, both in sheep

and swine, acute pulmonary hypertension develops simultaneously as the characteristic leukopenia which precedes the development of hypoxemia (Figure 1) [29,30]. A similar response occurs following infusion of autologous Zymosan activated plasma or C5a des Arg [22,30]. Therefore, it appears that the manifestations of complement activation that occur as a result of blood–foreign surface interaction consist of acute pulmonary hypertension, leukopenia and hypoxemia. Direct haemodynamic measurements performed during clinical haemodialysis in patients with acute renal failure have confirmed that increases in pulmonary vascular resistance do occur, including the development of acute pulmonary hypertension [31]. In addition, the animals which develop a severe pulmonary hypertensive response become tachypnoeic, and dyspnoeic, with evidence of myocardial ischaemia and arrythmias [29]. Therefore, it appears that a range of changes in pulmonary vascular tone may occur during the initial stages of haemodialysis and that the severity of the cardiopulmonary symptoms may reflect the degree of pulmonary hypertension.

The severity of the pressor response depends on the type of membrane used in animal experiments [29]. Injection of cupra ammonium cellulose activated autologous blood resulted in the development of significantly greater pulmonary hypertension in sheep when compared to injections of polyacrylonitrile activated blood [29]. During clinical haemodialysis, an improvement in adverse symptoms has been reported with the use of membranes which cause less complement activation such as polyacrylonitrile, polysulphone and polymethylmethacrylate as compared with the use of cupra ammonium cellulose [24–28]. In addition, intradialytic symptoms decrease and the hypersensitivity reaction is rare during reuse, where less complement activation develops, particularly when the reprocessing procedure is performed manually or using formaldehyde as the sterilizing agent [25,32–35]. The pulmonary vascular response is also abolished in animal studies during reuse with cupra ammonium cellulose activated blood using 2% formaldehyde or tetradecylbenzene sulphonate–hypochlorous complex as the sterilants [36].

Therefore, the amount of complement activated depends on the particular type of membrane used during dialysis. However, the development of the reaction is related to the quantity of anaphylotoxins generated, to the severity of pulmonary vascular response and, probably, to certain unexplained individual susceptibilitites.

Ethylene Oxide Sensitivity

Ethylene oxide is the commonly used sterilizing agent for disposable dialysis equipment and has been found in significant quantities in the rinsing fluid of sterilized artificial kidneys [37]. IgE Antibody conjugates of human serum albumen–ethylene oxide have been demonstrated in up to one-third of all patients on haemodialysis with adverse symptoms using a radioallergoabsorbent test (RAST) [38–42]. These antibodies occur more frequently in haemodialysis patients with a history of Atopy, symptoms of chronic asthma or the presence of peripheral eosinophilia. Ethylene oxide is trapped in the polyurethane potting material used in the manufacture of hollow fibre dialyzers and slowly released during dialysis [37]. This may account for the greater incidence of adverse reactions in hollow fibre dialyzers compared to flat plate artificial kidneys, which do not require any potting material during manufacture. In vitro studies have demonstrated that human albumen–ethylene oxide conjugates may induce IgE mediated degranulation of basophils in sensitized patients [40,43]. The reduction of adverse symptoms in ethylene oxide sensitized patients during dialysis with non-ethylene oxide sterilized equipment and

which recurred following re-exposure to ethylene oxide sterilized materials provides strong evidence for a central role for this agent in the etiology of certain of these reactions [40].

Alternatively, the IgE antibodies to ethylene oxide–human serum albumen may be an epiphenomenon. Ethylene oxide is capable of binding to other proteins rendering them antigenic. Certainly, contact between ethylene oxide and cupra ammonium cellulose results in the generation of a toxic residue, chloroethanol [44]. This may partly explain the disparity in cases where antibodies to ethylene oxide are undetectable. However, it is difficult to explain the few reports of the reaction as well as the reduction of adverse symptoms during dialysis with cellulose acetate, polyacrylonitrile, polysulphone or polymethylmethacrylate membranes which are sterilized with ethylene oxide unless one accepts that other factors must also be involved.

THE HAEMODYNAMIC MANIFESTATIONS

The initial event that occurs at the site of blood–foreign surface interaction is activation of the alternate pathway of complement which is now universally accepted as the cause of pulmonary leukosequestration with the development of leukopenia and hypoxemia. As previously stated, a third manifestation of complement activation is transient acute pulmonary hypertension. It has been suggested that it is the magnitude of this pressor response which results in the development of symptoms.

The haemodynamic consequences of this pulmonary vascular response need to be mentioned. In animal models, the acute pulmonary hypertension was accompanied by a fall in cardiac output [29,30] due to a decline in left ventricular preload as a consequence of failing right ventricular function [45]. The right ventricular ejection fraction, used as an indirect measurement of the pulmonary vascular response, decreases transiently during the initial stages of clinical haemodialysis in patients with end stage renal failure [46]. The peripheral resistance increases during experimental dialysis [30] to maintain the systemic pressure in the presence of a falling cardiac output [47]. The variable systemic pressure reported (hypo- or hyper-tension) in humans with adverse symptoms may, therefore, reflect the extent to which this response can occur.

It is necessary to examine what is known about the mechanisms of pulmonary hypertension and its relationship to the leukopenia and hypoxemia. Craddock et al. originally postulated that the complement induced pulmonary leukostasis resulting in pulmonary hypertension and hypoxemia. However, a temporal dissociation has been noted during experimental haemodialysis between the onset of the pressor response and the development of

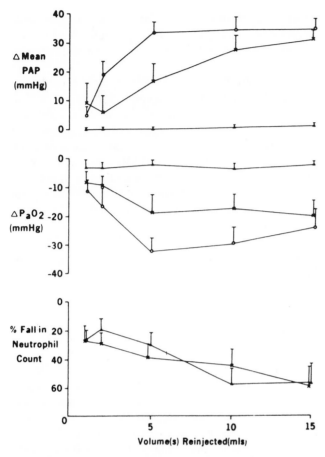

Figure 2. *Changes in mean pulmonary artery pressure (Mean PAP, mmHg), arterial oxygen tension (PaO2, mmHg) and % fall in neutrophil count in normal (x . . . x), Leukopenic (0 . . . 0) and Indomethacin pretreated (Δ . . . Δ) sheep. Results are expressed as mean ± SEM. Reproduced by permission of the editor of* Proc. EDTA-ERA *(from Ref. 52).*

peripheral leukopenia—the haemodynamic response precedes the leukopenia [30].

Certainly, the anaphylotoxins C3a and C5a that are produced are biologically active glycopeptides which are capable in vitro of causing smooth muscle contractions, increased vascular permeability and the release of histamine from mast cells [48–51]. Our studies in sheep, following injection of varying volumes of blood after static contact with a cupra ammonium cellulose hollow fiber artificial kidney, demonstrated that the use of the cyclo-oxygenase inhibitor, Indomethacin, abolished the pulmonary vascular response (Figure 2) [52]. The release of thromboxane A2, a potent vasoconstrictor, has been correlated with the pulmonary hypertension following infusion of cupra ammonium activated plasma [53] in swine and during experimental dialysis [54]. It appears that the anaphylotoxins result in pulmonary hypertension through a cyclo-oxygenase dependent mechanism with release of thromboxane A2. The source of the prostaglandin synthesis remains speculative.

Thromboxane A2 is known to be synthesized by stimu-

lated polymorphonuclear leukocytes [55,56], platelets [57,58], macrophages [56,59] and pulmonary endotheleum. Animal studies involving injections or infusions of cupra ammonium cellulose contacted blood and Zymosan activated plasma into leukopenic and thrombocytopenic sheep, respectively, caused a pulmonary vascular response similar to that in normal animals [52,60]. This leaves the pulmonary endothelium as the source of the vasoactive thromboxane A2.

It is interesting that the partial pressure of oxygen remained stable when the pulmonary vascular response was abolished by the use of the cyclo-oxygenase inhibitor, Indomethacin, following injection of varying volumes of autologous blood after static contact with a cupra ammonium cellulose hollow fiber artificial kidney in sheep without affecting the degree of leukopenia (Figure 2) [52]. Furthermore, the induction of leukopenia did not affect the magnitude of the pulmonary vascular response nor the degree of hypoxemia when compared to normal animals. Therefore, it appears that the hypoxemia is directly related to the pulmonary hypertensive response, probably as a result of acute changes in ventilation perfusion relationships, rather than intrapulmonary leukostasis as originally proposed by Craddock [22]. There is no doubt that acetate dialysate is a major factor in the pathogenesis of dialysis induced hypoxemia [60–63]. Blood–foreign surface interactions must also be considered in the etiology, particularly when it develops during the initial stages of haemodialysis. Clinical studies support this view: artificial kidneys containing membranes which activate less complement produce less hypoxemia, irrespective of the dialysate composition [64,65]. The direct consequence of complement activation during blood–foreign surface interaction is twofold: firstly, activated leukocytes with intrapulmonary leukostasis and peripheral leukopenia; secondly, pulmonary vasoconstriction mediated by Thromboxane A2 release with the development of pulmonary hypertension, which is responsible for the hypoxemia. It is possible that the leukocytes, once activated, may release further quantities of Thromboxane A2 or an intermediate such as leukotriene B4, which could aggravate this pulmonary vascular response [66].

It certainly appears that there is a wide variability in this pulmonary vascular response, ranging from no demonstrable effect in normal humans during mock dialysis [67] to the development of asymptomatic acute pulmonary hypertension [31]. In contrast, the peripheral leukopenia regularly accompanies complement activation, and apparently to the same extent. The severity of the cardiopulmonary response appears to depend on the particular membrane used in the extracorporeal circuit, the quantity of complement activated and Thromboxane generated, and the sensitivity of the pulmonary vascular bed. Undefined individual susceptibilities, such as the presence of pre-existing cardiopulmonary disease, may also be important.

TREATMENT

The therapy of adverse reactions currently is to try to modify the initial step(s) of blood–foreign surface contact, i.e., complement activation, by changing the chemical structure of the membrane and avoiding ethylene oxide sterilized dialyzers. However, the management of the severe hypersensitivity reaction is supported with the use of supplemental oxygen antihistamines, parental corticosteroids and administration of colloid. These measures remain unproven, as no clinical trial has been performed to determine their efficacy in this life-threatening situation. In view of the possibility of recurrence, it is advisable not to dialyze patients who have experienced adverse symptoms with the same dialyzer, but to use one which causes less complement activation and preferably which is not sterilized with ethylene oxide.

Certain precautions can be taken to minimize the risk of adverse symptoms. A 10 minute recirculation of the extracorporeal circuit followed by 1 liter of saline rinse on the blood side of the compartment prior to initiation of dialysis, as recommended by the dialyzer manufacturers, decreases the incidence [6]. Also, a gradual increase in the blood flow rate up to the maximum attenuates these symptoms. The use of newer membranes containing polyacrylonitrile, polysulphone or polymethylmethacrylate, which cause less activation of complement during dialysis, have been found to also cause a reduction in dialysis related symptoms. Alternatively, modification of complement activation in the extracorporeal circuit is a theoretical possibility. Both regional citrate anticoagulation and reduction of dialysate temperature to 20.5°C have resulted in reduction of peripheral leukopenia during clinical dialysis [68]. It seems reasonable to assume that these measures may also reduce the frequency of adverse reactions. Whether prophylactic therapy with cyclo-oxygenase inhibitor(s) is of any benefit (by diminishing the pulmonary haemodynamic response in vivo) remains unknown.

Ultimately, successful therapy will be developed as the mechanism(s) of this reaction become better understood. As a result, new equipment or techniques will result in more biocompatible devices being manufactured, thus avoiding this potentially life-threatening situation.

ACKNOWLEDGEMENTS

I greatly appreciate the advice and support of Dr. R. Lindsay, Dr. A. Linton and Dr. W. Sibbald, the technical assistance of Mr. Brian Dennis and Ms. Andrea Honan, and the secretarial assistance of Ms. Fiona Connolly.

REFERENCES

1 OGDEN, D. A. "New Dialyzer Syndrome." *N. Engl. J. Med.*, 302:1262–1263 (1980).

2 WELLS, S. "Possible Dialyzer Hypersensitivity. *Publisher*, 3:54–55 (1981).

3 POPLI, S, T. S. Ing, J. T. Daugirdas, A. L. Kheirbek, G. W. Viol, R. M. Vilbar and V. C. Gandhi. "Severe Reactions to Cuprophan Capillary Dialyzers." *Artif Organs*, 6:312–315 (1982).

4 KEY, J. M. Nahmias, S. Acchiardo. "Hypersensitivity Reactions on First Time Exposure to Cuprophan Hollow Fiber Dialyzer." *Am. J. Kidney Disease*, 2:664–666 (1983).

5 ING, T. S., J. T. Daugirdas, S. Popli and V. C. Gandhi. "First Use Syndrome with Cupra Ammonium Cellulose Dialyzers." *Int. J. Artif Organs*, 6:235–239.

6 NICHOLS, P. J. and M. M. Platts. "Anaphylactic Reactions Due to Haemodialysis, Haemofiltration or Membrane Plasma Separation." *Brit. Med. J.*, 285:1607–1609 (1982).

7 ZIROVANNIS, P., J. Thanon, K. Tsantoulis, E. Papathansion and N. Papadoyannakis. "Anaphylactic Reaction to Cuprophan and Cellulose Acetate Membranes." *Abstract EDTNA*, 21 (1983).

8 CESTERO, R. V. M., W. E. Hoy, R. B. Freeman. "Anaphylactoid Reactions and Eosinophilia in Patients Treated with Hollow Fiber Artificial Kidneys (HFAK). *Abstracts of the 20th Ann Mtg of American Soc. Artif Intern Organs*, Washington, DC: April 17–19 (1975).

9 AGAR, J. W., J. D. Hill, M. Kaplan and P. G. Pletka. "Acute Cardiopulmonary Decompensation and Complement Activation During Haemodialysis." *Ann Intern Med.*, 90:792 (1979).

10 WATHEN, R. L. and E. Klein. "Hypersensitivity in Haemodialysis." *Artif. Organs*, 8:270–272 (1984).

11 CESTRO, R. V. M., W. E. Hoy and R. B. Freeman. "Anaphylactoid Reactions and Eosinophilia in Patients Treated with Hollow Fiber Artificial Kidneys (HFAK)." *Abstracts of 20th Annual Mtg of American Society of Artificial Internal Organs*, 4:9 (1975).

12 MICHELSON, E. A., L. Cohen and R. E. Dankner. "Eosinophilia and Pulmonary Dysfunction During Cuprophan Haemodialysis." *Kidney Int*, 24:246–249 (1983)

13 VILLAROEL, F. and Ciarkowski. "A Survey on Hypersensitivity in Haemodialysis." *Artif Organs*, 9:231–238 (1985).

14 HENDERSON, L. W., A. K. Cheung and D. Chenoweth. "Choosing a Membrane." *Am. J. Kidney Disease*, 3:5–20 (1983).

15 FORET, M., F. Kuentz, T. Hachache, M. Christollet, R. Milongo, H. Meftahi, E. Dechelette and D. J. Cordonnier. "Hypersensitivity Reactions During Haemodialysis in France." *Proc. EDTA–ERA*, 22:181–186 (1985).

16 HAKIM, R. M., J. Breillant, J. M. Lazarus and F. K. Port. "Complement Activation and Hypersensitivity Reactions to Dialysis Membranes." *N. Engl. J. Med.*, 311:878–82 (1984).

17 POOTHULLIL, J., A. Shimizu, R. P. Day and J. Dolovich. "Anaphylaxis From the Product(s) of Ethylene Oxide Gas." *Ann. Intern. Med.*, 82:58 (1975).

18 MARSHALL, C., F. Pearson, M. Sagona, W. Lee, R. Watten, R. Ward and J. Dolovich. "Reactions During Haemodialysis Due to Allergy to Ethylene Oxide Gas Sterilization." *J. Allergy Clin. Immun.*, 75:563–567 (1985).

19 NICHOLLS, A. J. and M. M. Platts. "Anaphylactoid Reactions During Haemodialysis are Due to Ethylene Oxide Hypersensitivity." *Proc. EDTA*, 21:173–177 (1984).

20 RUMPF, K. W., A. Seubert, R. Valentin, H. Ippen, S. Seubert, H. D. Lowitz, H. Rippe and F. Scheler. "Association of Ethylene Oxide Induced IgE Antibodies with Symptoms in Dialysis Patients." *LANCET*, ll:1385–1387 (1985).

21 BOMMER, J., H. P. Barth, O. H. Wilhelms, H. Schindele and E. Ritz. "Anaphylactoid Reactions in Dialysis Patients: Role of Ethylene Oxide." *LANCET*, ll:1382–1385 (1985).

22 CRADDOCK, P. R., J. Fehr, K. L. Bryham, R. S. Kronenberg, H. S. Jacob. "Couplement and Leukocyte Mediated Pulmonary Dysfunc-

tion in Haemodialysis. *N. Eng. J. Med.*, 296:769–774 (1979).

23 CRADDOCK, P. R., J. Fehr, A. P. Dalmasso, K. L. Bryham and H. S. Jacob. "Haemodialysis Leukopenia: Pulmonary Vascular Leukostasis Resulting From Couplement Activation by Dialyzer Cellophane Membranes." *J. Clin INVEST*, 59:879–888 (1977).

24 CHENOWETH, D. E., A. K. Cheung and L. W. Henderson. "Anaphylotoxin Formation During Haemodialysis: Effects of Different Dialyzer Membranes." *Kidney Int.*, 24:764–769 (1983).

25 CHENOWETH, D. E., A. K. Cheung, D. M. Ward and L. W. Henderson. "Anaphylotoxin Formation During Haemodialysis: Comparison of New and Re-Used Dialyzers. *Kidney Int.*, 24:770–774 (1983).

26 HAKIM, R. M. and E. G. Lowrie. "Haemodialysis Associated Neutropenia and Hypoxemia–The Effect of Dialyzer Membrane Material Nephron." 32:32–39 (1982).

27 JACOB, A. I., G. Gavellas, R. Zarco, G. Perez and J. J. Bourgoinie. "Leukopenia, Hypoxia and Complement Functions with Different Haemodialysis Membranes." *Kidney Int.*, 18:505 (1980).

28 IVANOVICH, P., D. E. Chenoweth, R. Schmidt, H. Klinkman, L. A. Boxer, H. S. Jacob and D. E. Hammerschmidt. "Symptoms and Activation of Complement with Two Dialysis Membranes." *Kidney Int.*, 24:758–763 (1983).

29 WALKER, J. F., M. Lindsayr, S. D. Peters, W. J. Sibbald and A. C. Linton. "A Sheep Model to Examine the Cardiopulmonary Manifestations of Blood Dialyzer Interactions." *ASAIO J.*, 6:123–130 (1983).

30 CHEUNG, A. K., M. Lewinter, D. E. Chenoweth, W. Y. W. Lew and L. W. Henderson. "Cardiopulmonary Effects of Cuprophane-Activated Plasma in the Swine." *Kidney Int.*, 29:799–806 (1986).

31 WALKER, J. F., R. Lindsay, W. Sibbald, A. Lindon. "Changes in Pulmonary Vascular Tone During Early Haemodialysis." *Trans. Am. Soc. Artif Internal Organs*, 30:168–172 (1984).

32 BOK, D. V., L. Pascual, C. Herberjer, R. Sawyer and N. W. Levin. "Effect of Multiple Use of Dialyzers on Intradialytic Symptoms." *Proc. Clin. Dial. Transplant Forum*, 10:92–99 (1980).

33 KANTS, K. S., V. E. Pollack, M. Cathey, A. Goetz and R. Berlin. "Multiple Use of Dialyzers: Safety and Efficacy." *Kidney Int.*, 19:728–238 (1981).

34 HAKIM, R. M. and E. G. Lowrie. "Effect of Dialyzer Re-Use on Leukopenia, Hypoxemia and Total Haemolytic Complement System." *Trans Am. Soc. Artif Int Organs.*, 26:159–164 (1980).

35 IVANOVICH, P. "Re-use of Dialyzers and Blood Proc." *EDTA-ERA* 22:173–177 (1980).

36 LINDSAY, R. M., J. F. Walker. "The Cardiopulmonary Manifestations of Blood Dialyzer (New and Reused) Interactions in an Animal Model." (In press)

37 HENNE, W., W. Dietrich, Pelgerm et al. "Residual Ethylene Oxide in Willow Fiber Dialyzers." *Artif. Organs*, 8:306–310 (1984).

38 MARSHALL, C. P., F. C. Pearson, M. A. Sagona, et al. "Reactions During Haemodialysis Caused by Allergy to Ethylene Oxide Gas Sterilization." *J. Allergy Clin. Immun.*, 75:563–567 (1985).

39 NICHOLLS, A. J. and M. Platts. "Anaphylactoid Reactions During Haemodialysis are Due to Ethylene Oxide Hypersensitivity." *Proct EDTA*, 21:173–177 (1984).

40 BOMMER, J., H. P. Barth, H. Wilhemso, H. Schindelle H. and E. Ritz. "Anaphylactoid Reactions in Dialysis Patients: Role of Ethylene Oxide." *LANCET*, 2:1382–1384 (1985).

41 RUMPF, K. W., A. Seubert, R. Valentin, H. Ippen, S. Seubert, H. D. Lowitz, H. Rippe and F. Scheler. "Association of Ethylene-Oxide-Induced IgE Antibodies with Symptoms in Dialysis Patients." *LANCET*, 2:1385–1387 (1985).

42 DOLOVICH, J., C. P. Marshall, E. K. M. Smith, et al. "Allergy to Ethylene Oxide in Chronic Haemodialysis Patients." *Artif Organs*, 8:334–337 (1984).

43 BARTH, H., J. Bommer, H. Wilhelms, et al. "ETO-induced IgE Mediated Degranulation of Basophils of Dialysis Patients. *Abstracts of 22nd Congress of EDTA.* Brussels, June 28:98 (1985).

44 GUTCH, C. F., L. D. Eskelson, E. Ziegler, et al. "Chloro-ethanol as a Toxic Residue in Dialysis Supplies Sterilized with Ethylene Oxide." *Dial Transplant.*, 5:21–25 (1976).

45 SIBBALD, W. J. and A. A. Driedger. "Right Ventricular Function in Acute Disease States: Pathophysiologic Considerations." *Crit. Care Med.*, 11:334–345 (1983).

46 WALKER, J. F., R. M Lindsay, A. A. Driedger and A. L. Lindon. "Haemodialysis Commonly Causes Transient Acute Pulmonary Hypertension." *Kidney Int.*, 25:195 (1984).

47 McINTYRE, K. M. and Sasahara. "Determinants of Right Ventricular Dysfunction and Haemodynamics After Pulmonary Embolism." *Chest*, 65:534–543 (1974).

48 COCHRANE, C. G. and H. J. Muller-Eberhard. "The Derivation of Two Distinct Anaphylotoxin Activities From the Third and Fifth Components of Human Complement." *J. Exp. Med.*, 127:271–386 (1968).

49 JOHNSON, A. R., T. E. Hugli and H. J. Muller-Eberhard. "Release of Histamine from RAT MAST Cells by the Complement Peptides C3a and C5a." *Immunology*, 28:1067–1080 (1975).

50 FERNANDEZ, H. N., P. M. Henson, A. Otani and T. E. Hugli. "Chemotactic Response to Human C3a and C5a Anaphylotoxins. I. Evaluation of C3a and C5a Leukostasis in Vitro and Under Simulated Vivo Conditions." *J. Immunol.*, 120:109–115 (1978).

51 CHENOWETH, D. E. and T. E. Hugli. "Techniques and Significance of C3a and C5a Measurement." in *Further Perspectives in Clinical Laboratory Immunoassays.* R. M. Nakamura ed. New York: Alan R. Liss, 443–59 (1980).

52 WALKER, J. F., R. M. Lindsay, W. J. Sibbard and A. L. Linton. "Acute Pulmonary Hypertension, Leukopenia and Hypoxia in Early Haemodialysis." *Proc. EDTA-ERA*, 21:135–142 (1984).

53 CHEUNG, A. K. and R. L. Baranowski. "The Role of Thromboxane in Pulmonary Hypertension (PHTN) Induced By Cuprophane-Activated Plasma (CAP)." *Abstract Am. Soc. Nephrol.* p. 60A (1984).

54 WALKER, J. F., R. M. Lindsay, W. J. Sibbald, J. W. D. McDonald, G. A. Wells and A. L. Linton. "Thromboxane A2 Mediates Acute Pulmonary Hypertension During Early Haemodialysis in Sheep." (In press).

55 GOLDSTEIR, I. M., C. L. Halmstein, H. Kindahl, H. B. Kaplan, O. Radmark, B. Samuelson and G. Weissman. "Thromboxane Generation by Human Peripheral Blood Polymorphonuclear Leukocytes." *J. Exp. Med.*, 148:787–792 (1978).

56 MORLEY, J., M. A. Bray, R. W. Jones, D. H. Nugteren and D. A. Vandorp. "Prostaglandin and Thromboxane Production by Human and Guinea Pig Macrophages and Leukocytes." *Prostaglandins*, 17:730–736 (1979).

57 POLLEY, M. J., R. L. Nachman and B. B. Weksler. "Human Complement in the Arachidonic Acid Transformation Pathway in Platelets." *J. Exp. Med.*, 153:257–267 (1981).

58 HARTUNG, H. P., D. Bitter-Suermann and U. Hadding. "Induction of Thromboxane Release from Macrophages by Anaphylotoxic Peptide C3a of Complement and Synthetic Hexapeptide C3a." *J. Immunol.*, 130:1345–1349 (1983).

59 SCHULMAN, E. S., H. H. Newball, L. M. Demers, F. A. Fitzpatrick and N. F. Adkinson Jr. "Anaphylactic Release of Thromboxane

A2, Prostaglandin D2 and Prostacyclin from Human Lung Parenchyma." *Am. Rev. Respir. Dis.*, 124:402–406 (1981).

60 McDONALD, J. W. D., M. Ali, E. Morgan, E. R. Townsend and J. D. Cooper. "Thromboxane Synthesis by Sources Other than Platelets in Association with Complement Induced Pulmonary Leukostasis and Pulmonary Hypertension in Sheep." *Circ. Res.*, 52:1–6 (1983).

61 DOLAN, M. J., B. J. Whipp, W. D. Davidson, R. E. Weitzman and K. Wasserman. "Hypopnoea Associated with Acetate Haemodialysis: Carbon Dioxide-Flow-Dependent Ventilation." *N. Engl. J. Med.*, 305:72–75 (1981).

62 DAVIDSON, W. D., M. J. Dolan, B. J. Whipp, R. E. Weitzman and K. Wasserman. "Pathogenesis of Dialysis Induced Hypoxemia." *Artif Organs.*, 6:406–409 (1982).

63 QUEBBEMAN, E. J., W. J. Maierhofer and W. F. Pering. "Mechanisms Producing Hypoxemia During Haemodialysis." *Crit Care Med.*, 12:359–363 (1984).

64 HAKIM, R. M. and E. G. Lowrie. "The Relative Effect of Leukopenia and Dialysate Composition on the Dialysis-Associated Hypoxemia." *Proc. Dial, Transplant Forum*, 10:190–195 (1980).

65 DEBACKER, W. A., G. N. Verpooten, D. I. Borgonjon, P. A. Vermeire, R. R. Lins and H. E. DeRose. "Hypoxemia During Haemodialysis: Effects of Different Membranes and Dialysate Compositions." *Kidney Int.*, 23:738–743 (1983).

66 SIROIS, P., P. Borgeat, A. Jeanson, A. Roy and G. Girard. "The Action of Leukotriene B4 (LTB4) on the Lung." *Prostaglandin Med.*, 5:429–444 (1980).

67 BERGSTROM, J., A. Danielsson and U. Freyschuss. "Dialysis, Ultra-Filtration and Sham-Dialysis in Normal Subjects." (Abstracts) *Am. Soc. Nephrol.*, p. 59A (1984).

68 ENIA, G., C. Catalona, F. Pizzarelli, G. Creazzo, F. Zaccuri, A. Mundo, D. Iellamo and Q. Maguiore. "The Effect of Dialysate Temperature on Haemodialysis Leukopenia." *Proc. EDTA-ERA*, 21:167–171 (1984).

CHAPTER 16

Bioactive Ceramic Coatings for Orthopaedic and Dental Implant Applications

STEPHEN D. COOK, Ph.D.,[1] KEVIN A. THOMAS, Ph.D.,[1] and MARK R. BRINKER, M.D.[1]

ABSTRACT: Calcium phosphate ceramic coatings may be useful for promoting biological fixation of orthopaedic and dental implants. These materials are nontoxic, biocompatible and capable of direct bonding with bone as a result of their chemical similarity with bone mineral. The hydroxylapatite (HA) type of calcium phosphate coatings on metal implants have been shown to develop five to eight times the interface shear strength of identical uncoated metal surfaces. In addition, these coatings have been shown to support additional and earlier apposition of mineralized bone. With judicious use, calcium phosphate coating offers great promise in improving implant fixation.

INTRODUCTION

Orthopaedic and dental implants intended for biological fixation via tissue ingrowth or ongrowth have gained widespread popularity, resulting from advances in implant engineering, materials science, surgical technique and instrumentation.

Implant stabilization by bone growth into a microtextured (porous-coated) surface or by bone apposition to a macrotextured surface is generally considered feasible so long as certain criteria are met:

(1) The prosthetic material must be biocompatible.
(2) There must be no movement at the bone–implant interface.
(3) For porous-coated implants, the porous lattice must be of appropriate pore size and configuration [1–5].

DISCUSSION

Factors which tend to enhance the early biological response and bone–implant attachment (bone ingrowth or apposition) may increase the likelihood of biological stability and long-term success. In addition to implant design and material composition, meticulous site preparation and accurate fit between the implant and bone surfaces may be important factors for implant longevity and function [6,7]. An initial period with partial or no load bearing to minimize motion at the implant–bone interface appears to be important for clinical success [2,3,7–9].

Fixation via polymethylmethacrylate (PMMA) bone cement has been shown to loosen over time. Aseptic loosening rates for femoral hip components have been reported as approximately 20% two to seven years postoperatively and as high as 30–40% at ten year follow-up [10–13]. At least one study, however, has reported a loosening rate of 1.7% at 5 year follow-up in femoral components, where a medullary plug cementing technique was employed [14]. Cement fixation of a femoral component has the advantage over biologically fixed components of immediate postoperative stability. Long-term stable fixation is of particular concern because loosening results in the need for surgical revision. This is particularly important in younger patients who may require multiple surgical revisions over the course of their lives.

Porous-coated orthopaedic prostheses have proven to be a useful alternative to PMMA cement fixation. Revision of a noncemented component offers the advantage (over revision of a cemented component) of more bone stock available for stable fixation, regardless of the age of the patient. Short-term clinical studies indicate that results of noncemented, porous-coated hip implants are comparable to cemented prostheses [15]. Short-term findings of porous-coated knee prosthesis have shown similar results [16,17]. A further advantage of porous-coated implants is the enhancement of the implant–cement interface in cases where the surgeon chooses to use cement fixation with these type implants [18]. Disadvantages of porous-coated implants include more demanding surgical technique to

[1]Tulane University School of Medicine, Department of Orthopaedic Research, 1430 Tulane Avenue, New Orleans, Louisiana 70112, U.S.A.

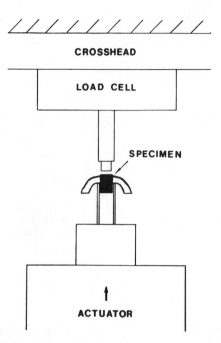

Figure 1. *Schematic representation of a specimen in the push-out test fixture.*

provide a precise fit of the prosthesis, and an initial non-weight-bearing period to minimize movement of the prosthesis while ingrowth occurs. Additionally, there is no immediate fixation of the prosthesis as there is with cement fixation. There is the added concern that the manufacturing techniques used to produce some porous implants may weaken the materials' resistance to fatigue. Cook et al. [19] have demonstrated the notch effect in porous-coated titanium devices. Also, metallic ion release may be potentiated as a result of increased surface area of porous-coated implants [19–23].

Anatomic constraints of structures involved in endosseous dental implants have precluded the use of bone cement. Here, too, biological fixation via bone apposition or ingrowth has enjoyed recent interest as a result of advances in implant materials, design and placement technique. The work of Brånemark and co-workers has demonstrated that endosseous dental implants are a useful treatment modality in the edentulous (or partially edentulous) patient [24]. In addition to specific implant design and material selection, meticulous site preparation and

proper implant placement are crucial for long-term stability and function with this particular implant [25]. Proper implant fit, followed by a two-stage placement procedure is of essential importance. The implant is positioned unloaded for a number of months before the functioning prosthesis is introduced.

Reports of histologic studies of retrieved porous-coated hip and knee prostheses have not been as encouraging as the short-term clinical follow-ups [26–31]. The majority of the porous material available for ingrowth has typically been filled with fibrous tissue, with or without a small percentage of bone. A fibrous tissue interface is not considered favorable for long-term fixation. Quite often, a fibrous membrane has separated the implant from the adjacent bone. In no case has extensive bony ingrowth, typical of that seen in animal studies, been observed in clinically retrieved implants. The effects of a fibrous interface on implant fixation remain obscure. Much interest in recent years has focused on methods to encourage bone ingrowth for long-term stable fixation.

Titanium and Ti–6A1–4V alloy are particularly attractive for use in orthopaedic and dental implants due to their light weight, resistance to corrosion, superior strength, and relatively low modulus of elasticity [21,32,33]. A number of titanium, porous-coated and macrotextured orthopaedic hip and knee prostheses, as well as dental implants, are currently in use.

Calcium phosphate ceramics may be useful in biological implants in that they are nontoxic, biocompatible, and capable of direct bonding with bone as a result of their chemical similarity with bone mineral [34–39]. The synthetic hydroxyapatite (HA) form of calcium phosphate is much like the apatitic bone mineral of vertebrate hard tissue which accounts for 60–70% of bone and 98% of dental enamel [34,40–42]. In appropriate forms, syn-

TABLE 2. Interface Shear Strength (MPa) Transcortical Macrotextured Implants

Weeks	HA-Coated Titanium Alloy	Uncoated CP Titanium
5	9.56	4.88
10	14.17	10.53
32	12.12	—

Taken from Thomas et al. [46].

TABLE 1. Interface Shear Strengths (MPa) of Transcortical Implants

Weeks	HA-Coated Titanium Alloy	Uncoated CP Titanium
5	6.96	0.93
10	7.27	0.98
32	6.07	1.21

Taken from Cook et al. [43].

TABLE 3. Transcortical Porous-Coated Implants

Weeks	HA-Coated Porous Titanium Alloy	Uncoated Porous CP Titanium
3	7.52	7.75
6	14.19	12.60
12	17.92	18.15

Taken from Cook et al. [44].

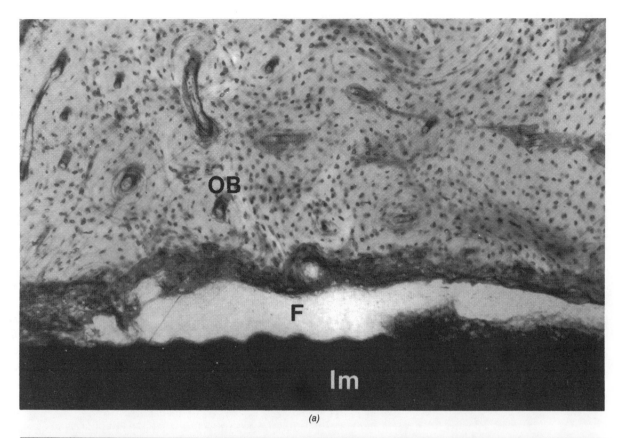

(a)

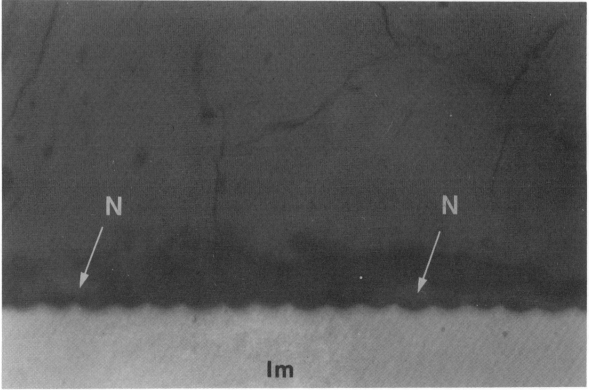

(b)

Figure 2. *Histologic section (a) and microradiograph (b) of the tissue–implant interface at five weeks implantation for bead-blasted CP titanium. Some areas of bone bridging to the implant surface are demonstrated, but mostly fibrous tissue is present at the interface. Im = implant; OB = original cortical bone; N = new bone; F = fibrous tissue. Magnification: 100×. Histologic section (c) and microradiograph (d) of the tissue–implant interface at five weeks implantation for HA-coated titanium alloy. Mineralization directly onto the implant surface is demonstrated in all areas with no intervening fibrous tissue present. Im = implant; H = hydroxyapatite coating; OB = original cortical bone; N = new bone. Magnification: 100×.*

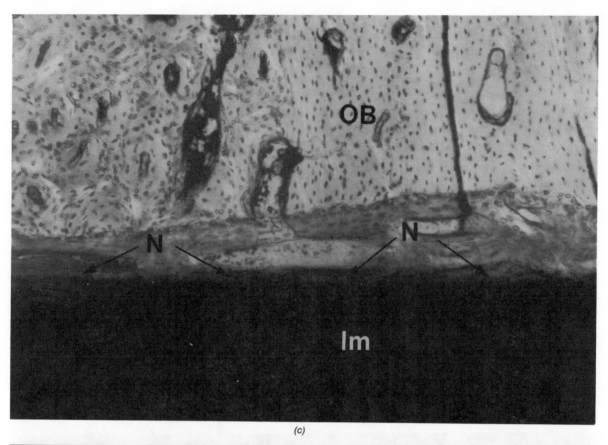

(c)

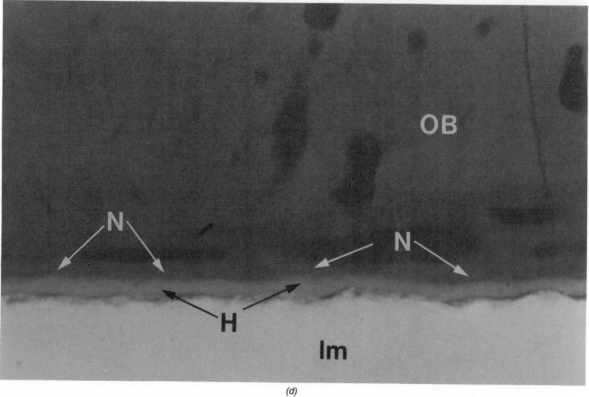

(d)

Figure 2 (continued). *Histologic section (a) and microradiograph (b) of the tissue–implant interface at five weeks implantation for bead-blasted CP titanium. Some areas of bone bridging to the implant surface are demonstrated, but mostly fibrous tissue is present at the interface. Im = implant; OB = original cortical bone; N = new bone; F = fibrous tissue. Magnification: 100×. Histologic section (c) and microradiograph (d) of the tissue-implant interface at five weeks implantation for HA-coated titanium alloy. Mineralization directly onto the implant surface is demonstrated in all areas with no intervening fibrous tissue present. Im = implant; H = hydrox-yapatite coating; OB = original cortical bone; N = new bone. Magnification: 100×.*

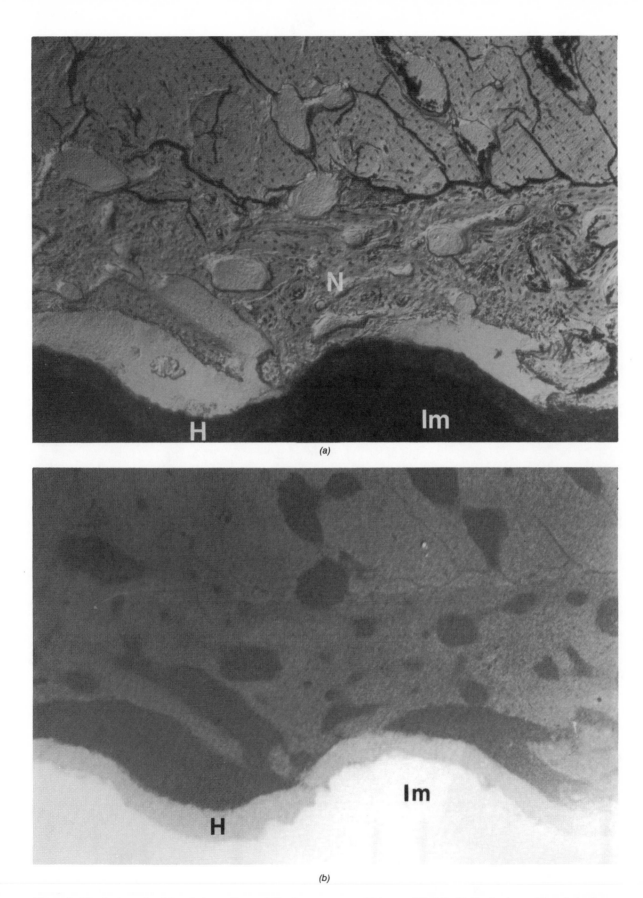

Figure 3. *Histologic section (a) and microradiograph (b) of a macrotextured HA-coated Ti–6Al–4V alloy implant at 32 weeks implantation. Section shown is from a mechanically tested sample demonstrating failure at the implant–HA interface, and minimal disruption of the bone within the recesses of the grooves. There is apparently no disruption at the bone–HA interface; the HA has been sheared off of the crest of the grooves (arrows). Im = implant; H = hydroxyapatite coating. Magnification: 80×.*

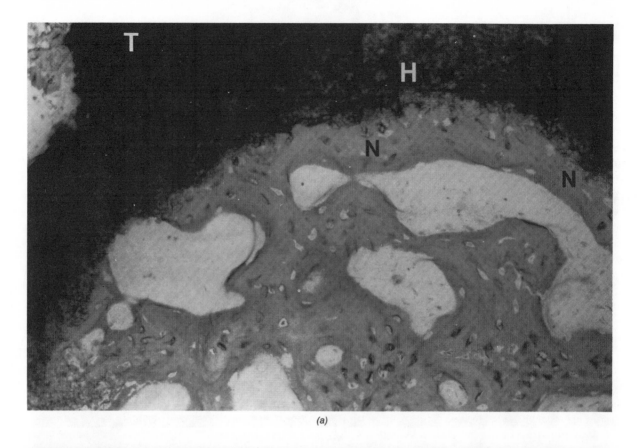

(a)

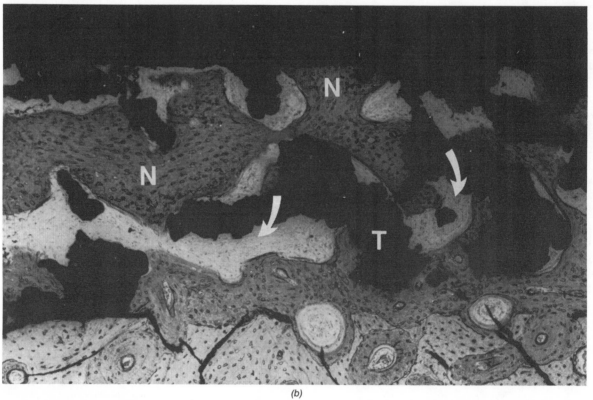

(b)

Figure 4. *Early histologic sections of porous titanium implants with (a) and without (b) HA coating. Figure 5(a) (HA-coated porous implant) demonstrates mineralization of the ingrowth bone within the porous structure directly onto the HA material. Magnification: 175×. Figure 5(b) (noncoated porous implant) demonstrates lack of extensive apposition of ingrowth bone to the titanium particles and the presence of an interposed fibrous layer (arrows). Magnification: 125×. H = hydroxylapatite coating; N = new bone, T = particle of titanium porous structure.*

thetic HA is not resorbed and is suitable for long-term clinical application in implants.

In recent years, our interest in HA-coated implants has focused on mechanical and histological testing in a transcortical implant model. Intact fresh long bone is retrieved and sectioned transversely at the implant site. Samples are tested for interface failure on a closed-loop hydraulic machine (i.e., MTS Systems, Inc.) (Figure 1). Interface shear strength may be calculated by dividing load at failure by bone–implant contact area. While the transcortical model fails to address performance as a function of specific implant design, it is an effective means of evaluating differences in interface shear strength for various materials and surface conditions. While the implants do not carry a physiological load, they are a valuable model for assessing biological fixation in implants that receive protective loading post-operatively.

Hydroxyapatite-coated (Calcitite® HA coating, Calcitek, Inc., San Diego, California) titanium alloy has been shown to develop five to eight times the interface shear strength of uncoated bead blasted (matte finish) CP titanium [43]. The establishment of significant interface strength in HA-coated titanum implants appears to occur rapidly, reaching a maximum at 10 weeks and not diminishing significantly thereafter (Table 1) [43]. The metallic substrate of CP titanium vs. Ti–6Al–4V vs Co–Cr–Mo does not appear to alter mechanical or histologic results in HA-coated implants [44,45]. HA-coated titanium alloy implants have been shown to support early mineralization of interface bone directly into implant surfaces [43]. This is in contrast to uncoated implants, where a thin fibrous interpositional layer limits direct apposition of bone to isolated area (Figure 2).

Surface macrotexture may be useful in preventing hydroxyapatite coating from being sheared off an implant when a load is applied. Push-out testing of HA-coated and uncoated macrotextured surfaces has revealed significantly greater surface shear strength in HA-coated implants at 5 and 10 weeks post-operatively (Table 2). Interface failure occurs at the bone–HA coating interface if tested early (at 5 weeks) [46]. Long-term (at 32 weeks) failure has been shown to occur at the hydroxyapatite– implant interface with minimal disruption of bone within the recesses of the grooves (Figure 3) [46].

Much like macrotextured implants, porous titanium implants coated with HA display mineralization of interface bone directly onto implant surfaces [44] (Figure 4). In porous implants not coated with HA, a fibrous layer has often been observed at the bone–implant interface [44] (Figure 4). A number of investigators have sought to define the role of porous-coated implants and their subsequent coating with HA in the spectrum of devices available.

Cook et al. reported a mean attachment shear strength of 18.7 megapascals (MPa) at 12 weeks implantation for porous-coated Co–Cr–Mo alloy devices [4]. Bobyn et al. reported values of 9.3 MPa at four weeks, and 15.2 MPa at 12 weeks in porous-coated implants [1]. Anderson et al. reported a mean shear strength of 21.9 MPa at 24 weeks in porous-coated titanium implants [47].

Ducheyne et al. [48] studied porous stainless steel intramedullary implants coated with HA and found enhancement in pull-out strength at two and four weeks, but no difference at 12 weeks. The enhanced shear strength seen by Ducheyne et al. may be explained by the increased biocompatibility of HA-coated, as opposed to noncoated, porous stainless steel. Additionally, differences for available pore size may be a factor when the thickness of HA coating is not accounted for. Rivero et al. [49] studied HA-coated fiber metal intramedullary components and found a significantly augmented attachment strength at only the four week interval. Samples tested at one, two and six weeks after implantation were found to exhibit no enhanced shear strength over uncoated samples. Finally, Cook et al. [44] found no enhancement in interface shear strength or rate of bone attachment by treating porous-coated implants with HA (Table 3).

HA coating in porous implants appears to offer no long-term advantage over uncoated porous implants. Furthermore, nearly equivalent fixation to porous devices can be achieved with macrotextured HA-coated implants. Macrotextured devices offer adequate fixation without the disadvantages of porous-coated implants: decreased resistance to fatigue, the notch effect, and metallic ion release.

CONCLUSIONS

(1) The use of hydroxyapatite coating in orthopaedic and dental implants may significantly augment biological fixation, imparting a chemical bonding to the surrounding tissue.

(2) HA coating appears to enhance the rate of attachment at the bone–implant interface in macrotextured and bead-blasted implants, but not in porous implants.

(3) The addition of HA coating appears to significantly improve shear strength in macrotextured and bead-blasted titanium implants, but not in porous implants.

(4) Histologic sections demonstrate direct mineralization of bone onto HA-coated implant surfaces with no interpositional fibrous tissue layer.

(5) Protection of HA coating is possible by surface macrotexture and microtexture and may be important in preventing HA coating from being pulled off components by physiologic loading.

REFERENCES

1 BOBYN, J. D., R. M. Pilliar, H. U. Cameron and G. C. Weatherly. "The Optimum Pore Size for the Fixation of Porous Surfaced Metal Implants by the Ingrowth of Bone," *Clin. Orthop.*, 150:263 (1980).

2 CAMERON, H. U., R. M. Pilliar and I. Macnab. "The Effect of Movement of the Bonding of Porous Metal to Bone," *J. Biomed. Mater. Res.*, 7:301 (1973).

3 CHANDLER, H. P.: "Postoperative Management and Follow-up Evaluation," in *Total Knee Arthroplasty: A Comprehensive Approach.* D. S. Hungerford, K. A. Krackow, and R. V. Kenna, eds. Baltimore: Williams & Wilkins, pp. 110–125 (1984).

4 COOK, S. D., K. A. Walsh and R. J. Haddad. "Interface Mechanics and Bone Growth into Porous Co-Cr-Mo Alloy Implants." *Clin. Orthop.*, 193:271 (1985).

5 HARRIS, W. H. and M. Jasty. "Bone Ingrowth Into Porous Coated Canine Acetabular Replacements: The Effect of Pore Size, Apposition and Dislocation," in *The Hip. Proceedings of the Thirteenth Open Scientific Meeting of The Hip Society.* St. Louis:C. V. Mosby, p. 214 (1985).

6 ENGH, C. A., J. D. Bobyn and A. H. Glassman. "Porous-coated Hip Replacement: The Factors Governing Bone Ingrowth, Stress Shielding, and Clinical Results." *J. Bone Joint Surg.*, 69B:45 (1987).

7 DUCHEYNE, P., P. DeMeester and E. Aernoudt. "Influence of a Functional Dynamic Loading on Bone Ingrowth into Surface Pores of Orthopedic Implants." *J. Biomed. Mater. Res.*, 11:811 (1977).

8 GALANTE, J. O. and D. P. Rivero. "The Biological Basis for Bone Ingrowth in Titanium Fiber Composites," in *Advanced Concepts in Total Hip Replacement.* W. H. Harris, ed. Thorofare, NJ: Slack, Inc., pp. 135–158 (1985).

9 HARRIS, W. H. "The Porous Total Hip Replacement System: Surgical Technique," in *Advanced Concepts in Total Hip Replacement.* W. H. Harris, ed. Thorofare, NJ: Slack, Inc., pp. 209–253 (1985).

10 AMSTUTZ, H. C., K. L. Marklof, G. M. McNeice and T. A. Gruen. "Loosening of Total Hip Components: Cause and Prevention," in *The Hip: Proceedings of the Fourth Open Scientific Meeting of The Hip Society.* St. Louis:C. V. Mosby, p. 102 (1976).

11 BECKENBAUGH, R. D. and D. M. Illstrup. "Total Hip Arthroplasty: A Review of Three Hundred and Thirty-Three Cases with Long-Term Follow-Up." *J. Bone Joint Surg.*, 60A:306 (1978).

12 STAUFFER, R. N. "Ten-year Follow-up Study of Total Hip Replacement, With Particular Reference to Roentgenographic Loosening of the Components. *J. Bone Joint Surg.*, 64A:983 (1982).

13 SUTHERLAND, C. J., A. H. Wilde, L. S. Borden and K. E. Marks. "A Ten-Year Follow-Up of One Hundred Consecutive Müller Curved-Stem Total Hip-Replacement Arthroplasties." *J. Bone Joint Surg.*, 64A:970 (1982).

14 HARRIS, W. H. and W. A. McGann. "Loosening of the Femoral Component After Use of the Medullary-Plug Cementing Technique." *J. Bone Joint Surg.*, 68A:1064 (1986).

15 ENGH, C. A. "Hip Arthroplasty With a Moore Prosthesis with Porous Coating: A Five-Year Study." *Clin. Orthop.*, 176:52 (1983).

16 HUNGERFORD, D. S. and K. A. Krackow. "Total Joint Arthroplasty of the Knee." *Clin. Orthop.*, 192:23 (1985).

17 LANDON, G. C., J. O. Galante and M. M. Maley. "Noncemented Total Knee Arthroplasty." *Clin. Orthop.*, 205:49 (1986).

18 COOK, S. D., N. Thongpreda, R. C. Anderson, K. A. Thomas, R. J. Haddad, C. D. Griffin. "Optimum Pore Size for Bone Cement Fixation." *Clin. Orthop.*, 223:296 (1987).

19 COOK, S. D., F. S. Georgette, H. B. Skinner and R. J. Haddad. "Fatigue Properties of Carbon- and Porous-Coated Ti-6A1-4V Alloy." *J. Biomed. Mater. Res.*, 18:497 (1984).

20 GEORGETTE, F. S. and J. A. Davidson. "The Effect of HIPing on the Fatigue and Tensile Strength of a Cast, Porous-Coated Co-Cr-Mo Alloy." *J. Biomed. Mater. Res.*, 20:1229 (1986).

21 WOODMAN, J. L., J. J. Jacobs, J. O. Galante and R. M. Urban. "Metal Ion Release from Titanium-Based Prosthetic Segmental Replacements of Long Bones in Baboons: A Long-Term Study." *J. Orthop. Res.*, 1:421 (1984).

22 MEMOLI, V. A., R. M. Urban, J. Alroy and J. O. Galante. "Malignant Neoplasms Associated with Orthopaedic Implant Materials in Rats." *J. Orthopaedic Research*, 4:346–355 (1986).

23 BUNDY, K. J., R. Luedemann. "Factors Which Influence the Accuracy of Corrosion Rate Determination on Implant Materials," in *Biomedical Engineering V: Recent Developments.* S. Saha, ed. Pergammon Press: New York (1986).

24 ADELL, R., U. Lekholm, B. Rockler and P.-I. Brånemark. "A 15 Year Study of Osseointegrated Implants in the Treatment of the Edentulous Jaw." *Int. J. Oral Surg.*, 10:387 (1981).

25 BRÅNEMARK, P.-I., B. O. Hansson, R. Adell, U. Breine, J. Lindstrom, O. Hallen, and A. Ohman. "Osseointegrated Implants in the Treatment of the Endentulous Jaw: Experience from a 10-Year Period." *Scand. J. Plast. Reconstr. Surg.*, [Suppl.] 16:1 (1977).

26 BOBYN, J. D. and C. A. Engh. "Human Histology of the Bone-Porous Metal Implant Interface." *Orthopedics*, 7:1410 (1984).

27 CAMERON, H. U. "Six Year Results With a Microporous-Coated Metal Hip Prosthesis." *Clin. Orthop.*, 208:81 (1986).

28 COLLIER, J. P., M. B. Mayor, C. O. Townley, J. B. Fening and F. F. Buechel. "Histology of Retrieved Porous-Coated Knee Prosthesis." *Abstracts, 53rd Annual Meeting, American Academy of Orthopaedic Surgeons*, New Orleans, LA, February, p. 41 (1986).

29 COOK, S. D., A. D. Scheller, R. C. Anderson and R. J. Haddad. "Histologic and Microradiographic Analysis of a Revised Porous Coated Anatomic (PCA) Patellar Component: A Case Report." *Clin. Orthop.*, 202:147 (1986).

30 HADDAD, R. J., S. D. Cook, K. A. Thomas, R. C. Anderson and J. O. Edmunds. "Histologic and Microradiographic Analysis of Noncemented Retrieved PCA Knee Components." *Abstracts, 53rd Annual Meeting, American Academy of Orthopaedic Surgeons*, New Orleans, LA, February, p. 41 (1986).

31 THOMAS, K. A., S. D. Cook, R. J. Haddad and K. L. Thomas. "Histologic Analysis of Tissue Growth into Retrieved Human Total Joint Components" in *Transactions, 33rd Annual Meeting, Orthopaedic Research Society*, 12:432 (1987).

32 LEMONS, J. E., M. W. Wiemann and A. B. Weiss. "Biocompatibility Studies on Surgical Grade Titanium, Cobalt and Iron-Based Alloys." *J. Biomed. Mater. Res.*, 7:549 (1976).

33 MEARS, D. C. *Materials and Orthopedic Surgery.* Baltimore:Williams & Wilkins (1979).

34 JARCHO, M. "Calcium Phosphate Ceramics as Hard Tissue Prosthetics." *Clin. Orthop.*, 157:259 (1981).

35 JARCHO, M. "Biomaterial Aspects of Calcium Phosphates: Properties and Applications." *Dent. Clin. North Am.*, 30:25 (1986).

36 JARCHO, M., J. F. Kay, K. I. Gaumaer, R. H. Doremus and H. P. Drobeck. "Tissue, Cellular, and Subcellular Events at a Bone Ceramic Hydroxyapatite Interface." *J. Bioeng.*, 1:79 (1977).

37 KAY, J. F., M. Jarcho, G. Logan and S. T. Liu. "The Structure and Properties of Hydroxyapatite Coatings on Metal." *Trans 12th Annual Meeting of the Society for Biomaterials*, Minneapolis, 9:13 (1986).

38 OGISO, M., S. Aikawa, T. Tabata and M. Inoue. "2-Step Apatite

Implant; Animal Experiment and Clinical Application" in *Trans 11th Annual Meeting Society for Biomaterials*, San Diego, 8:166 (1985).

39 TRACY, B. M. and R. H. Doremus. "Direct Electron Microscopy Studies of the Bone-Hydroxyapatite Interface." *J. Biomed. Mater. Res.*, 18:719 (1984).

40 ENGSTROM, A. "Aspects of the Molecular Structure of Bone" in *The Biochemistry and Physiology of Bone*, G. H. Bourne, ed. Vol. 1, ed. 2. New York: Academic Press, pp. 237–257 (1972).

41 HAM, A. W. and D. H. Cormack. Histology, ed. 8. Philadelphia: J. B. Lippincott, p. 399 (1979).

42 NEUMAN, W. F. "Bone Mineral and Calcification Mechanisms" in *Fundamental and Clinical Bone Physiology*, M. R. Urist, ed. Philadelphia: J. B. Lippincott, pp. 83–107 (1980).

43 COOK, S. D., J. F. Kay, K. A. Thomas and M. Jarcho. "Interface Mechanics and Histology of Titanium and Hydroxyapatite-Coated Titanium for Dental Implant Applications," *International Journal of Oral and Maxillofacial Implants,* 2:15 (1987).

44 COOK, S. D., K. A. Thomas, J. F. Kay and M. Jarcho. "Hydroxyapatite-coated Porous Titanium for Use as an Orthopedic Biologic Attachment System." *Clin. Orthop.*, 230:303 (1988).

45 COOK, S. D., K. A. Thomas, J. F. Kay and M. Jarcho. "Hydroxyapatite-coated Titanium for Orthopaedic Implant Applications." *Clin. Orthop.*, 232:225 (1988).

46 THOMAS, K. A., J. F. Kay, S. D. Cook and M. Jarcho. "The Effect of Surface Macrotexture and Hydroxyapatite Coating on the Mechanical Strengths and Histologic Profiles of Titanium Implant Materials." *J. Biomed. Mater. Res.*, 21:1395 (1987).

47 ANDERSON, R. C., S. D. Cook, A. M. Weinstein and R. J. Haddad. "An Evaluation of Skeletal Attachment to LTI Pyrolytic Carbon, Porous Titanium, and Carbon-Coated Porous Titanium Implants," *Clin. Orthop.*, 182:242 (1984).

48 DUCHEYNE, P., L. L. Hench, A. Kagan, M. Martens, A. Bursens and J. D. Mulier: "Effect of Hydroxyapatite Impregnation on Skeletal Bonding of Porous Coated Implants." *J. Biomed. Mater. Res.*, 14:225 (1980).

49 RIVERO, D. P., J. Fox, A. K. Skipor, R. M. Urban and J. O. Galante. "Calcium Phosphate-Coated Porous Titanium Implants for Enhanced Skeletal Fixation." *J. Biomed. Mater. Res.*, 22:191 (1988).

CHAPTER 17

Ceramic–Polyfunctional Carboxylic Acid Composites for Reconstructive Surgery of Hard Tissues

PRAPHULLA K. BAJPAI, Ph.D.[1]

ABSTRACT: Various types of composites and bone cements containing ceramic and, usually, polymeric materials have been developed for repairing bone defects. However, most of the polymeric materials used in these composites do not degrade in the host. A relatively quick-setting composite, consisting of a biodegradable setting agent and either a resorbable or a relatively nonresorbable ceramic would be ideal for replacing bone lost as a result of trauma or disease. Thus, a variety of biodegradable setting agents were tested with alumino calcium phosphorous oxide (ALCAP), hydroxyapatite, Ossoegraft (anorganic bone), tricalcium phosphate, or zinc calcium phosphorous oxide ceramics.

Both alpha-ketoglutaric and malic acids formed good composites with all the calcium phosphate based ceramic materials including: alumino calcium phosphorous oxide (ALCAP), Biorad hydroxyapatite (BHA), HA–1000 hydroxyapatite (HA), Osseograft (OG), tricalcium phosphate (TCP) and zinc calcium phosphorous oxide (ZCAP). By varying the acids and/or combining two different acids, setting times from 30 seconds to 10 minutes were achieved for hard-setting ceramic and polyfunctional carboxylic acid composites. Incorporation of calcium hydroxide in ceramic and polyfunctional carboxylic acid composites neutralized the acidity of the composites and made them alkaline. Implantation of most of these composites in animals successfully repaired experimentally traumatized bone. Addition of vitamin E succinate to the alkaline composites of TCP and malic acid delayed the resorbability of implanted composites in rats. Zinc sulfate containing zinc calcium phosphorous oxide ceramics (ZSCAP) provided a resorbable material which like Plaster of Paris® can set and harden on addition of deionized–distilled water.

INTRODUCTION

So far, modern technology has not been able to provide a bone substitute which equals or surpasses autogenous bone. However, autogenous bone cannot always be obtained in adequate quantities to repair severe bone trauma or large defects caused by various bone diseases. Complications associated with second surgery also act as a deterrent for generalized use of autogenous bone. In recent years, several calcium phosphate based synthetic ceramic particles, powders, and blocks have been used as fillers in oral and orthopaedic surgery. These materials include ceramics and glasses such as hydroxyapatite (HA), tricalcium phosphate (TCP), alumino calcium phosphorous oxide (ALCAP) and bioglass [1–9]. Of these materials, hydroxyapatite particles or powders have been used most extensively to correct oral and maxillofacial defects [3,5]. However, the ceramic particles have a tendency to migrate from the surgical site [3–5]. Thus, immobilization of these synthetic, particulate, bone-rebuilding materials is a major concern for both oral and orthopaedic surgeries [10–22].

Several approaches have been taken to achieve immobilization of both hydroxyapatite and tricalcium phosphate ceramic particles. These approaches involve preparation of composites of ceramic particles with inorganic salts, organic monomers, or polymers. However, an all-purpose composite for replacing defective, diseased, or traumatized hard tissue has not yet been developed.

GENERAL PROCEDURES

Alumino calcium phosphorous oxide (ALCAP) ceramic particles were prepared by routine procedures used in my laboratory [1,4,11–15]. Tricalcium phosphate was prepared by routine aqueous precipitation procedures [10,23,24]. Both zinc calcium phosphorous oxide (ZCAP) and zinc sulfate containing ZCAP (ZSCAP) ceramic particles were prepared by the procedures used in our laboratories [21,25–27]. Alumino calcium phosphorus oxide (ALCAP), tricalcium phosphate (TCP), Biorad hydroxy-

[1]Department of Biology, University of Dayton, Dayton, Ohio 45469, U.S.A.

apatite (Biorad Laboratories, Inc., Richmond, CA), Osseograft (reclaimed hydroxyapatite-rich bone meal from commercial bone flour), and HA-1000 hydroxyapatite (Orthomatrix, Inc., Dublin, CA) were each combined with ten different setting materials: orthophosphoric, lactic, citric, pyruvic, succinic, alpha-ketoglutaric, malic, fumaric and oxaloacetic acids, and water. ALCAP and TCP were also combined with bovine serum albumin, Carbopol®, polyvinyl pyrrolidone, or Hespan®. Because initial studies were conducted with ALCAP, we also combined ALCAP with fructose, dextrose, sesame seed oil, or rat blood. ZCAP ceramics were tested last, and only alpha-ketoglutaric or malic acid were used as setting agents. The particle size for all ceramic powders ranged from 10 to 400 um. However, in most trials, the size of the ceramic particles was 10–38 um.

Viscosity

Maximum viscosity of each mixture of ALCAP, Biorad hydroxyapatite (BHA), HA-1000 hydroxyapatite (HA), Osseograft (OG), or TCP and setting material in a water medium was estimated by observing the consistency of the mixture. Ratios of hydroxyapatite and various solutions or powders were varied to obtain maximum viscosities. Upon mixing acids with ceramic particles, care was taken to note if exothermic reactions were present, since initial experiments conducted with ALCAP and orthophosphoric acid generated substantial amounts of heat [10,13, 15,17].

Setting Hardness

For determining set time and set hardness, triplicates of one-gram samples of calcined ceramic particulate powders were mixed with either solutions or powders of the various test materials by means of a spatula in deep-well glass slides. Deionized–distilled water was added to each solid mixture to initiate the setting reactions. Gel time was monitored at 30-second intervals. Setting hardness was evaluated on a scale from zero to ten at 15-minute intervals. Nonsetting powder consistency was scored as 0, paste-like consistency as 3 and plaster-like consistency was scored as 10. Calcined zinc sulfate containing ZCAP particles (ZSCAP) was tested as such, in a similar manner by addition of deionized–distilled water [21]. All observations were made by the same technician and all triplicates had a similar rating. Thus, the standard deviations for all setting hardness values were zero.

pH Studies

Since ceramic–polyfunctional acid composites lowered the pH of neutralized saline, it was considered necessary to conduct pH studies with composites of ceramic and polyfunctional carboxylic acids [11,21,22]. Composite powders (200 mg) of TCP or ZCAP ceramic particles (10–35 μm) and alpha-ketoglutaric acid or malic acid, were placed in a dialysis bag, and the sealed bag was suspended in 50.0 ml of 0.9% saline (neutralized to a pH of 7.0) in a serum bottle. Each bottle was sealed, using teflon-coated septa, with the aid of a crimper. Triplicates of TCP or ZCAP and each composite in saline were incubated in an oscillating, deionized–distilled water bath at 37°C. The pH of saline was monitored by means of a digital pH meter at 1, 24, and 48 hours for TCP composites, and at 24 hours for ZCAP composites.

Scanning Electron Microscopy

Scanning electron micrographs of polyfunctional carboxylic acid composites, with or without calcium hydroxide, were taken after the composites had set and hardened. Mixtures of ceramic–polyfunctional acid, calcium hydroxide (250 mg), with or without DHCC or vitamin E succinate, and deionized–distilled water (40–100 μl) were set in a tuberculin syringe, squeezed out onto a glass plate in a cylindrical form, and allowed to harden overnight. These composites were then fractured by hand into two pieces and the best piece was mounted on an aluminum stub with the fractured surface up. The samples were sputter-coated with palladium in an Effa vacuum evaporator equipped with a sputtering head (E. F. Fullam, Inc., Latham, NY). Photographs of the mounted fractured surface were taken in the center of the specimen with a scanning electron microscope (Model 1000B, Amray, Inc., Bedford, MA) at 10 KV.

COMPOSITES

Bone is a composite of mineral apatite, salts and organic materials [23]. The success of both resorbable and nonresorbable synthetic calcium phosphate ceramics as bone scaffolds has had a tremendous impact in the area of oral and maxillofacial surgeries. However, ceramics, as such, are brittle and difficult to handle in particulate forms [3,5]. In order to prevent the migration of ceramic particles and overcome the brittleness of the ceramics, several investigators have attempted to develop composites of calcium phosphate ceramics and organic monomers or polymers including collagen [4,29–36]. Composites of some calcium phosphate ceramics and Plaster of Paris® are currently in clinical trials [37–39]. However, rapid resorption of the calcium sulfate phase in these composites may create problems in the future, when these composites are used in larger quantities in orthopaedic surgeries. According to Williams, development of a ceramic powder system which sets and hardens like gypsum may be of interest [40]. This narrative, in particular, reviews the development and uses of composites of calcium phosphate ceramics and agents which set in an aqueous environment [10,13,15–19].

Alumino Calcium Phosphorous Oxide Ceramics (ALCAP's)

In 1969, we reported the development of resorbable ceramics for future applications [9,41,42]. Two decades later, resorbable (redundant) ceramics seem to be the materials of choice for reconstructing hard tissues, since these synthetic materials are eventually replaced by endogenous bone. Eventually, we developed ALCAP ceramics and, by using an array of different procedures and tests, concluded that these biocompatible and biodegradable ceramics would be ideal for correcting various kinds of bone defects [41–59]. Although particulate forms of ALCAP have not been used extensively to repair bone, porous and resorbable blocks of ALCAP have been used to correct experimentally induced trauma in hard tissues of rats, rabbits, and nonhuman primates [1,8,45–47, 49–51,53–55]. However, ALCAP has had limited clinical use for correcting cleft palate defects and spinal fusion [5,8].

Nonresorbable cements composed of calcium fluoroaluminosilicate or calcium depleted aluminofluorosilicate glass powders, and polymers of polycarboxylic acids have been used as bandages and splints for joining two bones, and for attaching a device to bone [60,61]. However, these cements are nonporous and cannot be replaced by endogenous bone. ALCAP ceramics are nontoxic, biocompatible, nonmutagenic, and resorbable [1,8,9]. Use of fast setting ALCAP particulates in the form of composites could provide a slowly degradable synthetic material for repairing diseased or traumatized bones.

Viscosity of ALCAP Composites

A ratio of 7:4 was needed to attain maximum viscosity in composites of ALCAP combined with the following setting materials: bovine serum albumin (6%), dextrose (5M), fructose (5M), Hespan® (6%), lactic acid (85%), polyvinyl pyrrolidone (20%) and deionized–distilled water. Composites of ALCAP and fumaric or oxaloacetic acids in a ratio of 4:1 attained maximum viscosity on addition of deionized–distilled water. Maximum viscosity was attained with a 1:1 mixture of ALCAP with either sesame oil or Carbopol®. ALCAP ceramic particles, when mixed in a ratio of 5:4 with 10% orthophosphoric acid, also attained maximum viscosity. A 2:1 ratio was required to achieve maximum viscosity of ALCAP with alpha-ketoglutaric, citric, malic, pyruvic, or succinic acid powders, on addition of deionized–distilled water. If maximum viscosity was the only criterion for developing a bone composite, a toothpaste-like mixture could be produced by varying the ratio of ALCAP and the above setting agents.

Setting Hardness of ALCAP Composites

The setting hardness of ALCAP and deionized–distilled water (controls), and composites of ALCAP and rat blood, bovine serum albumin, Carbopol®, dextrose, fructose, Hespan®, polyvinyl pyrrolidone or orthophosphoric acid are shown in Table 1. The hardness profiles of composites of ALCAP and alpha-ketoglutaric, fumaric, malic, or oxaloacetic acids, after addition of deionized–distilled water to each gram of composite, are shown in Figure 1. The setting hardness of composites of ALCAP–ketoglutaric acid and citric acid are shown in Figure 2.

Composites of ALCAP and fumaric acid set almost instantaneously on addition of deionized–distilled water (0.4 ml/g). Composites of ALCAP and alpha-ketoglutaric acid set within 30 seconds on addition of deionized–distilled water (0.6 ml/g). However, by mixing different proportions of citric acid and alpha-ketoglutaric acid with ALCAP, setting times of three and five minutes were achieved on addition of deionized–distilled water (0.3 ml/g). Composites of ALCAP and malic acid took eight minutes to set, on addition of deionized–distilled water (0.3 ml/g), and reached maximum hardness within 15 minutes (Figure 1). ALCAP composites of either fumaric acid or alpha-ketoglutaric acid reached a maximum hardness of 10 within 45 minutes (Figure 1). By the end of the 60 minute test period, all other mixtures of ALCAP and setting agents (except orthophosphoric acid) failed to reach the hardness attained by composites consisting of ALCAP and alpha-ketoglutaric, fumaric, or malic acids. ALCAP and oxaloacetic acid composites showed the lowest degree of setting hardness for the entire 60 minutes (Figure 1). Composites of ALCAP and citric acid, lactic acid, pyruvic acid, succinic acid, or sesame oil did not set or harden within 60 minutes.

Examination of texture and brittleness of ALCAP–setting agent mixtures, 24 hours after initiation of the reaction, suggested that alpha-ketoglutaric acid, malic acid,

TABLE 1. Setting Hardness of Calcined ALCAP Ceramic Powder and Setting Agents (Test Material) at 15 Minute Intervals over a Duration of 60 Minutes.

	Time in Minutes			
	15	30	45	60
Setting Agents	Degree of Hardness			
D.D. water (control)	6	7	7	8
Fructose (5M)	2	2	3	3
Dextrose (5M)	2	2	3	3
Bovine serum albumin (6%)	5	6	7	8
Rat blood	3	4	5	6
Carbopol®	4	4	5	5
Polyvinyl pyrrolidone (20%)	3	3	4	5
Hespan® (6%)	4	6	6	7
Orthophosphoric acid (10%)	7	8	9	10

Modified from Bajpai, P. K., C. M. Fuchs and M. A. P. Strnat. Biomed. Engineering IV. Recent Developments, p. 24 (1985).

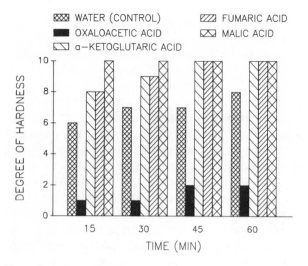

Figure 1. *Setting hardness of composites of calcined alumino calcium phosphorus oxide (ALCAP) particulate (10–38 μm) powder (1 g) and oxaloacetic (0.25 g), fumaric (0.25), alpha-ketoglutaric (0.5 g) or malic (0.5 g) acids on addition of deionized–distilled water (0.3–0.6 ml) over a duration of 60 minutes.*

and combinations of alpha-ketoglutaric and citric acid can be used successfully as bone composites (Figures 1 and 2). However, composites consisting of ALCAP and fumaric acid would be more suitable as powders for filling bleeding bone wounds. On setting to hardness, composites of ALCAP and orthophosphoric acid crumbled under application of the slightest amount of pressure. Thus, the usefulness of this mixture in bone healing applications is questionable. Since alpha-ketoglutaric, citric, fumaric, and malic acids are normal metabolic products of cells, it is likely that composites of ceramics and these acids

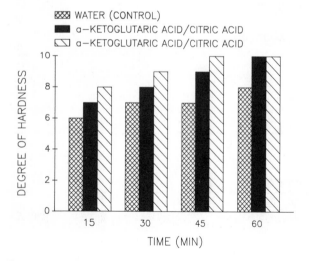

Figure 2. *Setting hardness of composites of calcined alumino calcium phosphorus oxide (ALCAP) particulate (10–38 um) powder (1 g) and alpha-ketoglutaric (0.35 g) and citric acid (0.15 g) or alpha-keto-glutaric (0.40 g) and citric acid (0.10 g) on addition of deionized–distilled water (0.3 ml) over a duration of 60 minutes.*

would not be toxic. However, their acidic properties could cause local irritation on implantation [11]. Thus, neutralization of the acidity of these composites is essential [11].

Strength of ALCAP Composite Plugs

Cylindrical plugs (1.25 cm in diameter) of ALCAP and alpha-ketoglutaric acid or malic acid were prepared by mixing 2.5 g cement with 0.8 ml deionized–distilled water. The compressive strength at failure when tested by a MTS Servo Hydraulic System, was 0.65 ± 0.7 MPa for ALCAP–alpha ketoglutaric acid cylindrical plugs and 1.3 ± 0.1 MPa for ALCAP–malic acid cylindrical plugs.

Scanning Electron Microscopy of ALCAP Composites

Scanning electron photomicrographs of cracked surfaces of hardened composites of ALCAP, alpha-ketoglutaric acid, and calcium hydroxide [Figure 3(a)], or ALCAP, malic acid, and calcium hydroxide, with or without vitamin E succinate [Figures 3(b) and 3(c)], show that these composites have both macro- and micro-pores between aggregates of ceramic particles bound by polyfunctional carboxylic acids [Figures 3(a), 3(b), and 3(c)]. The macropores should encourage ingrowth of new bone and the micropores should assist in the eventual degradation and replacement of the composite by the host's tissues. Vitamin E succinate was used to provide hydrophobicity to the composite and delay its degradation, on implantaton. The SEM of ALCAP, malic acid, calcium hydroxide, and vitamin E succinate shows that inclusion of vitamin E seems to decrease the size of the pores and increase the tightness between the ceramic particles.

Animal Studies on ALCAP Composites

Animal studies conducted to date suggest that surgically induced bone wounds in femur and calvarie of rats can easily be filled with ALCAP–alpha-ketoglutaric acid composites. Initial application of the composite powder to the bone wound acts as a hemostatic agent; the powder sets on reacting with blood. The highest dose of ALCAP–alpha-ketoglutaric acid composite (1 g), used in rats weighing 175 grams each, has not induced toxicity to date. Four weeks after surgery, ingrowth of both peri- and endo-steal trabecular bone was observed in ALCAP–alpha-ketoglutarate composite filled holes in the tibia of rabbits [13,15,19].

Recently, 12 Rhesus monkeys were implanted with composites of ALCAP, malic acid, and calcium hydroxide. Sintered ALCAP ceramic particles of 45–60 μm size were mixed with malic acid in a ratio of 2:1. The ceramic–malic acid mixture was then mixed with calcium hydroxide (15% by weight of the total composite). One-gram plugs of the ceramic, malic acid, and calcium hydroxide composites were obtained by adding 200 μl deionized–distilled water and compressing the composite in a tuberculin syringe. The plug was then extruded from the cut end of the syringe and allowed to harden. The extruded and hardened composites were then scraped with a scalpel blade to yield cylindrical plugs, each measuring 3.5 x 10 mm. Sterile composites were implanted in 3.5 mm holes drilled in the left femur and L-4 vertebra by means of a trephine. The bone wound was then troweled with freshly set sterile composite to insure continuity and a tight fit [59].

Blood was collected from each monkey prior to surgery, after injection of the bone labelling dyes, and at the time of euthanasia. Blood collected from each monkey on each occasion was analyzed for albumin, alkaline and acid phosphatase, aspartate aminotransferase, alanine aminotransferase, blood urea nitrogen (BUN), calcium, carbon dioxide, chlorine, creatine, glucose, globulin, phosphate, potassium, protein (total), sodium, uric acid, white blood cells (total counts), red blood cells, hemoglobin, hematocrit, MCV, MCH, MCHC, neutrophil, lymphocytes, monocytes, eosinophils, and basophils. Radiographs of all 12 monkeys were taken one day after recovery from surgery, and periodically at intervals of 1, 4, and 8 months and at the time of euthanasia [59].

Scanning electron photomicrographs of set and hardened composites, prior to implantation, confirmed the porosity of the hardened composite [Figure 3(b)]. Morphological examination of implantation sites 1, 4 and 8 months after implantation, showed tight apposition of the host tissue with the composites. Radiographs of ALCAP composites *in situ*, one day and 1, 4 and 8 months after implantation, showed that the composites did not induce inflammatory response and provided continuity for ingrowth of endogenous bone. Thus, the data obtained from tissue samples and blood chemistries indicated that ALCAP composites of malic acid and calcium hydroxide are biocompatible, and that the composite did not induce an inflammatory reaction, and provided continuity for ingrowth of bone [59].

Tricalcium Phosphate (TCP)

Plaster of Paris® was probably the first resorbable material used clinically to correct bone defects [5,62]. Tricalcium phosphate (TCP) ceramics are probably the second manmade materials which were approved for clinical trials in the U.S. Initial studies were conducted with TCP slurries [9]. Since these lacked mechanical strength, blocks of TCP were prepared for investigative research [9,63,64]. Since then, particulate, porous, and dense forms of TCP have been used to repair traumatized hard tissues in rats, dogs, and primates [5]. Tricalcium

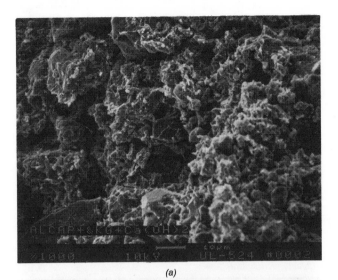

(a)

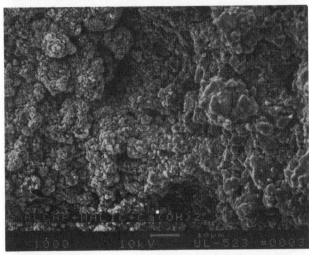

(b)

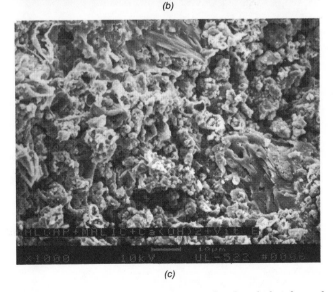

(c)

Figure 3. *Scanning electron photomicrographs of cracked surfaces of composites of alumino calcium phosphorus oxide (ALCAP) and (a) ketoglutaric acid and calcium hydroxide, (b) malic acid and calcium hydroxide, (c) malic acid, calcium hydroxide and vitamine E, after setting to maximum hardness.*

TABLE 2. Amounts of Setting Agent Solutions Required to Obtain Maximum Viscosity with One Gram of Tricalcium Phosphate

Setting Agent	Volume (ml)
D.D. water (control)	0.6
Bovine Serum Albumin (6%)	0.6
Carbopol®	1.0
Hespan® (6%)	0.6
Lactic acid (85%)	0.6
Orthophosphoric acid (10%)	0.8
Polyvinyl pyrrolidone (20%)	0.6

TABLE 3. Weights of Polyfunctional Carboxylic Acid Powders (g) and Amounts of Deionized–Distilled Water Required to Obtain Maximum Viscosity with 1.0 g Tricalcium Phosphate.

Polyfunctional Carboxylic acids	Weight (g)	D.D. Water (ml)
Alpha-ketoglutaric acid	0.50	0.5
Citric acid	1.00	0.3
Fumaric acid	0.25	0.6
Malic acid	0.50	0.4
Oxaloacetic acid	0.25	0.5
Pyruvic acid	0.50	0.6
Succinic acid	1.00	0.7

TABLE 4. Setting Hardness of Relatively Poor Tricalcium Phosphate Composites.

Setting Agent	Time in Minutes			
	15	30	45	60
	Degree of Hardness			
D. D. water (control)	1	2	3	5
Bovine Serum Albumin (6%)	2	2	2	4
Carbopol®	1	1	2	2
Hespan® (6®)	2	3	3	4
Polyvinyl pyrrolidone	2	2	3	3
Citric acid	7	8	8	8
Orthophosphoric Acid*	9	10	10	10

*Hardened composites of TCP and Orthophosphoric acid crumbled on application of pressure.

phosphate has been used clinically to fill periapical and marginal periodontal defects, open apexes, and augment alveolar ridge defects [5]. Currently, TCP is also in clinical trials in orthopaedic surgery.

Since Beta-TCP is a resorbable calcium phosphate (except for dense TCP) it may have limited use in rebuilding bone lost due to resorption. Thus, in contrast to development of composites containing hydroxyapatites, attempts to develop composites of TCP have been relatively few. One reason for this is that TCP in particulate form is just as inconvenient to handle as hydroxyapatite and has the same migration problems. Recently, a mixture of tricalcium phosphate (TCP) and Plaster of Paris® (1:2) was used to reconstruct alveolar rims [65]. Synergistic resorption of both tricalcium phosphate and Plaster of Paris® (calcium sulfate) could result in renal osteodystrophy [66]. However, the biodegradable properties of TCP may be ideal for developing a redundant synthetic ceramic–polyfunctional carboxylic acid composite for repairing traumatized or diseased hard tissues.

Viscosity of TCP Composites

The amounts of liquid setting agents (ml) required to obtain maximum viscosity with one gram of TCP are listed in Table 2. The amounts of polyfunctional carboxylic acid powders (g) and deionized–distilled water (ml) required to obtain maximum viscosity with one gram of TCP are presented in Table 3. Maximum viscosity was attained by TCP and Carbopol® in a ratio of 1:1 (Table 2). Beta-TCP, in combination with bovine serum albumin (6%), Hespan® (6%), lactic acid (85%), polyvinyl pyrrolidone or deionized–distilled water, in a ratio of 5:3, achieved maximum viscosity (Table 2). Maximum viscosity was also attained by a 5:4 mixture of TCP and orthophosphoric acid (Table 2).

Powders of TCP, mixed with pyruvic acid, alpha-ketoglutaric acid or malic acid, attained maximum viscosity in a ratio of 2:1 after the addition of deionized–distilled water (Table 3). Maximum viscosity was attained with a 1:1 mixture of TCP with citric or succinic acids after the addition of deionized–distilled water (Table 3). A ratio of 4:1 was required to attain maximum viscosity with mixtures of TCP and fumaric or oxaloacetic acids, on addition of deionized–distilled water (Table 3). Once again, if maximum viscosity was the only criterion for developing bone composites, a toothpaste-like composite could be produced by varying the ratio of TCP and the above setting agents [10].

3.2.2. Setting Hardness of TCP Composites

Setting hardness of relatively poor agents, including bovine serum albumin, Carbopol®, Hespan®, polyvinyl pyrrolidone, citric acid, orthophosphoric acid, or deionized–distilled water, are shown in Table 4. Hardness attained by composites of TCP and lactic, oxaloacetic, pyruvic, or succinic acids are shown in Figure 4. Setting hardness of composites of alpha-ketoglutaric, fumaric, malic or a combination of alpha-ketoglutaric and citric acids are shown in Figure 5.

Composites of TCP and orthophosphoric acid hardened within 30 minutes (Table 4). However, after drying, the composites crumbled on application of pressure. Composites of TCP and oxaloacetic, lactic, succinic, or pyruvic acids did not harden adequately within 60 minutes (Figure 4). In contrast, composites of TCP and alpha-ketoglutaric or malic acid attained maximum hardness within 60 minutes (Figure 5). However, composites of TCP and malic acid reached maximum hardness within 15 minutes (Figure 5). Although composites of TCP and alpha-ketoglutaric acid attained maximum hardness after 45 minutes, the gel could not be stirred within a minute. However, addition of citric acid to TCP–ketoglutaric acid composite delayed the gelling time to 2.5 minutes [10].

A composite which sets to hardness relatively quickly would have a better chance of staying in a wound than a nonsetting composite or a slow-setting composite. However, the composite must not set so quickly that the surgeon will not have adequate time to shape it within the wound. Taking these factors and the data collected into consideration, composites of TCP and Carbopol®, succinic acid, fumaric acid, citric acid, or pyruvic acid will not set adequately if a surgeon closes a wound within 45 to 60 minutes. At the other extreme, however, combinations of TCP and orthophosphoric acid or alpha-ketoglutaric acid set too quickly. These mixtures could be used as a powder to fill bleeding bone wounds. Probably by using combinations of orthophosphoric acid with other acids such as citric acid or oxaloacetic acid, the setting time can be delayed. In this investigation, alpha-ketoglutaric acid was combined with citric acid. The addition of citric acid delayed the setting time by two or three minutes. However, maximum hardness was never reached by TCP, ketoglutaric citric acid composites by the end of 60 minutes. Of the setting agents tested, the most promising seems to be malic acid. Composites of TCP and malic acid set in approximately seven to eight minutes and reach maximum hardness within 15 minutes. The compressive strength at failure for TCP–ketoglutaric acid cylindrical plugs was 4.2 MPa and for TCP–malic acid composite plugs was 6.2 MPa [10,19]. Average strength of trabecular bone is 5 MPa [67]. Thus, in comparison to composites of ALCAP and ketoglutaric or malic acid, composites of TCP–ketoglutaric or TCP–malic acid would be more desirable.

pH Studies of TCP Composites

Addition of calcium hydroxide (12, 15, 18, or 21% by weight of the composite) to either alpha-ketoglutaric or

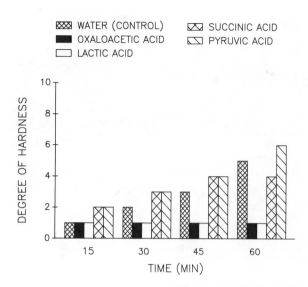

Figure 4. Setting hardness of composites of calcined tricalcium phosphate particulate (38–43 um) powder (1 g) and oxaloacetic (0.25 g), succinic (1.0 g) or pyruvic (0.5 g) acids on addition of deionized-distilled water (0.5–0.6 ml) or 85% lactic acid (0.6 ml) over a duration of 60 minutes.

malic acid composites of TCP increased the pH of the suspending medium toward the alkaline side [11]. The effect on pH of adding calcium hydroxide was almost linear [11]. Since alkaline pH encourages growth of bone [68], incorporation of calcium hydroxide (15–20% by weight) in TCP and polyfunctional carboxylic acid composites will not only neutralize the acidity of the composites but also provide an alkaline environment for growth of bone [11].

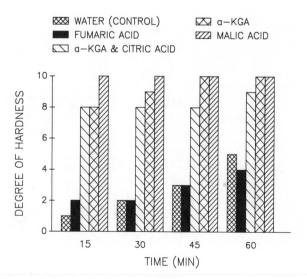

Figure 5. Setting hardness of composites of calcined tricalcium phosphate particulate (38–43 um) powder (1 g) and fumaric (0.25 g), malic (0.5 g) alpha-ketoglutraic (0.5 g) or mixtures of alpha-ketoglutaric (0.40 g) and citric (0.10 g) acids on addition of de-ionized-distilled water (0.5–0.6 ml) over a duration of 60 minutes.

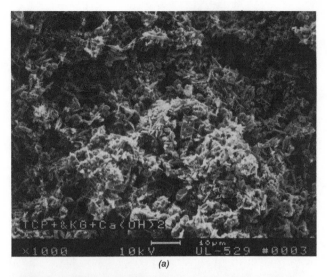

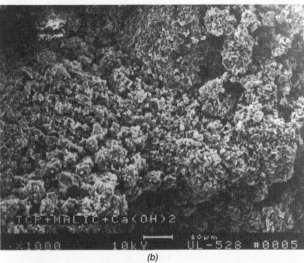

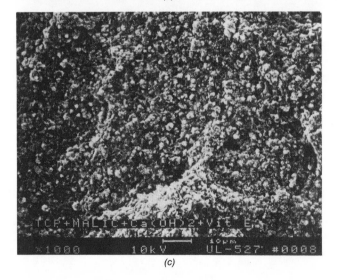

Figure 6. *Scanning electron photomicrographs of cracked surfaces of composites of tricalcium phosphate and (a) ketoglutaric acid and calcium hydroxide, (b) malic acid and calcium hydroxide, (c) malic acid, calcium hydroxide and vitamine E, after setting to maximum hardness.*

Scanning Electron Microscopy of TCP Composites

Scanning electron photomicrographs of cracked surfaces of hardened composites of TCP, alpha-ketoglutaric acid, and calcium hydroxide [Figure 6(a)], or TCP, malic acid, and calcium hydroxide with or without vitamin E succinate [Figures 6(b) and 6(c)], show that these composites have both macro- and micro-pores between aggregates of ceramic particles bound by polyfunctional carboxylic acids [Figures 6(a), 6(b), and 6(c)]. The macropores should encourage ingrowth of new bone and the micropores should assist in the eventual degradation and replacement of the composite by the host's tissues. Vitamin E succinate was used to provide hydrophobicity to the composite and delay its degradation on implantation. The SEM of TCP, malic acid, calcium hydroxide, and vitamin E succinate shows that inclusion of vitamin E seems to decrease the size of the pores and increase the tightness between the ceramic particles [Figure 6(c)]. The data obtained from recent studies conducted in rats with implants of TCP, malic acid, calcium hydroxide, and vitamin D_3 or vitamin E confirm the postulation that incorporation of these fat-soluble vitamins improves the handling of these composites and retention of these composites at the implantation site [69].

Animal Studies on TCP Composites

Animal studies with TCP–ketoglutaric or TCP–malic acid composites were conducted in both rats and rabbits. During surgery, it was observed that when initially applied to a bone wound the composite powder acts as a hemostatic agent and sets on reacting with blood. Studies conducted in rats showed that endogenous bone completely replaced TCP–ketoglutaric acid or TCP–Malic acid composites implanted in femurs [10]. Analysis of rat urine collected 24 hours post surgery showed that the alpha-ketoglutaric acid, resorbed from the TCP–acid composite, did not influence the metabolic status of the animals. Four weeks after implantation, TCP–ketoglutaric composite filled holes in the tibiae of rabbits showed ingrowth of large amounts of tetracycline labeled periosteal and endosteal trabecular bone and extensive resorption of the TCP composite [19]. The use of either acid as a setting agent did not cause deleterious effects in either rats or rabbits [10].

Recently, composites of TCP, polyfunctional acid (ketoglutaric or malic) and calcium hydroxide with and without vitamins (D or E), were used for repairing traumatized femurs in rats. One hundred and eight male white rats were equally distributed into six groups and implanted with TCP or composites, and autografts, in the contralateral leg. Body weights and radiographs were taken periodically, and blood was collected prior to euthanasia for measuring serum calcium, phosphorus, and alkaline phosphatase activity. Animals implanted with TCP or composites of TCP, polyfunctional acids, and calcium hydroxide, showed normal blood chemistry, healing of bone, and weight gain profile [69]. Animals implanted with any combination of 1,25-dihydrocholecalciferol (DHCC) showed weight loss and abnormal bone tissue [69]. Animals in the six week study group, implanted with vitamin D_3 (DHCC) containing composites, had significantly higher levels of serum calcium and significantly lower levels of serum phosphorus [68]. Substitution of DHCC with vitamin E succinate in the 12 week group allowed normal healing and weight gain profile [69]. The data obtained suggested that the addition of DHCC to TCP composites in the amount used in this investigation was undesirable, whereas composites of TCP, polyfunctional carboxylic acid, and calcium hydroxide with or without vitamin E succinate repaired traumatized bone in a normal manner without inducing deleterious side effects [69]. The animal studies conducted to date suggest that surgically induced bone wounds in rabbit tibiae or rat femurs can be repaired with TCP–ketoglutaric acid or TCP–malic acid composites [10,19,69].

Hydroxyapatite

Since synthetic hydroxyapatites are similar to natural mineral apatite, they seem to have a promising future in the area of hard tissue replacement [5,70]. Synthetic hydroxyapatites have shown good biocompatibility and bonding with bone [2,3,5,9]. Various forms of hydroxyapatites have been used in both oral and orthopaedic surgeries [5]. Of these, dense hydroxyapatites have been used primarily to repair bones lost due to resorption, since they show a very slow rate, or for all practical purposes, no degradation *in situ* [5]. Porous hydroxyapatites, particularly corraline hydroxyapatite, have had great success in repairing diseased or traumatized bone [9]. Use of resorbable hydroxyapatite is relatively new, but it should have the same success as resorbable TCP in correcting hard tissue defects.

The inconvenience of handling and the migration of hydroxyapatite particulates from the surgical site prompted the development of hydroxyapatite composites [5]. Currently, most of these composites are in the experimental stage while some have been used clinically to reconstruct diseased or traumatized hard tissues [3,5]. These defects can result from excision of donor bone or bone tumors, non-unions of comminuted fractures, and pathologic resorption of bone [17]. In contrast to the TCP–Plaster of Paris® mixtures, hydroxyapatite grouts, with or without Plaster of Paris®, seem to have been used with greater success in replacing bone lost due to trauma or resorption [3,17,32–34]. Thus, the development of a relatively fast setting hydroxyapatite bone grout, containing a resorbable

component, would be ideal for replacing bone lost due to resorption [17]. Three different forms of apatites, were used in our laboratory to develop composites of Biorad hydroxyapatite (BHA), HA-1000 hydroxyapatite (HA) and a bone meal apatite Osseograft (OG) [17].

Viscosity of Hydroxyapatite Composites

For Biorad hydroxyapatite (BHA), deionized–distilled water and a ratio of 2:1 Biorad hydroxyapatite to pyruvic acid or oxaloacetic acid was required to attain maximum viscosity. On addition of deionized–distilled water, composites of BHA and citric or succinic acids attained maximum viscosity in a ratio of 1:1. Biorad hydroxyapatite attained maximum viscosity on addition of either deionized–distilled water or 30% orthophosphoric acid in a ratio of 5:6. Maximum viscosity was attained by BHA and lactic acid (85%) in a ratio of 5:7. Composites of BHA and alpha-ketoglutaric acid attained maximum viscosity in a ratio of 1:3 upon the addition of deionized–distilled water. A ratio of 1:2 BHA and malic or fumaric acid was required to obtain maximum viscosity on addition of deionized–distilled water [17].

For Osseograft (OG), maximum viscosity was attained with a 1:1 mixture of Osseograft with citric, succinic, or alpha-ketoglutaric acid upon addition of deionized–distilled water. Composites of OG with deionized–distilled water, 50% orthophosphoric acid or 85% lactic acid achieved maximum viscosity in a ratio of 2:1. On addition of deionized–distilled water, composites of OG and pyruvic or malic acids attained maximum viscosity in a ratio of 2:1. Combining OG with either fumaric or oxaloacetic acid in a ratio of 4:1 yielded maximum viscosity on addition of deionized–distilled water [17].

For HA-1000 Hydroxyapatite (HA), upon the addition of deionized–distilled water, maximum viscosity was achieved with a 1:1 ratio of HA and citric acid. Composites of HA and pyruvic acid or alpha-ketoglutaric acid attained maximum viscosity in a ratio of 2:1 on addition of deionized–distilled water. Maximum viscosity was attained when HA-1000 hydroxyapatite was mixed with deionized–distilled water or 30% orthophosphoric acid in a ratio of 2:1. Composites of HA and succinic, fumaric, or oxaloacetic acids attained maximum viscosity in a ratio of 4:1 on addition of deionized–distilled water [17]. Maximum viscosity was achieved with a 10:3 mixture of HA and malic acid on addition of deionized–distilled water [17]. The viscous composites of HA and various acids probably could be used to fill sites which are not easily accessible and where setting to hardness is not critical.

Setting Hardness of Hydroxyapatite Composites

Setting hardness of composites of BHA, HA, or OG with citric acid, lactic acid, orthophosphoric acid,

TABLE 5. Setting Hardness of Composites of Biorad Hydroxyapatite (BHA), HA–1000 Hydroxyapatite (HA), or Osseograft (OG), and Various Setting Agents over a Duration of 60 Minutes.

Setting Agents		Hydroxy apatite (HA)	D.D. Water (ml/g HA)	Time in Minutes			
				15	30	45	60
					Degree of Hardness		
D. D. Water (Control)		BHA	1.2	1	3	3	4
		OG	0.5	5	6	7	8
		HA	0.5	1	1	1	1
Orthophosphoric	(30%)	BHA	1.2	8	9	9	9
Acid	(50%)	OG	0.5	4	5	6	7
	(30%)	HA	0.5	8	9	10	10
Lactic	(85%)	BHA	1.4	1	1	2	2
Acid		OG	0.5	3	3	3	3
		HA	0.6	1	1	1	1
Citric		BHA	0.8	1	1	1	2
Acid		OG	0.3	1	2	3	4
		HA	0.4	1	1	2	3
Pyruvic		BHA	1.2	1	1	2	2
Acid		OG	0.4	1	1	1	1
		HA	0.5	2	2	2	3
Succinic		BHA	1.6	1	2	3	4
Acid		OG	0.5	3	4	5	6
		HA	0.7	1	1	1	1
Composition #1		BHA	1.0	6	6	6	7
citric acid (0.15g)		OG	0.4	6	6	7	7
ketoglutaric (0.35g)		HA	0.3	7	8	8	9
Composition #2		BHA	1.0	7	7	7	8
citric acid (0.10g)		OG	0.4	6	7	7	8
ketoglutaric (0.40g)		HA	0.3	8	9	10	10

Modified from Bajpai, P. K. and C. M. Fuchs, Acad. Surg. Res., 1:50–54, 1985.

pyruvic acid, succinic acid, combinations of alpha-ketoglutaric and citric acids, or deionized–distilled water are shown in Table 5. The hardness profiles of composites of Biorad hydroxyapatite and oxalacetic, alpha-ketoglutaric, fumaric, oxaloacetic, or malic acids are shown in Figure 7. Setting hardness profile of composites of Osseograft and oxaloacetic, fumaric, alpha-ketoglutaric, or malic acids are shown in Figure 8. The hardness profile of composites of HA-1000 hydroxyapatite and oxaloacetic, fumaric, alpha-ketoglutaric, or malic acids are shown in Figure 9.

BHA and alpha-ketoglutaric acid mixtures set in 30 seconds after the addition of deionized–distilled water. Maximum hardness was achieved in 60 minutes by composites of BHA and alpha-ketoglutaric acid on addition of deionized–distilled water (Figure 7). Slower setting times of two to five minutes were achieved by adding citric acid to composites of BHA and alpha-ketoglutaric acid. Composites of BHA and 30% orthophosphoric acid set in two minutes and generated substantial amounts of heat. Composites of BHA and malic acid set in 10 minutes on addition of deionized–distilled water. All other BHA and setting agent mixtures failed to reach the maximum hardness within 60 minutes (Table 5, and Figure 7). The data suggest that BHA, in combination with either alpha-keto-

glutaric acid or malic acid, can be used as a bone grout [17].

Composites of OG and alpha-ketoglutaric acid set after one minute on addition of deionized–distilled water, and attained maximum hardness within 45 minutes (Figure 8). The addition of citric acid (composition #1 and #2) to composites of OG and alpha-ketoglutaric acid extended the setting time from one to four and eight minutes, respectively. Composites of Osseograft and malic acid set in approximately four minutes on addition of deionized–distilled water, and attained maximum hardness within 60 minutes (Figure 8). Composites of OG and deionized–distilled water or orthophosphoric acid (50%) did not attain maximum hardness within 60 minutes (Table 5). All other Osseograft and setting agent mixtures failed to achieve maximum hardness within 60 minutes (Table 5, and Figure 8). The data suggest that OG, in combination with either alpha-ketoglutaric acid or malic acid, can be used as a bone grout [17]. Since composites of OG and orthophosphoric acid generated substantial amounts of heat on addition of deionized–distilled water, their use as in situ bone grouts may be undesirable [17].

Composites of HA and fumaric acid set in 30 seconds after the addition of deionized–distilled water. Composites of HA and alpha-ketoglutaric acid took 90 seconds to

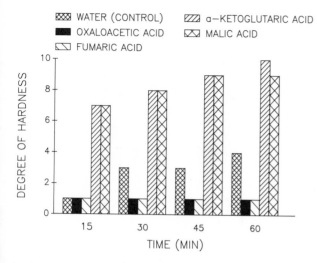

Figure 7. Setting hardness of composites of calcined Biorad hydroxyapatite particulate (10–38 um) powder (1 g) and fumaric (2.0 g), malic (2.0 g) oxaloacetic (0.5 g) or alpha-ketoglutraic (3.0 g) acids on addition of deionized–distilled water (1.0–2.0 ml) over a duration of 60 minutes.

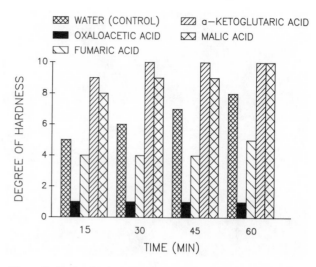

Figure 8. Setting hardness of composites of calcined Osseograft particulate (10–38 um) powder (1 g) and fumaric (0.25 g), malic (0.5 g) oxaloacetic (1.0 g) or alpha-ketoglutraic (0.5 g) acids on addition of deionized–distilled water (0.4–0.6 ml) over a duration of 60 minutes.

set after the addition of deionized–distilled water. Slower setting times of three to five minutes were achieved by adding citric acid to composites of HA and alpha-ketoglutaric acid. On addition of deionized–distilled water, composites of HA and malic acid set in 10 minutes. Composites of HA and alpha-ketoglutaric, malic, fumaric, or alpha-ketoglutaric and citric acids (Composition #2) set to maximum hardness on addition of deionized–distilled water (Table 5 and Figure 9). Composites of orthophosphoric acid (30%) and HA–1000 hydroxyapatite generated heat, but attained maximum hardness within 45 minutes (Table 5). All other composites of HA and setting agents failed to reach maximum hardness within 60 minutes (Table 5 and Figure 9).

The compressive strength at failure for HA–1000 hydroxyapatite (420–1200 μm particles) and alpha-ketoglutaric acid cylindrical plugs was 0.7 ± 0.09 MPa. The data suggest that mixtures of HA–1000 hydroxyapatite and alpha-ketoglutaric, fumaric, malic, or combinations of alpha-ketoglutaric and citric acids can be used as grouts to repair bone. To date, composites of HA–1000 and alpha-ketoglutaric or malic acids have been used successfully to repair experimentally traumatized bones [17,18].

Scanning Electron Microscopy of Hydroxyapatite Composites

Hydroxyapatite is relatively insoluble. Thus, the size of pores between aggregates of hardened HA particles have to be large enough to allow ingrowth of new bone. Scanning electron microscopy of hardened HA, alpha-ketoglutaric acid, and calcium hydroxide [Figure 10(a)], or HA, malic acid, and calcium hydroxide [Figure 10(b)],

show that these composites have both macropores and micropores between aggregates of ceramic particles bound by polyfunctional carboxylic acids [Figures 10(a), and 10(b)]. These large macropores should encourage ingrowth of new bone within the composite.

Animal Studies

Animal studies conducted to date suggest that surgically induced bone wounds in femur and calvarie of rats can easily be filled with HA–1000 hydroxyapatite and polyfunctional carboxylic acid grouts. Four weeks after sur-

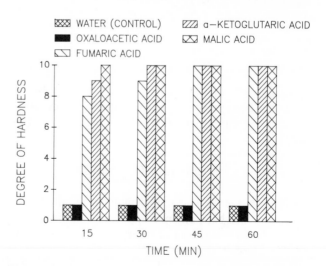

Figure 9. Setting hardness of composites of HA–1000 hydroxyapatite particulate (400 um) powder (1 g) and fumaric (0.25 g), malic (0.30 g) oxaloacetic (0.25 g) or alpha-ketoglutraic (0.5 g) acids on addition of deionized–distilled water (0.3–0.4 ml) over a duration of 60 minutes.

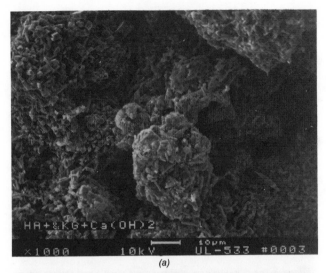

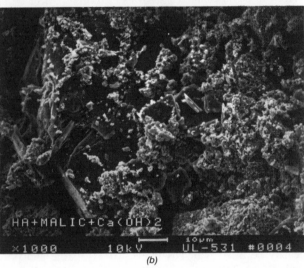

Figure 10. *Scanning electron photomicrographs of cracked surfaces of composites of hydroxyapatite and (a) ketoglutaric acid and calcium hydroxide, (b) malic acid and calcium hydroxide, after setting to maximum hardness.*

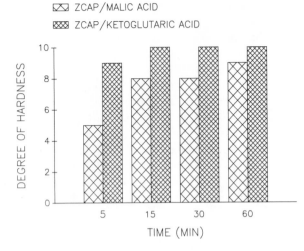

Figure 11. *Setting hardness of (2:1) composites (300 mg) of zinc calcium phosphorus oxide (ZCAP) ceramic particles and malic or alpha-ketoglutraic acids on addition of deionized–distilled water (200 ul) over a duration of 60 minutes (Modified from Gromofsky, J. R., Arar, H. and Bajpai, P. K. Digest of Papers, Seventh Southern Biomedical Engineering Conference. D. D. Moyle, ed., Washington, D.C.:Mc-Gregor and Werner, p. 22 (1988).*

cumulate in the tissues. Although zinc deficiency is quite common in both animals and humans, its toxicity has not been reported in man [72]. A biodegradable and porous ZCAP ceramic was developed recently by Bajpai and co-workers for correcting bone defects and delivering chemicals and biologicals [25–27,74]. Rather than being toxic, implanted ZCAP ceramics are likely to correct zinc deficiency. Hence, it was also considered desirable to develop ZCAP composites of polyfunctional carboxylic acids and zinc sulfate containing ZCAP ceramics for use in bone repair.

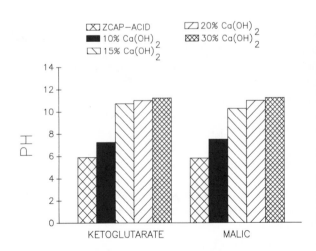

Figure 12. *Effect of adding 10, 15, 20 or 30% calcium hydroxide to composites of zinc calcium phosphorus oxide (ZCAP) ceramic particles and malic or alpha-ketoglutaric acids at 37°C (Modified from Gromofsky, J. R., Arar, H. and Bajpai, P. K. Digest of Papers, Seventh Southern Biomedical Engineering Conference. D. D. Moyle, ed., Washington, D.C.:McGregor and Werner, p. 22 (1988).*

gery, ingrowth of both peri- and endo-steal trabecular bone has been observed in HA-1000 hydroxyapatite-alpha-ketoglutaric grout filled holes in the tibia of rabbits [18].

Zinc Calcium Phosphorous Oxide (ZCAP)

Zinc is one of the 14 essential elements required by the body. Zinc has been claimed to promote wound healing [71,72]. It is a component of several metalloenzymes, including alcohol dehydrogenase, alkaline phosphatase, carbonic anhydrase, and leucine aminopeptidase [25–27,71–73]. Zinc has been isolated from bone, eye, heart, kidney, lung, liver, muscle, pancreas, and prostate. It is excreted regularly and does not have a tendency to ac-

Setting Hardness of ZCAP Composites

Setting hardness of ZCAP ceramic particles (10–38 μm) and alpha-ketoglutaric acid or malic acid are shown in Figure 11. Both alpha-ketoglutaric and malic acid composites of ZCAP hardened relatively quickly on addition of 200 μl of deionized–distilled water to 300 mg of the composite [21]. ZCAP and alpha-ketoglutaric acid composites attained maximum hardness within 15 minutes of addition of water. In contrast, composites of ZCAP and malic acid attained adequate, but not maximum, hardness in 60 minutes. The rapidity with which hardness is achieved by ZCAP composites of either ketoglutaric or malic acid suggests that both of these composites can be used successfully in repairing traumatized bone if the final composition is not highly acidic [21]. Strnat observed that implantation of ZCAP composites of alpha-ketoglutaric or malic acids caused inflammatory reactions on implantation in bone [22]. The hardness characteristics of ZCAP ceramics containing 15, 30 or 45% zinc sulfate (ZSCAP) are shown in Figure 12. All ZSCAP ceramic calcined particles hardened on addition of water, and their consistency was similar to that of set and hardened Plaster of Paris®. However, incorporation of more than 15% zinc sulfate in the ceramic had a deleterious effect in terms of hardness achieved on addition of water [21]. Since ZSCAP ceramic particles containing 15% zinc sulfate set and harden like Plaster of Paris® on addition of water, they can be used, as such, for repairing traumatized bone. This achieves the goal of developing another ceramic powder which sets and hardens like gypsum, on addition of water.

pH Studies of ZCAP Composites

The changes in pH of neutral saline, containing suspensions of composites of ZCAP and alpha-ketoglutaric or malic acids with and without calcium hydroxide (10, 15, 20 or 30% by weight of the composite), for a total duration of 24 hours are shown in Figure 13. Addition of 10% calcium hydroxide to ZCAP–polyfunctional carboxylic acid composites increased the pH of neutral saline to 7.0–7.5 [21]. Addition of higher amounts of calcium hydroxide (15–30%) to ZCAP and polyfunctional carboxylic acid composites increased the pH of neutral saline toward the alkaline side (Figure 13). Since alkaline pH encourages growth of bone [67], composites of ZCAP, polyfunctional carboxylic acids, and calcium hydroxide should be suitable for repairing traumatized bone.

CONCLUSIONS

Monomers of low molecular weight polyfunctional carboxylic acids, in particular alpha-ketoglutaric and malic acids, formed good composites with all the calcium

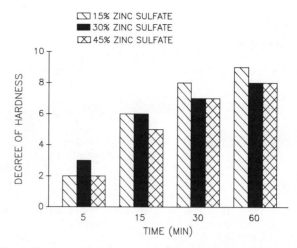

Figure 13. *Setting hardness of zinc calcium phosphorus oxide (ZCAP) ceramic powder containing 15, 30 or 45% zinc sulfate on addition of deionized–distilled water over a duration of 60 minutes [Reproduced from Gromofsky, J. R., Arar, H. and Bajpai, P. K. Digest of Papers, Seventh Southern Biomedical Engineering Conference. D. D. Moyle, ed., Washington, D.C.: McGregor and Werner, p. 21 (1988)].*

phosphate based ceramic materials, including: alumino calcium phosphorous oxide (ALCAP), Biorad hydroxyapatite (BHA), HA–1000 hydroxyapatite (HA), Osseograft (OG), tricalcium phosphate (TCP), and zinc calcium phosphorous oxide (ZCAP). By varying the acids and/or combining two different acids, setting times from 30 seconds to 10 minutes were achieved for hard-setting ceramic and polyfunctional carboxylic acid composites. Incorporation of calcium hydroxide in ceramic and polyfunctional carboxylic acid composites neutralized the acidity of the composites and made them alkaline. Development of zinc sulfate containing zinc calcium phosphorous oxide ceramic composite (ZSCAP) provided a resorbable material which can set and harden like Plaster of Paris®, on addition of deionized–distilled water. Implantation in animals of most of these composites successfully repaired experimentally traumatized bone.

ACKNOWLEDGEMENTS

Acknowledgements are due to: Dan Palomino and Brian Granite for technical assistance in preparation of this manuscript, S. Sgt. Joseph Maslanka (AAMRL/THD, WPAFB, Dayton, OH) for providing the scanning electron photomicrographs, and Robin Bajpai for editing the manuscript.

REFERENCES

1 Mattie, D. R. and P. K. Bajpai. "Analysis of the Biocompatibility of ALCAP Ceramics in Rat Femurs." *J. Biomed. Maters. Res.*, 22:1101–1126 (1988).

2 Lemons, J. E., P. K. Bajpai, P. Patka, G. Bonel, L. B. Starling, T. Rosenstiel, G. Muschler, S. Kampner and J. Timmermans. "Sig-

nificance of the Porosity and Physical Chemistry of Calcium Phosphate Ceramics: Orthopedic Uses," in *Bioceramics: Material Characteristics Versus In Vivo Behavior; Annals of New York Academy of Sciences,* 523:278–282 (1988).

3 PARSONS, J. R., J. L. Ricci, H. Alexander and P. K. Bajpai. "Osteoconductive Composite Grouts for Orthopaedic Use," in *Bioceramics: Material Characteristics Versus In Vivo Behavior,* Annals of New York Academy of Sciences, 523:190–207 (1988).

4 BAJPAI, P. K., G. A. Graves, Jr., D. R. Mattie and F. B. McFall. "Resorbable Porous Alumino–Calcium–Phosphorous Oxide (ALCAP) Ceramics," in *Quantitative Characterization and Performance of Porous Implants for Hard Tissue Applications,* ASTM STP 953; J. E. Lemons, ed., Philadelphia, PA:American Society for Testing and Materials, pp. 389–398 (1988).

5 ALEXANDER, H., J. R. Parsons, J. L. Ricci, P. K. Bajpai and A. B. Weiss. "Calcium-based Ceramics and Composites in Bone Reconstruction." *CRC. Crit. Rev. Biocompatibility,* 4:43–77 (1987).

6 BAJPAI, P. K. "Bioceramics: Future Role in Implant Technology and Regeneration," in *Less Invasive/Innovative Surgical Technologies,* R.A. Prosek, ed., Tustin, CA:Information International Resources, Inc., 4.1–4.12 (1984).

7 HENCH, L. L. "Bioceramics and the Origin of Life," *J. Biomed. Maters. Res.,* 23:685–703 (1989).

8 BAJPAI, P. K., G. A. Graves, Jr., L. G. Wilcox and M. J. Freeman. "Use of Resorbable Alumino-Calcium-Phosphorous Oxide Ceramics in Health Care," *Trans. Soc. Biomat.,* 7:217 (1984).

9 BAJPAI, P. K. "Biodegradable Scaffolds in Orthopedic, Oral and Maxillo-Facial Surgery," in *Biomaterials in Reconstructive Surgery,* L. R. Rubin, ed., St. Louis, MO:C. V. Mosby Co., pp. 312–328 (1983).

10 BAJPAI, P. K., C. M. Fuchs and D. E. McCullum. "Development of Tricalcium Phosphate Ceramic Cements," in *Quantitative Characterization and Performance of Porous Implants for Hard Tissue Applications,* ASTM STP 953, J. E. Lemons, ed., Philadelphia, PA:American Society for Testing and Materials, pp. 377–388 (1988).

11 GEISELMAN, E., P. Delli and P. K. Bajpai. "Effect of Calcium Salts on Ceramic-Organic Acid Composites," in *Digest of Papers, Seventh Southern Biomedical Engineering Conference,* D. D. Moyle, ed., McGregor and Werner: Washington, DC., pp. 24–27 (1988).

12 GEISELMAN, E., Lisa M. Morris and P. K. Bajpai. "Resorbable Ceramic Amine and Vitamin Composites for Repairing Bone," in *Digest of Papers, Seventh Southern Biomedical Engineering Conference,* R. C. Eberhard, ed., Washington, DC.: McGregor and Werner, pp. 182–185 (1987).

13 BAJPAI, P. K. "Surgical Cements." Patent No. 4,668,295. U.S.A. (1987).

14 BAJPAI, P. K. and E. Geiselman. "Ceramic Amine Composites for Repairing Traumatized Hard Tissues," in *Digest of Papers, Seventh Southern Biomedical Engineering Conference,* R. C. Eberhart, ed., Washington, DC.: McGregor and Werner, pp. 174–177 (1987).

15 BAJPAI, P. K., C. M. Fuchs and M. A. P. Strnat. "Development of Alumino-Calcium-Phosphorus Oxide (ALCAP) Ceramic Cements," in *Biomedical Engineering IV. Recent Developments,* B. W. Sauer, ed., New York, NY: Pergamon Press, pp. 22–25 (1985).

16 SUTOR, S. D., M. A. P. Strnat and P. K. Bajpai. "Biocompatibility of ALCAP Polyfunctional Acid Cements," *Trans. Soc. Biomat.,* 9:113 (1986).

17 BAJPAI, P. K. and C. M. Fuchs. "Development of a Hydroxyapatite Bone Grout," *Academy of Surgical Research,* 1:50–54 (1985).

18 RICCI, J. L., H. Alexander, J. R. Parsons, R. Salsbury and P. K. Bajpai. "Partially Resorbable Hydroxylapatite Based Cement for Repair of Bone Defects," in *Biomedical Engineering V. Recent Developments,* S. Saha, ed., New York, N.Y.: Pergamon Press, pp. 469–474 (1986).

19 RICCI, J. L., P. K. Bajpai, A. Berkman, H. Alexander and J. R. Parsons. "Development of a Fast-Setting Ceramic Based Grout Material for Filling Bone Defects," in *Biomedical Engineering V. Recent Developments,* S. Saha, ed., New York, N.Y.: Pergamon Press, pp. 475–481 (1986).

20 BAJPAI, P. K. "Ceramic Amino Acid Composites for Repairing Traumatized Hard Tissues," *Trans Soc. Biomat.,* 11:465 (1988).

21 GROMOFSKY, J. R., H. Arar and P. K. Bajpai. "Development of Zinc Calcium Phosphorous Oxide Ceramic-Organic Acid Composites for Repairing Traumatized Hard Tissue," in *Digest of Papers, Seventh Southern Biomedical Engineering Conference,* D. D. Moyle, ed., Washington, D.C.:McGregor and Werner, 20–23 (1988).

22 STRNAT, M. A. P. "Development of a Zinc Calcium Phosphorous Oxide (ZCAP) Ceramic Bone Replacement Composite," *M.S. Thesis.* University of Dayton, Dayton, Ohio (1987).

23 FUCHS, C. M., S. R. Jenei and P. K. Bajpai. "Biocompatibility of Ceramic/Polycarboxylic Acid Composites," *Ohio J. Sci.,* 86:16 (1986).

24 JARCHO, M. "Calcium Phosphate Ceramics as Hard Tissue Prosthetics," *Clin. Orthop. Rel. Res.,* 157:259–278 (1980).

25 BINZER, T. D. "The Use of Zinc-Calcium-Phosphate (ZCAP) Ceramics in Reconstructive Bone Surgery," *B.Sc. Honors Thesis.* Dayton, OH:University of Dayton (1987).

26 BINZER, T. D. and P. K. Bajpai. "The Use of Zinc-Calcium-Oxide (ZCAP) Ceramics in Reconstructive Bone Surgery," in *Digest of Papers, Sixth Southern Biomedical Engineering Conference,* R. C. Eberhart, ed., Washington, D.C.:McGregor and Werner, 178–179 (1987).

27 BAJPAI, P. K. ZCAP Ceramics, Patent No. 4,778,471. U.S.A. (1988).

28 KATZ, J. L. "Hard Tissue as a Composite Material, Part 1: Bounds on the Elastic Behavior," *J. Biomech.,* 4:455–473 (1971).

29 LIN, T. C. and S. Krebs. "Synthetic Bone Composite Material," *Trans. Soc. Biomat.,* 9:207 (1986).

30 TURNER, D. I. "Dental Applications for Composites: A Review," *Trans. Soc. Biomat.,* 9:213 (1986).

31 CLAE, L. E. "Composites in Orthopaedics," *Trans. Soc. Biomat.,* 9:214 (1986).

32 BLOCK, M. S., J. N. Kent, C. A. Homsy, J. A. Maxwell and M. S. Anderson. "The Tissue Response of Hydroxyapatite-PTFE Composites," *Trans. Soc. Biomat.,* 11:467 (1988).

33 DOYLE, C. "Composite Materials in Orthopaedic Surgery," *Trans. Soc. Biomat.,* 11:26 (1988).

34 WADA, M., S. Imura, Y. Otashi, T. Ozaki, S. Sasahara and Y. Abe. "New Bone Formation in Porous Calcium Phosphate Glass Ceramic and Its Composite Materials," *Trans Soc. Biomat.,* 11:182 (1988).

35 WILSON, J., A. Fetner, M. S. Hartigan and A. E. Clark. "Bioactive Paste for Craniofacial Repairs," *Trans. Soc. Biomat.,* 11:464 (1988).

36 STUPP, S. I., J. A. Eurell, J. A. Hanson and G. W. Ciegler. "Organoapatites as Artificial Bone," *Trans. Soc. Biomat.,* 12:108 (1989).

37 TERRY, B. C., R. D. Baker, M. R. Tucker and J. S. Hanker. "Alveolar Ridge Augmentation with Composite Implants of Hydroxylapatite and Plaster for Correction of Bony Defects, Deficiencies and Related Contour Abnormalities," *Mat. Res. Soc. Symp. Proc.,* 110:187–198 (1989).

38 CARNEVALE, R. A., G. W. Greco, C. M. Bullard and J. S. Hanker.

"Hydroxylapatite/Plaster Implantation for the Treatment of Severe Periodontal Osseous Defects," *Mat Res. Soc. Symp. Proc.*, 110:247–256 (1989).

39 LEWIS, R. D., R. A. Carnevale, B. L. Giammara and J. S. Hanker. "Composite Hydroxylapatite/Plaster Implants for Complex Endodontic Periapical Defects and Lesions," *Mat. Res. Soc. Symp. Proc.*, 110:301–310 (1989).

40 WILLIAMS, D. F. *Biocompatibility of Clinical Implant Materials*, Boca Raton, Fl:CRC Press Inc. (1981).

41 HENTRICH, R. L., G. A. Graves, Jr., H. G. Stein and P. K. Bajpai. "An Evaluation of Inert and Resorbable Ceramics for Future Clinical Applications," *J. Biomed. Mater. Res.* 5:25–51 (1971).

42 GRAVES, Jr., G. A., R. L. Hentrich, Jr., H. G. Stein and P. K. Bajpai. "Resorbable Ceramic Implants in Bioceramics," in *Engineering and Medicine (Part 1).* C. W. Hall, S. F. Hulbert, S. N. Levine and F. A. Young, ed., New York, N.Y.:Interscience Publishers, 91–115 (1972).

43 CARVALHO, B. A., G. A. Graves, Jr. and P. K. Bajpai. "Calcium and Inorganic Phosphate Contents of Implanted Resorbable Porous Calcium Aluminate Ceramics," *IRCS. Med. Sci.*, 3:185 (1975).

44 WYATT, D. F., P. K. Bajpai, G. A. Graves, Jr., and P. A. Stull. "Remodelling of Calcium Aluminate Phosphorous Pentoxide Ceramic Implants in Bone," *IRCS. Med. Sci.*, 4:421 (1976).

45 CARVALHO, B. A., P. K. Bajpai and G. A. Graves Jr. "Effect of Resorbable Calcium Aluminate Ceramics on Regulation of Calcium and Phosphorous in Rats," *Biomedicine Express*, 25:130–133 (1976).

46 BAJPAI, P. K., D. F. Wyatt and G. A. Graves, Jr. "Effect of Calcium Aluminate Ceramics on the pH of Distilled Water, Phosphate Saline and Human Plasma," *IRCS. Med. Sci.*, 5:288 (1977).

47 FREEMAN, M. J., P. K. Bajpai, G. A. Graves, Jr. and D. E. McCullum. "Use of Alumino-Calcium-Phosphorous-Oxide Ceramics for Rebuilding the Mandible," *Ohio J. Sci.*, 80:99 (1980).

48 BAJPAI, P. K. and G. A. Graves, Jr. "Porous Ceramic Carriers for Controlled Release of Proteins, Polypeptide Hormones and Other Substances within Human and/or Mammalian Species," Patent No. 4,218,255. U.S.A. (1980).

49 BAJPAI, P. K., S. N. Khot, G. A. Graves, Jr. and D. E. McCullum. "Effect of Particle Size and Time and Temperature of Sintering on the Density of Partially Resorbable Porous Alumino-Calcium-Phosphorous-Oxide Ceramics," *IRCS. Med. Sci.*, 9:696–697 (1981).

50 FREEMAN, M. J., D. E. McCullum and P. K. Bajpai. "Use of ALCAP Ceramics for Rebuilding Maxillo-Facial Defects," *Trans. Soc. Biomat.*, 4:109 (1981).

51 MATTIE, D. R., S. N. Khot, C. J. Ritter and P. K. Bajpai. "A Dissolution Study of Alumino-Calcium-Phosphorous-Oxide (ALCAP) Ceramics," *Ohio J. Sci.*, 82:105 (1982).

52 McFALL, F. B., C. J. Ritter, D. R. Mattie and P. K. Bajpai. "A Continuous Flow-Through System for Studying the Dissolution Characteristics of Resorbable Ceramics," in *Biomedical Engineering II. Recent Developments*, C. W. Hall, ed., New York, N.Y.:Pergamon Press, pp. 357–360 (1983).

53 MATTIE, D. R., P. K. Bajpai, D. E. McCullum, R. S. Thompson, J. R. Lattendresse and T. J. Foster. "Biocompatibility and Toxicology of Alumino-Calcium-Phosphorous-Oxide (ALCAP) Ceramics," *Trans. Soc. Biomat.*, 6:5 (1983).

54 MATTIE, D. R., F. B. McFall, P. K. Bajpai and J. Gridley. "ALCAP Ceramic: A Nontoxic Aluminum, Calcium and Phosphorous Oxide Biomaterial," *Fed. Proc.*, 43:327 (1984).

55 MATTIE, D. R., C. J. Ritter and P. K. Bajpai. "Use of Alumino-Calcium-Phosphorous-Oxide (ALCAP) Ceramics for Reconstruction of Bone," *Trans. Soc. Biomat.*, 7:353 (1984).

56 McFALL, F. B. and P. K. Bajpai. "Effect of Resorbable Alumino-Calcium-Phosphorous-Oxide (ALCAP) Ceramic Implant in Rats," *Trans. Soc. Biomat.* 7:354 (1984).

57 MATTIE, D. R., P. K. Bajpai and J. R. Lattendresse. "The Effect of ALCAP Ceramics on Erythrocytes and Muscle," *IRCS. Med. Sci.*, 13:420–421 (1985).

58 MATTIE, D. R. and P. K. Bajpai. "Biocompatibility Testing of ALCAP Ceramics," *IRCS. Med. Sci.*, 14:641–643 (1986).

59 BAJPAI, P. K. "Ceramic Composites for Studying Bone Ingrowth and Remodeling," in *Final Report, 1988 – USAF/UES Summer Faculty Research Program* (Contract No.: F49620-87-R-0004), (1988).

60 POTTER, W. D., A. C. Barclay, R. Dunning and R. J. Parry. "Curable Composition Comprising a Calcium Fluoro-Alumino Silicate Glass and Poly(carboxylic acid) or Precursor Thereof," Patent No. 4,123,416. U.S.A. (1978).

61 SCHMITT, W. R., P. J. Purrman and O. Gasser. "Calcium Fluorosilicate Glass Powder for Use in Dental or Bone Cements," Patent No. 4,376,835. U.S.A. (1983).

62 PELTIER, L. F. "The Use of Plaster of Paris to Fill Defects in Bone," *Clin. Orthop. Rel. Res.*, 21:1–31 (1961).

63 BHASKAR, S. N., J. M. Brady, L. Getter, M. F. Grower and T. D. Driskell. "Biodegradable Ceramic Implants in Bone," *Oral. Surg.*, 32:336 (1971).

64 SIGNS, S. A., C. G. Pantano, T. D. Driskell and P. K. Bajpai. "*In vitro* Dissolution of Synthos® Ceramics in an Acellular Physiological Environment," *Biomat. Med. Dev. Art. Org.*, 7:183–190 (1979).

65 VIECO, E. B. "Conservation of the Alveolar Bone with a Mixture of Tricalcic Phosphate Plaster of Paris and Blood," *Implantologist*, 2:56–62 (1981).

66 MICHALK, D., B. Klare, F. Manz and K. Scharer. "Plasma Inorganic Sulfate in Children with Chronic Renal Failure," *Clin. Nephrol.*, 16:8–12 (1981).

67 GERHART, T. N., A. A. Renshaw and C. W. Hayes. "Quantitative Histology and Mechanical Testing of a Biodegradable Bone Cement," *Mater. Res. Soc. Symp. Proc.*, 110:229–232 (1989).

68 BINDERMAN, I., M. Goldstein, I. Horowitz, N. Fine, S. Taicher, A. Ashman and A. Shtayer. "Grafts of HTR Polymer Versus Kiel Bone in Experimental Long Bone Defects in Rats," in *Quantitative Characterization and Performance of Porous Implants for Hard Tissue Applications*, ASTM STP 953. J. E. Lemons, ed., Philadelphia, PA:American Society for Testing and Materials, 370–376 (1987).

69 EVELAND, E. S., T. Mayer, J. Maslanka, P. K. Bajpai. "Alkaline Tricalcium Phosphate-Polyfunctional Acid Composites for Repairing Traumatized Bone," in *Digest of Papers, Eighth Southern Biomedical Engineering Conference. Richmond, VA. October 15–16, 1989*, W. A. Krause, ed., Richmond, VA:Medical College of Virginia, pp. 193–198 (1989).

70 HASTINGS, G. W. "Biomdical Engineering and Materials for Orthopedic Implants," *J. Phys. Eng. Sci. Instrum.* 13:599 (1980).

71 PREVITE, J. J. *Human Physiology*, New York, N.Y.:McGraw-Hill Book Co. (1983).

72 PORIES, W. J. and W. H. Strain. "Zinc and Wound Healing," in *Zinc Metabolism.* A. S. Prasad, ed., Springfield, IL:Thomas Inc., 378–394 (1970).

73 UNDERWOOD, E. J. *Trace Elements in Human and Animal Nutrition*, Third Edition. New York, N.Y.:Academic Press, Inc. (1971).

74 BAJPAI, P. K. and M. A. P. Strnat. "Zinc Based Ceramics for Rebuilding Bone," *J. Invest. Res.*,1:234 (1988).